Disorders of Ventilation

Disorders of Ventilation

JOHN SHNEERSON

MA DM (Oxon) MD (Cantab) FRCP
Director
Assisted Ventilation Unit
Newmarket General Hospital
Consultant Physician
Newmarket General, Papworth,
Addenbrooke's and
West Suffolk Hospitals

Blackwell Scientific Publications

OXFORD LONDON EDINBURGH

BOSTON PALO ALTO MELBOURNE

© 1988 by
Blackwell Scientific Publications
Editorial offices:
Osney Mead, Oxford OX2 0EL
  (*Orders*: Tel. 0865 240201)
8 John Street, London WC1N 2ES
23 Ainslie Place, Edinburgh EH3 6AJ
3 Cambridge Center, Suite 208, Cambridge,
  Massachusetts 02142, USA
667 Lytton Avenue, Palo Alto
  California 94301, USA
107 Barry Street, Carlton
  Victoria 3053, Australia

First published 1988

Photoset by Enset (Photosetting)
Midsomer Norton, Bath, Avon
Printed and bound in Great Britain
by William Clowes Limited
Beccles and London

DISTRIBUTORS

USA
  Year Book Medical Publishers
  200 North LaSalle Street
  Chicago, Illinois 60601
  (*Orders*: Tel. 312 726-9733)

Canada
  The C.V. Mosby Company
  5240 Finch Avenue East
  Scarborough, Ontario
  (*Orders*: Tel. 416-298-1588)

Australia
  Blackwell Scientific Publications
  (Australia) Pty Ltd
  107 Barry Street
  Carlton, Victoria 3053
  (*Orders*: Tel. (03) 347 0300)

British Library
Cataloguing in Publication Data

Shneerson, J.
  Disorders of ventilation.
  1. Respiratory insufficiency
  I. Title
  616.2   RC732

ISBN 0-632-01668-X

Contents

Part 4 · **Treatment of Ventilatory Failure**

Preface

The exchange of oxygen and carbon dioxide within the lungs is as dependent on the respiratory pump to inflate the lungs as it is on the functioning of the lungs themselves. Respiratory failure can develop even when the lungs are capable of working normally. The respiratory pump comprises the neurological respiratory control mechanisms, the peripheral nerves, respiratory muscles and the bones and soft tissues of the chest wall. The disorders of these important structures and their effects on ventilation are the subject of this book.

The many causes of respiratory pump or ventilatory failure cross the boundaries of the conventional medical specialties. It is virtually impossible when working within a single discipline to see the whole range of these conditions. Specialists in intensive-care medicine primarily look after patients during acute exacerbations of their respiratory failure, chest physicians usually care for the more severely affected patients, neurologists for those with previously recognized neurological disorders, and referral to sleep laboratories is biased towards patients with symptoms referable to sleep. I have tried to overcome this problem by bringing together these various approaches to provide an overview of ventilatory failure and its physiological basis.

The study of the disorders of ventilation and their treatment has been neglected to a remarkable extent until recently. This is now changing, largely due to the development of non-invasive techniques of monitoring respiration. New methods of ventilatory assistance that are effective and more acceptable to the patient than many of the older treatments have now become available. The balance between over-enthusiasm for the new techniques and continuing with what is outdated is delicate. I have endeavoured to create not only a wider awareness of recent developments but also a sense of perspective of their value.

The theme of this book is the physiological interpretation of the clinical aspects of disorders of ventilation and how this should guide the choice of treatment. The text is divided into four main parts. Part 1 describes the physiological and anatomical components of the respiratory pump. Details of pulmonary physiology are not included since they are already well described in other accounts. Emphasis is laid particularly on the control of respiration, especially in sleep, and on the function of the respiratory muscles, including the muscles of the upper airway. This leads on to Part 2, where the clinical features and the methods of investigating the functioning of the respiratory pump are reviewed. These chapters do not contain technical details of the tests since this is not a practical manual. The aim is to provide the reader with an understanding of the principles of the tests that link Part 1 with the later chapters.

The individual disorders of ventilation are discussed in Part 3. They are considered as far as possible according to the anatomical site of the abnormality since this is very important in determining the physiological effects and is often the starting point for the clinician. The pathophysiology of lesions at each site is described in each chapter before the individual conditions are discussed. Part 4 deals with the management of ventilatory failure, laying particular emphasis on the mechanical forms of ventilatory assistance. The conventional medical aspects of the treatment of respiratory failure are mentioned only briefly since they are adequately covered elsewhere. Each chapter discusses the physiological effects of treatment, as well as the clinical aspects. Guidance on how to select the best form of treatment for any individual patient is given in Chapter 26, and the problems of organizing an assisted ventilation service and its value are considered in the final chapter.

From these four parts a picture emerges of the interactions of the disorders of each of the components of the respiratory pump. Their complexity may seem daunting but, wherever possible, flow charts or line diagrams have been included to illustrate the interrelationships. The text is thoroughly referenced since, although many readers will consult none of the references, others may wish to trace the original publications.

This book should be of value, particularly to chest physicians, those involved in intensive-care units and sleep laboratories, anaesthetists, neurologists and physiologists interested in ventilation. Many of the most important recent advances in physiology have been stimulated by observations of disordered function. The conditions that are described are not confined to these specialties but overlap with cardiology, orthopaedic surgery, rheumatology and physiotherapy. The text is directed primarily at postgraduates, but the inclusion of the physiology sections and the chapters on special investigations should help to make the subject understandable to those without specialist knowledge.

This account is largely based on my experience in the Assisted Ventilation Unit at Newmarket General Hospital, and it could not have been written without the help of both the patients and the staff of the Unit. I would also like to thank Drs John Scadding and Don Bethune for their helpful comments on the neurological and intermittent positive pressure ventilation sections, respectively. I am indebted to Marcia Thorburn and Nicola Townley of Addenbrooke's Hospital Medical Photographic Department for the preparation of the illustrations. I owe especial gratitude to Doris Sibbons who has unerringly typed each draft of the text and the references, and to whom no amount of dictation appeared to pose any problems. To my wife, Anne, I would like to express my debt for her encouragement at each stage of the preparation of this book and for her tolerance over the last two years which has enabled it to be completed.

List of Abbreviations

bd	twice daily
C_{cw}	chest wall compliance
C_l	lung compliance
C_{rs}	total respiratory compliance
cmH_2O	centimetres of water
CPAP	continuous positive airway pressure
CSF	cerebrospinal fluid
DRG	dorsal respiratory group
ECG	electrocardiogram
EEG	electroencephalogram
EMG	electromyogram
EOG	electro-oculogram
ERV	expiratory reserve volume
f	respiratory frequency
FEV_1	forced expiratory volume in 1.0 sec
FRC	functional residual capacity
FVC	forced vital capacity
h	hour
HCO_3^-	bicarbonate
Hz	Hertz
IPPB	intermittent positive pressure breathing
IPPV	intermittent positive pressure ventilation
kg	kilogram
kPa	kilopascal
l	litre
mg	milligram
min	minute
mmHg	millimetres of mercury
msec	millisecond
MSVC	maximal sustainable ventilatory capacity
MVV	maximum voluntary ventilation

NREM	non-rapid eye movement
$P_{0.1}, P_{0.15}$	mouth occlusion pressure 0.1 or 0.15 sec after onset of inspiratory effort
P_{abd}	intra-abdominal pressure
P_{di}	transdiaphragmatic pressure
P_{pl}	pleural pressure
PE_{max}	maximal expiratory pressure
PI_{max}	maximal inspiratory pressure
P_{CO_2}	partial pressure of carbon dioxide
P_{O_2}	partial pressure of oxygen
Pa_{CO_2}	arterial carbon dioxide pressure
Pa_{O_2}	arterial oxygen partial pressure
$P_{A_{CO_2}}$	alveolar carbon dioxide pressure
$P_{ET_{CO_2}}$	end tidal carbon dioxide pressure
PEFR	peak expiratory flow rate
R	respiratory exchange ratio
REM	rapid eye movement
RV	residual volume
Sa_{O_2}	arterial oxygen saturation
sec	second
SLE	systemic lupus erythematosus
tds	three times daily
T_E	expiratory time
T_I	inspiratory time
T_{TOT}	duration of a single breath
TLC	total lung capacity
UPPP	uvulopalatopharyngoplasty
V_D	dead space
V_T	tidal volume
VC	vital capacity
VRG	ventral respiratory group
$\dot{V}_{E_{max}}$	maximal exercise ventilation
$\dot{V}_{O_{2max}}$	maximal oxygen uptake

Part I
Physiology of Ventilation

Chapter 1
Ventilatory Control

The act of respiration depends entirely on the stimulation of the respiratory muscles by the central nervous system. Information received from chemoreceptors sensitive to hypoxia and hypercapnia and from mechanoreceptors is integrated in the brain stem and spinal cord. The brain stem respiratory centres are closely linked with the reticular formation and with the spinal cord. Impulses to and from the cerebral cortex connect it with both the brain stem respiratory centres and the spinal cord (Fig. 1.1).

Despite these complex anatomical interrelationships, it has proved useful to divide the functioning of the respiratory control system into a voluntary (behavioural) system and an automatic (reflex) system. The voluntary system adapts respiration to rapidly changing environmental factors and enables it to be modified for important functions, including speech, eating and expression of emotions such as anger or fear. The automatic system coordinates the chemoreceptor and mechanoreceptor input and adjusts ventilation according to the metabolic requirements and the mechanical properties of the lungs, chest wall and respiratory muscles. The blood gases are thereby kept constant and the work of breathing is minimized [1995, 2390].

This division has been valuable in analysing respiratory patterns, particularly during sleep, and in various disorders of the brain and spinal cord (Chapters 10 and 11). It is, however, important to realize that it is a functional description of respiratory control and that anatomical correlations cannot be precise because of the complex interrelationships of the cerebral cortex, brain stem and spinal cord.

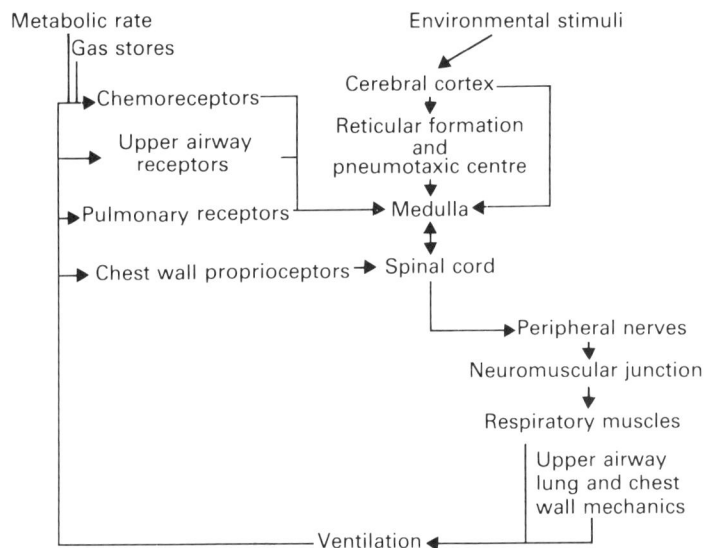

Fig. 1.1. *Schematic representation of the respiratory control system.*

VOLUNTARY CONTROL OF VENTILATION

Studies of hemiplegic subjects have indicated that respiratory movements are represented bilaterally in the cerebral cortex (p. 112), but most of the information concerning cortical control of respiration in man has been gained from electrical stimulation studies. These have shown both excitatory and inhibitory areas. An increase in respiratory frequency can be elicited by electrical stimulation, particularly around the precentral gyrus, which contains the motor cortex [435, 1600, 2435, 2988, 3015]. In contrast, bradypnoea or even prolonged apnoeas are seen with stimulation of other areas of the cerebral cortex, especially the temporal cortex and the limbic system [344, 435, 1601–1603, 2292, 2518, 3015, 3324]. Apnoea occurs with the chest wall in the expiratory position [1601, 1602], indicating that both inspiratory and expiratory muscle activity is inhibited [1600]. Glottic closure can also be induced [700].

Apnoea induced by electrical stimulation of the cerebral cortex is only one aspect of a more generalized inhibition of somatomotor activities. It is often associated with tameness and loss of fear in monkeys [3324] and tiredness and sleepiness in man [1602], and illustrates how respiratory control is integrated into the overall behavioural pattern [1601, 2593].

The descending fibres from the cerebral cortex pass both to the brain stem and to the spinal cord. They travel through the internal capsule and remain close together in the upper brain stem [1786, 2711]. They inhibit the medullary respiratory centres directly and also indirectly through the reticular formation. Corticospinal fibres enter the pyramidal tracts and travel in the dorsolateral spinal cord to the motor nuclei of the respiratory muscles, particularly the phrenic nerve (Fig. 1.2). Most fibres decussate in the medulla and are anatomically distinct in the spinal cord from the descending fibres leaving the medullary respiratory centres. The coordination of corticospinal impulses with the other respiratory influences in the motor nuclei of the respiratory muscles is described on p. 11.

AUTOMATIC CONTROL OF VENTILATION

The early investigators of the automatic control of respiration proposed a variety of interrelated respiratory centres in the brain stem on the basis of ablation experiments and electrical stimulation. Ablation experiments not only destroy parts of the brain but also induce compensatory reactions in other areas. This was not adequately taken into account when interpreting the results and with electrical stimulation it is often uncertain whether a respiratory centre or the afferent or efferent fibres have been stimulated. Most of the models of respiratory control built up on the basis of these experiments have been shown to be misleading and have been discarded [252, 1644, 2187–2189]. Electrical recording of the activity of individual neurons has proved more

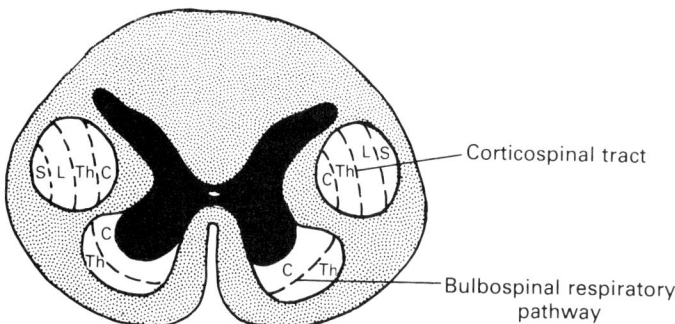

Fig. 1.2. *Cross-section of spinal cord to show position of corticospinal tract and bulbospinal respiratory pathway. Fibres terminating on motor neurons in cervical, thoracic, lumbar and sacral cord are represented by C, Th, L and S, respectively.*

reliable and has led to a reappraisal of the functioning of the respiratory centres [444, 865, 2758]. Modern views are more in line with the conclusions drawn from the early studies of comparative anatomy [1412].

Anatomy of respiratory centres and spinal cord

The origin of the respiratory rhythm has long been thought to be located in the medulla because breathing ceases after transection of the spinal cord whereas it persists if the medulla is left intact. Two main groups of neurons have been identified. The dorsal respiratory group (DRG) is situated in the ventrolateral nucleus of the tractus solitarius, rostral to the obex. The ventral respiratory group (VRG) is composed of three parts, one close to the nucleus ambiguus, another adjacent to the nucleus retroambigualis, and the third comprising the nucleus retrofacialis (Botzinger complex).

The DRG receives afferent impulses, particularly from the glossopharyngeal and vagus nerves, and integrates information from the chemoreceptors and lung receptors [936] (Fig. 1.3). The respiratory rhythm generator and the inspiratory 'off-switch' mechanism may also be located in the DRG. This thereby controls the respiratory pattern. It also projects both to the VRG and to the phrenic nerve nuclei in the cervical cord.

The VRG, which extends throughout the length of the medulla, receives no afferent impulses directly but is driven by the DRG. Its rostral area is predominantly inspiratory and the caudal area expiratory. It innervates the inspiratory and expiratory intercostal muscles, the abdominal muscles and, to a certain extent, the diaphragm. Some fibres run in the vagus nerve and coordinate the activity of the pharynx, larynx and possibly the trachea and bronchi with the contraction of the other respiratory muscles. The nucleus retrofacialis projects to the contralateral DRG and ipsilaterally to the other VRG nuclei, as well as to the respiratory muscles.

Most of the bulbospinal fibres connecting the medullary respiratory centres to the respiratory motor nuclei in the spinal cord are crossed [252, 278, 600, 2187, 2188]. The inspiratory fibres appear to decussate higher than the expiratory fibres, but the majority cross between the obex in the medulla and the upper cervical cord [154,

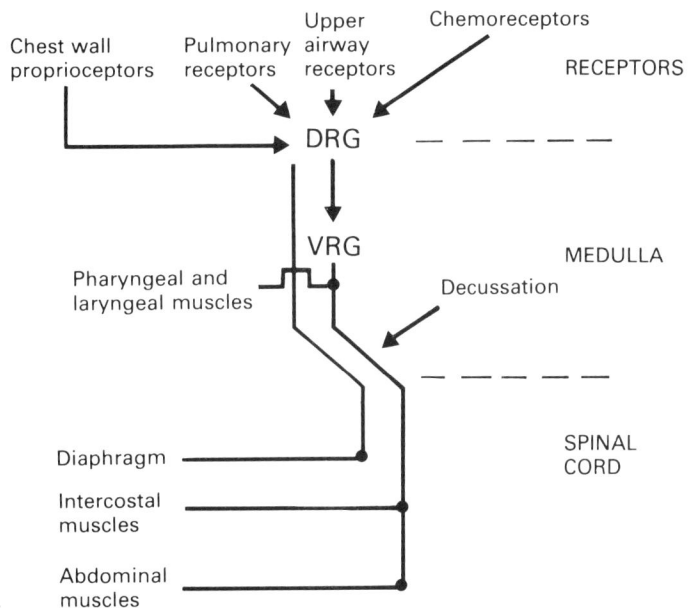

Fig. 1.3. *Diagrammatic representation of neural connections of DRG and VRG.*

598]. A few fibres decussate lower in the cervical cord [598]. This pattern explains the crossed phrenic phenomenon whereby following a unilateral cord section leading to an ipsilateral muscle weakness section of the contralateral phrenic nerve increases the activity of the initially damaged side [2521]. The phrenic section leads to an increase in respiratory drive, which is transmitted to the side of the spinal cord section by fibres that decussate below the level of the damage [1886].

The bulbospinal fibres change from being ventrolateral to dorsolateral as they descend in the spinal cord [1493]. In the upper spinal cord they are more than 3 mm from the margin of the cord [236, 1438] and they lie just lateral to the exit of the ventral root [2279] (Fig. 1.2). The inspiratory and expiratory fibres are next to each other [237] and are closely related to the spinothalamic tract [1026, 1438].

The fibres from the brain stem to the spinal cord, serving reflex non-rhythmic respiratory activities such as sighing, coughing and hiccoughing, travel in anatomically separate tracts from the fibres controlling the rhythmic respiratory movements. Either pathway can be selectively interrupted [2301]. The descending pathway for the abdominal component of the cough reflex lies in the ventral column. Coordination of these reflexes with the rhythmic respiratory movements occurs mainly within the spinal cord.

The nucleus of the phrenic nerve forms a discrete column of longitudinally orientated cells in the ventromedial part of the ventral horn of the cervical cord [1658, 3261]. This column of cells usually extends from the upper border of C3 to C5 but occasionally into the upper region of C6 or even lower [1658]. This histological finding has been confirmed by the observation of diaphragmatic spasms in some C5 quadriplegics, indicating that the phrenic nerve nucleus extends below this level [2930].

Respiratory rhythmicity and timing

The origin of the respiratory rhythm in the brain stem is still uncertain [278]. It has been proposed that inspiration is due to a cyclic activity in an inspiratory centre or, conversely, that it arises from a continuous inspiratory discharge that is periodically inhibited. This inhibition has been variously attributed to vagal afferent impulses, to the pneumotaxic centre in the pons or to activity of the reticular formation. A variant of this theory is that there is continuous expiratory activity, which is periodically inhibited by the inspiratory centre [252]. Spontaneously depolarizing pacemaker cells or similarly acting neural networks have been proposed to explain the cyclic activity of the respiratory centre. Several types of network have been put forward, including a bi-stable oscillator in which there is reciprocal inhibition of the inspiratory and expiratory centres [2757], inhibitory phasing [2188] and networks whose activity is self-limiting in other ways.

The duration of inspiration and expiration is controlled by the medullary centres. The concept of inspiratory and expiratory on- and off-switches has not been fruitful since these are purely descriptive terms and do not explain the alternation of the phases of respiration.

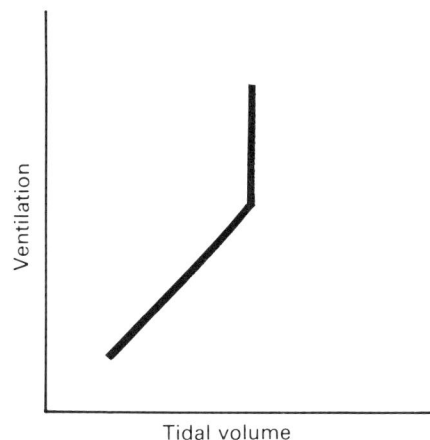

Fig. 1.4. *Simplified diagram of the tidal volume change with increase in ventilation. At the inflexion point, further increase in tidal volume is achieved by an increase in respiratory frequency.*

Inspiration is terminated in certain circumstances by afferent impulses from pulmonary stretch receptors [935], but mechanoreceptors in the chest wall and chemoreceptors may also play a part. The factors determining the termination of expiration are less certain, but this can be influenced by the carotid bodies [358, 359].

When ventilation increases, the tidal volume (V_T) initially rises and this is followed by an increase in respiratory frequency [1417] (Fig. 1.4). The expiratory time (T_E) shortens more than the inspiratory time (T_I) [1417, 2302]. The rise in V_T despite a fall in T_I implies that the mean inspiratory flow rate (V_T/T_I) becomes more rapid when V_T increases. The mean inspiratory flow rate is determined by the mechanical properties of the lungs and chest wall, the intensity of stimulation of the inspiratory muscles and their strength [2157]. It reflects a different aspect of the functioning of the respiratory centres to the timing of inspiration and expiration.

Control of T_I, T_E and V_T/T_I enables any combination of V_T and respiratory frequency to be achieved. The chemoreceptors ensure that alveolar ventilation is sufficient to maintain normal blood gases, and experimental work has shown that the pattern of ventilation is adjusted to minimize the work of breathing [1995, 2390].

Control of medullary respiratory centres

The respiratory function of the medullary centres is not fixed. They can adapt to changes in the P_{O_2} and P_{CO_2}, respiratory mechanics and the environment [251]. Integration of these influences is carried out in the medulla and at other levels in the central nervous system, particularly the spinal cord. The most important areas that alter the behaviour of the medullary respiratory centres are:

CEREBRAL CORTEX

The descending impulses from the cerebral cortex have a predominantly inhibitory action on the medullary centres and limit, for instance, the ventilatory response to hypercapnia.

BRAIN STEM

The region of the nucleus parabrachialis medialis and the Kolliker–Fuse nucleus are particularly important. They probably correspond to the pneumotaxic centre in the rostral dorsolateral pons, which was postulated from ablation experiments [252, 600, 2188]. They appear to inhibit the DRG either by influencing the termination of inspiration or by changing the threshold for the response of the DRG to chemoreceptor and mechanoreceptor stimulation [2185].

The hypothalamus appears to have relatively little control over respiration. An increase in the temperature due to hypothalamic activity may increase ventilation [278]. Experimentally induced lesions diminish inspiratory activity, and electrical stimulation increases respiratory frequency [2558, 2583, 2584]. These experimental findings may be due to interruption or stimulation of descending paths to the medulla rather than to areas within the hypothalamus that have a specifically respiratory function.

Lesions in the brain stem reticular formation may influence respiration by altering the level of consciousness and the emotional state. The descending fibres from the cerebral cortex may be interrupted by brain stem lesions so that the medulla is released from this inhibitory influence. Ablation experiments in cats have shown that destruction of areas of the midbrain slows respiration and diminishes the ventilatory response to hypercapnia [599, 986]. Electrical stimulation causes apnoea in the expiratory position [3199].

The effect of the cerebellum on respiration has hardly been studied. It appears to have a tonic inhibitory influence on inspiration similar to that of the pneumotaxic centre [1138, 2225, 3042, 3043]. Both α and γ respiratory motor neurons are inhibited on the side of the cerebellar stimulation to a greater extent than the inhibition of purely postural muscles [645, 2133]. Stimulation of the vermis of the cerebellum may, however, lead to an increase in ventilation and particularly the respiratory frequency [3043]. The outputs from the cerebellum and the medullary respiratory centres are coordinated in the spinal cord.

CHEMORECEPTORS

Hypoxia

Carotid bodies. The aortic bodies have little influence on respiration in man, the effect of hypoxia on respiration being mediated almost entirely through the carotid bodies. The receptors are probably the nerve endings that synapse with the neurosecretory type I (glomus) cells [1986]. The type II (sheath or sustentacular) cells are probably equivalent to Schwann cells. The afferent nerve fibres are both myelinated and non-myelinated. They run in the carotid sinus nerve, which is a branch of the glosso-pharyngeal nerve, and synapse in the DRG. The cell bodies of the afferent neurons lie mainly in the petrosal ganglion.

The receptors are sensitive to slight changes in the P_{O_2} of arterial blood, but not to changes in oxygen saturation or content. The discharge frequency of the nerve fibres leading from the carotid body increases hyperbolically as the P_{O_2} falls [295], but cyclic fluctuations in P_{O_2} are probably important in controlling ventilation during exercise [296].

The carotid body is very vascular and is supplied by the carotid body artery, which is a branch of the external carotid artery. Receptor activity increases if the blood flow to the carotid body falls. This may be due to hypotension, to vasoconstriction due to increased sympathetic activity, or to respiratory or metabolic acidosis. The discharge frequency increases in the same fibres that respond to hypoxia [295]. The carotid body can also be stimulated pharmacologically by acetylcholine and nicotine and by carbon monoxide and cyanide, which block the cytochrome systems [2337].

Ventilatory response to hypoxia. Ventilation rises approximately hyperbolically as the P_{O_2} falls,

although this relationship can be equally well described by an exponential function. The ventilation increases almost linearly with the fall in oxygen saturation, not because of any causal relationship but because the shape of the oxyhaemoglobin dissociation curve is similar to that of the ventilatory response to the P_{O_2}. The contribution of the carotid bodies to respiratory control in normal subjects is thought to be small, except during exercise, but it becomes important in the presence of hypoxia or hypercapnia [2337].

The ventilatory response to oxygen varies considerably between subjects. It correlates with height, weight and the ventilatory response to carbon dioxide [1436], and decreases with age [1769]. A diminished hypoxic response has been noted in several members of the same family [1486, 2206], and twin studies have suggested that this has a genetic basis [613]. The response is greater if the metabolic rate is increased, for instance by feeding [117, 1034, 3410]. Conversely, starvation [805, 3345] and hypothyroidism [2081, 2174, 3409] decrease the ventilatory response to hypoxia. It may also be reduced in athletes [457], sleep deprivation [825, 3311] and in chronic hypoxia, whether this is due to chronic lung or chest wall disease or congenital heart disease [321, 879] or altitude [1793]. The blunting of the response is greatest if the first two years of life are spent at altitude [3003, 3004, 3006]. Relief of hypoxia by correction of congenital heart disease may not improve the ventilatory response to hypoxia [3005]. Similarly, adults who have moved to high altitude hardly alter their hypoxic responses, suggesting that adaptation of the carotid bodies or their central connections occurs only slowly in adult life [1019, 3275].

Hypercapnia

Carbon dioxide receptors and CSF bicarbonate. The ventilatory response to hypercapnia is due to receptors both in the carotid body and near to the surface of the medulla. The same fibres in the carotid body respond to hypercapnia and hypoxia. Their firing frequency increases almost linearly with the P_{CO_2} [295].

The central CO_2 receptors probably lie in three bilaterally symmetrical zones within 0.5 mm of the ventrolateral surface of the medulla [320]. They appear to be distinct from the area within the medulla that integrates the chemoreceptor inputs [253]. The receptors are sensitive to the pH of either the intracellular or extracellular fluids within the brain or to the gradient across the cell membrane. The extracellular fluid equilibrates with the cerebrospinal fluid (CSF). The pH of the CSF changes slowly when the arterial P_{CO_2} is altered, because the blood–brain barrier is permeable to CO_2 but not to bicarbonate or to the hydrogen ion. The brain is therefore largely protected from acute metabolic acid-base changes.

A rise in the arterial P_{CO_2} increases the CSF P_{CO_2} and this equilibrates with the CSF bicarbonate. Bicarbonate is the only CSF buffer, and its pH change for any given increase in P_{CO_2} is inversely related to the concentration of bicarbonate in the CSF [1177, 1400]. This concentration increases in chronic hypercapnia and in metabolic alkalosis due, for instance, to diuretic treatment, and blunts the reduced ventilatory response to hypercapnia. Conversely, chronic hyperventilation increases the ventilatory response to hypercapnia [978].

The reaction to a raised P_{CO_2} is also determined by the cerebral blood flow. Cerebral blood flow is normally regulated so that the rate of oxygen delivery is kept constant [417]. It is not related to the P_{O_2} or to the oxygen content, the viscosity of the blood, haemoglobin concentration, age or blood pressure [417]. Hypercapnia is a cerebral vasodilator and, above a threshold value for P_{CO_2} [2417], increases the blood flow [964, 1659]. The capillary–brain P_{CO_2} gradient falls when the cerebral blood flow increases, so that the ventilatory response to CO_2 is reduced. This homeostatic mechanism reduces the variation in CSF pH relative to arterial pH and P_{CO_2}.

Ventilatory response to hypercapnia. The ventila-tory response to hypercapnia has a threshold, but above this the increase in ventilation is linearly related to the P_{CO_2} (Fig. 1.5). In the presence of hypoxia, the threshold is reduced and the slope of the response rises [2311]. Similarly, the ventilatory response to hypoxia is greater in the presence of hypercapnia than when the P_{CO_2} is normal [646] (Fig. 1.6). Both chronic hypoxia [3275] and acute hypoxia have a depressant effect on the hypercapnic response if they are severe, probably by a direct action on the metabolism of the medullary neurons.

The wide variation in ventilatory response to hypercapnia between individual subjects is partly explained by its correlation with height, weight [1436], and age [1769]. A diminished hypercapnic drive is sometimes familial [2206, 2235]. Twin studies have suggested that the increase in V_T in the presence of hypercapnia is genetically determined, but that the increase in respiratory frequency depends on environmental factors and personality [101]. Sleep depriva-

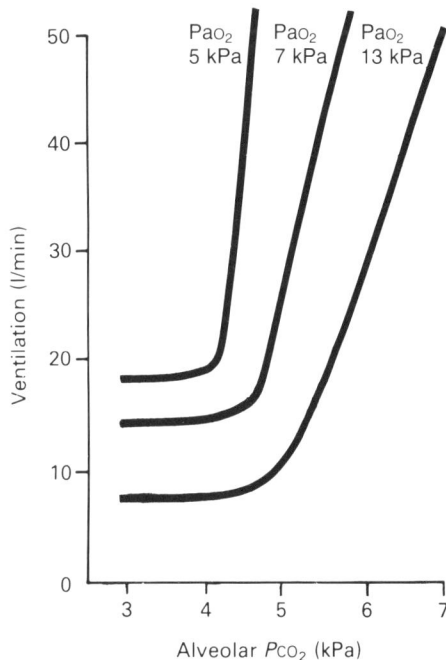

Fig. 1.5. *Ventilatory response to CO_2 in the presence of different Pa_{O_2}. As Pa_{O_2} falls, the threshold of the ventilatory response to hypercapnia falls, and the slope increases.*

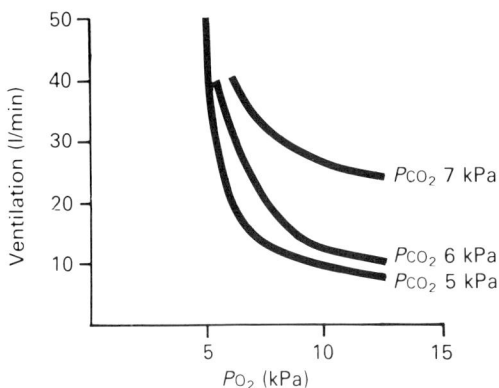

Fig. 1.6. *Ventilatory response to hypoxia at different* P_{CO_2}.

tion may also be important in limiting the response to hypercapnia [643, 825, 3311], as may mechanical abnormalities of the chest wall and lungs, even if the respiratory drive itself is normal [646, 1251].

MECHANORECEPTORS

The mechanoreceptors that can influence respiration are best considered according to their anatomical sites.

Upper airway receptors

Receptors in the nose respond to both chemical and mechanical stimuli. Their innervation is complex [3328] but the afferent fibres travel mainly in the olfactory and trigeminal nerves. Impulses from receptors in the pharynx and larynx pass in the 9th and 10th cranial nerves [3205] to the medulla. Efferent fibres to the muscles of the soft palate, pharynx and larynx originate in the nucleus ambiguus.

In experimental animals, a negative pressure in the upper airway leads to an increase in the activity in the hypoglossal nerve [1513] and in the electrical activity of the pharyngeal dilators, such as the genioglossus [2083, 3328]. The rate of rise of diaphragmatic contraction is diminished [1966]. These responses all tend to preserve the patency of the upper airway (p. 31). Nasal occlusion also increases the electromyogram (EMG) activity of the genioglossus

[2084], which would tend to open the upper airway. Both T_I and T_E are prolonged [2085], and inhibition of involuntary inspiratory movements during breath-holding is seen if air passes through the nose, particularly if the air is cool [1975]. This inhibition is abolished by applying local anaesthetic to the nose. These observations suggest that upper airway receptors have a role in inhibiting or terminating inspiration, as well as in stabilizing the upper airway. Activity of the dilator muscles is diminished when the stimulation of the receptors is decreased by the construction of a tracheostomy [2780].

The receptors also initiate protective reflexes. Stimulation of the nose causes sneezing and the diving response comprising apnoea, bradycardia, a decrease in the cardiac output and vasoconstriction [3328]. The larynx closes and the secretion of tracheal mucus is increased [2470]. Pharyngeal stimulation leads to sniffing or gasping and inhibition of inspiration, bronchodilatation and hypertension [3327]. Laryngeal irritant receptors lead to cough, apnoea, bronchoconstriction, hypertension and an increase in the secretion of tracheal mucus [2470, 3176].

Lung receptors

Stretch receptors. These receptors are located in the airways, and afferent impulses travel in myelinated fibres via the vagus nerve to the medulla. They are stimulated by inflation of the lungs and inhibited by hypercapnia. They are also responsible for the Hering–Breuer inflation reflex, whereby lung inflation inhibits inspiration. The importance of this has been overemphasized in the past, and it is more prominent in experimental animals than in man. In cats, T_I increases hyperbolically as V_T falls, but in man this relationship only appears when V_T exceeds 1.5–2.0 litres [583]. Vagal block does not alter the respiratory frequency or V_T during quiet breathing in man [1313]. Stimulation of these receptors also causes bronchodilatation, tachycardia and vasoconstriction. The Hering–Breuer deflation reflex probably does not exist in man [1311, 1315].

Irritant receptors. These are located in the large airways and respond particularly to chemical stimuli. Their impulses travel in myelinated fibres in the vagus nerve and cause cough, rapid shallow breathing, bronchoconstriction and an increase in the frequency of sighing. Their activity is increased if the lung compliance falls [3327], which may be of significance in restrictive chest wall disorders.

Juxtapulmonary capillary (J) receptors. The J receptors are located in the pulmonary capillary wall and are thought to respond particularly to an increase in the extracellular fluid volume of the lungs. Their impulses travel in non-myelinated vagal fibres and lead to apnoea or shallow breathing, together with bradycardia and hypotension.

Chest wall receptors

The most important chest wall receptors appear to be the muscle spindles and the tendon organs. The diaphragm and the parasternal intercostal muscles are unusual in having very few muscle spindles [644, 864, 865] and are the only respiratory muscles that do not appear to have a postural function. The afferent fibres from the receptors synapse in the spinal cord and, by segmental and intersegmental reflexes [2594], adjust the firing frequency and recruitment of motor neurons of the respiratory muscles to achieve the ventilatory level set by the higher centres. Impulses from the receptors may also influence respiratory timing. Reflexes from the intercostal muscles shorten inspiration [775] and may even inhibit inspiration in neonates [1328, 1708]. Sensory information from the muscle spindles probably leads to the awareness of a disparity between the length and tension developed by the respiratory muscles and the sensation of breathlessness.

Other receptors

Respiration can also be modified by impulses from, for instance, cutaneous receptors, proprioceptors outside the respiratory muscles, and by pain.

Spinal cord physiology

Both the medullary respiratory centres and the spinal cord coordinate the respiratory movements, but in different ways. The rhythm and duration of inspiration and expiration, and possibly the mean inspiratory flow rate, are determined in the medulla. In the spinal cord, the timing and coordination of contraction of the individual muscles are finalized both for respiratory acts and for non-respiratory acts such as vomiting or defaecation.

The descending respiratory impulses from the brain are capable of simultaneously exciting and inhibiting different groups of α motor neurons. For instance, during inspiration the motor neurons to the inspiratory muscles are activated, while those to the expiratory muscles are inhibited. This prevents the stretch reflex, which is mediated by muscle spindles, from increasing the activity of antagonist muscles that would obliterate the respiratory pattern generated in the medulla. This inhibition has not been detected in the phrenic nerve nucleus [2188], probably because the diaphragm has very few muscle spindles [644, 865]. The effect of the stretch reflex is also minimized by direct inhibition of the γ motor neurons supplying the muscle spindles. The stretch reflex is also modified by reciprocal inhibition of inspiratory and expiratory motor neurons via segmental interneuronal networks [2594], which are largely independent of the descending impulses [72].

The motor nuclei in the spinal cord are the final site of integration of the voluntary and automatic control systems. The voluntary system is able to override the metabolic control of respiration for short periods in order to adapt to environmental changes, but the sensory information from the mechanoreceptors largely determines which respiratory muscles are activated during each breath. The frequency of impulses in the α motor neurons rises, and more motor neurons are recruited when the force of contraction increases [1127]. The neurons supplying the fatigue-resistant type 1 muscle fibres have a lower threshold for depolarization than those innervating type 2 fibres, and they become active at lower intensities of work [1259, 2759]. Type 2 fibres are recruited for short periods of more intense contraction [1184].

Chapter 2
Respiratory Movements and Muscles

Much more attention has been paid to the functioning of the lung than to the respiratory muscles and the movements of the chest wall. The early observations of Duchenne [849] and others have largely remained neglected. Interest in the respiratory pump and particularly the respiratory muscles has, however, re-awakened and there have been several recent reviews [262, 430, 480, 519, 741, 775, 1239–1241, 1952, 2006, 2671, 2672, 2675, 2716, 2717, 2719–2721].

The chest wall functions as an air pump with a variable stroke volume and frequency [2391 (a)]. It is required to work continuously and is as essential to life as the cardiac pump (Fig. 2.1). Gas exchange across the alveolar capillary membrane is entirely dependent on the chest wall pump.

In this chapter, the details of the skeletal anatomy of the thorax are not described since they are available in standard anatomy textbooks. The terms 'chest wall' and 'rib cage' are given wider meanings in physiological discussion than their anatomical definitions would suggest. The rib cage is usually taken to include the soft tissues of the thorax and the spine, as well as the ribs themselves, and the chest wall includes not only the rib cage but also those parts of the abdomen that move during respiration.

MOVEMENTS OF RIB CAGE AND ABDOMEN

Inflation of the lungs is achieved either by expansion of the rib cage or by depression of the diaphragm (Fig. 2.2). The rib cage and abdomen act as two compartments in series that are coupled hydraulically. During quiet breathing,

the abdominal expansion is usually less than that of the rib cage while sitting [257, 1255, 1727], but it increases in the supine position [2880, 3227]. It also increases as V_T rises [480] and during exercise [1255] when the end expiratory volume may be less than the functional residual capacity (FRC) because of contraction of the abdominal muscles during expiration.

Analysis of the expansion of the rib cage is complex because of the multiplicity of muscles that are inserted onto the ribs and spine and the differences in length, obliquity and types of joint of the individual ribs [1592]. The first seven 'true' ribs articulate via their costal cartilages with the sternum, whereas the remaining 'false' ribs do not. The 8th–10th ribs articulate anteriorly with the costal cartilages of the rib above, but the 11th and 12th ribs lie free (floating ribs). The head of each rib articulates posteriorly with the body of the vertebra, and the tubercle of the rib with the transverse process. Movement of the ribs occurs along the axis of the neck of the rib, which lies between the head and the tubercle [1591].

When the rib cage expands it is deformed by the force of the muscles. Its shape does not follow the pattern that would be predicted solely from its elastic properties. The extent of this deformation varies with the pattern of inspiratory muscle activity and the lung volume. Expansion can take place in the longitudinal, anteroposterior and transverse diameters. The length of the rib cage is increased by elevation of the 1st rib, extension of the spine and descent of the diaphragm. The anteroposterior diameter is also increased by elevation of the 1st rib. The upper ribs slope downwards and as the sternum rises with the 1st rib it moves forward and the

(a) Respiratory pump

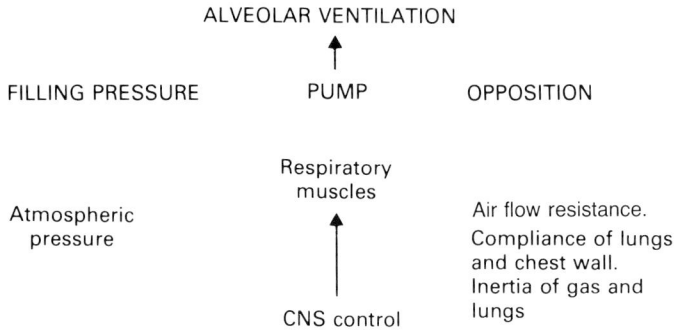

ALVEOLAR VENTILATION

↑

FILLING PRESSURE   PUMP   OPPOSITION

Respiratory
muscles

Atmospheric
pressure
     ↑

Air flow resistance.
Compliance of lungs
and chest wall.
Inertia of gas and
lungs

CNS control

(b) Cardiac pump

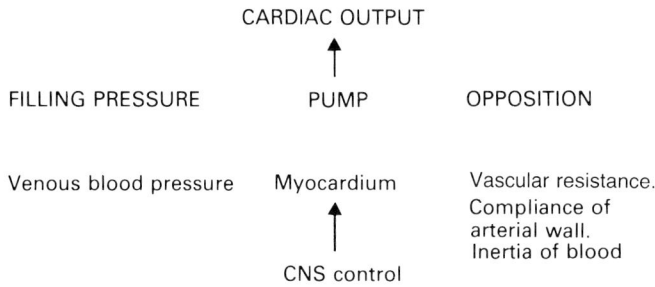

CARDIAC OUTPUT

↑

FILLING PRESSURE   PUMP   OPPOSITION

Venous blood pressure   Myocardium

Vascular resistance.
Compliance of
arterial wall.
Inertia of blood

↑

CNS control

Fig. 2.1. *Main components of (a)
respiratory pump and
(b) cardiac pump.*

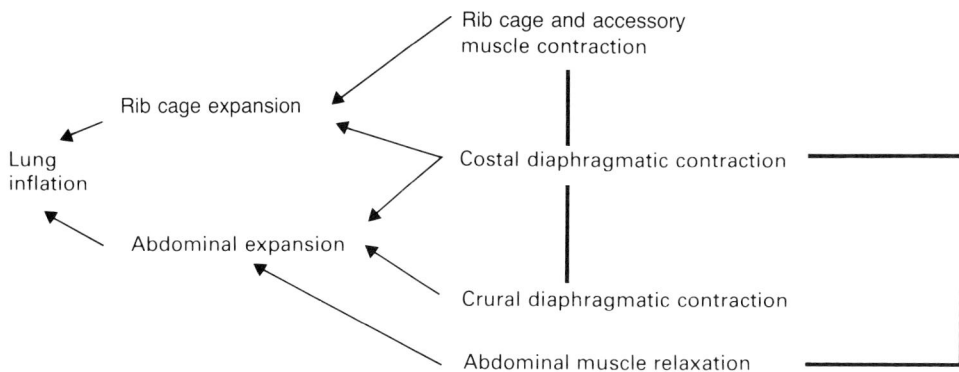

Rib cage and accessory
muscle contraction

Rib cage expansion

Lung
inflation

Costal diaphragmatic contraction

Abdominal expansion

Crural diaphragmatic contraction

Abdominal muscle relaxation

Fig. 2.2. *Diagrammatic representation of the relationships of the rib cage, abdomen and the respiratory muscles. Heavy lines
indicate main interactions between muscle groups.*

lower ribs become more horizontal (pump handle movement). The increase in the transverse diameter, which is usually less than the anteroposterior expansion, is most marked over the lower ribs. This is partly due to the oblique angle of the axis of the neck of the ribs and partly to the fact that the ribs slope downwards. The transverse as well as the anteroposterior diameter increases as they rise. Elevation of the ribs also leads to rotation around their anterior and posterior extremities, which are relatively fixed, because of the shape of the ribs and their downward slope. This rotation increases the transverse diameter of the rib cage, particularly at the costal margin (bucket handle movement), and is seen particularly at high tidal volumes.

Analysis of the abdominal movements during respiration usually assumes that the abdominal contents are incompressible and that pressure changes are conducted throughout the abdomen. Neither of these assumptions is true. The abdomen contains a considerable quantity of gas, the volume of which changes as the abdominal pressure alters. Direct measurement of the abdominal pressure in different areas has shown wide variations during respiratory movements [761, 2007]. The pressure immediately beneath the diaphragm may be quite different to that elsewhere in the abdomen.

In general, however, a fall in the abdominal pressure may be due to contraction of the intercostal or accessory muscles, or relaxation of the diaphragm or abdominal muscles. The last causes the abdominal wall to protrude but the others retract it. Abdominal expansion may also be due to contraction of the diaphragm. The extent to which the abdomen expands depends on the compliance of the abdominal wall, which is largely determined by the degree of contraction of the abdominal muscles. Their contraction will increase the abdominal pressure for any given diaphragmatic contraction and cause the diaphragm to remain higher and the ratio of abdominal to rib cage movement to fall. Normally, the compliance of the abdomen is approximately the same as the compliance of the rib cage [1725], so that diaphragmatic contraction

causes both abdominal and rib cage expansion [1176].

MECHANICAL PROPERTIES OF CHEST WALL

The contraction of the inspiratory muscles inflates the lungs by overcoming the elastic properties of the lungs and chest wall, the air flow resistance and the relatively small viscosity and inertia of the tissues. The elastic recoil of the chest wall is closely related to its volume (Fig. 2.3). The relationship is approximately linear at volumes used during quiet breathing, and the slope of the relationship is the compliance. The distensibility of the chest wall falls at both high and low lung volumes, so that more energy is required to inflate and deflate the lungs. The compliance of the chest wall is determined by the soft tissues, including fat, the skeleton, and muscle tension. There is some postural tone in the muscles of the chest wall but the activity varies considerably during each breath. The compliance of the chest wall falls with age [2196], probably because of degenerative changes in the costovertebral and other joints.

If the chest wall is separated from the lungs, the volume that it assumes because of its elastic recoil and in the absence of muscle tension is considerably greater than the volume assumed by the lungs. The volume at which these two opposite forces are balanced, when the lungs and chest wall are in contact, is the FRC. This is the end expiratory volume if there is no respiratory muscle activity.

The factors determining total lung capacity (TLC) and residual volume (RV) are more complex. The force of the inspiratory muscles falls as the lung volume increases [2549] because they become shorter and are at a mechanical disadvantage. The compliance of the lungs and chest wall also decreases and abdominal muscle contraction may limit further lung expansion [472]. The diaphragm is elevated so that the end expiratory volume is less than the FRC. Inspiration is consequently aided by elastic recoil and

(a) Sitting

(b) Supine

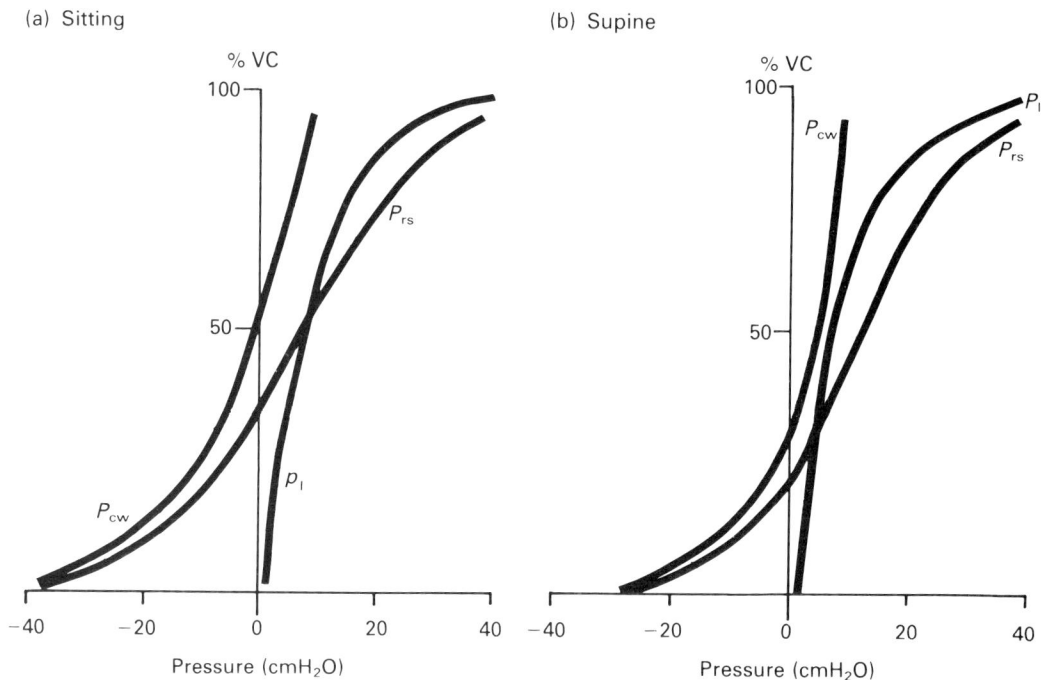

Fig. 2.3. *Static volume–pressure curves for chest wall, lung and total respiratory system in (a) sitting and (b) supine positions. The pressures contributed by the chest wall (P_{cw}), lungs (P_l) and the combination of both of these (P_{rs}) are separately identified.*

the diaphragm is lengthened so that its force is increased. Conversely, near the RV the expiratory muscles are shortened and are working at a mechanical disadvantage. Reflex diaphragmatic contractions may also appear [35]. The compliance of the chest wall and lungs is reduced and the upper airway may be occluded by laryngeal or pharyngeal closure due to reflexes initiated by pulmonary stretch receptors. In older subjects, airway closure may limit the degree of expiration [1860, 3387] and contribute to the rise in RV.

CONTRACTILE PROPERTIES OF RESPIRATORY MUSCLES

Contraction of the respiratory muscles provides the energy to expand the lungs. In common with all other skeletal muscles, they are composed of longitudinally aligned muscle fibres enmeshed in connective tissue. The fibres are activated when an impulse reaches the neuromuscular junction and releases acetylcholine from the presynaptic membrane. This depolarizes the muscle fibre membrane, with the loss of its internal negative potential of about 75 mV.

The group of muscle fibres that is innervated by a single axon constitutes a motor unit [2897]. All the fibres within each motor unit contract simultaneously. The fibres within each motor unit are all of the same type (see below), although they may be scattered throughout the muscle [886]. The number of muscle fibres comprising a motor unit varies, but in general is larger if the fibres are fast-contracting and smaller if they are slow-contracting. Their activity is controlled not only by the α motor neurons but by feedback from muscle spindles.

The force developed by the respiratory muscles depends on several factors, the most important of which are listed below.

Types of muscle fibre

The fibres within each muscle have different structural, histochemical, and contractile properties. Two main types have been recognized. Type 1 (red) have a smaller diameter, have more oxidative enzymes, a lower phosphorylase activity, more mitochondria and fat droplets, and a higher myoglobin content than type 2 (white) fibres. The type 2 fibres have been subdivided into 2A and 2B: the 2A fibres are intermediate between type 1 and type 2B fibres.

The physiological properties of the fibre types appear to correlate with the ultrastructural and biochemical features. The type 1 fibres have a longer twitch time, measured as the interval between the onset of contraction and the moment of maximum tension following a single nerve impulse. They are also more resistant to muscle fatigue, presumably because of their predominantly oxidative metabolism. Type 1 fibres are depolarized by lower impulse frequencies in the motor neurons that supply them than type 2 fibres [1259]. These fatigue-resistant fibres are therefore active for longer periods than type 2 fibres, which are recruited during more intensive contraction when the firing frequency rises.

All the respiratory muscles contain both type 1 and type 2 fibres. Their proportions and the elastic properties of the muscle itself determine the contraction time of the muscle.

Contractile mass

The force developed by a muscle depends on its mass or cross-sectional area and the proportion of fibres that have been activated. Skeletal muscles can hypertrophy and increase their strength with appropriate training schedules (p.287). The mass is also influenced by the nutritional state, age (which is associated with a loss of α motor neurons and motor units) and pathological disorders of the muscles (Chapter 15). The mass of contracting muscle employed to cope with any applied load can be increased by recruiting new muscle groups. This enables the firing frequency of the motor neurons to the muscles to fall, which prevents or relieves muscle fatigue. Failure to recruit muscles may be due to a lack of motivation or an impairment of the respiratory control. The force of contraction can also be increased by recruiting extra motor units within each muscle, as described above.

Frequency of stimulation

At birth, the respiratory muscles consist predominantly of type 2 fibres [886, 1634, 1635]. Respiratory muscle fatigue readily occurs [1942, 2251], even in physiological circumstances such as during rapid eye movement (REM) sleep. Postnatally, the differentiation of these fibres into type 1 fibres largely depends on their frequency of stimulation. Low frequency motor units develop type 1 fibres and high frequency units remain as type 2 fibres. This has been confirmed by experiments in which the electrical stimulation frequency was controlled [2759], and by cross-innervation [2702], which induced both ultrastructural and biochemical changes in the fibres. Similar alterations can be produced by physical training [1456, 1457] (p. 287) and by low frequency stimulation [575, 2760, 2761] (p. 273).

The tension developed during a single muscle twitch is less than that seen with rapid repeated stimulation (tetanus). After a single stimulation, the muscle fibre relaxes before its elastic properties have allowed the maximal tension to be attained. This is the basis of the frequency–force relationship (Fig. 2.4). The exact relationship between the frequency and the force of muscle contraction depends on the fibre type composition of the muscle and factors that affect its contractility, such as fatigue. In general, the force developed is about 25% maximum at a stimulation frequency of 10 Hz, 70% maximum at 20 Hz, 95% maximum at 50 Hz, and maximal at 100 Hz.

Length

Muscle fibres readily adapt to changes in their length. It has been shown in cats that if the

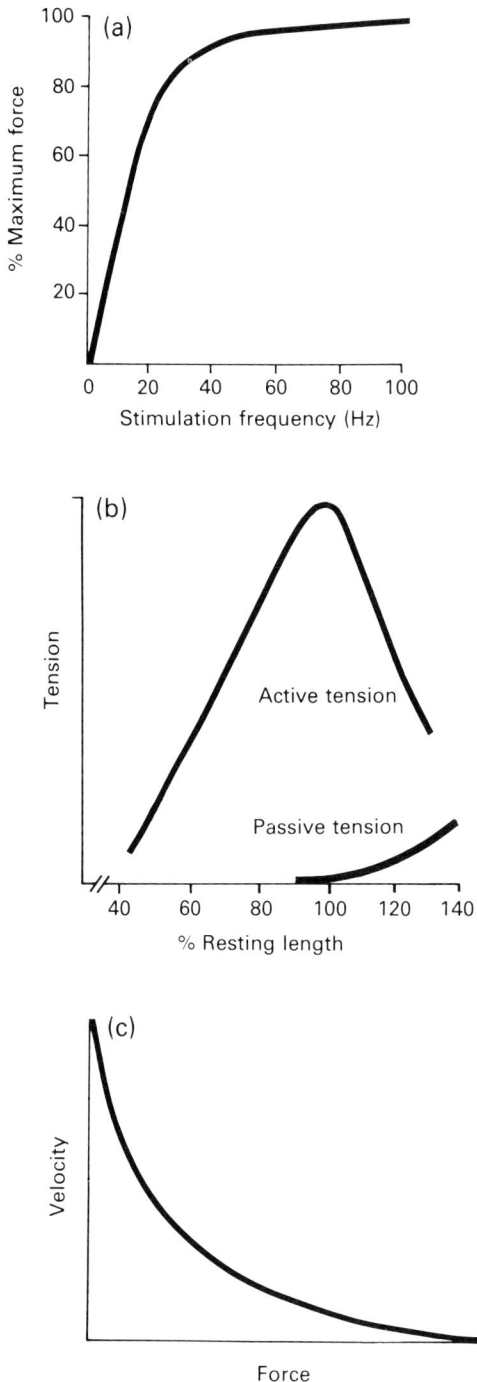

soleus muscle is kept extended, the muscle fibres develop more sarcomeres in series and more changes in their length–tension curve within four weeks [3131]. In general, unless the muscle is overstretched, the greater its initial length, the more force it can develop during tetanic stimulation. The relationship between the length of the muscle and muscle tension is illustrated in Fig. 2.4.

The muscle length is an important determinant of the force generated by the respiratory muscles. The inspiratory muscles are more effective near the RV when they are longest, and the expiratory muscles at TLC when they are stretched. The volume of the lungs is, however, only a rough guide to the length of the muscles. At any lung volume, the configuration of the rib cage depends on the amount that it has been deformed by muscle contraction from its shape predicted by its elastic properties. The length of the respiratory muscles may, therefore, vary from breath to breath, even at the same lung volume.

Velocity of contraction

When muscle fibres are activated the muscle may shorten (isotonic contraction), or tension may be developed with no change in length (isometric contraction). The more rapidly the muscle shortens, the less is the tension that can be maintained. This is illustrated by the force–velocity curve (Fig. 2.4). More muscle energy is required if the muscle shortens rapidly than if its length remains constant. The velocity of shortening of the respiratory muscles is hard to analyse in any detail, but it has been shown that muscle fatigue is more likely if the mean inspiratory flow rate is rapid [582, 1981].

Contractility

The contractility of skeletal muscle is decreased by hypoxia [1562], hypercapnia [1594], lack of bicarbonate [681], and hypokalaemia and other metabolic and nutritional factors (p. 176). It is also decreased by muscle fatigue (see below).

Fig. 2.4. *Properties of skeletal muscle: (a) frequency–force curve, (b) length–tension relationship, (c) force–velocity curve.*

Fatigue

Weakness of a muscle is the inability to generate the expected force, but fatigue is the inability to sustain a force. It is the opposite of muscle endurance and can be regarded as the development of weakness during sustained or repeated contraction.

It is important to distinguish the fatigue arising in the muscle or neuromuscular junction from the failure to generate a force because of an insufficient drive from the central nervous system or because of mechanical inefficiency of the muscle (see below). Early studies in which subjects breathed through a resistance demonstrated 'fatigue', but this was attributed to a defect in the respiratory centres rather than to the respiratory muscles [729]. The possibility of true respiratory muscle fatigue was realized later [1666]. When muscle fatigue is developing, there is normally a compensatory increase in the firing frequency and in the number of active motor neurons supplying the muscle [2240]. The adequacy of the respiratory drive, therefore, has to be assessed in the light of the presence or absence of fatigue.

Two types of muscle fatigue have been demonstrated [889].

HIGH-FREQUENCY FATIGUE

High-frequency fatigue is thought to be due to fatigue at the neuromuscular junction or to impaired depolarization of the muscle cell membrane. It is characteristic of myasthenia gravis. The force generated by the muscle is particularly reduced during stimulation at high frequencies (60–100 Hz) (Fig. 2.5). Recovery from high-frequency fatigue may be complete in about 10 min [127, 891].

LOW-FREQUENCY FATIGUE

Low-frequency fatigue is thought to occur within the muscle fibre and to be due to a fault in the excitation–contraction coupling. It is seen in primary muscle disorders such as the myopathies. A change in the frequency–force curve is induced by stimulation at low frequencies (10–30 Hz) (Fig. 2.5). Low-frequency fatigue takes a few minutes to develop and may last for up to 24 h [127, 891].

Muscle fatigue develops when the energy demands outstrip the supplies [2004, 2009]. It therefore depends on the following factors.

Blood supply and energy stores

Initially, the myoglobin stores in the muscle may be adequate to maintain oxidative metabolism, particularly of type 1 fibres. Muscle glycogen may also be metabolized [1184]. Most of the energy supply is, however, dependent on

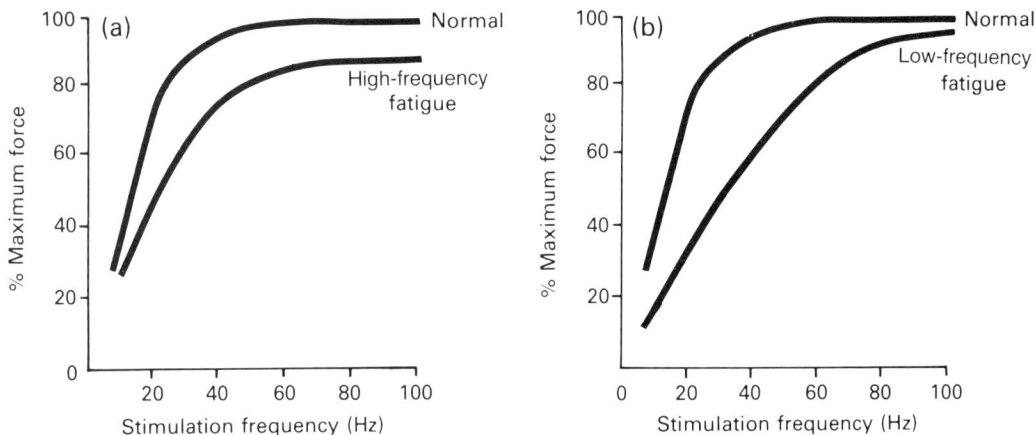

Fig. 2.5. *Muscle fatigue: (a) high-frequency fatigue, (b) low-frequency fatigue.*

the blood flow to the muscle and on its content of oxygen and other nutrients. The cardiac output increases during exertion, when the energy demands of the respiratory muscles increase. There is very little data on the changes in regional blood flow to the respiratory muscles during exercise, but it appears that the blood flow to the diaphragm rises as ventilation increases [519, 2652,2653, 2677, 2682, 2721]. In normal subjects, this is unlikely to be the factor determining when diaphragmatic fatigue appears. This may, however, be precipitated by a fall in cardiac output, hypotension, anaemia or hypoxia [2722], and be relieved by oxygen administration [2401].

Muscle work

The amount of energy required by the contracting muscles depends on the efficiency of contraction (p. 21), the proportion of each fibre type and the force of contraction. Type 1 fibres have a predominantly oxidative metabolism and are more resistant to fatigue than type 2 fibres (see above). The limit of endurance is also set by the ratio of the force developed to the maximal force that can be developed. This implies that fatigue is related to muscle strength and that weaker muscles fatigue more easily. Muscle fatigue is probably a major factor in contributing to the development of ventilatory failure in neuromuscular disorders.

In general, skeletal muscles can maintain an isotonic force of over 40% of their maximal force, if the duration of contraction and relaxation is equal, and an isometric force of over 15% of the maximal force [2009]. A transdiaphragmatic pressure at the FRC of about 40% of the maximal transdiaphragmatic pressure can be indefinitely sustained [2722], whereas higher pressures cause fatigue. A similar relationship holds for the maximal inspiratory pressure (P_{Imax}), of which about 60% can be sustained [2718].

Fatigue can be more accurately predicted when the duration of contraction is taken into account; for inspiratory muscles, this is the ratio

of inspiratory time to the duration of the breath; (T_I/T_{TOT}). The period of contraction is known as the duty cycle, which increases as the respiratory frequency increases, because T_E shortens, and predisposes to fatigue independently of any effect of the respiratory frequency itself [582]. The duty cycle can be taken into account by calculating the 'tension time index'. This is the product of the T_I/T_{TOT} ratio and the percentage of the maximal transdiaphragmatic pressure attained. Fatigue usually occurs in normal subjects if this index is greater than 0.15 [227–229] (Fig. 2.6). Fatigue is also more likely if the mean inspiratory flow rate is increased, since the energy consumption is greater if the velocity of contraction increases [582, 1981].

Muscle fatigue is uncommon in normal subjects but it has been demonstrated in runners who have completed a marathon [1933] and after breathing through an inspiratory resistance [1261, 2238]. It has been recognized for many years that the maximum voluntary ventilation (MVV) manoeuvre over 15 sec cannot be sustained indefinitely, and that the longer the test the smaller the fraction of the MVV that can be maintained [1040, 1041, 1896, 2070, 2895, 3148, 3400]. About 50% of the MVV can be

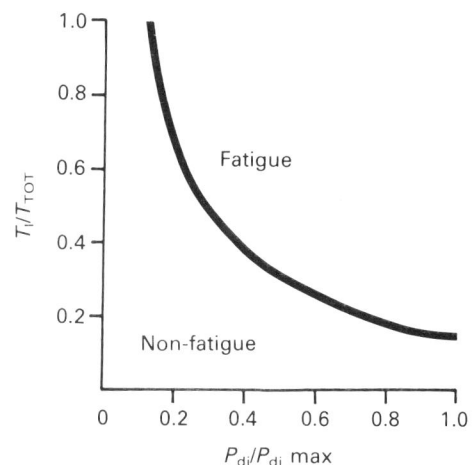

Fig. 2.6. *Respiratory muscle fatigue. Fatigue is likely to develop if the product of T_I/T_{TOT} and $P_{di}/P_{di\,max}$ lies above the line indicated on the graph.*

indefinitely sustained [1041] without muscle fatigue developing.

EFFICIENCY AND WORK OF RESPIRATION

Energy is used by the inspiratory muscles to overcome the resistance to air flow, elastic forces of the chest wall and lungs and, to a much smaller extent, the viscosity and inertia of the lungs and chest wall. Inspiration occurs passively only if the end expiratory volume is less than the FRC, in which case elastic recoil initiates the inflation of the lungs.

Some of the energy spent during inspiration is stored as potential energy and released during expiration when the lungs and chest wall return towards the FRC. The time constant of the respiratory system is short and expiration would proceed rapidly if it were due purely to elastic recoil [1100] (Fig. 2.7). This would favour basal airway closure and hinder gas exchange. Electromyogram studies have shown that expiration is actively 'braked' by a persisting contraction of 'inspiratory' muscles during the early part of expiration [2890] and, probably more importantly, by constriction of the upper airway at various sites. This prolongs expiration, prevents basal airway closure and facilitates mixing of the inspired gas in the lungs and the exchange of gas across the alveolar capillary membrane. Expiratory braking is achieved by contraction of the diaphragm [34, 2450], of the intercostal muscles [3143], larynx [2565], velopharyngeal sphincter [2685] and, particularly in emphysema, by pursed lip breathing. When ventilation increases, e.g. during exercise, T_E shortens since expiratory braking is removed. The rate of expiration can be increased further by abdominal muscle contraction [472, 480].

The external work performed by a muscle is the product of the force developed and the distance moved. This is hard to estimate for any of the respiratory muscles except for the sternomastoid [895, 2239]. Work is, however, the product of the force and the distance the object is moved, so that an approximation to the external work carried out is the product of the pressure developed and the volume change. The efficiency of ventilation is of the order of 10% [480], but this varies with the length and velocity of shortening of the muscle. Both of these factors change continuously during inspiration and expiration. The relationship of lung volume to muscle length has been discussed on p. 18, but the lung volume has two other effects on the efficiency of ventilation. Firstly, the air flow resistance decreases and the compliance of the respiratory system falls as the lung volume approaches TLC. Near the RV, air flow resistance increases and the compliance falls. Secondly, the dimensions of the chest wall determine the mechanical advantage of the muscle independently of its length. Laplace's law states that for a cylinder the pressure developed is proportional to the wall tension divided by the radius.

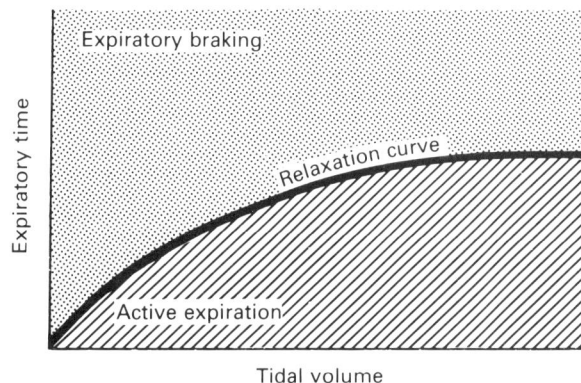

Fig. 2.7. *Relationship between expiratory time and tidal volume. In the absence of respiratory muscle activity, expiratory time follows the relaxation curve as tidal volume increases. If expiration is braked, expiratory time lies above this line, whereas if it is assisted by expiratory muscle contraction it falls below this line.*

As the lungs inflate and the radius of curvature of the inspiratory muscles, e.g. the diaphragm, increases, the pressure required to achieve a given change of volume also increases. The mechanical effects of volume changes are more complex if the thorax is asymmetrical, as in scoliosis or following a thoracoplasty, but the same principles apply.

The oxygen cost of breathing has been estimated to be about 0.25 ml/l ventilation during quiet breathing [486]. It increases approximately linearly with increasing ventilation up to a point, but then rises more rapidly. It may even exceed the quantity of oxygen taken up by the lungs, in which case hypoxaemia rapidly develops.

The oxygen cost of breathing reflects both the external work carried out by the respiratory muscles and their efficiency. There is an optimal frequency and tidal volume for any given ventilation, which are determined by the mechanical properties of the lungs and chest wall (Fig. 2.8). In general, the optimal respiratory frequency falls and the tidal volume increases as air flow obstruction worsens; the opposite is seen with restrictive defects. The work of breathing and the intrapleural pressure swings are minimized at optimal frequency and tidal volume [1995, 2390]. The T_I/T_{TOT} ratio, the mean inspiratory flow rate and T_E are probably also adjusted to minimize the work of the respiratory muscles.

COORDINATION OF RESPIRATORY MUSCLES

Normal respiration is the result of the coordinated action of the respiratory muscles. The importance of the diaphragm is often emphasized but, to be effective, it requires the activity of other muscles. For instance, abdominal muscle contraction during expiration elevates the diaphragm into an optimal position for its contraction during inspiration. The intercostal muscle activity stabilizes the rib cage and prevents paradoxical movement due to the negative intrapleural pressure generated by diaphragmatic contraction, and the inspiratory activity of the abdominal muscles decreases the compliance of the abdomen and enables it to act as a fulcrum so that the diaphragm can expand the rib cage. Conversely, the intercostal and accessory muscles lower the intrapleural pressure and would cause the diaphragm to move into the chest during inspiration unless its contraction opposed this paradoxical movement.

The division between the primary and accessory respiratory muscles is artificial. The scalene muscles have been thought to be accessory muscles, but EMG studies have shown them to be active during quiet inspiration in normal subjects. Other 'accessory' muscles, such as the sternomastoids, become active as the tidal volume increases [2559]. It is better to regard the respiratory muscles as being capable of recruitment according to the pattern of ventilation, posture, wakefulness or stage of sleep, muscle strength, air flow resistance, and compliance of the lungs and chest wall.

The muscles of the upper airway are often overlooked, but are as much respiratory muscles as those of the chest wall they preserve the patency of the airway and control the rate of expiration, and their activation is closely coordinated with the chest wall muscles.

Most of the respiratory muscles also have a

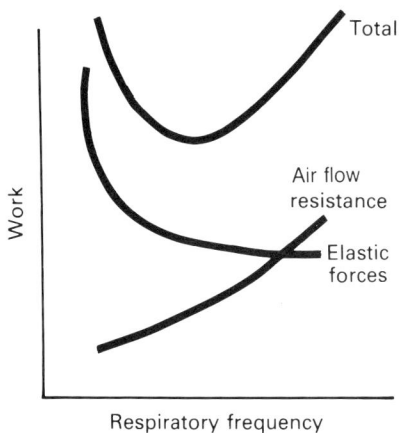

Fig. 2.8. *Changes in the relative contributions of air flow resistance and elastic forces to the work of the respiratory muscles at different respiratory frequencies.*

postural function. They all contain plentiful muscle spindles, except for the diaphragm and the parasternal intercostal muscles. These two sets of muscles are almost purely respiratory, but the electrical activity of the other muscles correlates with postural activity as well as with respiration [864]. Some respiratory muscles, particularly the accessory muscles, are also used for arm movements, and this may hinder the coordination of their contraction with the other respiratory muscles (p. 28).

INDIVIDUAL RESPIRATORY MUSCLES (Table 2.1; Figs 2.9, 2.10)

Diaphragm

ANATOMY

The diaphragm is conventionally considered as a single muscle or as being composed of a right and left hemi-diaphragm, but there is some evidence that its costal and sternal fibres should be regarded as a single muscle and the crural fibres as a separate muscle [757, 758]. All the muscle fibres run radially and converge on the aponeurotic central tendon, but only the costal and sternal fibres have an origin on the rib cage. The costal fibres arise from the inner aspect and upper margin of the lower six ribs, and interdigitate with those of the transversus abdominis. The sternal fibres originate from the back of the xiphoid process. In contrast, the crural fibres arise on the right from the 1st–3rd and on the left from the 1st and 2nd lumbar vertebrae, and from the medial and lateral arcuate ligaments. They have no direct attachment to the rib cage and their origin is less mobile than that of the costal and sternal fibres.

The embryological origin of the components of the diaphragm is complex [1837]. The central tendon is derived from the septum transversum.

Table 2.1. *Actions of individual respiratory muscles in isolation*

	Muscle	Pressure changes	Actions
1	Upper airway dilators	↓ Upper airway pressure	Opening or dilatation of upper airway
2	Upper airway constrictors	↑ Upper airway pressure	Constriction or occlusion of upper airway
3	'Accessory' muscles	↓ Pleural pressure ↓ Abdominal pressure	Rib cage expansion Diaphragm elevation Abdominal indrawing
4	Inspiratory intercostal muscles	↓ Pleural pressure ↓ Abdominal pressure	Rib cage expansion Diaphragm elevation Abdominal indrawing
5	Expiratory intercostal muscles	↑ Pleural pressure ↑ Abdominal pressure	Rib cage compression Diaphragm depression Abdominal expansion
6	Diaphragm	↓ Pleural pressure ↑ Abdominal pressure	Upper rib cage indrawing Zone of apposition reduction Diaphragm depression Abdominal expansion
7	Abdominal muscles without rib cage attachment	↑ Pleural pressure ↑ Abdominal pressure	Rib cage expansion Diaphragm elevation Abdominal compression
8	Abdominal muscles with rib cage attachment	As for (7) plus further ↑ pleural pressure	As for (7) plus rib cage compression

(a)

INSPIRATORY   EXPIRATORY
MUSCLES   MUSCLES

Sternomastoid

Scalenes

                                          Internal
                                          intercostals

External
intercostals

Diaphragm

                                          External oblique
                                          Rectus abdominis
                                          Internal oblique

                                          Transversus
                                          abdominis

(b)

Serratus
posterior
superior

Erector spinae

Serratus
posterior
inferior

                                          Latissimus dorsi

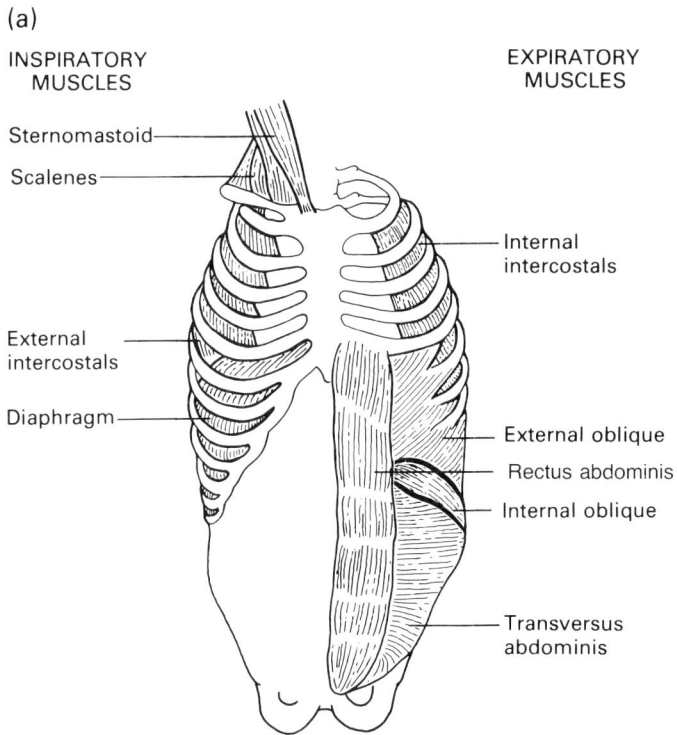

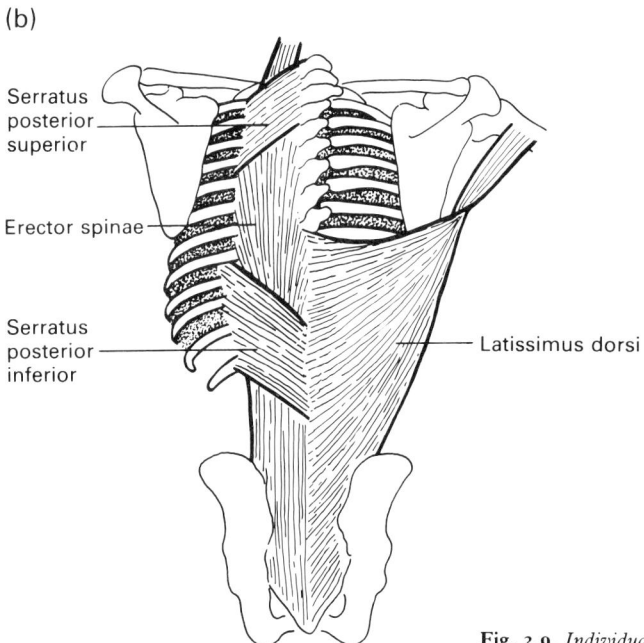

Fig. 2.9. *Individual respiratory muscles: (a) anterior, (b) posterior.*

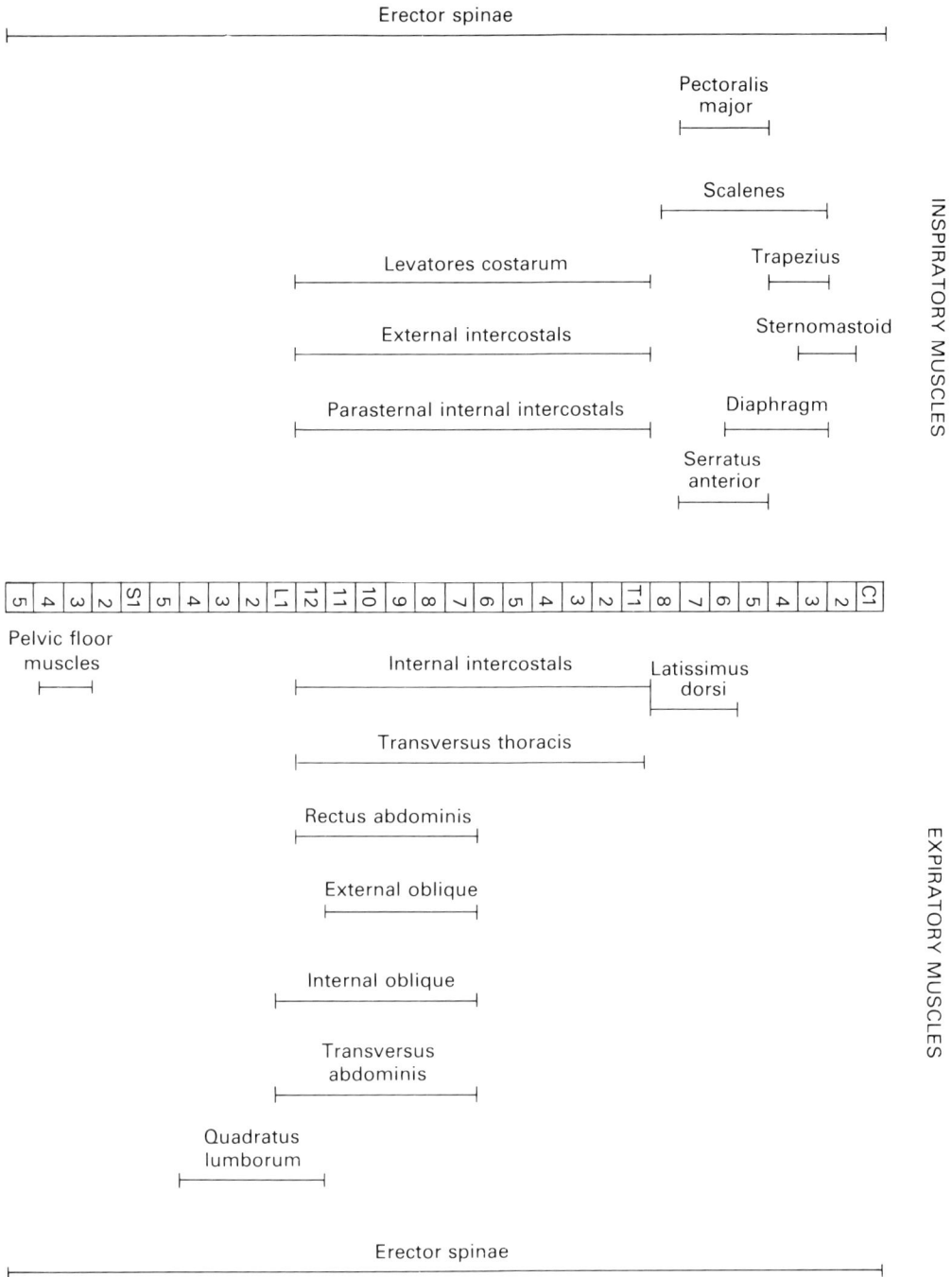

Fig. 2.10. *Level of spinal cord innervation of respiratory muscles.*

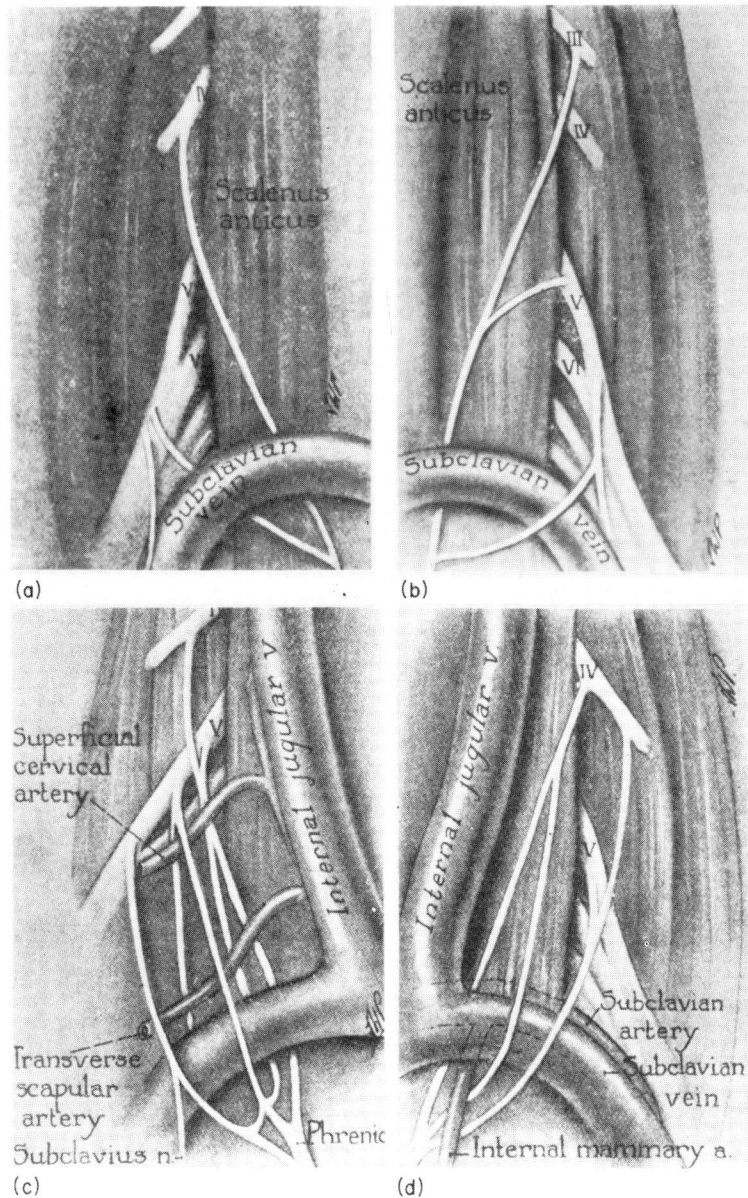

Fig. 2.11. *Examples of the variations in the anatomy of the phrenic nerves in the neck. (a) Main phrenic nerve trunk and accessory nerve passing behind subclavian vein. (b) Accessory phrenic nerve passing anterior to subclavian vein. (c) Complex arrangement of nerves that form a single phrenic nerve below the subclavian vein. (d) Phrenic nerve rootlets arising mainly from C4 but remaining separate until below the subclavian vein. Reproduced, with permission, from Davies HM.* Pulmonary Tuberculosis. Medical and surgical treatment. *Macmillan Publishing Company, 1933: 323–6.* (Originally published in the UK by Cassell.)

The costal fibres are homologous to the transversus abdominis muscle but the crural fibres have a different origin and grow into a derivative of the primitive mesentery.

INNERVATION

The cell bodies of the motor neurons supplying the diaphragm are situated in the phrenic nerve nuclei (p. 6). The cell bodies of the fibres supplying the crural part of the diaphragm in cats are situated more caudally than those reaching the costal fibres [2779], and in monkeys the cranial part of the nucleus supplies the fibres in the centre of the diaphragm [350]. In man, the phrenic nerve usually forms a single trunk only after it enters the thorax, and the anatomical details are often complex [728] (Fig. 2.11). The nerve rootlets from C3–C5 or C6 join to form a main trunk, but an accessory phrenic nerve is present in around 75% of subjects [1642]. This accessory nerve is formed largely from C5 and usually joins the main phrenic nerve trunk behind the sternal end of the 1st rib [55, 1642, 2088, 2221]. The nerve to the subclavius muscle may also give off a medial branch to join the phrenic nerve [1642].

It has been proposed that motor fibres reach the diaphragm through the intercostal nerves as well as the phrenic nerve [350, 2705], but this is unlikely [2779]. Most of the sensory fibres from the diaphragm also travel in the phrenic nerve, but some afferent impulses from the margin of the diaphragm may pass in the lower six intercostal nerves [55, 2705]. The phrenic nerve also contains sensory fibres from the diaphragmatic pleura, peritoneum and mediastinal structures, such as the pericardium. There is some evidence that within the phrenic nerve the motor and sensory fibres are arranged in discrete strands [1690].

The phrenic nerve divides within the diaphragm into an anterior, lateral, and a larger posterior division. These branches run intramuscularly and form anastomosing neural arcades [2837]. Some fibres cross over, particularly from the left to the right side of the diaphragm [2779]. The diaphragm contains few muscle spindles [644, 865] but most of those that are present are located in the crura [428], which may have a postural as well as a respiratory function. The costal and sternal parts of the diaphragm appear to be inhibited to a lesser extent during REM sleep than the postural muscles, which have a higher muscle spindle density (p. 37).

FIBRE TYPES

The proportion of type 1 muscle fibres in the diaphragm is greater in smaller mammals, which have a higher metabolic rate and respiratory frequency [1098]. Man is intermediate in this respect, but there is considerable variation in the proportion of fibre types in different areas of the diaphragm [2625]. Overall, about 55% of fibres are type 1, 20% type 2A and 25% type 2B [1896]. The resistance to fatigue of the diaphragm [957, 1843] appears to be due to this high proportion of fatigue-resistant fibres and also to the ability of the blood flow to the diaphragm to increase approximately in step with the ventilation (p. 20).

ACTIONS

The action of both the costal and crural fibres decreases the intrapleural pressure and raises the abdominal pressure. In the absence of intercostal muscle contraction, the upper rib cage is drawn in, but the lower rib cage is exposed to the intra-abdominal pressure and, like the abdomen, expands. Except at high lung volumes, the costal diaphragmatic fibres run almost vertically and parallel to the interior of the lower rib cage. This 'zone of apposition' [2099] decreases as the diaphragm descends [757]. The ratio of abdominal to rib cage expansion depends on the compliance of these two compartments. However, the costal fibres also directly expand the rib cage because of their origin from the lower six ribs. Contraction of these vertical fibres elevates the lower ribs, leading to an increase in both the anteroposterior and transverse diameters. The crural fibres do not have this action.

The effectiveness of diaphragmatic contraction depends on the length of the diaphragm, its shape and the velocity of shortening. The tension developed by the diaphragm increases with its length up to a critical point [2178]. In dogs, the range of lengths over which the diaphragm is effective is greater than in other skeletal muscles [1670]. It is able to generate force at as little as 40% of its resting length and a maximal force at 125% of the resting length. For most other skeletal muscles, the figures are 50% and 105%, respectively. The diaphragm is, therefore, able to generate tension over a wide range of lung volumes, although if hyperinflation is severe the transdiaphragmatic pressure does fall [2436, 2676].

In normal subjects, the diaphragm is approximately a hemispherical dome at the end of expiration, but as the central tendon descends and the zone of apposition decreases it approximates to a flattened sheet. Its radius of curvature therefore increases and, by Laplace's law, less pressure is generated for any given muscular tension. Experimental work both in dogs [1670] and in humans [388] has, however, indicated that the change in the radius of curvature is less than might be expected, although accurate measurements are difficult because of the changes in the zone of apposition. If the thorax is asymmetrical, as in scoliosis, the shape and mechanical efficiency of the right and left hemidiaphragms may differ considerably.

The transdiaphragmatic pressure is less if the length of the diaphragm changes rapidly [2003, 2436]. The rate of shortening largely depends on the contraction of the abdominal muscles [1175] and on the intensity of stimulation of the diaphragm.

COORDINATION OF ACTIVITY

The contraction of the diaphragm cannot be viewed in isolation, and is only one component of respiratory muscle activity. An important function of this coordination is to prevent excessive shortening of the diaphragm so that it is unable to generate adequate tension during the next inspiration [2880]. The length of the diaphragm is not fixed at any given lung volume because the rib cage and abdomen act in series and the configuration of both can be altered by muscular contraction [388, 1229]. If, however, abdominal expansion predominates, the diaphragm shortens and the maximal transdiaphragmatic pressure falls [1175].

The diaphragm has long been recognized as the most important inspiratory muscle [849], particularly in the supine position [2005, 3249, 3258]. It is probably responsible for 60–75% of V_T during quiet breathing [3248, 3258] but a smaller percentage at higher V_T. If the intercostal muscles do not contract during inspiration, the fall in intrapleural pressure caused by diaphragmatic contraction will lead to paradoxical movement of the rib cage and a reduction in the V_T.

Electrical activity of the diaphragm is detectable throughout inspiration, but it also persists early into expiration [34, 2450]. The importance of this has been discussed on p. 21. End expiratory activity is also detectable close to the RV [35]. It contracts during expulsive efforts such as parturition, defaecation, vomiting, coughing and sneezing, in conjunction with the abdominal muscles so that the abdominal pressure is raised.

Intercostal and other rib cage muscles

ANATOMY

There are three layers of rib cage muscles. The external intercostals extend from the tubercles of the ribs to the costochondral junctions, where they become continuous with the anterior intercostal membrane. Their fibres slope obliquely downwards and forwards from the upper rib to the rib below. The internal intercostals extend from the sternum to the angles of the ribs posteriorly, where they become continuous with the posterior intercostal membrane. Their fibres slope obliquely downwards and backwards from the upper rib to the rib below. The fibres that lie between the costal cartilages (interchondral or parasternal muscles) have fewer muscle spindles [864] and slightly different functions to the remainder of the internal intercostals. Both layers of intercostal muscles are supplied from T1–T12 segments by the intercostal nerves.

Inside the internal intercostal muscles is the thin layer of the transversus thoracis group of muscles. This can be divided into the anterior sternocostal muscle, the lateral intercostales intimi and the posterior subcostales. This group of muscles is expiratory in function [3143]. The only other rib cage muscles of any respiratory significance are the levatores costarum, which arise from the transverse processes of C7–T11 vertebrae and insert between the tubercle and angle of the rib immediately caudal to the vertebra from which they arise. They probably have an inspiratory action.

ACTIONS

The respiratory functions of the intercostal muscles have been disputed for many years. Their arrangement has suggested that the external intercostals and the parasternal muscles would elevate the ribs and that the interosseous internal intercostals would lower the ribs. Electrical recordings have confirmed that the external intercostals are active only during inspiration [3143]. The parasternal muscles are also active during inspiration, even at rest [749, 751, 755, 3143]. Other intercostal muscles are recruited as the tidal volume increases and as the rate of inspiration becomes more rapid [1713]. Studies of rib cage mechanics in dogs have shown that the ribs are more readily displaced upwards if an equal force is applied both above and below the rib and have suggested that even the interosseous internal intercostal muscles are inspiratory [755].

Contraction of the intercostal muscles also stabilizes the rib cage if the intrapleural pressure is lowered by diaphragmatic or accessory muscle contraction. This is particularly important in infants, in whom the chest wall is very compliant [2222]. Expiratory activity of the internal intercostal muscles can be detected particularly over the lower lateral chest wall during quiet breathing, and this may help brake expiration [3143]. The end expiratory position of the diaphragm is also partially determined by intercostal activity, which regulates the degree of expansion of the rib cage [1508(b)].

The parasternal intercostal muscles probably have a purely respiratory function [864], but the other intercostal muscles also have a postural role. This may conflict with their function as respiratory muscles and, like other postural muscles, their tone is markedly reduced during REM sleep.

Abdominal muscles

ANATOMY

The most important abdominal muscles that are active during respiration are:

Rectus abdominis

This muscle arises from the pubic symphysis and crest and joins the 5th–7th costal cartilages.

External oblique

This arises from the outer surfaces of the lower eight ribs. The dorsal fibres pass downwards to the iliac crest but the rest of the muscle merges into the linea alba anteriorly.

Internal oblique

This muscle arises from the lumbar fascia, the iliac crest and the lateral part of the inguinal ligament. The dorsal fibres pass vertically to join the last three ribs and the rest of the muscle merges into fibrous tissue anteriorly.

Transversus abdominis

This innermost muscle arises from the costal cartilages of the lower six ribs, the lumbar fascia, the iliac crest and the lateral part of the inguinal ligament. It passes horizontally to join the internal oblique anteriorly.

The rectus abdominis is supplied by T7–T12, the external oblique by T7–T11 and the internal oblique and transversus abdominis by T7–L1.

ACTIONS

All four muscles reduce the compliance of the abdomen and increase the intra-abdominal pressure when they contract. This reduces the degree of abdominal expansion during inspiration but enables the abdomen to act as a fulcrum so that the rib cage can expand. The raised intra-abdominal pressure is transmitted directly to the lower rib cage over the zone of apposition of the diaphragm, particularly at low lung volumes. The position of the diaphragm and its mechanical efficiency are influenced by the degree of contraction of the abdominal muscles [2146].

The rectus abdominis and the external oblique muscles also change the dimensions of the rib cage directly, because they are inserted into the ribs. The internal oblique and transversus abdominis muscles lack this action. Contraction of the rectus abdominis displaces the sternum caudally in dogs and diminishes the anteroposterior and transverse diameters of the rib cage [756].

The abdominal muscles normally contribute little to expiration unless the ventilation is greater than about 40 l/min [472, 480]. They are not readily activated by an increase in the expiratory air flow resistance since this is usually compensated for by extra inspiratory muscle effort [474] and a reduction in expiratory 'braking'. Expiratory contraction of the abdominal muscles during exercise lowers the end expiratory volume below the FRC, so that the start of inspiration is aided by elastic recoil and the diaphragm is lengthened and able to generate high inspiratory pressures [1255]. The abdominal muscles also become active when the lung volume approaches TLC and may limit further inflation of the lungs [472].

Electromyogram studies have indicated that the abdominal muscles have a tonic postural action in the erect but not in the supine position. This prevents the abdominal wall from protruding and maintains the diaphragm in an effective position [740]. They are able to generate high abdominal pressures during expulsive manoeuvres such as coughing, parturition, vomiting and defaecation [484].

'Accessory' muscles

SCALENE MUSCLES

There are three scalene muscles, of which the middle is the largest. The anterior scalene arises from the transverse processes of the 3rd–6th cervical vertebrae and inserts into the 1st rib anteriorly. The middle scalene arises from the transverse processes of the 2nd–7th cervical vertebrae and inserts into the 1st rib, whereas the posterior scalene muscle arises from the transverse processes of the 5th–7th cervical vertebrae and inserts posteriorly into the 2nd rib. The scalene muscles are supplied by C3–C8.

Their contraction elevates the upper rib cage [480, 754, 3153] in a similar manner to the other accessory muscles and the intercostal muscles. They counteract the action of the parasternal muscles on the sternum and increase the anteroposterior diameter of the upper rib cage [741, 751]. They decrease the intrapleural pressure and may lead to paradoxical movement of the rib cage if the intercostal muscles are inactive [754].

Electrical activity in the scalene muscles can be detected in most subjects, even during quiet inspiration [473, 749, 2559] and they should be regarded as primary muscles of respiration rather than 'accessory' muscles. Their contraction is prolonged and more forceful if V_T increases, as inspiration becomes more rapid, or in the presence of hyperinflation [2559, 3153].

STERNOMASTOID MUSCLES

The sternomastoid muscles arise from the sternum and the medial part of the clavicle and insert into the mastoid process and occipital bone. They are supplied mainly by the 11th cranial nerve, but also by the 2nd cervical nerve. Contraction elevates the sternum and increases the anteroposterior diameter of the thorax. Electrical activity is seen less frequently during quiet inspiration than in the scalene muscles [473], but the sternomastoids are recruited as the tidal volume increases [2559]. Like the scalene muscles, the sternomastoids are particularly important when the lungs are hyperinflated, since this puts the diaphragm and intercostal muscles at a mechanical disadvantage.

OTHER MUSCLES

A large number of other muscles of the rib cage and shoulder girdle may have a respiratory action in certain circumstances. These include the trapezius, pectoralis major and minor, latissimus dorsi, serratus anterior and posterior, quadratus lumborum and erector spinae [480, 1713].

Upper airway muscles

The upper airway is surrounded by about twenty-four muscles, which function as a unit

Table 2.2. *Muscles of upper airway and their functions. Reproduced, with permission, from Proctor D.F.* Eur. J. Respir. Dis. *1983;* **64:** *Suppl 128, 89–96*

Section of airway	Dilators	Action uncertain	Constrictors
1 Nasal valve	Dilator naris		
2 Main nasal passage		Vascular smooth muscle	
3 Velopharyngeal sphincter			Tensor veli palatini Levator veli palatini Palatopharyngeus
		Salpingopharyngeus	
4 Oropharynx	Muscles of lips and tongue		
5 Pharynx	Masseter Pterygoids Genioglossus Hyoglossus		
			Pharyngeal constrictors Styloglossus
	Digastric Mylohyoid Geniohyoid Stylohyoid		
		Omohyoid Thyrohyoid Sternohyoid Sternothyroid	
6 Larynx	Posterior cricoarytenoid		
			Aryepiglottic Interarytenoid Lateral cricoarytenoid Thyroarytenoid
		Cricothyroid	

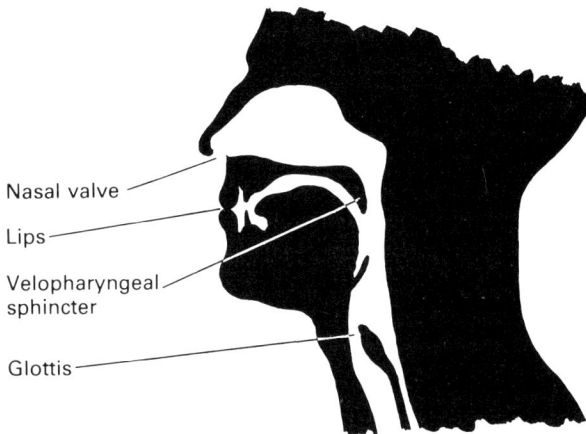

Nasal valve

Lips

Velopharyngeal
sphincter

Glottis

Fig. 2.12. *Sites at which the flow of air through the upper airway can be controlled.*

even though they are anatomically separate [1967, 2533, 2534, 2685]. The details of the individual muscles are shown in Table 2.2. The upper airway is a respiratory conduit that warms, humidifies and filters the inspired air, but the muscles also have to assist swallowing, coughing, speech and abdominal expulsive efforts. The contraction and relaxation of the upper airway muscles is closely linked to that of the chest wall muscles. Respiration is dependent on their ability to maintain a patent upper airway and to regulate the air flow resistance.

The upper airway consists of a nasal and an oral route, which converge in the pharynx to form a single conduit to the larynx (Fig. 2.12). Air flow resistance is less during mouth breathing but the inspired air is less adequately warmed, humidified and filtered than during nasal breathing. The consequence of exposing a large surface area to the inspired air in the nose is that the resistance to air flow is high and the air flow is turbulent. In normal subjects, the nasal resistance is more than half of the total resistance to air flow [451, 3011], although there is considerable variation between individuals. The nasal resistance is partly due to contraction of the muscles of the alae nasi and partly to vascular erectile tissue within the nose. The nasal cavity is rigid in its bony and cartilaginous parts but collapsible at the nares and particularly

near the inferior turbinates [396]. Collapse of the upper airway may also occur in the oropharynx at a critical transmural pressure that is influenced by the compliance and diameter of the airway (Chapter 6). Collapse is favoured by a low intra-airway pressure due to inspiratory activity of the chest wall muscles, narrowing of the airway and a reduction in the tone of the dilator muscles. The muscular activity of the upper airway largely controls these potentially flow-limiting segments and stabilizes the airway [1784, 2534, 2595].

The alae nasi prevent collapse at the nares and near the inferior turbinates (nasal valve) [395]. Their activity is related to the volume of nasal air flow and is absent during mouth breathing [607]. Their contraction decreases the compliance of the nares and counteracts the narrowing of the airway due to the vascular tissue within the nose. This dilates and constricts in a regular 2–4 hourly 'nasal cycle', which is controlled both by the autonomic nervous system and by local release of chemicals [3207]. The nasal resistance varies with posture [606, 1377], exercise [2367], mechanical and chemical irritation, and the temperature of inspired air [605, 3328].

The velopharyngeal sphincter, as well as the lips, determine whether air is inspired through the mouth or through the nose [2685]. In infants, apposition of the soft palate and epiglottis frequently prevents mouth breathing, and in adults the velopharyngeal sphincter is able to brake expiration [2685].

The soft tissues of the hypopharynx are supported by the hyoid bone. The patency of the airway is maintained by postural muscles [2893], and by pharyngeal dilators such as the genioglossus and geniohyoid that pull the tongue and hyoid forwards in inspiration [1217, 2194].

The muscular control of the laryngeal aperture is complex [84]. The sole dilator is the posterior cricoarytenoid muscle and the main constrictor is the thyroarytenoid muscle. Normally, the glottis widens during inspiration and narrows during expiration [384], with corresponding changes in the air flow resistance [200]. There is some tonic activity in the intrinsic muscles of the larynx [985] but the activity of the abductors increases during inspiration [2273], particularly when the tidal volume increases [384]. Adduction of the cords during expiration is mainly due to relaxation of the posterior cricoarytenoid muscle rather than contraction of the adductors [2255]. Glottic narrowing during expiration slows the deflation of the lungs and is more marked if expiration proceeds through the low resistance pathway to the mouth rather than through the higher resistance nasal airway [2565].

The contraction of each of these groups of upper airway muscles is coordinated and occurs just before the contraction of the chest wall muscles. The dilator muscles of the alae nasi show EMG activity before the onset of inspiratory air flow [3081], and this is followed by activity in the genioglossus and then the diaphragm [408, 2372]. In general, the contraction of the upper airway muscles is more sudden in onset than the diaphragm and is maximal in mid-inspiration [3333].

The upper airway muscle activity is modified by the degree of inflation of the lungs and the blood gases. They are inhibited by stimulation of the pulmonary stretch receptors, whose afferent fibres travel in the vagus nerve. Both the genioglossus and the abductor muscles of the larynx have been shown to be inhibited [1238, 1967]. The glottic size is related to lung volume [384], and a similar relationship has been shown for the pharynx [1446, 1449].

Reflex changes in the activity of the upper airway muscles are discussed on p. 10. The contraction of both the upper airway and the chest wall muscles increases during hypoxia and hypercapnia or occlusion of the airway [408, 1217, 2371, 2372, 3279]. The vocal cords abduct during inspiration, and when expiratory braking is removed [200]. These adaptations enable ventilation to be increased and the blood gases to return to normal. The nasal resistance also falls, probably by reflex sympathetic vasoconstriction due to hypercapnia [1976]. There is no change when hypoxic gas mixtures are inhaled, except at very low concentrations [1976].

Chapter 3
Respiration during Sleep

The changes in respiration during sleep have received considerable attention over the last few years and have been the subject of several reviews [820, 1757, 2466]. It is now recognized that observations of respiration during wakefulness cannot be extrapolated to sleep. During wakefulness there is greater dependence on the higher centres, particularly the cerebral cortex [984, 2860]. Some behavioural activities that affect respiration, such as laughing, only occur during wakefulness, and environmental stimuli, particularly visual, may cause respiratory stimulation in a way that could not take place during sleep [121]. The activity of the cerebral cortex and of the brain stem is very different during sleep and this affects the control of all of the skeletal muscles, including the respiratory muscles.

SLEEP STAGES

The early studies of sleep assumed that it was a homogeneous state and it was described purely by behavioural criteria (behavioural sleep). Analysis of electroencephalogram (EEG) recordings during sleep subsequently revealed two main stages of sleep; non-rapid eye movement (NREM) and rapid eye movement (REM) sleep [109]. An extensive terminology to describe the physiological changes during these stages of sleep has been developed [788].

Cerebral cortical activity is inhibited during NREM sleep by the reticular formation of the brain stem. This largely controls the metabolic rate and activity of the skeletal muscles. In contrast, cerebral cortical activity is prominent in REM sleep but both the sensory and motor functions of the central nervous system are different to those seen during wakefulness.

NREM sleep predominates at the onset of sleep. Rapid changes between wakefulness and the lighter stages of NREM sleep may be seen initially ('unsteady' sleep). The first phase of REM sleep usually appears about 90 min after the onset of sleep and it then alternates with NREM sleep at approximately 90-min intervals, although it may become more frequent and prolonged towards the end of the night. The proportions of NREM and REM sleep also vary with age. In neonates, REM sleep accounts for a high proportion of sleep time; NREM sleep only appears at the age of 3–4 months. It increases to a maximum of about 75% of sleep time prepubertally and then decreases steadily with age. The pattern of sleep is also influenced by factors such as sleep deprivation, sleep fragmentation and sedative drugs, including alcohol.

The diagnosis of NREM and REM sleep is based primarily on EEG criteria. These have been used to subdivide NREM sleep into four stages.

STAGE 1

This is the lightest stage of NREM sleep and is a transitional phase between wakefulness and sleep. It represents about 5% of total sleep time and is characterized by low-voltage, high-frequency θ waves and the presence of a $\propto$ waves for $<$ 50% of the time.

STAGE 2

This accounts for about 50% of sleep time and is marked by the appearance of low-voltage waves of mixed frequencies. Specific EEG complexes, including sleep spindles (bursts of waves with a frequency of 12–14 Hz) and K complexes (large independent waves with a voltage > 75 μV), are seen.

STAGE 3

This represents about 5% of sleep time and is characterized by low-frequency δ waves with a high voltage (> 75 μV). These features are present for 20–50% of this sleep stage.

STAGE 4

The EEG criteria of this phase of sleep are similar to those of stage 3 NREM sleep, except that the diagnostic features are present for $> 50\%$ of sleep time. About 15% of total sleep time is spent in stage 4 sleep.

Stages 1 and 2 NREM sleep are sometimes grouped together as light sleep, in contrast to slow-wave sleep that comprises stages 3 and 4 NREM sleep. The EEG recording during REM sleep is similar to that of stage 1 NREM sleep but of lower voltage and with the addition of random saw-tooth waves that coincide with EMG activity in the extraocular and other muscles.

RESPIRATION DURING SLEEP

Respiration is influenced by physiological changes occurring during sleep that are common to all stages of sleep (Fig. 3.1). These include a decrease by about 10–20% in the metabolic rate [2466, 3313] and changes in cardiac output and cerebral blood flow. Respiration increases when the subject arouses from sleep in response to various respiratory stimuli such as hypoxia, hypercapnia, laryngeal stimulation or upper airway obstruction. Arousal is a protective mechanism that relieves the sleep-induced respiratory abnormality and, if appropriate, enables a behavioural response to be made to the cause of the stimulus [2469]. Lesser degrees of stimulation may lead to protective reflexes, such

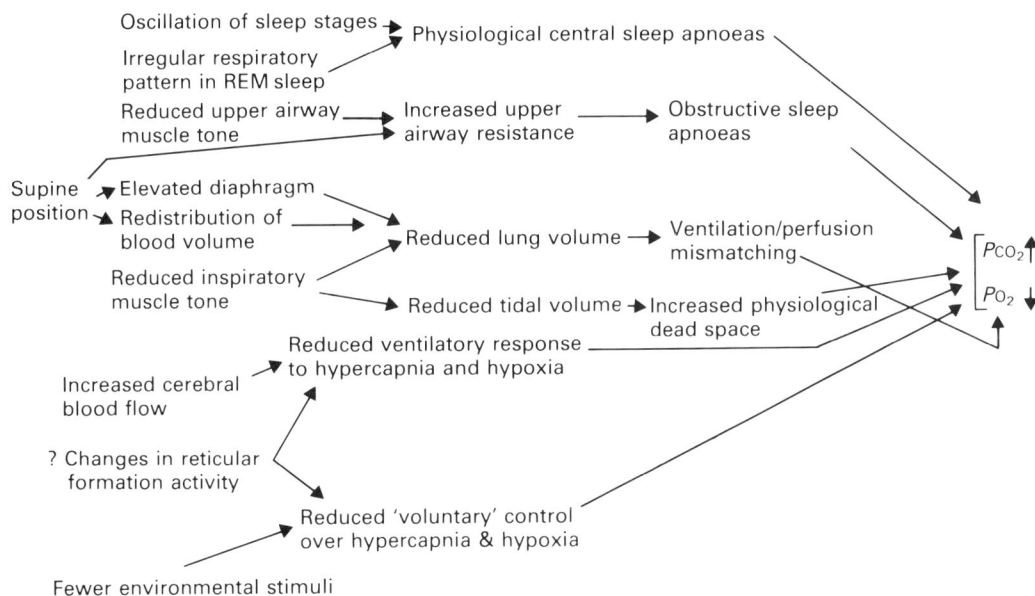

Fig. 3.1. *Flow chart to show the interactions of physiological changes during sleep that may contribute to hypoxia or hypercapnia.*

as coughing, without arousal [3101]. Failure to arouse with hypoxia is particularly important because of the risk of serious complications such as cardiac dysrhythmias. The threshold for arousal to hypoxia appears to rise if hypercapnia is also present [91]. The carotid bodies mediate arousal from hypoxia [3094] (p. 120) but not arousal from other causes such as laryngeal stimulation [360]. Sleep deprivation probably depresses the arousal response [361, 2468].

Many of the features of respiration during sleep are specific to the particular sleep stage (Fig. 3.1). NREM and REM sleep represent two different stages of neurophysiological organization and have distinct effects on respiration. The early observations of respiration during sleep did not take into account the effects of sleep stage and are hard to interpret [2177, 2659]. Automatic control of ventilation predominates during NREM sleep, whereas many of the respiratory features of REM sleep are due to cerebral cortical activity. This coincides with periods of dreaming and changes in the autonomic nervous system, such as an increase in parasympathetic activity, causing, for example, a bradycardia. Rapid changes in cerebral cortical activity lead to bursts of activity in the extraocular and other muscles, which may be manifested as irregular respiratory movements. These periods of phasic muscle contraction alternate with periods in which the tone in all the postural muscles is reduced. The diaphragm and, to a lesser extent, the parasternal intercostal muscles are the only non-postural respiratory muscles and they largely escape this reduction in activity. The irregular muscle contractions of phasic REM sleep are absent during tonic REM sleep and the respiratory pattern is much more regular.

NREM sleep

RESPIRATORY PATTERN

Many normal subjects oscillate between wakefulness and stages 1 and 2 NREM sleep at the onset of sleep. The control of respiration differs in each of these three states and this causes a fluctuation in the ventilatory pattern. A regular waxing and waning of V_T, which may be indistinguishable from Cheyne-Stokes respiration or Cheyne-Stokes variant (periodic breathing), or have an abrupt onset and termination, appears in 40–80% of subjects [438]. It is particularly frequent in infants, normal subjects at altitude and in older age groups [1765, 3268], in which the duration of these lighter stages of sleep is increased. The upper airway narrows and may close towards the end of the apnoeic phase [1448]. The length of the cycle of this Cheyne-Stokes respiration varies between 30 and 120 sec and the apnoeic phase is usually 10–40 sec. It therefore falls within the definition of a sleep apnoea and failure to recognize that this is a physiological finding, particularly in older subjects, has led to errors in interpretation of many of the reports of ventilation during sleep (p. 61).

The blood gases oscillate during Cheyne-Stokes respiration during sleep in the same way as during wakefulness. Hypoxia and hypercapnia are most marked at the end of the apnoeic phase. The threshold for the ventilatory response to hypercapnia is, however, different during wakefulness and stages 1 and 2 NREM sleep. This leads to oscillations in the P_{CO_2} and ventilation, as the stage of sleep changes. These oscillations are particularly marked if the sleep stages change frequently, if there is a large difference in the thresholds between wakefulness and each sleep stage, or if the slope of the ventilatory response to hypercapnia is steep.

In contrast, many subjects show little oscillation in sleep stage at the onset of sleep. Their respiratory pattern is more regular and Cheyne-Stokes respiration is not seen. The ventilation and tidal volume are probably less than during wakefulness and the P_{CO_2} may rise slightly. These trends are more marked in stages 3 and 4 NREM sleep [3066]. The P_{CO_2} rises by about 0.4–1.0 kPa and P_{O_2} falls by 0.5–1.25 kPa [1757], despite a decrease in the metabolic rate. The respiratory pattern is remarkably regular, in keeping with its control by the medullary respiratory centres and the relative inactivity of the cerebral cortex. The tidal volume and mean inspiratory flow rate are reduced but there is no change in the inspiratory muscle duty cycle [1757].

UPPER AIRWAY RESISTANCE

The upper airway resistance increases during NREM sleep. This is probably due to a loss of activity in the pharyngeal dilator muscles and particularly in the tensor palati which normally prevents the soft palate from occluding the airway. The ability to compensate for an increase in air flow resistance is less than during wakefulness [1517] and the time taken to arouse in the presence of airway obstruction is very variable [1543]. Nevertheless, the intercostal muscle activity appears to increase during NREM sleep, in response to the increase in upper airway resistance, and the ratio of rib cage to abdominal expansion increases [3066].

VENTILATORY DRIVE

The ventilatory responses to hypoxia and hypercapnia are diminished during NREM sleep. In men, the hypoxic drive is about two-thirds that of wakefulness but little change is seen in women [824]. This difference may reflect the greater waking hypoxic drive in men [820]. The slope of the ventilatory response to hypercapnia is about half that seen during wakefulness [826], and there is no difference between this response in men and women [820].

REM sleep

RESPIRATORY PATTERN

The respiratory pattern during phasic REM sleep is very irregular. This has made it hard to assess any overall changes in tidal volume, respiratory frequency or arterial blood gases. In the tonic phase of REM sleep, the activity of all the respiratory muscles except the diaphragm and parasternal intercostal muscles is reduced [866, 1327, 3203]. The diaphragm has very few

muscle spindles [644, 865, 866] so that supraspinal inhibition of muscle spindles has less effect than in other muscles [2466]. This decrease in muscle tone lowers the FRC and leads to collapse of basal airways and ventilation/perfusion mismatching. The loss of the stabilizing action of the intercostal muscles leads to paradoxical movement of the rib cage, particularly in infants. The inspiratory muscle duty cycle remains unchanged but the tidal volume probably falls. Diaphragmatic fatigue may appear, particularly in infants, and if the diaphragm is paralysed, prolonged periods of hypoventilation mimicking central sleep apnoeas appear. True central sleep apnoeas are also common in normal subjects during REM sleep, particularly in the older age groups [1765].

UPPER AIRWAY RESISTANCE

The reduction in muscular activity in tonic REM sleep is also seen in muscles of the upper airway, including the laryngeal abductor muscles [2375]. The air flow resistance increases [1485, 2374] and the airway becomes unstable and may close (Chapter 6).

VENTILATORY DRIVE

The ventilatory responses to hypoxia and hypercapnia are less than in NREM sleep. The hypoxic drive is approximately one-third that of wakefulness [824] and is slightly more diminished in men than in women [820]. Hypoxia increases the mean inspiratory flow rate and tidal volume, but there is relatively little increase in respiratory frequency [269]. The slope of the ventilatory response to hypercapnia is reduced to a similar extent [826]. The arousal threshold for hypoxia and hypercapnia may be set at more abnormal levels than during NREM sleep [269] and there appears to be little compensation for an increase in air flow resistance [820]. The response to pulmonary receptors, such as irritant receptors, is diminished so that clearance of tracheobronchial secretions may be impaired [2466].

Part 2
Ventilatory Failure and Dysrhythmias and their Assessment

Chapter 4
Ventilatory Failure

The function of respiration is to maintain the arterial P_{O_2} and P_{CO_2} within narrow limits, and respiratory failure is defined by abnormalities of the blood gases. The arbitrary criteria of P_{O_2} < 6.7 kPa (50 mmHg) or 8.0 kPa (60 mmHg) and a P_{CO_2} of > 6.0 kPa (45 mmHg) or 6.7 kPa (50 mmHg) are usually taken. Respiratory failure due to inadequacy of the ventilatory pump should be distinguished from failure caused by an impairment of gas exchange across the alveolar capillary membrane. In pump or ventilatory failure, the alveolar ventilation is insufficient for normal gas exchange to take place, even if the lungs are normal.

It is a characteristic of ventilatory or pump failure that both hypercapnia and hypoxia are present, since alveolar ventilation is inadequate for exchange of either of these gases. With abnormalities of the lungs themselves, hypoxia is usually the only abnormality (Fig. 4.1). The sigmoid shape of the oxyhaemoglobin dissociation curve prevents the well-perfused alveoli from adequately compensating for blood that is shunted through the lungs past poorly ventilated alveoli. Hypoxia inevitably results. Carbon dioxide can still be adequately eliminated since it is readily diffusible and the P_{CO_2} is related almost linearly to the carbon dioxide content of the blood.

Alveolar ventilation depends both on the total ventilation and on the volume of the dead space. The anatomical dead space is approximately 2.2 ml/kg body weight. In normal subjects the physiological dead space is only slightly greater, but if the lungs are abnormal it may increase considerably. The pattern of respiration also influences the dead space. If the tidal volume is small, the proportion that reaches the alveoli is reduced and ventilatory failure may develop.

Hypoventilation affects the arterial P_{O_2} and P_{CO_2} in different ways. The body stores of oxygen are much less than those of carbon dioxide. The lungs contain about 0.5 litre, the blood 1.2 litre and the tissues 0.3 litre [545]. Changes in arterial P_{O_2} therefore occur rapidly if ventilation becomes inadequate, and when metabolism becomes anaerobic, lactic acidosis develops. About 100 litres of carbon dioxide are available in bone as carbonates and a further 20 litres in the soft tissues and blood [545, 953]. In the blood, carbon dioxide is carried mainly as bicarbonate but also as carbon dioxide in solution and as carbamino groups bound to proteins, including haemoglobin. The arterial P_{CO_2} changes slowly when ventilation falls [3104] and this has led to the concept of slow and fast compartments, the former represented mainly by carbonates in bone. The response to an acute rise in P_{CO_2} is renal bicarbonate retention and loss of chloride. This induces a metabolic alkalosis, which compensates for the respiratory acidosis so that the

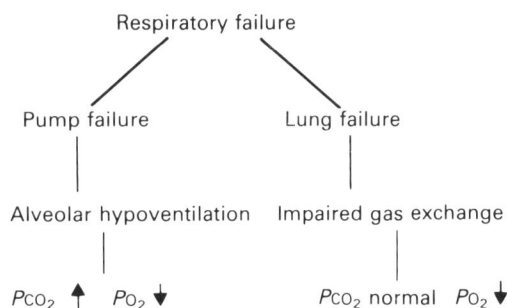

Fig. 4.1. *Comparison of respiratory pump and lung failure.*

pH returns towards normal [2656]. Treatment with diuretics and glucocorticoid drugs promotes the loss of potassium and contributes to the metabolic alkalosis.

INTERMITTENT VENTILATORY FAILURE

Respiratory failure is conventionally defined by the blood gas abnormalities at rest, breathing air at sea level while awake. The P_{O_2} and P_{CO_2} are, however, the result not only of the alveolar ventilation and transfer of gas across the alveolar capillary membrane but also of the metabolic rate and respiratory exchange ratio. These determine the oxygen consumption and the production of carbon dioxide. Blood gas abnormalities may be present intermittently during physiological activities such as exercise, eating and sleep, or in certain positions.

Exercise

During exercise, the metabolic rate increases and this places greater demands on ventilation. Alveolar ventilation is increased and ventilation/perfusion matching improves because of changes in the pulmonary circulation. New vessels are recruited and this reduces the pulmonary vascular resistance so that there is only a slight increase in pulmonary artery pressure. Perfusion to the apices of the lungs increases and the net result is that in normal subjects the arterial P_{O_2} remains constant and the P_{CO_2} may fall slightly. However, if the ability to increase ventilation is limited or if pulmonary hypertension is present in association with mismatching of ventilation and perfusion, the P_{CO_2} may rise and the P_{O_2} may fall during exercise.

Eating

The P_{O_2} and P_{CO_2} may deteriorate during eating, partly because of the increased metabolic rate and partly because swallowing interrupts the normal pattern of respiration [418] (p. 84).

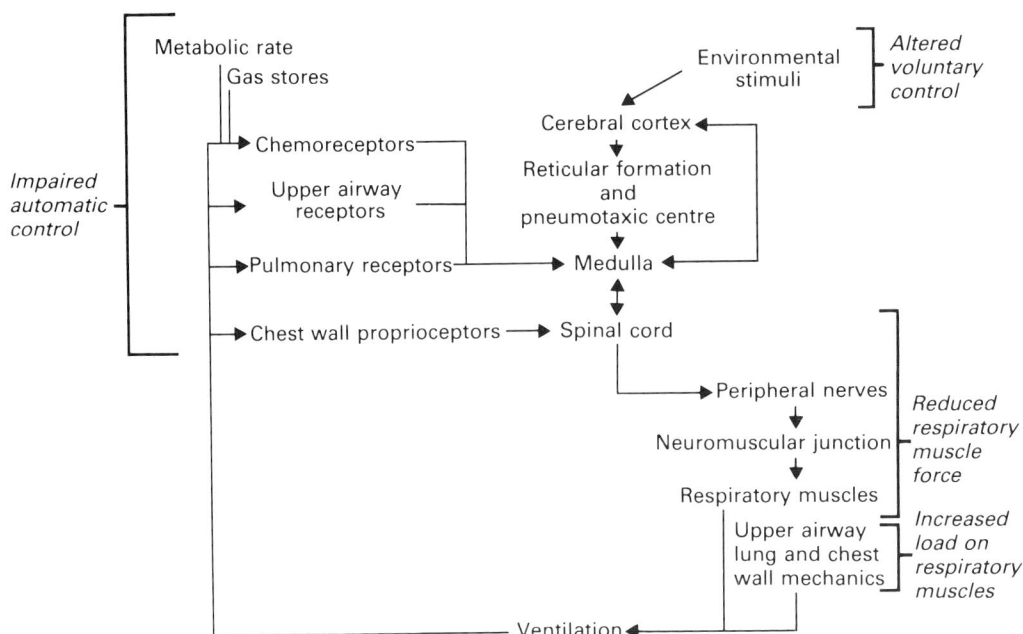

Fig. 4.2. *Diagram to show the main causes of ventilatory failure and their relationship to the normal control of ventilation.*

Sleep

The changes in respiration during sleep described in Chapter 3 in normal subjects are not accompanied by any deleterious consequences. However, in the presence of a disorder of any component of the respiratory pump, serious hypoxia or hypercapnia may appear because these physiological responses are accentuated. The most important of these are:

CHANGES IN SLEEP STRUCTURE

The majority of the physiological changes in respiration during sleep (Fig. 3.1) and the pathological alterations seen in disorders of the respiratory pump (Fig. 4.3) are related to the stage of sleep. Alterations in the total sleep time and the structure of sleep, therefore, have a major effect on the frequency with which these problems occur. REM sleep is reduced by many factors, including drugs such as tricyclic antidepressants, amphetamines and alcohol. Stages 3 and 4 NREM sleep and REM sleep are usually reduced if sleep is fragmented, e.g. by frequent arousals due to hypoxia or hypercapnia. Conversely, when sleep returns to normal, a rebound in the amount of REM sleep is seen.

AROUSAL

The threshold for arousal to hypoxia is lower and to hypercapnia is higher in REM sleep than in NREM sleep. This allows more severe and prolonged changes in blood gases to occur before the subject wakens. Arousal may also be due to obstruction of the airway, particularly the upper airway.

AUTOMATIC RESPIRATORY CONTROL

The ventilatory responses to hypoxia and hypercapnia are less during sleep than wakefulness and lowest during REM sleep. Any minor defect in ventilatory drive is, therefore, magnified during sleep and, consequently, ventilatory failure usually develops during sleep before it is apparent during wakefulness.

UPPER AIRWAY RESISTANCE

This increases both during NREM and REM sleep, probably due to a reduction in the tone of the upper airway dilator muscles. This predisposes to upper airway obstruction and obstructive apnoeas. The continuing contraction of the inspiratory chest wall muscles contributes to the

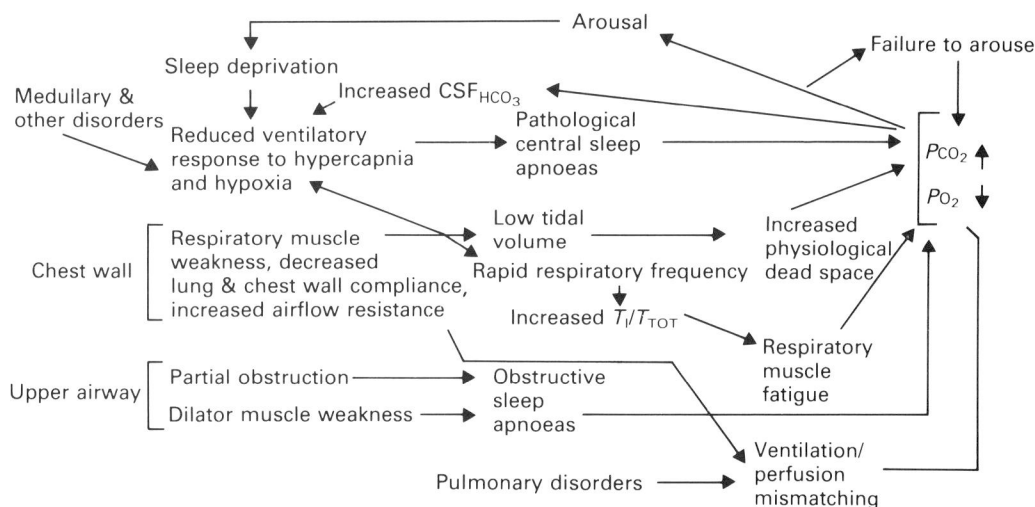

Fig. 4.3. *Flow chart to show the effect of neuromuscular and skeletal disorders on respiration during sleep.*

maintenance of the upper airway obstruction by lowering the pressure within the lumen of the airway.

CHANGE IN LUNG VOLUME

The lung volume normally falls during sleep. The diaphragm ascends in the supine position and blood is redistributed into the lungs from the lower limbs. A reduction in lung volume is linked, probably reflexly, to the reduction in the upper airway diameter in the supine position [1446, 1449]. The nasal resistance is also greater in the supine position [606, 1377]. During REM sleep the tone of the postural muscles, which include all the respiratory muscles of the chest wall except for the diaphragm, is reduced. The fall in lung volume is most marked in infants, in whom intercostal paradoxical movement may appear. The basal airways close at low lung volumes, worsening the matching of ventilation and perfusion and lowering the oxygen saturation.

CHANGE IN TIDAL VOLUME

In NREM sleep, the tidal volume falls and the ratio of dead space to tidal volume (V_D/V_T) increases. Alveolar ventilation is therefore reduced to a greater extent than would be anticipated from the small reduction in overall ventilation.

CIRCULATORY CHANGES

The metabolic rate is usually decreased during sleep and this lessens the oxygen requirements and carbon dioxide production. Although the cardiac output falls, cerebral perfusion increases, particularly in REM sleep, and may fluctuate considerably. The increase in cerebral perfusion lessens the arterial–CSF P_{CO_2} gradient and thereby reduces the ventilatory response to hypercapnia.

CAUSES OF VENTILATORY FAILURE

The most common cause of acute ventilatory failure in the presence of neuromuscular or skeletal disorders is a chest infection. This may precipitate ventilatory failure by several mechanisms. A pneumonia or pleural effusion causes a restrictive defect, secretions retained in the airways increase air flow resistance, the level of consciousness and thereby the respiratory drive may fall, a rise in body temperature increases the metabolic rate, and the catabolic effect of the infection and hypoxia reduce respiratory muscle strength and predispose to fatigue.

A fault at any level of the respiratory pump interacts with other abnormalities so that, for instance, a slightly reduced respiratory drive or skeletal abnormality of the thorax will precipitate ventilatory failure at an early stage if there is also mild respiratory muscle weakness. Lung disease also increases the mechanical load on the respiratory muscles. Hyperinflation is particularly important since it decreases the length of the inspiratory muscles, puts the inspiratory muscles at a mechanical disadvantage, and decreases the compliance of the chest wall and lungs. Ventilation/perfusion matching is usually impaired in pulmonary disorders and this reduces the oxygen saturation both during wakefulness and sleep. If the oxygen saturation lies on the steep part of the oxyhaemoglobin dissociation curve, even a minor physiological change in alveolar ventilation or ventilation/perfusion matching during sleep may be sufficient to cause severe hypoxic dips, usually with only a minor increase in P_{CO_2}.

Ventilatory failure may be caused by an inadequate ventilatory drive, weakness of the respiratory muscles or a fall in chest wall or lung compliance, or increase in air flow resistance (Fig. 4.2). The disorders that cause chronic ventilatory failure are discussed in Chapters 10–16 and are listed in Table 4.1. Physiological changes with age also predispose to ventilatory failure. For instance, in neonates the chest wall

Table 4.1. *Major non-pulmonary causes of ventilatory failure*

Disorder	Reduced automatic ventilatory drive	Upper airway obstruction	Reduced chest wall compliance	Respiratory muscle weakness
Carotid body disorders	+ +			
Pontine and medullary haemorrhage, infarct, trauma and tumours	+ +	+		
Encephalitis	+ +	+		
Disorders of autonomic nervous system	+ +	+		
Central alveolar hypoventilation	+ +	?+		
Central sleep apnoeas	+ +			
Sedative drugs	+ +	+		
Metabolic alkalosis	+ +			
High cervical cordotomy	+ +			
Syringobulbia	+	+ +		
Syringomyelia		+ +		+
Poliomyelitis	+ +	+	+	+ +
Traumatic quadriplegia				+ +
Motor neuron disease		+		+ +
Spinal muscular atrophy				+ +
Tetanus		+	+ +	
Acute idiopathic polyneuropathy		+		+ +
Miller Fisher syndrome				+ +
Porphyria	+			+ +
Myasthenia gravis		+		+ +
Botulism				+ +
Muscular dystrophies		+		+ +
Congenital myopathies				+ +
Myositis				+ +
Malnutrition				+ +
Electrolyte disturbances				+ +
Acromegaly		+ +		+
Obesity		+ +	+	+
Asphyxiating thoracic dystrophy			+ +	
Chest trauma			+ +	+
Thoracoplasty			+ +	+ +
Kyphosis			+ +	
Scoliosis			+ +	

+ + = The most important or common effect; + = less common or important effect.
Changes in chest wall compliance due to reduced lung volume and restricted range of respiratory movements and reduction in muscle strength purely because of alterations in length or configuration are omitted.

is very compliant so that paradoxical movement readily occurs. There are few fatigue-resistant muscle fibres and ventilation is more dependent on the diaphragm and, therefore, more vulnerable during REM sleep than in older children. In adults, the ventilatory drive, chest wall compliance [2196] and respiratory muscle strength all decline with age.

The individual disorders of the respiratory pump fall into the following groups.

Disorders of voluntary respiratory control

Defects in the voluntary respiratory control would not be anticipated to be of importance in NREM sleep since the cerebral cortex is largely inactive. This in itself does, however, contribute to the appearance of Cheyne-Stokes respiration (p. 56). The influence of the voluntary control system on breathing during REM sleep is uncertain.

Disorders of automatic respiratory control

The rarer ventilatory dysrhythmias due to defects in automatic respiratory control may persist from wakefulness into sleep, e.g. ataxic or cluster respiration. Hypoventilation is, however, more common and is related to the reduction in ventilatory response to hypoxia, hypercapnia and, probably, to airway obstruction. Ventilation is least in NREM sleep, during which the voluntary respiratory drive is virtually absent. Pathological central sleep apnoeas are particularly common in stages 3 and 4 NREM sleep, when the chemoreceptor drive is at its least, and during phasic REM sleep.

Disorders of spinal cord peripheral nerve, neuromuscular junction and respiratory muscles

In these conditions, the fall in lung volume predisposes to ventilation/perfusion mismatching and a drop in the oxygen saturation during sleep. Alveolar ventilation is reduced because the tidal volume decreases, often with an increase in respiratory frequency so that the dead space increases and inspiratory muscle fatigue is provoked. In REM sleep, the activity of the respiratory muscles other than the diaphragm is reduced and ventilatory failure is most marked. If the diaphragm is paralysed there are no effective inspiratory muscles, and 'pseudo-central' sleep apnoeas appear (p. 77).

Skeletal abnormalities and obesity

The effect of these conditions is similar to that of respiratory muscle weakness, but the chest wall compliance is more reduced. In the obese, in addition to the falls in the FRC and ventilation/perfusion matching, which are greater than normal because of the weight of the abdominal contents, diaphragmatic function is impaired. This leads to 'pseudo-central' sleep apnoeas, and the small upper airway predisposes to obstructive apnoeas.

Upper airway disorders

Any condition that narrows the upper airway will predispose to obstructive apnoeas, particularly during REM sleep when the muscle tone is decreased. Anatomical lesions or paralysis of the pharyngeal dilator or vocal cord abductor muscles are important factors. The upper airway diameter is also determined by the lung volume. This is reduced by respiratory muscle weakness and skeletal abnormalities of the thorax, and decreases further during sleep (Chapter 3).

EFFECTS OF VENTILATORY FAILURE

Ventilatory failure has the advantage that carbon dioxide can be excreted with less energy expended by the respiratory muscles. The carbon dioxide concentration in the expired gas is greater than normal or, conversely, the carbon dioxide load is excreted with a lower alveolar ventilation. This adaptive mechanism enables more of the inspired oxygen to be available for non-respiratory purposes and lessens the risk of respiratory muscle fatigue [181, 2630]. These advantages are, however, outweighed by the largely deleterious consequences of hypercapnia and hypoxia.

Hypercapnia

Hypercapnia has three main consequences.

VENTILATORY STIMULATION

Acute hypercapnia is a potent stimulus to ventilation until the P_{CO_2} reaches levels above approximately 12.0 kPa. In the presence of chronic hypercapnia, bicarbonate retention diminishes the ventilatory response to carbon dioxide (p. 9).

CARDIOVASCULAR CHANGES

An increase in cardiac output, heart rate and blood pressure is seen with a rise in P_{CO_2} of about 1.0 kPa [1265]. Hypercapnia causes reflex vasoconstriction in the visceral circulation and sweating due to an increase in sympathetic activity, but it has a direct vasodilator action on the cutaneous and cerebral circulation. The intracranial pressure rises even as high as 600 mm H_2O [1984] as the P_{CO_2} increases [723, 811, 853, 3302], probably because of an increase in the intracranial blood volume. Changes in the intracranial pressure occur too rapidly for an increase in the secretion or decrease in the reabsorption of the CSF to be responsible. Autopsy studies have shown venous congestion and even coning of the cerebellum due to the raised intracranial pressure [2945].

Hypercapnia shifts the oxyhaemoglobin dissociation curve to the right, so that although the oxygen saturation at any given partial pressure is diminished, oxygen is released more readily in the tissues. This, together with the circulatory changes, increases the oxygen delivery to the tissues.

NEUROLOGICAL EFFECTS

Neurological changes are induced by higher levels of P_{CO_2} than are required to cause the circulatory changes. The commonest manifestations are:

Motor changes

Motor changes, particularly fine facial tremor, myoclonus and asterixis are frequent [3303] and usually occur when the P_{CO_2} rises by about 2.0 kPa [1265]. Myoclonus is the presence of irregular twitches, often of the large joints, and occurs particularly when the muscles are at rest. Asterixis is the inability to maintain a posture and is due to intermittent failure of excitation of the muscles. It is best elicited by dorsiflexing the wrist and is indistinguishable from asterixis due to hepatic or renal failure.

Generalized muscle weakness and hypertonia may appear, but occasionally the neurological signs are focal. They include unilateral pupillary abnormalities, asymmetrical weakness and even Jacksonian epileptic fits [622, 623, 2483]. They are probably due to a combination of hypercapnia and local vascular abnormalities, but unless this is realized, a cerebral tumour or other space-occupying lesion may be suspected. Hypercapnia diminishes the tendon reflexes and causes extensor plantar reflexes and small pupils that hardly react to light.

Headache

The headache of carbon dioxide retention is characteristically frontal, constant, and occurs immediately after waking, particularly if sleep has been deep or prolonged. It lasts about 20 min. It is probably due to stimulation of meningeal and cerebrovascular receptors, which are stretched by the changes in the intracranial blood volume. The fall in P_{CO_2} on waking, rather than the level of the P_{CO_2} itself, may be responsible [844].

Papilloedema

Papilloedema is uncommon but can lead to optic atrophy [1039, 2304]. It is not closely related to the level of the P_{CO_2} [2304] or to the intracranial pressure [2158], but it may improve when ventilatory failure is treated [2587, 2978]. The combination of a rise in the CSF and venous pressure has been postulated as a cause of papilloedema [140], but it rarely occurs with superior vena caval obstruction or pure right heart failure [2944]. It may be partly due to the increase in cerebral blood flow [140], but there may be specific retinal vessel abnormalities [1039, 2544, 2931]. Papilloedema appears to be commonest in acute on chronic respiratory failure [623, 853] if the P_{CO_2} rises by about 4.0 kPa [1265].

Mental changes

Carbon dioxide narcosis was first noticed in animals as long ago as 1820 [579]. In man, confusion, irritability and loss of memory are common if the P_{CO_2} rises by about 2.0 kPa [1265], particularly in the presence of acidosis [967]. As the P_{CO_2} rises further, disorientation and even coma may occur [368, 853]. Coma (carbon dioxide 'narcosis') is usually seen when the P_{CO_2} is > 12.0 kPa and the pH is < 7.25 [1662, 2589, 2922, 3303], or if the P_{CO_2} rises by about 4.0 kPa [1265]. A deterioration in the level of consciousness, fits, hemiplegia and even coma may follow from lowering the P_{CO_2} too rapidly, and these features may not be reversible [1338, 2714]. They are probably due to acute cerebral hypoxia caused by a combination of cerebral vasoconstriction, when the P_{CO_2} falls, and a low arterial P_{O_2}.

Hypoxia

ACUTE HYPOXIA

The most important effects of acute hypoxia are:

Ventilatory stimulation

Hypoxia increases ventilation, particularly in the presence of hypercapnia, but generalized central nervous system depression with a reduction in respiratory drive occurs if it is severe. This subject is discussed more fully on p. 8.

Cardiovascular changes

There are several adaptive changes to hypoxia, which promote the oxygen delivery to the tissues. The cardiac output, heart rate and blood pressure increase and, although there is visceral vasoconstriction, the coronary and cerebral blood flow increases (p. 9). Hypoxia causes pulmonary vasoconstriction and thereby increases the pulmonary vascular resistance and the pulmonary artery pressure.

Tissue damage

The susceptibility of the tissues to hypoxia varies considerably. Skeletal muscle function is largely retained despite severe hypoxia, whereas renal and hepatic function is more readily impaired. The brain is the most easily damaged since its metabolism is almost purely aerobic. Acute hypoxia causes impairment of judgement at around a saturation of 65% and loss of consciousness at around 55% [1444]. Confusion and intellectual impairment [1506] are common.

Cyanosis

The most important physical sign of hypoxia is central cyanosis. This is usually apparent when the oxygen saturation falls to about 80% [618, 1965, 2107, 2850]. The absolute quantity of reduced haemoglobin, rather than the saturation, determines whether cyanosis is detectable; 5 g/100 ml of reduced haemoglobin can be recognized. Chronic hypoxia may lead to polycythaemia, which enables cyanosis to be seen at higher saturations than normal.

There is considerable interobserver variation in the detection of cyanosis. The quality of the lighting is important, but physiological factors such as the number and size of capillaries, thickness of the epidermis and the presence of pigmentation also influence its detection. It is best sought in the tongue, on the inside of the lips and in the conjunctivae, where vasoconstriction is least likely [2107]. The concentration of reduced haemoglobin depends not only on the arterial Po_2, total haemoglobin concentration and the amount of oxygen extracted by the tissues, but also on the oxygen uptake in the tissue capillaries. A relatively low blood flow and high oxygen uptake account for the occasional false positive diagnosis of central cyanosis.

CHRONIC HYPOXIA

Chronic hypoxia causes:

Ventilatory stimulation

This is discussed in Chapters 1 and 9.

Pulmonary hypertension

Hypoxia causes vasoconstriction in the pulmonary circulation directly, although the exact mechanism is uncertain [3243]. There may be an individual variation in vascular reactivity to hypoxia, which would explain why only some hypoxic subjects develop pulmonary hypertension. A progressive rise in the pulmonary artery pressure during repeated hypoxic episodes may occur even if the severity of hypoxia is unchanged [3209]. This is particularly relevant to sleep apnoeas, in which episodes of hypoxia recur frequently (Chapter 6). Structural changes, particularly hypertrophy of smooth muscle, develop with chronic hypoxia [1379], but vasoconstriction still contributes to pulmonary hypertension since it may be rapidly, although only partially, reversed by oxygen [2908]. There may be a further fall in pulmonary artery pressure over a period of months if relief of hypoxia is maintained, suggesting that some of the structural changes are also reversible [1267].

The relationship between pulmonary hypertension and chronic hypoxia has been demonstrated in normal subjects breathing hypoxic gas mixtures [3298], at altitude [1267], in emphysema [667] and scoliosis [2908]. The mean pulmonary artery pressure is said to be approximately 34 mmHg with an oxygen saturation of 80%, and 55 mmHg when the saturation falls to 60% [969] (Fig. 4.4). These published figures are falsely precise since the degree of hypoxia varies, for instance, between sleep and wakefulness and rest and exercise. In rats, intermittent hypoxia as well as continuous hypoxia can induce right ventricular hypertrophy [2282], and in humans it is the mean oxygen saturation during sleep that is most closely linked to the mean pulmonary artery pressure during wakefulness [2800].

Pulmonary hypertension in neuromuscular and skeletal disorders is often largely due to hypoxia but also partly to other factors that diminish the size of the pulmonary vasculature. These include congenital hypoplasia of the lung or failure of the lungs to develop to a normal size, as in scoliosis, and resection of lung tissue or damage to the pulmonary circulation by lung diseases such as chronic bronchitis or tuberculosis. Pulmonary hypertension increases the work of the right ventricle and, in time, leads to right ventricular hypertrophy and failure. The symptoms of pulmonary hypertension are discussed on p.78. The most important physical signs are a small-volume arterial pulse, the presence of a right ventricular heave in the parasternal region, a prominent 'a' wave in the jugular venous pulse with or without a raised venous pressure, a 4th heart sound, a loud pulmonary 2nd sound and occasionally an early systolic pulmonary ejection click or signs of pulmonary or tricuspid regurgitation.

Polycythaemia

The stimulus to haemoglobin production is erythropoietin liberated by the kidneys in response to hypoxia [164, 1366, 3069]. The degree of hypoxia is determined by the renal metabolism and the oxygen transport to the kidney, which depends on the cardiac output, the regional blood flow to the kidneys, the haemoglobin con-

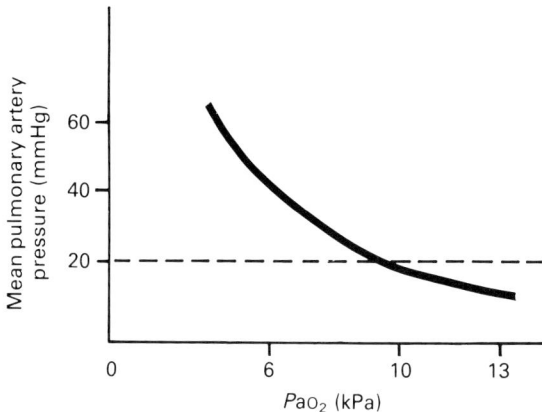

Fig. 4.4. *Relationship between mean pulmonary artery pressure and Pa_{O_2} in subjects with normal lungs. Dashed line indicates upper limit of normal mean pulmonary artery pressure.*

centration, arterial P_{O_2} and the shape of the oxyhaemoglobin dissociation curve. It is surprising that there is a close relationship between hypoxia and polycythaemia when so many factors determine the erythropoietin production (Fig. 4.5).

Polycythaemia is an adaptive mechanism that tends to increase the oxygen delivery to the tissues in the presence of hypoxaemia. The haemoglobin concentration itself may be misleading, since polycythaemia may be masked by an increase in the plasma volume [2259] or falsely suspected if plasma volume is decreased, for instance, by diuretics. The relationship between oxygen saturation and hypoxia was suggested by early studies of polycythaemia at altitude [1507] and was confirmed in lung diseases such as chronic bronchitis [1368]. Some of the variability in erythropoietic response is due to smoking, which produces carboxyhaemoglobin, chronic inflammation that impairs iron utilization and lowers the haemoglobin concentration, and unrecognized intermittent hypoxia. This has been shown in humans [1507] and in rats to be capable of increasing the red cell mass [2210, 2282], and polycythaemia is a frequent finding in subjects with hypoxia during sleep [2212].

The most important deleterious effect of polycythaemia is the increase in the blood viscosity [1368]. This predisposes to venous and arterial thromboses, raises the pulmonary artery pressure and the systemic vascular resistance, and thereby leads to left and right ventricular hypertrophy. Cerebral blood flow diminishes [3388]; this is not a specific effect of the viscosity but reflects the changes in oxygen transport to the brain (p. 9).

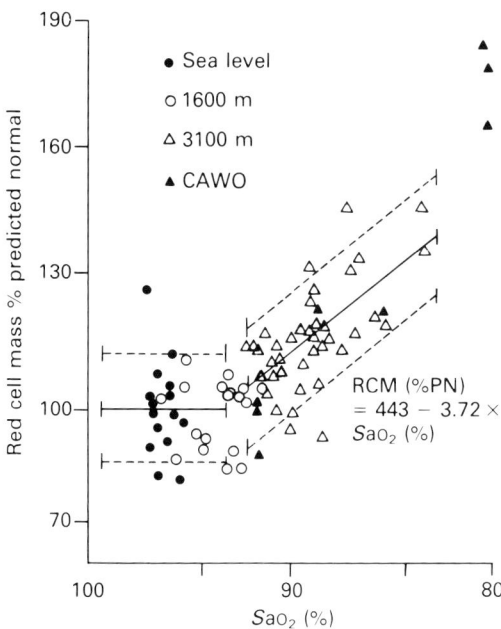

Fig. 4.5. *Relationship between % predicted red cell mass and oxygen saturation in normal subjects at sea level and at altitude and in patients with chronic air flow obstruction (CAWO). Broken lines represent 95% confidence limits. Reproduced, with permission, from Stradling J.R. & Lane D.J. Thorax 1981; 36: 321–5.*

Hypoxic polycythaemia should be treated by relieving the hypoxia. The haemoglobin concentration does not fall immediately since the life span of the red cells is over 100 days, but an improvement is detectable in six weeks [526]. If the hypoxia cannot be corrected, venesection, preferably with simultaneous infusion of Dextran 40 [1247], should be considered if the haematocrit is greater than about 60% [1368]. Plasmapheresis is an alternative [3272]. A haematocrit of about 50% should be reached [3285], at which level exercise ability, mental alertness and pulmonary hypertension may all improve [3272]. Iron supplements should be given if venesection or plasmapheresis needs to be repeated.

Systemic hypertension

Systemic hypertension may develop because of prolonged sympathetic vasoconstriction in response to hypoxia. The systemic vascular resistance is also increased by polycythaemia. Fluid retention, due to increased secretion of antidiuretic and adrenocorticotrophic hormones may contribute to hypertension. The left ventricle may fail as a consequence, but hypoxic impairment of contractility may also contribute to this. Severe hypertrophy of the right ventricle can mechanically impede the contraction of the left ventricle and worsen pulmonary oedema.

Chapter 5
Respiratory Dysrhythmias

The respiratory pattern normally adapts to environmental stimuli and sustains a sufficient alveolar ventilation to maintain normal blood gas tensions. There are, however, several discernible patterns of respiration that are not closely related to environmental changes or to the balance of alveolar ventilation and the metabolic rate. These abnormal rhythms may occur both during wakefulness and sleep and, in certain cases, when the level of consciousness is pathologically lowered. The details of the abnormalities underlying most of these dysrhythmias have remained elusive because of the complexity and close interrelationships of the components of respiratory control [2489–2491, 2494, 2496, 2498]. Some of the dysrhythmias are purely due to a deranged automatic control of respiration, but others involve voluntary control as well.

Most of the dysrhythmias discussed in this chapter do not cause chronic hypoventilation. Central, mixed and obstructive sleep apnoeas are briefly mentioned but are more fully discussed in Chapter 6. Some abnormalities of respiratory rhythm are due to factors other than alterations in respiratory drive; these are included in this chapter since it is the characteristic respiratory pattern that leads to their recognition.

RESPIRATORY DYSPRAXIA

Respiratory dyspraxia is a disorder in which the voluntary control of the depth and frequency of respiration is impaired. It is a specific motor dyspraxia of respiration and can only be diagnosed if the patient understands the instructions and there is no sensory or motor respiratory defect. It is characteristic that the ability to obey a command, such as to hold the breath or take a deep breath, to mimic the examiner [1394] or to match the tidal volume or respiratory frequency to a target, is impaired, although speech and cough may be normal. This abnormality is thought to be due to a bifrontal abnormality in the cerebral cortex. The arterial blood gases are usually normal but in one study a respiratory dyspraxia appeared to contribute, with a defect in automatic respiratory control, to ventilatory failure [3367]. The mechanism is uncertain but the respiratory dyspraxia may have reduced the tidal volume and thereby increased the physiological dead space and decreased alveolar ventilation.

CHEYNE-STOKES RESPIRATION (PERIODIC BREATHING) (Fig. 5.1)

Cheyne-Stokes respiration was recognized by John Hunter in 1781 before the classical descriptions of Cheyne in 1818 and Stokes in 1854 [3259]. It is characterized by a regular waxing and waning of ventilation. Periods of apnoea alternate with periods of breathing, during which the tidal volume steadily increases to a maximum before it progressively falls again. A similar respiratory pattern without an apnoeic phase is also recognized (Cheyne-Stokes variant) and a more abrupt change in tidal volume is characteristic of stages 1 and 2 NREM sleep. The arterial P_{O_2} and P_{CO_2} fluctuate during each cycle of Cheyne-Stokes respiration. The P_{O_2} is lowest and the P_{CO_2} highest at the end of the apnoea.

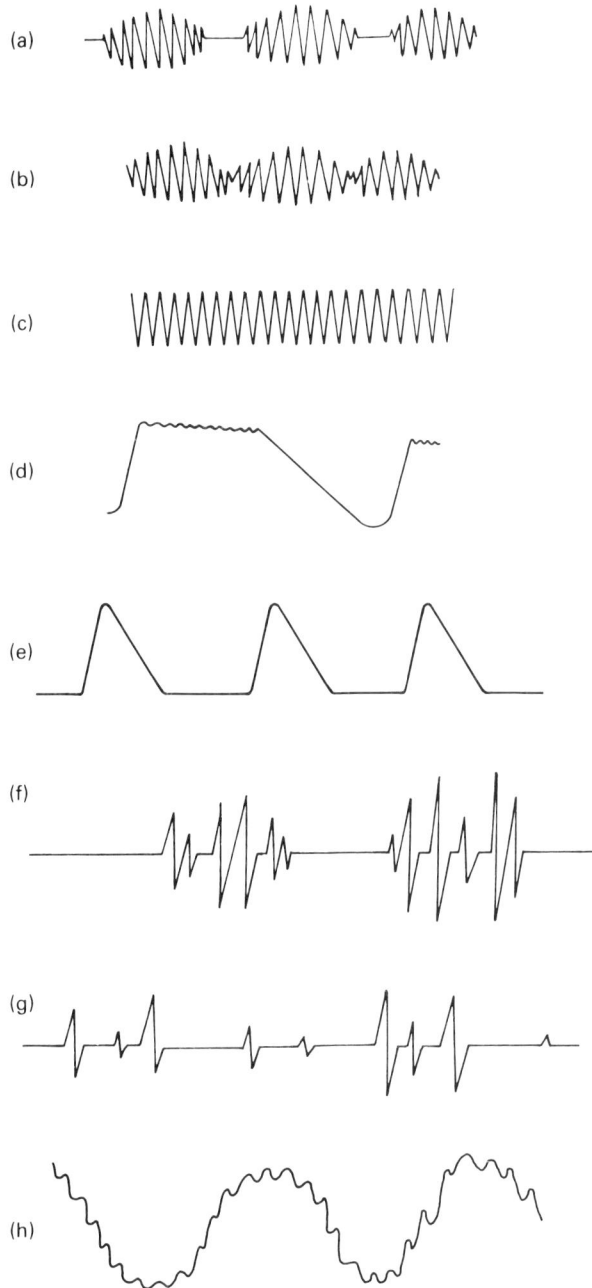

Fig. 5.1. *Abnormal patterns of respiration: (a) Cheyne-Stokes respiration, (b) Cheyne-Stokes variant, (c) central neurogenic hyperventilation, (d) apneusis, (e) gasping, (f) cluster respiration, (g) ataxic respiration, (h) respiratory myoclonus.*

Pathogenesis

Cheyne-Stokes respiration reflects the cyclic changes in activity of the automatic respiratory control. These fluctuations are normally insignificant, but in Cheyne-Stokes respiration the control system becomes unstable [540–542, 544, 546, 1660, 1936, 2496, 2498, 3172]. Ventilation is normally controlled by chemoreceptor activity through a feedback loop, whose reaction time is the interval between the blood leaving the lungs and reaching the chemoreceptors. Instability can be introduced into this control system by increasing the gain of the ventilatory response to chemoreceptor stimulation, by decreasing the damping of the ventilatory response, or by increasing the reaction time (Fig. 5.2).

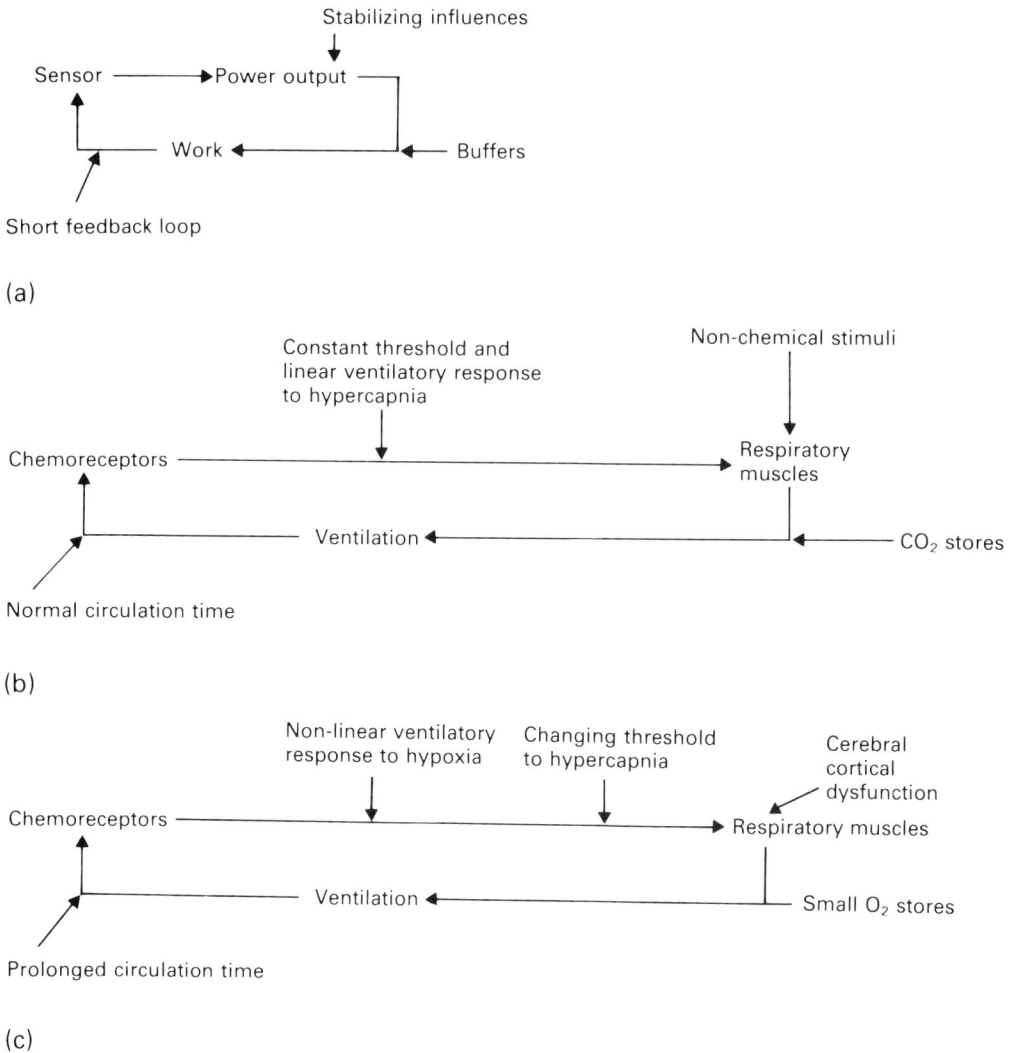

Fig. 5.2. *Cheyne-Stokes respiration: (a) principles of stable control system, (b) schematic representation of normal respiratory control to show how it remains stable, (c) respiratory control system in Cheyne-Stokes respiration showing features contributing to instability.*

The chemical control of ventilation is, in normal circumstances, dominated by the hypercapnic drive. The ventilatory response increases linearly with the P_{CO_2}. Instability appears if the hypoxic drive becomes relatively more important. The ventilatory response to hypoxia increases hyperbolically as the P_{O_2} falls, so that the ventilatory response becomes progressively greater as hypoxia worsens. This increase in the gain of the ventilatory response is an important factor in initiating Cheyne-Stokes respiration. The maximal tidal volume during the hyperpnoeic phase is related to the degree of hypoxia and hypercapnia at the end of the apnoeic phase [829] and to the magnitude of the ventilatory response to hypoxia and hypercapnia.

Damping of respiratory control is normally achieved by the large body stores of carbon dioxide (p. 41), which minimize the breath-to-breath variations in arterial P_{CO_2}. The stores of oxygen are much smaller, so that the damping of blood gas oscillations diminishes when the hypoxic drive becomes more prominent. The oxygen present as gas within the lungs is an important component of the body's oxygen content and this is reduced if the FRC falls, as, for instance, in many neuromuscular and skeletal disorders.

Instability of respiratory control is also exacerbated by a delay between the blood leaving the lungs and reaching the chemoreceptors. A delay introduces an overcorrective reaction, which causes the ventilation and blood gases to fluctuate. The response time of the carotid body chemoreceptors and the medullary receptors is much shorter than the circulation time between the lungs and the receptors, and for practical purposes can be disregarded. Cheyne-Stokes respiration can be induced experimentally by prolonging the circulation time [1310]. In general, the slower the circulation time the longer the cycle of Cheyne-Stokes respiration [2496]. The cycles are approximately twice the lung-to-brain circulation time.

These considerations explain the hyperpnoeic phase of Cheyne-Stokes respiration, but the apnoeic phase depends on the arterial P_{CO_2} and the threshold of the ventilatory response to P_{CO_2}. The P_{CO_2} remains below the threshold for longer if the threshold is high and if cerebral cortical activity does not maintain ventilation in the absence of a chemical drive to breathe. The apnoeic phase of Cheyne-Stokes respiration is therefore analogous to post-hyperventilation apnoea [2498]. Apnoea was thought to follow hyperventilation in normal waking subjects [1331, 2227], but this has not been confirmed by other studies [2176, 2495]. Ventilation is maintained, except during sleep, unless cerebral cortical function is deranged [2493, 2495]. In these situations, apnoea follows a period of hyperventilation and the release of the tonic cortical inhibition of the ventilatory response to hypercapnia also increases the gain of the ventilatory response to hypercapnia during the hyperpnoeic phase [1419, 2493, 2494].

Aetiology

There has been considerable debate as to whether or not Cheyne-Stokes respiration is primarily caused by neurological or circulatory abnormalities. An understanding of the pathogenesis indicates, however, that several factors may interact to produce this respiratory pattern. The most important of these factors are:

HYPOXIA

Hypoxia from any cause predisposes to Cheyne-Stokes respiration by increasing the importance of the hypoxic drive relative to the hypercapnic drive. Cheyne-Stokes respiration is seen in normal subjects at altitude, as well as in pulmonary and cardiac conditions causing hypoxia [1561]. Metabolic alkalosis also predisposes to Cheyne-Stokes respiration by reducing the hypercapnic drive.

REDUCED FRC

A reduction in the FRC lowers the body stores of oxygen and may also cause hypoxia if there is basal airway closure and ventilation/perfusion mismatching. This may be seen in restrictive chest wall disorders, left ventricular failure and in normal subjects during sleep. The FRC, which normally buffers the effects of the apnoeic phase on the Po_2 and Pco_2, and the threshold of the ventilatory response to CO_2, which initiates the hyperpnoeic phase, determine the duration of the apnoea. Stretch receptors in the lungs, which are activated by the lung volume changes, also appear to determine the respiratory frequency during the hyperpnoeic phase [544]. This is faster if the lungs are smaller at the end of the apnoea. The duration of each inspiration shortens as ventilation wanes [544].

PROLONGED CIRCULATION TIME

Cheyne-Stokes respiration is a feature of conditions in which the circulation time is increased, either because the cardiac output is low or the blood volume is increased [437, 1009, 1807, 2540]. Cardiac disease may also predispose to Cheyne-Stokes respiration if left ventricular failure develops. This leads to hypoxia, which destabilizes respiration, hypocapnia, which diminishes the body stores of carbon dioxide, and a lowering of the FRC.

Cheyne-Stokes respiration may also appear if there is cerebrovascular disease. Hypercapnia normally causes cerebral vasodilatation and increases the cerebral blood flow. This reduces the capillary–CSF Pco_2 gradient and lessens the ventilatory response. This reactivity to CO_2 may be lost if there is cerebrovascular disease. Together with a prolonged circulation time, it may be responsible for the frequent appearance of Cheyne-Stokes respiration in otherwise normal older subjects.

CEREBRAL CORTICAL DYSFUNCTION

Cheyne-Stokes respiration is frequently seen in any situation in which the function of the cerebral hemispheres or the diencephalon is diminished [2498]. Cheyne-Stokes respiration is common in sleep, particularly in stages 1 and 2

NREM sleep [2525] and in subjects over the age of about forty-five [3268]. The control of the cerebral cortex over respiration is reduced and, as the sleep stages fluctuate, the threshold for the ventilatory response to hypercapnia changes [770]. Upper airway obstruction is unusual in Cheyne-Stokes respiration during sleep but it may be present [51, 3068] and is probably due to a reduction in upper airway muscle activity [2369]. Sedative drugs and any disorder that reduces the level of consciousness may also precipitate Cheyne-Stokes respiration.

In premature infants, the cerebral cortical function is not fully developed and Cheyne-Stokes respiration may appear. It is also a feature of other disorders such as encephalitis, strokes [1845, 1846, 2723], head injury [3221], metabolic disorders [2498], raised intracranial pressure [829] and pseudobulbar palsy [412, 2525]. It is occasionally a feature of bilateral midbrain or pontine damage [1845]. Both Cheyne-Stokes respiration and, in particular, Cheyne-Stokes variant, indicate a good prognosis in acute cerebral disorders [2723] but the pattern in which there are only 3–4 breaths between apnoeic intervals has a poor prognosis [993].

Symptoms

Cheyne-Stokes respiration rarely causes breathlessness [1394] but may do so if the respiratory mechanics are abnormal. Occasionally, the hyperpnoeic phase wakes the patient during sleep [2585]. This should be distinguished from orthopnoea due to bilateral diaphragmatic paralysis, nocturnal left ventricular failure, and hyperventilation following arousal from obstructive or central sleep apnoeas.

Physical signs

The most important observation is the regular waxing and waning of the tidal volume with an almost constant respiratory frequency. The period of hyperventilation is usually longer than the period of apnoea and may not be able to be altered by the patient if there is an underlying neurological disorder [1394, 2498]. The cycle length is usually < 50 sec if the cause is primarily neurological, but greater than this if circulatory factors are more important [1806, 2333].

Cheyne-Stokes respiration is often accompanied by circulatory and neurological changes. Hypoxia increases the sympathetic activity reflexly through the carotid body chemoreceptors but may depress medullary function directly if it is severe. Hypercapnia increases cerebral blood flow and the intracranial pressure [2067], causing a bradycardia, hypertension and other effects on medullary function. If Cheyne-Stokes respiration is due to a neurological disorder, the heart rate falls [993] and the blood pressure rises [2510] during the apnoeic phase. The close coupling of the respiratory and cardiovascular medullary centres [3215], together with the changes in intracranial pressure, may be responsible for the bradycardia, and the increase in sympathetic activity contributes to the hypertension. Opposite changes may occur with circulatory disorders [192, 1009, 2510]. Dysrhythmias such as atrial fibrillation, ventricular ectopics and atrioventricular block appear [192, 980] and may be abolished by atropine, suggesting that they are mediated by the parasympathetic nervous system [192].

The neurological features that appear during the apnoeic phase include eye closure and upward rotation of the eyes, conjugate gaze deviation, hyporeflexia, upgoing plantar reflexes, pupillary constriction, a reduction in tone of the limb muscles and a diminished level of consciousness [829, 993]. During the hyperpnoeic phase the pupils dilate [3102, 3103], abnormal movements may appear, tendon reflexes increase and the patient may become agitated [829].

Treatment

Treatment is rarely required for Cheyne-Stokes respiration unless breathlessness proves troublesome or cardiac dysrhythmias appear. It is important to treat the cause of the ventilatory instability by, for instance, increasing the cardiac output or treating any cause of cerebral cortical dysfunction. Cheyne-Stokes respiration can also be abolished by any measure that stabilizes ventilatory control. The balance between the chemical drive due to hypoxia and hypercapnia can be swung towards the stabilizing influence of hypercapnia by administering oxygen [1561, 3103] or even by breathing gas containing carbon dioxide [3134]. Respiratory stimulants may be effective if they lower the threshold of the ventilatory response to CO_2. They may, however, increase the gain of the control system by raising the slope of the ventilatory response. Doxapram can be used in the short term. Acetazolamide induces a metabolic acidosis and may abolish Cheyne-Stokes respiration or at least increase the length of the cycle and diminish the maximal tidal volume [980, 1322, 3117, 3178]. Aminophylline is also effective [830] since it lowers the threshold of the ventilatory response to CO_2 and increases the cardiac output.

CENTRAL NEUROGENIC HYPERVENTILATION (Fig. 5.1)

This respiratory pattern is characterized by rapid, regular respirations of a consistent tidal volume [2500]. The respiratory frequency is usually between 40 and 115 breaths per minute and Ti/TTOT increases. The regularity of the rhythm suggests that it is determined purely by the automatic control of respiration. Inhibitory influences on the medullary centres, including those from the cerebral cortex, appear to be damaged so that the response to respiratory stimuli is exaggerated. The threshold of the ventilatory response to hypercapnia falls [2494] (Fig. 5.3) and the arterial PCO$_2$ is low. The ventilatory pattern can be modified by other stimuli such as supraorbital pressure [2500].

Central neurogenic hyperventilation is probably less common than used to be thought since a similar pattern can be due to pulmonary disorders such as oedema or aspiration pneumonia. Central neurogenic hyperventilation can only be

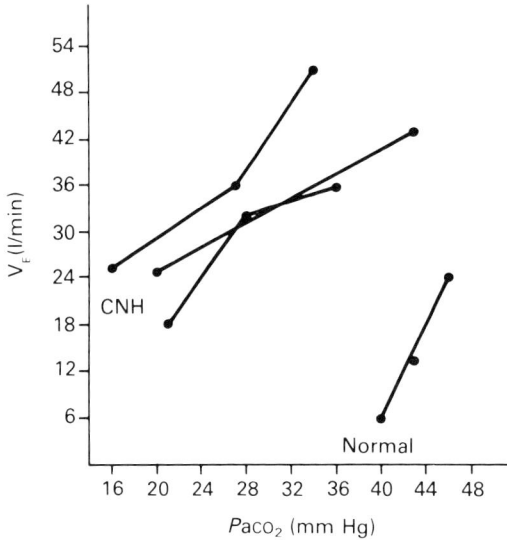

Fig. 5.3. *Ventilatory response to carbon dioxide in normal subjects and central neurogenic hyperventilation (CNH3). Reproduced, with permission, from Plum F. Ann. N.Y. Acad. Sci. 1963;* **109**: *926.*

diagnosed with any certainty if there is no evidence of pulmonary damage and if the arterial P_{O_2} is normal. It is usually due to extensive damage in the central tegmentum of the mid-brain and rostral pons. This may be due to cerebral infarction [1845, 2723], sepsis, encephalitis, head injury or cerebral tumours [1805]. The damage to the central nervous system is usually extensive. Most patients are comatose and show pupillary, ocular muscle signs and upgoing plantar reflexes.

APNEUSIS (Fig. 5.1)

Apneustic respiration is an uncommon pattern in which inspiration is prolonged at a volume close to the TLC. There is often some rhythmicity superimposed on the prolonged inspiratory 'spasm' and there may be small irregular inspirations during the often prolonged expiration between the inspiratory spasms. Milder forms, in which there is a brief end inspiratory pause, are more common [2492]. Apneusis appears to

be due to a disorder of respiratory timing and is accentuated by breathing gas containing carbon dioxide. It is associated with lesions in the dorsolateral, mid or caudal pons at or below the level of the pneumotaxic centre. This centre influences the respiratory rhythm and when it is damaged the ability to inhibit a sustained inspiration is abolished. Pontine lesions that are associated with apneusis include encephalitis lethargica [1442, 3200], rabies encephalitis [3260], Reye's syndrome [1756], meningitis, infarction [1755, 2492], haemorrhage [1697, 3037], posterior fossa surgery [1750], multiple system atrophy [171] and respiratory myoclonus [3168].

GASPING RESPIRATION (Fig. 5.1)

The appearance of infrequent deep respirations is probably the reciprocal of apneusis in that expiration is prolonged and inspiration occasionally breaks through. The anatomical site of the abnormality has not been determined but it has been recognized in conditions such as poliomyelitis [2787], which affect predominantly the medulla.

CLUSTER RESPIRATIONS (Fig. 5.1)

Respirations of a very variable tidal volume occur in groups or clusters at irregular intervals and are followed by an apnoea or a few respirations, usually of a low tidal volume. This pattern of breathing is seen when the lower pons or upper medulla is damaged [1442, 2498], such as in multiple system atrophy [1924] and poliomyelitis [2787].

ATAXIC (IRREGULAR) RESPIRATION (Fig. 5.1)

This pattern of slow and irregular respirations, first described by Biot in 1876 [286], indicates a disruption of the normal medullary rhythmicity of respiration. The ventilatory response to carbon dioxide and oxygen is usually impaired. This type of breathing is seen in a wide variety of medullary disorders, including head injury [2333], meningitis [625, 626], poliomyelitis [415, 1904, 2787] and medullary compression from, for instance, pontine haematomas or cerebello-tonsillar herniation. It is commonest with central medullary lesions and, therefore, is rare in cerebral ischaemia, which has to be bilateral to infarct the central medulla. Other features, such as depression of the lower jaw with each inspiration and an end expiratory cough-like movement, carry a poor prognosis [993].

CENTRAL APNOEA

Central apnoeas are more fully discussed in Chapter 6. They are commonest with lesions in the caudal medulla, particularly close to the obex where the descending fibres from the medullary respiratory centres decussate. Similar features are seen following high cervical cordotomy (p. 129). The ventilatory response to hypercapnia and hypoxia is usually diminished, confirming that the automatic control of respiration is disrupted.

OBSTRUCTIVE AND MIXED APNOEAS

These respiratory dysrhythmias are primarily due to occlusion of the upper airway rather than to an abnormality of respiratory rhythmicity (Chapter 6).

SHALLOW RESPIRATIONS

A pattern of regular respirations of a small tidal volume is frequently seen, particularly in neuromuscular and skeletal disorders. It may be present during wakefulness but also during sleep, particularly NREM sleep [373, 2145]. The physiological dead space is increased and this may lead to alveolar hypoventilation. This pattern of respiration usually indicates respiratory muscle weakness or fatigue, or abnormal respiratory mechanics, which limit the tidal volume and increase the respiratory frequency. Respiratory control is usually normal. This respiratory pattern may be a more important cause of nocturnal hypoventilation than has been recognized.

RESPIRATORY MYOCLONUS (DIAPHRAGMATIC FLUTTER, PALATOPHARYNGEAL MYOCLONUS) (Fig. 5.1)

This uncommon condition was first described by van Leuwenhoek in 1723, who noticed that his own respiratory rate was rapid and independent of the cardiac pulsations [1870]. He ascribed this to contractions of the diaphragm but it is now recognized that respiratory myoclonus may affect any of the respiratory muscles. The palate and pharynx are most commonly involved but the tongue, larynx, intercostal muscles and diaphragm [837, 3049, 3385], and occasionally other muscles, including the facial and external ocular muscles, may exhibit myoclonus. Diaphragmatic contraction has even been recorded synchronously with that of the biceps [3200]. Both halves of the diaphragm usually contract simultaneously, but myoclonus may be unilateral [837].

The origin of the rapid myoclonic contractions is not the medullary respiratory centres but damage to the olive, and dentate and associated nuclei [1272]. In many cases there is also a psychogenic element, and the myoclonus is worse with stress [2458]. It often [3138], but not always [1005, 3385], improves during sleep. In the past, damage to the olive was most frequently due to encephalitis, particularly encephalitis lethargica [832, 1083, 3200], but strokes are now a more common cause. There may also be local precipitating factors, such as a cervical rib [1502] or pressure on the xiphoid cartilage [292], and unilateral myoclonus of the diaphragm may even be synchronous with the heart beat [2996].

The frequency of respiratory myoclonus is 40–300 but usually 60–200 breaths per minute. The myoclonic movements are occasionally forceful and lead to a sensation of pounding in the chest and even to audible clicks in the chest

[678, 3126]. Similar noises in the head are due to rapid opening and closing of the Eustachian tubes [3049]. The myoclonic movements may completely suppress the normal respiratory activity but, more often, they are superimposed on the slower respiratory rate. Rapid undulations are apparent within the normal respiratory movements. A similar pattern has been termed dirhythmic breathing [1005, 3138]. The tidal volume of the myoclonic movements is usually small, particularly at high lung volumes [837]. The normal respiratory rate, but not the myoclonic movements, can be suppressed by respiratory-depressant drugs such as pethidine [3138].

Respiratory myoclonus is usually diagnosed by the observation of two separate respiratory rhythms, rapid movements of the upper airway muscles or the appearance of epigastric pulsations. It can be confirmed by, for instance, diaphragmatic fluoroscopy [2996, 3168], a sawtooth appearance in flow volume loops [340], or EMG studies [2458]. The arterial $P\text{CO}_2$ [1083] and ventilatory response to hypercapnia [2458] are normal.

Respiratory myoclonus may last for only a few seconds or minutes and reassurance may be sufficient. Drug treatment is not very effective. Topical ethylchloride spray has been used successfully [832, 1083, 2996] and droperidol and diazepam [3138], phenytoin [2458] and possibly quinidine [2458, 3126] may be of value. Phrenic nerve block has been reported to be ineffective [3138] but there may be some benefit from unilateral [1188, 2621] or even bilateral [1244] phrenic nerve section. The respiratory complications of the latter procedure outweigh the advantages, except in extreme cases. Diaphragmatic pacing has also been attempted [3323].

NON-RHYTHMIC RESPIRATORY ACTIONS

The respiratory muscles are used for a variety of non-rhythmic respiratory actions, such as coughing (p. 83), sighing (p. 283), yawning and hiccoughing. Hiccough can be precipitated by a wide variety of thoracic and abdominal conditions [3007], but appears to be essentially a gastrointestinal reflex [2296]. An abrupt contraction of the diaphragm and intercostal muscles is followed by closure of the upper airway at or near the larynx. The hiccoughing frequency is usually 10–60 per minute, but it is occasionally synchronous with the heart beat [1863]. The frequency of hiccough is reduced by rebreathing CO_2 [2296]. Hiccough may be induced by lesions in the floor of the 4th ventricle in the medulla, but the muscular contractions are largely coordinated within the spinal cord [2296].

Chapter 6
Sleep Apnoeas

The patterns of respiration described in Chapter 5 may occur during sleep as well as during wakefulness. Most of these respiratory rhythms were identified before modern methods of recording respiratory movements were introduced. These identify the pauses between respirations more clearly than the periods of normal or increased ventilation, and have led to the introduction of new terminology. The most important concept is the sleep apnoea. This is conventionally defined as a cessation of air flow for at least 10 sec. Apnoeas are heterogeneous and two main types have been recognized. In central apnoeas there is no respiratory muscle activity, whereas in obstructive apnoeas the diaphragm and other chest wall respiratory muscles are active but the upper airway is obstructed. In mixed apnoeas a period resembling a central sleep apnoea is followed by respiratory movements against an obstructed airway (Fig. 6.1).

Unfortunately, many of the newer terms have not been clearly defined and are used in different ways by various authors. A further problem is that the overlap between normal and abnormal breathing patterns has not been clarified for most of the types of breathing during sleep that have been identified.

The abnormal patterns of respiration during sleep are readily apparent and have been the subject of several review articles [322, 323, 882, 1758, 2409, 2595, 2799, 3064, 3071, 3098, 3309]. The respiratory pattern is, however, less important than its physiological consequences. The degree and duration of hypoxia, hypercapnia and sleep deprivation and fragmentation largely determine the clinical and physiological significance of ventilatory changes during sleep.

DEFINITIONS OF RESPIRATORY PATTERNS

An apnoea is usually regarded as a cessation of air flow for 10 sec or more but this is, strictly speaking, inaccurate since expiratory air flow can often be detected in obstructive sleep apnoeas [1784, 2775]. It is better defined as the absence of inspiratory air flow for a given period of time. The term 'hypopnoea' is used less precisely than apnoea to imply a decrease in the tidal volume, usually to less than a half or a third of the previous breath, with or without a fall of 4% or more in Sao_2. There are two sources of confusion with these definitions. Firstly, the errors in quantitating tidal volumes during sleep are considerable and the diagnosis of hypopnoea is often made incorrectly. Secondly, the fall in oxygen saturation during a period of hypoventilation depends largely on the initial oxygen saturation because of the curvilinear oxyhaemoglobin dissociation curve. The same change in ventilation may or may not qualify as a hypopnoea simply because of a different baseline oxygen saturation. The term hypopnoea is, therefore, of little value.

'Sleep disordered breathing' is often used to encompass both apnoeas and hypopnoeas, but since the latter concept is so vague, sleep disordered breathing is equally unsatisfactory. 'Periodic breathing' has been used synonymously with Cheyne-Stokes respiration for many years, but more recently its meaning has been broadened so that it is often almost equivalent to sleep disordered breathing.

Cheyne-Stokes respiration may also cause confusion because it is recorded as a central

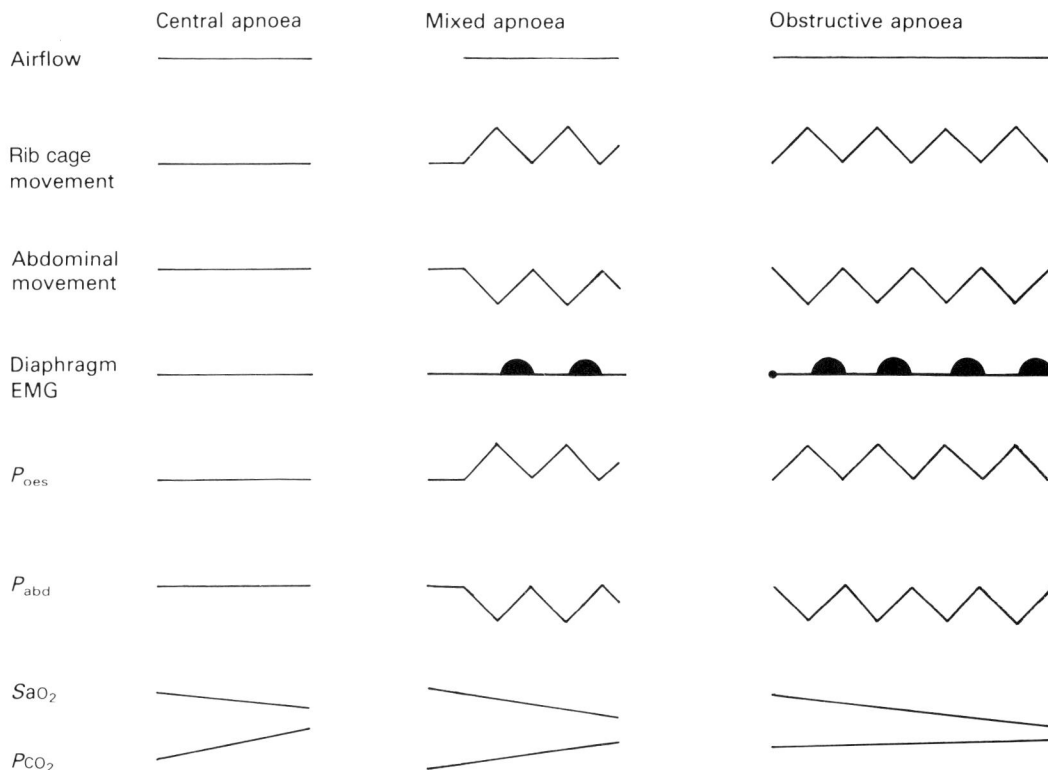

Fig. 6.1. *Schematic representation of events during central, mixed and obstructive apnoeas.*

apnoea by the conventional criteria if the apnoeic phase is 10 sec or longer. The underlying Cheyne-Stokes pattern may not be recognized and this normal respiratory rhythm may be erroneously interpreted as representing pathological central apnoeas. Conversely, Cheyne-Stokes variant, which is physiologically similar to Cheyne-Stokes respiration, does not have an apnoeic phase. It may pass unrecognized by conventional methods of sleep analysis or be interpreted as periods of regular 'hypopnoeas'.

RANGE OF NORMALITY

The selection of 10 sec as the duration of an apnoea was based on a small number of normal subjects [1280, 1282, 1302]. It has not been subjected to adequate further study since it was introduced. It would seem unlikely that a 10-sec apnoea would have the same physiological con-

sequences, for instance, from the neonatal phase to old age. Longer periods, such as 25 sec [2968], have been used as criteria to separate normal from abnormal apnoeas but have not gained acceptance. It might be more appropriate to relate, for instance, the length of the apnoea to the duration of the previous respiratory cycle rather than to regard any fixed duration as abnormal [1106].

The 'apnoea index' has been defined as the number of apnoeas per hour or over a period of seven hours sleep. This has been widely, but uncritically, used. It was originally suggested that an index of more than five apnoeas per hour [1280] or thirty over seven hours [1282, 1302] was abnormal, but there is very little data to support these suggestions. Subjects who have less than thirty sleep apnoeas per night are unlikely to have any symptoms or arousals from sleep [302], but many subjects, particularly over the age of forty, also have no symptoms or other apparent abnormalities even with an 'abnormal' apnoea index [78, 267, 504, 514, 2969]. Symptoms are unusual if there are less than about twenty apnoeas per hour [2870, 3071], but even if they are more frequent they correlate poorly with the presence of symptoms. Neither the development of respiratory failure while awake [376, 1084] nor the appearance of right heart failure [2829] are related to the frequency of apnoeas.

A similar index using the sum of the apnoeas and hypopnoeas has also been recommended to distinguish patients who have abnormally frequent disordered breathing during sleep. This index has never been validated and also has the disadvantage of the uncertainty of what a hypopnoea really represents.

A new set of terms is required to describe the respiratory patterns during sleep and this should be based on modern views of the physiology of respiratory control and of respiratory mechanics. A description in terms of observations such as the respiratory frequency, tidal volume, inspiratory and expiratory time and their fluctuations over a given period of time would be of value. These patterns should ideally be analysed statistically and related to arterial blood gases, the sleep stage and established normal values.

SLEEP APNOEA SYNDROME

A source of confusion in the study of breathing during sleep has been the introduction of the term 'sleep apnoea syndrome' and its many subsequent variants, such as the obstructive sleep apnoea syndrome and primary sleep apnoea syndrome. The sleep apnoea syndrome was initially defined purely by the presence of an 'abnormal' apnoea index, without necessarily any symptoms or evidence for oxygen desaturation [1282, 1302]. This term should be abandoned since the criteria for an abnormal apnoea index are still unsettled. Many subjects who are designated as having the sleep apnoea syndrome have

no detectable abnormalities and have a normal prognosis.

Somnolence was later added to the criteria for the diagnosis of sleep apnoea syndrome by some authors, but there seems no reason to single out this particular complication of sleep apnoeas to define the disorder. It would, perhaps, be preferable to indicate the severity of sleep apnoeas by including respiratory failure during the day, or right heart failure, in any definition. These physiological consequences of hypoventilation during sleep are more important than the frequency of the apnoeas.

RELATIONSHIP OF CENTRAL, MIXED AND OBSTRUCTIVE APNOEAS

There has been considerable debate regarding the relationship between central, mixed and obstructive apnoeas. Mixed apnoeas have been generally considered to be closely related to obstructive apnoeas, but there are diverging opinions as to whether or not central and obstructive apnoeas are fundamentally similar or represent two completely different abnormalities.

This problem is best approached by dissecting the apnoeas into their components. A central apnoea comprises a period without any respiratory activity in the muscles of the upper airway or chest wall. This is terminated by arousal or by stimulation of ventilation because of hypercapnia or hypoxia. In a typical central sleep apnoea, the airway is not occluded but if this does occur there is no ventilatory response to it. In obstructive apnoeas the upper airway is blocked but, unlike central apnoeas, there is a ventilatory response to this. The biochemical respiratory drive is normal, at least until chronic hypercapnia develops, and the apnoea is terminated when arousal occurs. The obstruction to the upper airway does not necessarily imply that there is a fault in respiratory control, since it may be precipitated by local abnormalities of the upper airway (see below).

The essence of a central apnoea is therefore that the drive to the respiratory muscles temporarily fails, whereas in obstructive apnoeas there is a normal ventilatory response to upper airway obstruction. A loss of upper airway muscle tone may be associated with the failure of the respiratory drive to the chest wall muscles during central apnoeas, so that the airway closes when inspiratory efforts restart. This results in a mixed apnoea [51, 1518]. The cycle is repeated if hyperventilation after the apnoea lowers the $P\text{CO}_2$ sufficiently to suppress respiratory efforts [1519].

Central sleep apnoeas are heterogeneous and there is therefore no single explanation for the association of central and obstructive apnoeas in the wide variety of conditions in which they coexist. Some central apnoeas are physiological (p. 75) and their association with obstructive apnoeas may be fortuitous. In other conditions, such as hypothyroidism and acromegaly, there appears to be a more definite relationship. Central apnoeas can be converted into obstructive apnoeas if a metabolic acidosis is induced, for instance, by acetazolamide [2876, 2877, 2909]. The increase in the ventilatory response to hypercapnia due to the acidosis is responsible for this change. Conversely, after treatment of obstructive apnoeas by tracheostomy and other methods, central apnoeas frequently appear [492, 594, 1279, 1397, 3163]. The mechanism is uncertain but may involve upper airway reflexes initiated by changes in nasal air flow [2780].

SLEEP APNOEAS AND CENTRAL ALVEOLAR HYPOVENTILATION

The concept of central alveolar hypoventilation (p. 124) was developed before the importance of sleep apnoeas was realized. In the 1950s, it became apparent that ventilatory failure could occur without any abnormality of the lungs, pleura, chest wall, respiratory muscles or peripheral nerves, and without obesity. Similar features were recognized after high cervical cor-

dotomy, to which the term 'Ondine's curse' was applied [2861]. Ondine was a mythological water spirit revived in Jean Giraudoux's play. Ondine's husband, Hans, was cursed so that he could no longer breathe if he fell asleep. Ondine tried to prevent this happening but was not herself cursed. The term Ondine's curse is therefore inaccurate. Central alveolar hypoventilation and Ondine's curse came to be used almost synonymously but the latter is best avoided [3089].

Central alveolar hypoventilation is a descriptive term for ventilatory failure due to a defective automatic ventilatory drive. It is more marked during sleep than during wakefulness and there is considerable overlap between this condition and patients with frequent sleep apnoeas. Unfortunately, very few studies of central alveolar hypoventilation included a description of the respiratory pattern during sleep. It is likely that most of the published case reports would now be diagnosed as having obstructive sleep apnoeas in the absence of obesity, or as having frequent central apnoeas. Both types of apnoea have been documented in a few patients with central alveolar hypoventilation [536, 1141, 1428, 1645]; other respiratory patterns, particularly shallow respirations that would increase the physiological dead space and decrease alveolar ventilation, have also been recorded [193, 2404] (p. 125). Similarly, patients with frequent central apnoeas [377] and obstructive apnoeas may develop respiratory failure, which is indistinguishable from central alveolar hypoventilation.

The relationship between central alveolar hypoventilation and sleep apnoeas is close but it could arise purely through a persistently small tidal volume without any true apnoeas. Conversely, not all patients with frequent apnoeas develop ventilatory failure. Factors other than the apnoeas themselves are important. These have not yet been accurately identified but may include the severity of desaturation during the apnoea [377], the degree to which the blood gases return to normal between the apnoeas, the ease with which the ventilatory response is blunted by consistently high $P\text{CO}_2$, the presence of other lung diseases that would lower the P_{O_2} and perhaps raise the P_{CO_2}, and the degree of sleep deprivation and fragmentation. Central alveolar hypoventilation does not, therefore, equate exactly with any recognized respiratory pattern during sleep.

OBSTRUCTIVE SLEEP APNOEAS

A clear description of obstructive sleep apnoeas was provided as long ago as 1877 by Broadbent [399]. Their importance gradually became recognized between about 1955 and 1970, particularly in explaining respiratory failure in the obese (p. 181). Since then, they have been recognized increasingly frequently, particularly in countries such as the USA where obesity is prevalent, but elsewhere they have received less attention. This probably reflects both a true geographical difference in prevalence but also a lack of awareness and an inability to diagnose upper airway obstruction during sleep.

Site of upper airway obstruction

In obstructive sleep apnoeas, respiratory efforts, particularly of the diaphragm, continue despite occlusion of the upper airway. Gastaut's investigations around 1965 [1093, 1094] indicated

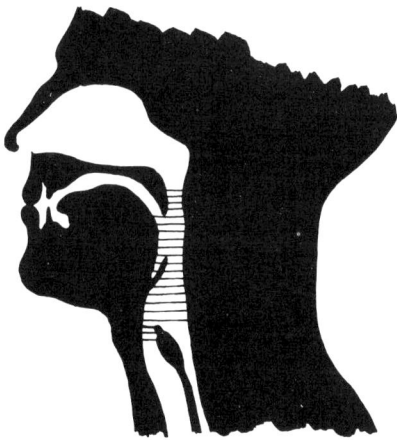

Fig. 6.2. *Diagram to illustrate the usual area of occlusion of the upper airway during obstructive sleep apnoeas (hatched area).*

that the obstruction occurred in the pharynx. This has been largely confirmed by subsequent observations particularly fibre-optic endoscopy, (Fig. 6.2). The lateral or posterior wall of the pharynx invaginates early in inspiration to block the airway [1273, 1289, 1425, 1821, 3255]. The airway closes circumferentially and the collapsed segment may lengthen during the progressively stronger inspiratory efforts during the apnoea [2697, 2970, 3288]. In some cases the hypopharynx is the first to invaginate but in other subjects the airway closes initially at the velopharyngeal level [346, 3139, 3288] or even near the glottis [1759]. Velopharyngeal closure has been shown by videofluoroscopy to be associated with upward and posterior movement of the tongue to meet the palate [346]. This may be particularly important in mandibular abnormalities, macroglossia and acromegaly (see below).

The larynx remains patent during obstructive sleep apnoeas, possibly because the negative pressure in the upper airway reflexly activates the abductors of the vocal cords [3328]. However, if the vocal cords are paralysed or if there is a pathological lesion in the larynx, the airway may become occluded. Obstructive apnoeas due to vocal cord adduction may also be induced by diaphragmatic pacing (p. 275) or negative pressure ventilation (p. 227). These methods of treatment may prevent normal synchronization of upper airway muscle activity or inhibit the laryngeal muscle activity as part of a generalized inhibition of respiratory muscles.

Pathogenesis of upper airway obstruction

The maintenance of the patency of the upper airway depends on the balance between the pressure inside and outside the airway and on the physical properties, particularly the compliance and the diameter of the airway itself (Fig. 6.3). The balance of these forces changes during the apnoea because of factors such as the progressive increase in diaphragmatic activity [1274].

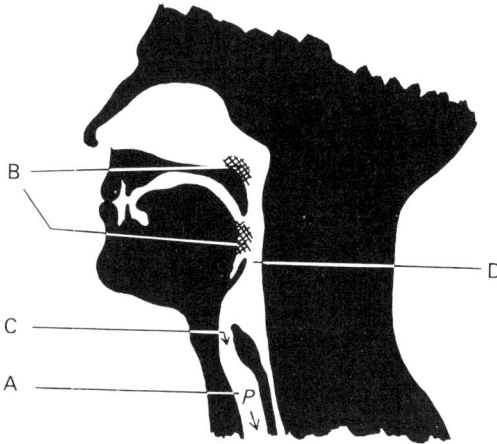

Fig. 6.3. *Causes of pathological obstruction to upper airway:
A = excessive chest wall inspiratory muscle contraction
leading to a fall in intra-airway pressure (P ↓), B = partial
obstruction of upper airway, C = laryngeal lesion or vocal
cord palsy, D = decreased pharyngeal dilator muscle tone.*

TRANSMURAL UPPER AIRWAY PRESSURE

The pressure within the upper airway falls
during inspiration. The pressure in the tissues
surrounding the airway is approximately atmospheric. Consequently, the greater the
inspiratory effort the greater is the transmural
pressure gradient and the tendency of the upper
airway to collapse. The diaphragmatic activity
increases during the apnoea, probably in
response to hypoxia, hypercapnia and to the
increased upper airway resistance. This maintains the closure of the airway throughout the
apnoea.

COMPLIANCE OF UPPER AIRWAY

The compliance of the upper airway is thought
to largely depend on the muscle tone, but individual variations in the detailed anatomy of the
mandible, hyoid, and related structures may be
important. Most attention has been paid to the
genioglossus muscle because of its accessibility,
but other muscles controlling, for example, the
movement of the palate [2685] and the anterior
movement of the hyoid [1217] are probably
equally important.

Theoretically, the upper airway might collapse if the activity of the constrictor muscles
increased or the activity of the dilator muscles
was reduced. Electromyogram studies have,
however, shown that there is no change in the
function of the pharyngeal constrictor muscles
during obstructive sleep apnoeas [1273, 1289].
It is the loss of tone in dilator muscles such as
the genioglossus that accompanies the apnoea
[1289, 1425, 2597]. This is particularly prominent during REM sleep when the tone of all the
postural muscles is reduced [2797] (p. 36). Diaphragmatic contraction continues even during
REM sleep, and the loss of pharyngeal dilator
activity lowers the pressure within the pharynx
that is required to close the upper airway [407,
2407]. The pharyngeal dilator muscles remain
inactive throughout the obstructive apnoea
[1545]. The airway only opens when the patient
arouses, causing voluntary control of ventilation
to return and pharyngeal dilator muscle activity
then increases rapidly [326, 2597, 3241].

SIZE OF UPPER AIRWAY

The patency of the upper airway is greatly influenced by its size at the onset of the apnoea. By
Laplace's law, the tension in the wall of a cylinder is the product of the pressure and the radius.
If the radius decreases, the tension required to
maintain it is less than previously. The tension
in the wall of the pharynx is largely controlled
by the muscle tone and if this does not adjust
immediately to changes in diameter, the airway
will progressively narrow until it closes. It is
therefore unstable and, like small blood vessels,
has a critical closing pressure at any given wall
tension. Conversely, once the airway has closed,
a high pressure within the lumen is required to
open it (critical opening pressure). This has been
documented experimentally [3353]. A lack of
appreciation of Laplace's law has led to various
explanations involving, for instance, the adhesive properties of the pharyngeal mucosa [326]
to explain these observations.

When the upper airway is narrowed the flow
rate at the point of the constriction increases,

the pressure falls by Bernouilli's principle and airway closure becomes more likely. The resistance to air flow increases at the point of narrowing and gas flow may become turbulent. This further increases the resistance. A greater negative pressure is required to overcome the resistance of the narrowing itself and the added effect of turbulent air flow. The negative pressure within the upper airway downstream from the obstruction falls and this predisposes the airway to collapse. Upper airway narrowing can, therefore, lead to occlusion either at the point of narrowing or downstream from it.

A small upper airway is also more vulnerable to other factors that may block it, such as the backward movement of the tongue in the supine position [510, 1631]. The pharyngeal cross-sectional area is closely related to the FRC in the supine position, particularly during REM sleep when the postural muscle tone is reduced. The FRC falls and the pharyngeal cross-sectional area also decreases [1446, 1449]. Obstructive apnoeas become more frequent [2368], particularly if the initial diameter of the upper airway was small.

Physiological studies have demonstrated that the upper airway resistance is increased in subjects with frequent obstructive sleep apnoeas, particularly if they are obese [75, 77, 3071]. This has been confirmed by analysis of flow volume loops [1346, 2628]. A saw-tooth pattern is common [535, 1351] and has been correlated with direct observation of airway occlusion by fibre-optic endoscopy [2772, 3139]. The upper airway inspiratory flow rates increase after appropriate surgical treatment [1351].

Disorders causing obstructive sleep apnoeas

Obstructive sleep apnoeas may be initiated purely by physiological changes. Upper airway resistance may increase, for instance, by constriction of the alae nasi and, particularly during REM sleep when muscle tone is decreased, the airway may collapse. The diameter of the upper airway varies considerably in normal subjects and it appears that those with the narrowest

airway are predisposed to obstructive apnoeas (p. 71).

Several techniques have been used to assess the size of the upper airway. Cephalometry is a technique in which a lateral radiograph of the head and neck is taken under carefully standardized conditions. A variety of measurements of the upper airway can be made [1298, 2628, 2638]. This technique is particularly valuable for showing abnormalities of the mandible and hyoid, which appear to be common in obstructive apnoeas [2639]. It has, however, been largely superseded by computerized tomography (CT) scanning. This shows the cross-sectional dimensions of the upper airway at different levels and, like cephalometry, is of particular value when surgical treatment for obstructive apnoeas is being considered (Fig. 6.4). Acoustic reflection techniques in which high-frequency sound waves are reflected from interfaces in the neck are also of value [868, 1037]. Cinefluoroscopy shows the changes in upper airway dimensions during apnoeas, and fibre-optic endoscopy allows direct observation of the movements of the airway. These and other techniques have demonstrated obstructive apnoeas in the following conditions.

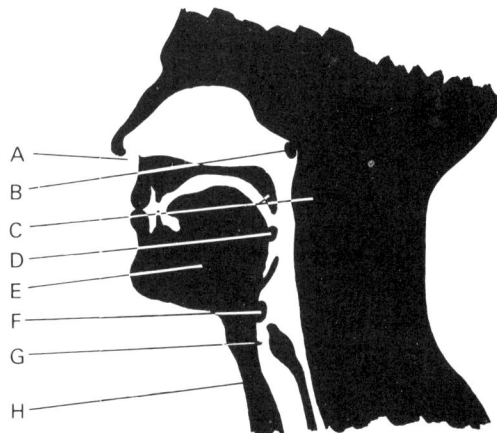

Fig. 6.4. *Surgical procedures that may abolish obstructive sleep apnoeas: A = relief of nasal obstruction, B = adenoidectomy, C = uvulopalatopharyngoplasty (UPPP), D = tonsillectomy, E = mandibular advancement, F = hyoidoplasty, G = laryngeal surgery, H = tracheostomy.*

INCREASED TRANSMURAL UPPER
AIRWAY PRESSURE

The normal ventilatory response to an increase
in upper airway resistance is to increase the
strength of the contraction of the inspiratory
muscles. This will lower the pressure within the
pharynx and increase the transmural pressure.
The inspiratory activity of the chest wall muscles
increases during the apnoea as hypoxia and
hypercapnia develop, and this sustains the occlusion of the airway. This normal response
therefore induces an obstructive apnoea and any
abnormality would lessen rather than increase
the risk of apnoeas appearing.

INCREASED COMPLIANCE OF UPPER AIRWAY

The upper airway tends to collapse if its compliance is increased. In practice, any factor that
decreases the tone of the dilator muscles will
predispose to obstructive apnoeas. It has been
proposed that obstructive apnoeas are due to
failure to activate the pharyngeal dilator muscles
when the diaphragm and other chest wall
muscles contract. This could explain the occlusion of the upper airway, particularly if this
was initially narrowed, but direct evidence in
support of this theory is lacking. Sleep deprivation, however, lessens the EMG activity in
genioglossus and leads to airway occlusion
[1857].

Alcohol diminishes muscle tone and increases
the upper airway resistance [2664]. In women,
the loss of genioglossus activity is greater after
consuming alcohol in the follicular than in the
luteal phase of the menstrual cycle [1856]. The
neural output to the upper airway muscles decreases to a greater extent than the stimulation
to the diaphragm [2750]. Alcohol also influences
the reticular formation so that the threshold for
arousal to hypoxia and hypercapnia is lowered
and it changes the sleep pattern so that the sleep
latency is shorter, stages 3 and 4 NREM sleep
occur earlier and there is an increase in the
amount of REM sleep during the second half
of the night [3130]. The frequency and severity

of obstructive sleep apnoeas increase [1274,
1542, 2839, 3130].

Marijuana [1421] and opiates [2666] have
relatively slight effects but other sedative drugs
such as flurazepam, many of which are also
muscle relaxants, increase the frequency and
severity of obstructive apnoeas [807, 2127]. In
cats, diazepam reduces the stimulation of the
upper airway muscles more than that of the diaphragm [343]. These drugs also diminish the
ventilatory response to hypercapnia [1103].
General anaesthetic and muscle-relaxant drugs
have similar effects [1421]. Post-operative
obstructive apnoeas are partly due to these drugs
and partly to the influence of the supine position
[2338].

SMALL SIZE OF UPPER AIRWAY

The most important abnormalities of the upper
airway that predispose to obstructive sleep
apnoeas are:

Nasal obstruction

The significance of nasal obstruction causing
somnolence and other features of sleep abnormalities has been recognized since the nineteenth century [1825, 3290]. The regular changes
in air flow resistance during the nasal cycle,
and the changes with posture, lead to intermittent complete nasal obstruction even if the
anatomical abnormality is only unilateral. The
nasal cycle is more marked in allergic rhinitis
than in normal subjects and this exacerbates the
tendency towards nasal obstruction [1377].

Most neonates and infants are virtually unable
to breathe through the mouth because the soft
palate is long and the epiglottis large and high
[1097]. When the nose is obstructed, efforts to
breathe continue but air only enters through
narrow slits between the lips. The respiratory
movements are also influenced by reflexes initiated by the cessation of nasal air flow. Stimulation of nasal receptors is reduced and this decreases the activity of the respiratory muscles
and leads to central apnoeas. It may also cause
selective inhibition of the dilator muscles of the

upper airway and predispose to obstructive apnoeas [3380]. Obstructive apnoeas can also be induced in adults by application of local anaesthetic to the nose and oropharynx without any nasal obstruction [2022].

In some children the P_{O_2} can be maintained, but in others hypoxia develops and the V_T falls or a pattern of periodic breathing appears [1726]. Ventilation and respiratory frequency are reduced, particularly during REM sleep [2541]. This contrasts with the response in awake adults to an increase in air flow resistance, in whom the respiratory frequency decreases but the V_T rises [729, 1995]. The importance of a patent nasal airway in children is illustrated by the problems that follow the surgical construction of a pharyngeal flap to improve velopharyngeal incompetence. This obstructs the nasal airway and causes frequent arousals from sleep and blood gas abnormalities [1741].

Nasal obstruction is also of importance in adults. Occlusion of the nares by nasal plugs leads to nocturnal oxygen desaturation, an increase in the frequency of arousal from sleep, loss of stages 3 and 4 NREM sleep and an increase in the frequency of apnoeas [3408]. Conversely, an increase in nasal air flow in NREM sleep increases ventilation [2021]. The apnoeas are mainly central and mixed rather than obstructive [3408], suggesting that the reflex mechanisms described above may be of more importance than the changes in intrapharyngeal pressure. Lignocaine applied to the nasal mucosa during sleep also increases the frequency of central apnoeas [3310].

Similar changes have been observed in subjects whose nostrils are blocked [1827, 2365, 3113] and following the insertion of nasal packs after nasal surgery [3129]. In allergic rhinitis, both periodic breathing [1828] and obstructive sleep apnoeas [1890, 2024] occur. Daytime somnolence associated with nocturnal central apnoeas and frequent arousals has been reported with a deviated nasal septum [1830] and nasopharyngeal carcinoma [2229]. Nasopharyngeal stenosis secondary to pemphigoid may also cause obstructive apnoeas [2366]. The resistance

of the upper airway increases in obesity when this is associated with obstructive apnoeas, and improves following a nasal decongestant [76, 77, 3112]. This nasal obstruction is additional to and independent of the narrowing of the pharynx seen in obesity (p. 182).

Correction of these abnormalities by, for instance, submucosal resection or nasal polypectomy often relieves the apnoeas. These procedures should be considered even if the nasal obstruction is only minor, since it may be sufficient to precipitate obstructive apnoeas in combination with an anatomically narrowed oropharynx. Daytime somnolence and sleep quality can be improved [1397, 1830, 2726] and the frequency and duration of apnoeas diminished [1397, 2091]. Central apnoeas may, however, appear [1397].

Enlargement of tonsils and adenoids

Enlargement of the tonsils during acute infections is well known to cause acute obstruction of the airway [3010] but around 1965 it was recognized that chronic air flow obstruction was associated with enlargement of the tonsils or adenoids, or both [2125, 2329]. In severe cases, the clinical picture shows several characteristic features: daytime somnolence, nocturnal snoring and noisy breathing, which may stimulate asthma, are frequent. The air flow obstruction may be severe enough to cause respiratory arrest [3135] but, more commonly breathlessness is worse lying flat than sitting up [801, 2080]. This is probably due to a gravitational effect of the enlarged tonsils and adenoids but, in severe cases, left ventricular failure may contribute to the orthopnoea [38, 1963].

The chest radiograph may show an enlarged heart and the electrocardiogram (ECG) may reveal features of right ventricular hypertrophy due to pulmonary hypertension [1881, 2329, 2858, 3338]. The P_{O_2} and P_{CO_2} are abnormal, both during wakefulness and sleep [1189, 1740], and the pulmonary artery pressure rises during sleep [2125]. Arousals and apnoeas, which are predominantly obstructive, are frequent [2091,

2865]. They occur particularly during REM sleep but are most prolonged during stages 3 and 4 NREM sleep [1740]. Ventilation may be severely depressed by oxygen [2125] and by respiratory-depressant drugs [1740].

This clinical picture is commonest in children between the ages of two and six years, but may be seen in older children [1285]. In milder cases only snoring and sleep apnoeas may be present [910] together, in some cases, with somnolence [2052]. Obstructive sleep apnoeas may be more common than is usually recognized. In a prospective study of children selected for tonsillectomy and adenoidectomy, about 3% showed right-sided ECG changes, which were reversed after surgery [3338].

Tonsillectomy and adenoidectomy are usually required [2091], but occasionally tonsillectomy alone [2080] or adenoidectomy alone [1042, 1881, 1963] is effective. If there is doubt whether the tonsils and adenoids are the cause of the upper airway obstruction, a nasopharyngeal tube can be inserted. This quickly improves the clinical condition if the obstruction to air flow is at this level [884, 1740]. Improvement also occurs rapidly after surgery: somnolence disappears [317, 2080], the sleep pattern improves [2052], apnoeas become less frequent [910, 2052], arterial blood gases improve [1881, 2478], pulmonary artery pressure falls [317, 1189, 1881, 1963, 2125] and right heart failure is relieved [884]. The ventilatory response to hypercapnia may not return to normal after surgery [1530]. This suggests that the effect of chronic upper airway obstruction is irreversible or that the hypercapnic response was abnormal even before the tonsillar enlargement.

Enlargement of the tonsils in adults is much less common than in children, but it can occasionally cause chronic upper airway obstruction. Recurrent upper airway infections are the usual cause of enlarged tonsils but other conditions, such as a lymphoma [1674, 2382] or Down's syndrome [317, 1821], should be considered. The whole of the upper airway should be assessed and other abnormalities, such as a deviated nasal septum, may need to be corrected in addi-

tion to removing the tonsils [3062]. Somnolence [2382, 3062], snoring [2382] and the frequency of obstructive apnoeas [3062] are all reduced by tonsillectomy.

Mandibular abnormalities

A small (micrognathia) or posteriorly positioned (retrognathia) mandible may cause upper airway obstruction during sleep. Cinefluoroscopy has demonstrated that the tongue lodges against the posterior pharyngeal wall [634], and sleep studies have confirmed that apnoeas are obstructive rather than central [634, 730, 2440]. These mandibular abnormalities are usually present from birth or childhood, but respiratory failure is uncommon [3016] and does not usually develop until adult life [634]. Occasionally, micrognathia acquired in adult life due, for instance, to rheumatoid arthritis can cause sleep apnoeas [730]. Micrognathia may be associated with other abnormalities of the upper airway, such as pharyngeal hypoplasia in the Treacher–Collins syndrome, which contribute to the appearance of obstructive apnoeas [2641].

The dimensions of the oropharynx can be increased by mandibular advancement. This involves a mandibular osteotomy, which moves the tongue forwards and lessens the risk of it obstructing the airway. Mandibular advancement also corrects the cosmetic deformity of the poorly developed chin and improves dental occlusion. Mandibular advancement is often sufficient to improve symptoms such as somnolence and snoring [209, 1781, 2524, 3020] and to lessen the number of apnoeas [1781] and nocturnal desaturation [2524]. Tracheostomy is effective in these subjects [592, 634, 730, 1525, 2440, 3216] but has been largely replaced by mandibular advancement.

Macroglossia

Obstructive sleep apnoeas may be due to enlargement of the tongue, which blocks off the pharynx, particularly in the supine position [492]. Enlargement of the tongue is one feature of several conditions, such as acromegaly (see below) which affects much of the upper respiratory tract and conditions such as amyloid in which the tongue is selectively enlarged. Amyloid may also cause ventilatory failure by infiltrating the diaphragm [3075]. Both obstructive and mixed apnoeas appear and, while a tracheostomy is effective [492], a tongue-retaining device may be sufficient [509, 511].

Pharyngeal narrowing

In the majority of subjects with frequent obstructive apnoeas, there is no obvious anatomical abnormality of the upper respiratory tract. Investigation of such subjects, particularly with CT scans and acoustic reflection, have, however, shown that the cross-sectional area of the pharynx is narrower than in normal subjects [337, 370, 1350, 2638, 2639, 3111]. The narrowest region appears to be in the oropharynx posterior to the soft palate, but other constricted areas, particularly in the nasopharynx and hypopharynx, have been detected. The airway is narrowed circumferentially, possibly because of an increase in the thickness of the mucous membrane, particularly the lymphoid tissue. Obesity predisposes to obstructive apnoeas but fat is not seen around the upper airway. It is largely subcutaneous and probably narrows the airway by displacing the other tissues in the neck medially.

A large soft palate and a long uvula are often seen in patients with frequent obstructive apnoeas. It is uncertain whether these features predispose to apnoeas or are a consequence of them. In pycnodysostosis, the long uvula has been shown fluoroscopically to obstruct the airway [3392]. Myotonia of the pharyngeal constrictors may narrow the airway and cause obstructive apnoeas in dystrophia myotonica [3076].

Two operations have been proposed to enlarge the pharynx and to prevent obstructive sleep apnoeas:

Hyoidoplasty. Hyoidoplasty can be achieved by transecting the hyoid and moving the greater cornua laterally, together with the middle constrictor and hyoglossus. The body of the hyoid is moved anteriorly with the geniohyoid and genioglossus. This operation increases the dimensions of the superior hyopharynx by pulling the epiglottis and the anterior pharyngeal wall forwards. Volume–pressure studies in dogs have given encouraging results using this technique [2418], with few problems with swallowing and laryngeal competence. It has not been widely used in man, but a slight improvement in snoring, somnolence and frequency of apnoeas has been recorded [1632, 2629].

Uvulopalatopharyngoplasty (UPPP). This operation has been devised to remove 'redundant' oropharyngeal tissue, which may predispose to obstructive sleep apnoeas. The uvula is amputated or shortened, the posterior margin of the soft palate is removed, the mucosa is stripped from the posterior pharyngeal wall and tissue is removed from the lateral aspect of the pharynx. This widens the oropharynx and also causes scar tissue to form, which may diminish the compliance of the pharynx and its tendency to collapse during inspiration. The separation of the soft palate from the posterior pharyngeal wall might be expected to cause velopharyngeal insufficiency, with a nasal voice and nasal regurgitation of fluids. These complications are usually only temporary [1060]. Palatal stenosis is uncommon post-operatively [657].

Several studies have shown that UPPP is highly effective in treating snoring [657, 1059, 1411, 2933]. Resection of part of the soft palate prevents it from vibrating and thereby abolishes snoring (p. 80). Uvulopalatopharyngoplasty is less satisfactory for treating daytime somnolence [631, 1060, 1411] and even less so in improving objective rather than subjective complications of obstructive apnoeas. Apnoeas are diminished in frequency in only about 50% of subjects [630, 631, 1060, 1288, 1411, 3405] and oxygen desaturation is improved in a smaller percentage [630, 631, 1060, 1288]. The quality of sleep, including the sleep latency time, may improve [1060, 3405] and this correlates better with the improvement in somnolence than any changes in nocturnal oxygen desaturation [3405].

The criteria for selecting patients for UPPP have not been settled. The response appears to be best in milder cases [1288] but is very variable [1060, 3405]. There is conflicting evidence as to whether or not obesity is an indication or a contraindication to surgery. In one study, poor results were obtained in massively obese patients [1288], but a subsequent report has shown good results [1060]. Uvulopalatopharyngoplasty appears to be most effective if there is an oropharyngeal abnormality such as a large uvula, wide tonsillar pillars and palatoglossal folds, excessive posterior pharyngeal mucosa or a low arched palate. In contrast, non-responders frequently have hypopharyngeal abnormalities such as a large base of the tongue, an omega-shaped epiglottis and 'redundant' aryepiglottic folds, often in addition to oropharyngeal abnormalities [1060]. A careful anatomical assessment of the upper airway is therefore essential before UPPP is considered, and this should include techniques such as cephalometry, rhinometry and a CT scan of the pharynx [657]. A disadvantage of UPPP is that it prevents nasal continuous positive airway pressure (CPAP) from being effective, if this is subsequently required (Chapter 21).

Laryngeal obstruction

Stridor is a well-recognized feature of laryngeal obstruction, but obstructive sleep apnoeas also occur and may be severe. They have been described in vocal cord palsy due to achondroplasia [3150], following neurosurgery and neck surgery [1448], syringobulbia (p. 122), multiple system atrophy (p. 123), poliomyelitis (p. 143), and the lateral medullary syndrome (p. 121). Organic disorders of the larynx may also cause obstructive apnoeas. These include congenital laryngeal webs or cysts [2366, 2932] and thickening of the laryngeal tissues as in hypothyroidism and acromegaly (see below). Obstructive sleep apnoeas due to a failure of contraction of the vocal cord abductors are also

a feature of negative pressure ventilation and diaphragmatic pacing. Tracheostomy is usually required [694, 1448] but laryngeal surgery is indicated in selected cases.

Other conditions

Acromegaly. Somnolence and other features of nocturnal respiratory disorders are now well recognized in acromegaly, but have in the past been confused with narcolepsy [1290]. Snoring is frequent and sleep apnoeas may be of the obstructive, mixed or central types [1374, 2142, 2441]. They are longer and cause more severe oxygen desaturation during REM sleep [2142]. They may contribute to hypertension and even cardiomegaly, which are common in acromegaly.

The exact cause of the sleep apnoeas is uncertain. The changes in the thorax are probably of little significance. The ribs lengthen and thicken [3039] and, despite a kyphosis, the lung volumes increase in males although possibly not in females [937]. The tissues of the upper airway, including the nose, mandible, tongue, epiglottis and larynx, are diffusely thickened, and enlargement of the thyroid may also compress the trachea. The laryngeal mucosa hypertrophies, often irregularly, so that the glottis is narrowed and stridor may be heard [277, 852, 937, 1701, 2701]. The ventilatory response to hypercapnia is normal in both active and inactive acromegaly [1374], but sleep apnoeas are particularly common in the presence of a high growth hormone level [1374, 2441].

Endoscopy during sleep has shown that the lateral and posterior hypopharyngeal walls invaginate during inspiration [675] and that the enlarged tongue bulges into the pharynx and obliterates the airway [2142]. It is also possible that the myopathy of acromegaly decreases the tone of the upper airway muscles and predisposes to upper airway occlusion. Examination of flow volume loops [2441] and maximal expiratory and inspiratory flow rates [937] has confirmed the presence of upper airway obstruction. Tracheostomy is effective [459, 852] but is rarely necessary since the symptoms improve and sleep apnoeas become less frequent when the acromegaly is treated [530, 852, 2142].

Hypothyroidism. Obstructive sleep apnoeas are well recognized in hypothyroidism [2081, 2381, 2553, 2958, 3383]. Thickening of the vocal cords [281] predisposes to obstructive apnoeas but usually presents with hoarseness of the voice. Obesity secondary to the hypothyroidism is probably the most important factor, but there may also be a localized thickening of the soft tissues of the tongue and upper airway as part of the hypothyroidism. Removal of a goitre compressing the trachea has been reported to lessen the frequency of obstructive apnoeas [3028].

Achondroplasia. Obstructive sleep apnoeas are present in up to 10% of subjects with achondroplasia [1814, 3058]. The mechanism is uncertain but vocal cord palsy may be important in some cases [3150]. Fluoroscopy has also demonstrated occlusion of the airway at the base of the tongue extending down towards the epiglottis [2986]. The small foramen magnum and associated skeletal abnormalities may cause hydrocephalus and cervical cord compression. Automatic control of ventilation may be impaired so that central sleep apnoeas [1043] and cyanosis after, for instance, crying [3058] are seen. Decompression of the foramen magnum may be required [3382].

Hurler and Hunter syndromes. These mucopolysaccharidoses may be complicated by obstructive sleep apnoeas. Nasal abnormalities, enlargement of tonsils and adenoids, macroglossia, an omega-shaped epiglottis and laryngeal oedema may all contribute to these. Tracheostomy may be required [2872].

Neoplasia. A variety of tumours may obstruct the upper airway and cause obstructive apnoeas. Infiltration in the neck by a lymphoma [3406], and a submandibular lipoma [1728] and a neurofibroma compressing the pharynx [3068] have been reported. High-dose irradiation for head and neck carcinomas may induce extensive fibrosis in the neck, causing severe obstructive sleep apnoeas [163, 2511]. Tracheostomy may be required since the airway is narrowed over a considerable length.

Clinical features

Obstructive sleep apnoeas can occur neonatally or in childhood but become increasingly common with age [78, 324, 504, 2969]. It has been thought that they are commoner in males, particularly under the age of about fifty [324, 504, 2969], and that this might have an endocrine basis [2778, 3086]. However, recent studies have shown no sex difference in the frequency of apnoeas when allowance is made for obesity and other factors [514]. Apnoeas may be frequent and severe in premenopausal women [3335]. Occasionally a family history of obstructive sleep apnoeas is obtained [2712, 3084].

Obstructive sleep apnoeas occur most frequently during REM and stages 1 and 2 NREM sleep [2370]. They are rare in stages 3 and 4 NREM sleep but these sleep stages are uncommon since most of the subjects have frequent arousals, which prevent these deeper sleep stages from being attained. The duration of the apnoeas is longer in REM than in NREM sleep [981, 1829], but they become more prolonged in NREM sleep later in the night [1829]. This may be due to a fall in the arousal threshold to hypoxia or hypercapnia, secondary to sleep deprivation.

The most prominent symptoms of obstructive apnoeas are snoring and daytime somnolence. The relationship of snoring to obstructive apnoeas is discussed on p. 79. Somnolence was initially thought to be due to a raised $P\text{CO}_2$ during the daytime, but this is often normal. A primary defect within the brain, particularly within the reticular formation, causing somnolence or a lack of arousal is unlikely since they improve rapidly after tracheostomy or when other effective treatment is given. There is some evidence that the severity of hypoxia correlates with somnolence [2380, 2383, 2948], but it is more likely that the degree of sleep deprivation and fragmentation is the main factor. Fragmentation of sleep is due to arousal at the end of each apnoea. The subject may awaken or change into a lighter stage of sleep. This increases the ventilatory response to hypoxia and hypercapnia so that there is often a period of hyperventilation after the apnoea.

Obstructive apnoeas follow an expiration and are terminated by an inspiration [2074]. The respiratory movements of the chest wall muscles persist after the upper airway closes. The rib cage and abdomen move in opposite directions since no air can enter the lungs. This is an important physical sign of obstructive apnoeas. The apnoea often terminates with a loud snort as arousal occurs and the upper airway opens.

The two most important complications of obstructive sleep apnoeas are:

RESPIRATORY FAILURE

Temporary abnormalities of the blood gases occur during obstructive apnoeas. The severity of the blood gas disturbance depends on the P_{O_2} and P_{CO_2} before the apnoea, the FRC (since the lungs hold a considerable proportion of the body oxygen stores), the metabolic rate (which controls the rate of oxygen uptake and carbon dioxide production) and the duration of the apnoea. The duration of the apnoea is itself governed by the arousal threshold for hypoxia and hypercapnia, and the rate of fall of P_{O_2} and rate of rise of P_{CO_2}.

Hypercapnia during wakefulness is not related to the frequency or severity of the obstructive apnoeas or to the degree of sleep deprivation or fragmentation. It is more closely linked to the severity of the hypoxaemia [377] and is more common if there is coexisting lung or chest wall disease such as obesity [375, 3098]. These conditions may prevent the P_{O_2} from returning to normal levels between apnoeas, and thereby greatly prolong the overall period of hypoxia. The CSF bicarbonate increases once hypercapnia becomes established, and the hypercapnic drive becomes reset at a different level, perpetuating the hypercapnia (p. 9).

CARDIOVASCULAR EFFECTS

The most common cardiac dysrhythmia during obstructive sleep apnoeas is a sinus arrhythmia. This has been used as a screening test for obstructive apnoeas, but is not sufficiently reliable. Over 30 beats/min variation between inspiration and expiration may be recorded [2171] and extreme sinus bardycardia and even sinus arrest are well recognized [1278, 1524, 3407]. Following the sinus bradycardia, there is usually an abrupt sinus tachycardia when breathing resumes [1277], but this does not occur if there is an underlying abnormality of the autonomic nervous system [1303]. The cardiac index falls during and rises after the apnoea, in parallel with the changes in heart rate [1297].

Sinus bradycardias appear if the apnoea is prolonged and oxygen desaturation is severe, but are not related specifically to any stage of sleep [3407]. The bradycardia can be blocked by prior administration of atropine, suggesting that it is mediated by an increase in parasympathetic activity [1277, 3164]. It can also be prevented by oxygen administration. Hypoxia presumably increases the parasympathetic activity, but the apnoea itself has some similarities to breath-holding and there may be direct reflex effects that slow the heart rate [3407]. The tachycardia after the apnoea is the result of increased sympathetic activity.

More serious dysrhythmias appear if the hypoxic dips are severe [2894, 3163]. Tachydysrhythmias, including short runs of ventricular tachycardia, ventricular ectopics and atrial fibrillation, develop together with first- and second-degree atrioventricular block [763, 1278, 2171, 2894, 3170]. These are more likely to occur if there is hypertension or heart disease, which would be expected to raise the hypoxic threshold for initiating dysrhythmias [2384]. These dysrhythmias may be responsible for sudden death during sleep.

There is normally a periodicity in the pulmonary artery and systemic blood pressure during sleep [1957], but during apnoeas associated with oxygen desaturation both of these pressures rise transiently [593, 2826, 3162]. The highest pulmonary artery pressure is seen in REM sleep, when hypoxia is most severe [594]. Hypoxia causes vasoconstriction in the pulmonary circulation by a direct action on vascular smooth muscle, and systemic vasoconstriction through an increase in sympathetic activity. Persistent hypertension is also a feature of subjects with frequent obstructive sleep apnoeas [3162], and nocturnal hypoxia may be partly responsible for this.

Right heart failure, secondary to pulmonary hypertension, is well recognized but occurs only in a small percentage of subjects who have frequent obstructive apnoeas. It is not related to the number or duration of apnoeas but to the mean oxygen saturation during sleep and while awake, and also to the $P\text{CO}_2$ while awake [375, 2828]. The factors that determine the severity of the blood gas abnormalities have been discussed on p. 64. Obesity and air flow obstruction increase the likelihood of right heart failure.

CENTRAL SLEEP APNOEAS

Central sleep apnoeas were clearly described by Mitchell in 1890 [2193] in a patient who later died during his sleep. They received little attention for many years and even recently more emphasis has been placed on obstructive apnoeas.

Central apnoeas are due to an inhibition of all of the respiratory muscles of the chest wall. The T_E of the breaths preceding the apnoea lengthens gradually, but there are no changes in T_I or in the amplitude of the EMG activity of the respiratory muscles [2174, 2370]. The apnoea occurs in the expiratory position [1784] and can be regarded as a prolonged expiration. It is terminated by a deep inspiration and usually by a period of hyperventilation if sufficient hypoxia or hypercapnia has developed.

Pathogenesis (Fig. 6.5)

Central sleep apnoeas may be seen in normal sleep. The activity of the respiratory and other muscles is particularly irregular in phasic REM sleep and the intervals between muscle contractions may be sufficient to qualify as apnoeas by conventional criteria. In many subjects the fluctuations in sleep stage at the onset of sleep (unsteady sleep) lead to frequent changes in the threshold of the ventilatory response to carbon dioxide and the appearance of Cheyne-Stokes respiration. The apnoeic phase is usually > 10 sec so that it is classified as a central apnoea. These physiological apnoeas are more frequent in the presence of an alkalosis and at altitude [1815, 3117] (p. 126).

Central sleep apnoeas may also be initiated by stimulation of receptors in the upper airway. They initiate protective reflexes, including the diving reflex (p. 10), of which one feature is apnoea. A negative pressure in the upper airway reduces the diaphragmatic activity [1966] but increases that of the dilator muscles of the upper airway, such as genioglossus [2083, 3328]. Nasal occlusion has similar effects on the genioglossus [2084], prolongs both T_I and T_E [2085] and may even induce central apnoeas [1546]. Pharyngeal [3327] and laryngeal [3176] receptors cause similar reflexes. The threshold for at least the laryngeal reflexes is higher during REM than stages 3 and 4 NREM sleep [3101].

Central sleep apnoeas may occur if the ventilatory response to hypoxia or, more commonly, to hypercapnia is pathologically reduced. These central apnoeas are seen particularly in stages 3 and 4 NREM sleep, when control of ventilation is almost solely automatic. The voluntary control is absent and unable to compensate for any defect in automatic control. The normal ventilatory response to the hypoxia and hypercapnia that develops during the apnoea is absent. If the threshold for a response is reached before arousal occurs, breathing will commence without any awakening, but arousal is often necessary to terminate the apnoea. Its threshold, together with the initial blood gas tensions and their rate of fall, determine the severity of the apnoea. Central apnoeas have been reported to be shorter than obstructive apnoeas [1546, 1772], but this probably reflects

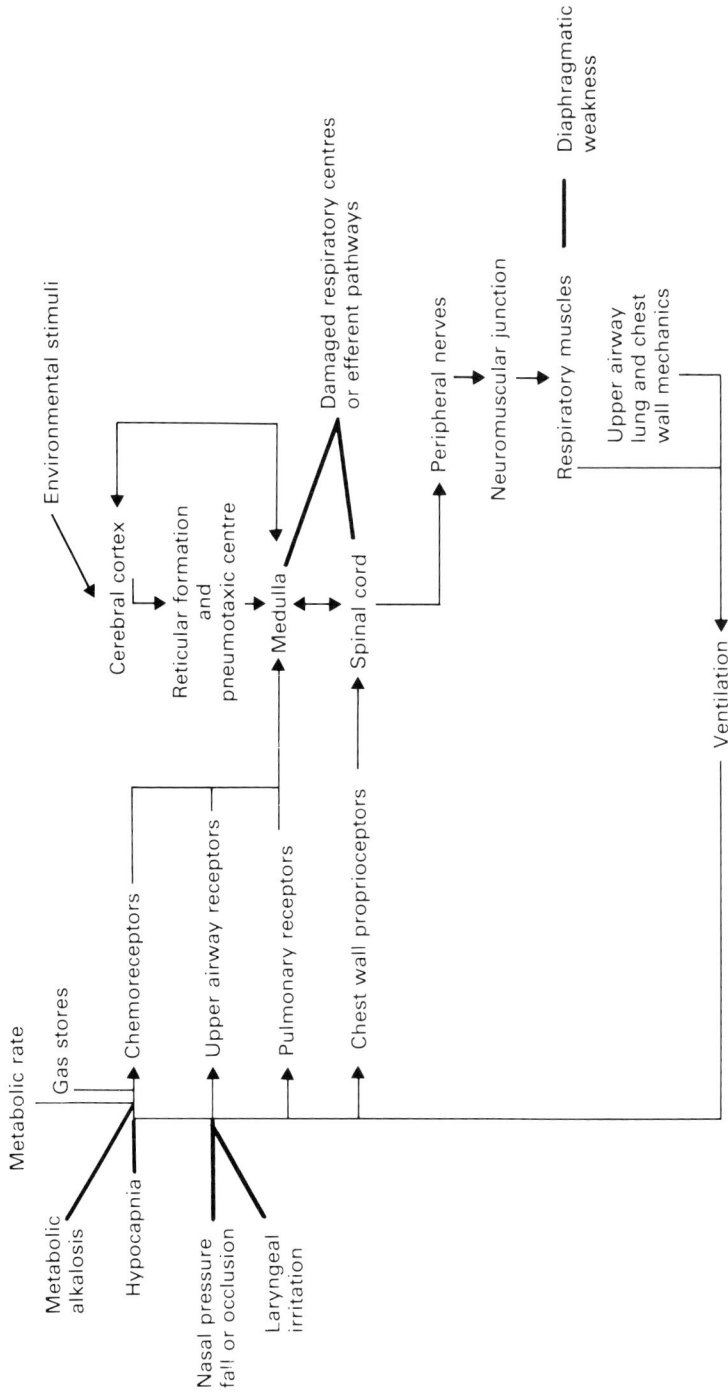

Fig. 6.5. Diagram to show the main causes of central sleep apnoeas (indicated by thick lines) and their relationship to the normal control of ventilation.

the differing severity of the populations studied rather than any true difference.

Diaphragmatic paralysis can mimic central sleep apnoeas, even if the ventilatory drive is normal. During REM sleep the tone of the respiratory muscles other than the diaphragm and, to a lesser extent, the parasternal intercostal muscles is greatly reduced. If the diaphragm is completely paralysed, no residual muscle activity will be seen and a pseudocentral sleep apnoea results.

Aetiology

'Physiological' central apnoeas may therefore occur in normal subjects or as a normal reaction to stimulation of upper airway receptors, e.g. by fluid reflux into the pharynx from the stomach [374].

'Pathological' central apnoeas should be distinguished from these. They are not a feature of cerebral cortical disorders [2969], although they are recognized in Jakob-Creutzfeldt disease [2050]. They usually indicate a disorder of:

CHEMORECEPTORS OR AFFERENT PATHWAYS

This may be more frequent than is commonly realized. Disorders of the carotid body or stretching of the 9th cranial nerve, e.g. in the Arnold-Chiari malformation, may be responsible.

MEDULLARY RESPIRATORY CENTRES

These may be damaged by a variety of conditions such as poliomyelitis, syringobulbia, autonomic nervous system disorders, encephalitis, Leigh's disease [21] and neurosurgery. A decrease in the blood flow to the brain stem [2138] may be responsible for the central apnoeas in polycythaemia rubra vera [2284]. Sedative drugs, secondary diminution in ventilatory drive due to chronic hypercapnia, sleep deprivation and occasionally severe hypoxia may also lead to central apnoeas.

EFFERENT PATHWAYS FROM MEDULLARY RESPIRATORY CENTRES

These may be involved either in the medulla or in the cervical cord, particularly by high cervical cordotomy.

DIAPHRAGM WEAKNESS

Diaphragmatic weakness or paralysis from any cause predisposes to pseudocentral apnoeas in REM sleep.

Clinical features

Central apnoeas are often asymptomatic and may be a normal finding, particularly in older subjects [78, 504, 2969]. Confusion between physiological apnoeas and those indicating a failure of automatic respiratory control has led to errors in assessing the significance of the apnoeas. The symptoms of pathological central apnoeas are similar to those of obstructive apnoeas. Somnolence is common and probably reflects the number of arousals and the extent of sleep deprivation. Observation of the lack of respiratory movements enables central apnoeas to be clearly distinguished from obstructive apnoeas.

Complications

Central sleep apnoeas may lead to respiratory and right heart failure by mechanisms that are probably similar to those of obstructive apnoeas. The relationship of central alveolar hypoventilation to such apnoeas is discussed on p. 64.

Chapter 7
History

A skilfully taken history provides information about the severity of ventilatory failure and its causes that cannot be obtained in any other way. It is often necessary to talk to relatives or friends, particularly if the patient is somnolent or confused. It may be difficult to obtain an accurate description of the respiratory abnormalities during sleep, but the patient's partner should be carefully questioned.

The time course of the symptoms is important. In many of the neuromuscular and skeletal disorders there is a longer period of clinical stability, despite a severe restrictive defect, before a phase in which deterioration occurs quite rapidly. The stable phase may appear before respiratory failure has developed, but may often be prolonged even after blood gas abnormalities are present. Ventilatory failure may be precipitated by an acute illness, particularly a chest infection, and evidence for this should be sought.

The history of the underlying neurological or skeletal disorder may date back to infancy or childhood, particularly with the congenital myopathies and congenital scoliosis. Adolescent idiopathic scoliosis frequently worsens at puberty. A careful medical history may provide other clues to the cause of the ventilatory failure, such as an episode of encephalitis or poliomyelitis. A recent increase in weight raises the possibility of obstructive sleep apnoeas. The family history should be carefully taken into account since many neurological diseases are genetically determined and scoliosis is often familial.

SYMPTOMS

The symptoms of the respiratory complications of neuromuscular and skeletal disorders are different from those encountered with lung diseases. Pulmonary and pleural symptoms such as cough, haemoptysis, wheeze and chest pain are uncommon. The symptoms reflect the abnormalities of the blood gases, the changes in respiratory pattern during sleep and the alterations in respiratory muscle function and mechanics of the chest wall.

Symptoms due to abnormal blood gases

The symptoms due particularly to acute changes in arterial blood gases are discussed in Chapter 4. Chronic hypoxia also leads to pulmonary hypertension and polycythaemia. There are no pathognomonic symptoms of these complications, but they may cause:

CHEST PAIN

Both polycythaemia and pulmonary hypertension predispose to pulmonary infarction, which may present as chest pain. Pulmonary hypertension may also cause angina, particularly on exertion. Cardiac ischaemia occurs because the right ventricle is unable to increase its output during exertion and blood flow is diverted away from the heart to the active skeletal muscles. Chest pain may also develop, particularly in spinal deformities because of nerve root pain and occasionally when the ribs rub on the upper margin of the pelvis.

FATIGUE

This is a feature of severe pulmonary hypertension in which the cardiac output is limited but may also be due to respiratory abnormalities during sleep.

SYNCOPE

The patient may lose consciousness, particularly during exertion, if pulmonary hypertension is severe and cerebral perfusion is inadequate.

HAEMOPTYSIS

This is a feature of pulmonary hypertension.

ANKLE SWELLING

Ankle swelling is a common symptom of right heart failure secondary to hypoventilation. It may also appear in chronic respiratory failure in the absence of any other feature of right heart failure, probably due to an increase in capillary permeability caused by hypoxia or possibly hypercapnia.

Symptoms due to respiratory abnormalities during sleep

SNORING, SNORTING AND GRUNTING

The inspiratory vibrating noise of a snore should be distinguished from snorts and grunts. Snorts occur at the end of an obstructive sleep apnoea when arousal occurs and the upper airway opens suddenly. It is often loud and, unlike a snore, does not occur with each breath. Grunting is heard during expiration and is the result of air escaping through the glottis in association with the strong expiratory contraction of the abdominal muscles. The high intrathoracic pressure during expiration reduces the venous return to the right atrium and helps to prevent pulmonary oedema [180, 1370]. Grunts are also heard in the presence of diaphragmatic paralysis. The

high abdominal pressure raises the end expiratory position of the diaphragm so that inspiration occurs passively by elastic recoil [2667].

Snoring is very common, particularly in older subjects and males [1954, 2334]. It is caused by vibration of the soft palate and often of the posterior faucial pillars [2662, 3074]. This instability of the upper airway is analogous to the vibration of bronchi, which is responsible for wheezing. It is most frequent and loudest in REM and stages 1 and 2 NREM sleep [1567, 1956, 2608]. The inspiratory noise during obstructive sleep apnoeas is often mistaken for snoring. It usually has a higher frequency and is probably due to turbulent air flow through a narrow pharyngeal or, occasionally, laryngeal orifice.

The same factors predispose to snoring and to obstructive sleep apnoeas (Chapter 6). Strong inspiratory efforts that decrease the intrathoracic and intrapharyngeal pressure make snoring more likely and louder [576]. A reduction in the tone of the upper airway muscles [371], for instance by alcohol [1544], predisposes to snoring and it is also more common if the upper airway is narrowed. Complete obstruction of the nasopharynx prevents snoring since air cannot be inspired through the nose. Partial obstruction from any cause is associated with snoring and the cross-sectional pharyngeal area of snorers has been shown to be less than that of normal subjects [370].

The exact relationship between snoring and obstructive apnoeas is still uncertain. Snoring is common in subjects with frequent apnoeas but only a few persistent snorers have a significant number of apnoeas. It is uncertain how many snorers eventually develop frequent apnoeas and whether this is simply related to the degree of airway obstruction, loss of muscle tone or the intrapharyngeal pressure.

Snoring is a symptom of the listener rather than the snorer. However, there is some epidemiological data to suggest that snoring may be harmful. It has been associated with hypertension [1954, 2334]; the blood pressure rises transiently during sleep in snorers [1956] and

epidemiological surveys have suggested that angina, myocardial infarction and strokes are more
frequent in snorers [1736, 2334]. These complications may be due to hypertension but further
investigation is required before this is accepted
as the cause of these complications. A completely independent factor, such as excessive
alcohol intake, which may cause hypertension
and snoring, could be responsible for the
observed associations.

Even loud snoring is often tolerated without
treatment being required, but it is occasionally
necessary either to protect the listener from the
noise with earplugs or to treat the snorer. Advice
about losing weight, avoiding sleeping in a
supine position or taking alcohol or muscle-
relaxant drugs may be sufficient. A tongue
retainer [509, 511] may be helpful and a chin
strap may be of benefit. Injection of a sclerosing
agent into the pharynx to cause fibrosis and to
decrease its compliance has been recommended
[3074] and UPPP is also effective (p. 71). These
surgical treatments are nowadays rarely
required since nasal CPAP with pressures as
low as 2–6 cmH$_2$O [1546] is effective in patients
who do not respond to simpler measures [268,
1544].

INSOMNIA

Insomnia is a symptom of both obstructive and
central sleep apnoeas [1, 1283, 1284, 2692].
When the hypoxia and hypercapnia reach the
threshold for arousal, the level of consciousness
rises and the subject may awaken. The arousal
threshold determines the degree of oxygen desaturation and hypercapnia that occurs during
the apnoeas. Arousal protects against the
physiological consequences of the blood gas abnormalities, but it fragments sleep so that sleep
deprivation occurs. Sleep deprivation reduces
the ventilatory response to hypercapnia [643,
825, 3311] and raises the threshold for arousal
[361, 2468] so that the blood gas abnormalities
become more severe later in the night.

Insomnia may also be due to breathlessness
during sleep (p. 56).

NOCTURNAL SOMATIC SYMPTOMS

Abnormalities of respiration during sleep lead
to a variety of somatic symptoms. Abnormal
movements of the limbs are common during
apnoeas [1275, 1291] and should be distinguished from nocturnal myoclonus and nocturnal epilepsy which can be induced or worsened
by sleep deprivation or by hypoxia during sleep
[17, 1004, 1515, 2670, 2861, 3379]. Night
sweats frequently accompany sleep apnoeas and
appear to be due to increased sympathetic activity or possibly an increased sensitivity to
catecholamines due to the hypoxia [584]. Nocturnal polyuria and enuresis has also been reported [1291].

CHANGES IN PERSONALITY AND INTELLECT

Personality changes are common if sleep apnoeas are frequent [266, 275, 1286, 1291]. Intellectual deterioration, an inability to concentrate,
depression and a decrease in libido are frequently observed. It was initially proposed that
these symptoms were more common in obstructive than central sleep apnoeas [1280, 1282], but
this has not been confirmed. The changes in
personality and intellect are probably due to
sleep fragmentation and deprivation, but in
severe cases abnormalities of the blood gases
may be responsible.

DAYTIME SOMNOLENCE

This common symptom should be distinguished
from tiredness and is characterized by the subject falling asleep against his will. This may present as an inability to successfully carry out work
or with recurrent road traffic accidents due to
falling asleep while driving. There is often a
long delay before patients with daytime somnolence seek medical help [1275]. Daytime somnolence has also been confused with narcolepsy in
the past, but this has specific diagnostic features.

Somnolence is particularly common in
obstructive sleep apnoeas [1, 1767] in which the
multiple sleep latency time is reduced [767].

This objective measure of somnolence correlates with the frequency of arousal during sleep [3045] and it is probably the sleep fragmentation and sleep deprivation that are responsible for the daytime somnolence. It was initially thought that hypercapnia was responsible, but somnolence is common in the absence of a raised P_{CO_2}. Some studies have suggested that nocturnal hypoxia is the cause [2380, 2383, 2948], but this is unlikely unless hypoxia is very severe. Somnolence is probably not due to central nervous system disease, except in the occasional patient who has had encephalitis, since it can be reversed quickly by treatment such as nasal CPAP or tracheostomy. Sedative drugs may predispose to somnolence by lowering the level of consciousness, diminishing the ventilatory drive and decreasing the tone of the upper airway and predisposing to obstructive apnoeas.

Symptoms due to abnormalities of respiratory muscles and mechanics

BREATHLESSNESS

The physiological basis of breathlessness is still uncertain. Breathlessness probably represents more than one type of sensation [479, 485]. Tightness in the chest may be due to afferent impulses from pulmonary receptors that travel in the vagus nerve, but the more common distressing sensation of difficulty in breathing appears to originate in chest wall receptors [2720]. The intensity of breathlessness is related to the fraction of the maximal inspiratory pressure that is developed during inspiration rather than to muscle fatigue [372, 775, 1584, 1665] (Fig. 7.1). The disparity between the length of the respiratory muscles and the tension that they develop may also contribute to the sensation of breathlessness [485].

Breathlessness is not closely related to the arterial blood gases, and may even be relieved by breathing hypoxic gas mixtures [1024]. It is unusual when ventilation increases either because of metabolic acidosis or Cheyne-Stokes respiration [1394]. If breathlessness is present, it usually indicates lung or pleural disease.

Breathlessness on exertion is a common feature of neuromuscular and skeletal disorders. Their ventilatory capacity is limited either by respiratory muscle dysfunction or a low chest wall compliance. Exercise testing usually confirms that it is ventilatory rather than cir-

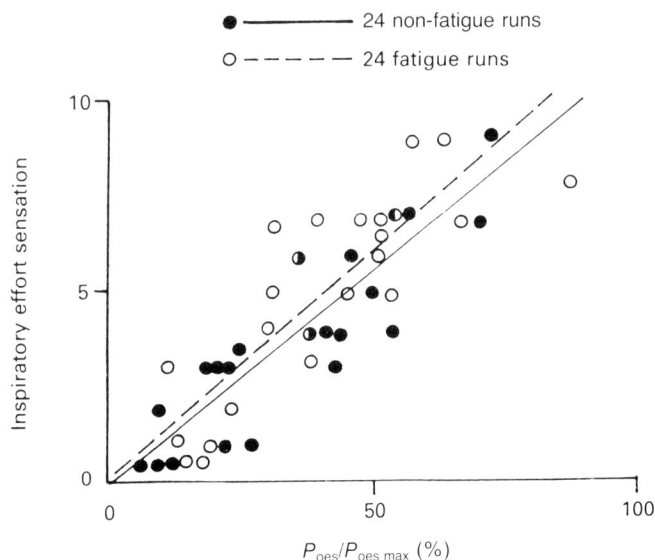

Fig. 7.1. *Relationship between breathlessness and oesophageal pressures (P_{oes}) in the presence and absence of respiratory muscle fatigue. The severity of breathlessness is closely related to the percentage of the maximum oesophageal pressure generated but muscle fatigue has no independent effect on breathlessness. Reproduced, with permission, from Bradley T.D., et al. Am. Rev. Respir. Dis. 1986; 134: 119–24.*

culatory factors that limit maximal exercise. These subjects often have other disabilities, such as weakness of their leg muscles, which prevent intense exercise from being achieved. Breathlessness is, therefore, often an inconspicuous symptom. Some degree of exertional breathlessness may be present for many years, but a change may signify the development of a complication such as respiratory muscle fatigue. Breathlessness is absent or inappropriately mild in disorders of the carotid body and medullary respiratory centres or cervical cord [2294] because the pathways to the cerebral cortex are damaged or absent. Dangerous hypoxia and hypercapnia may result, particularly during sleep, at altitude and during underwater swimming.

Orthopnoea is well recognized as a symptom of pulmonary oedema and, less frequently, of air flow obstruction, but it is also a prominent feature of bilateral diaphragmatic paralysis (Fig. 7.2) (p. 162). In contrast to pulmonary oedema, the orthopnoea of diaphragmatic paralysis may become apparent within a few seconds of lying flat and is relieved immediately when the upright position is resumed. The subject may also be breathless while standing in water, since the passive inspiratory descent of the diaphragm due to gravity is prevented by the raised extra-abdominal pressure [2151]. Diaphragmatic paralysis may present as breathlessness during sleep. The differential diagnosis includes the hyperpneic phase of Cheyne-Stokes respiration, which presents in a similar way [2585], and the

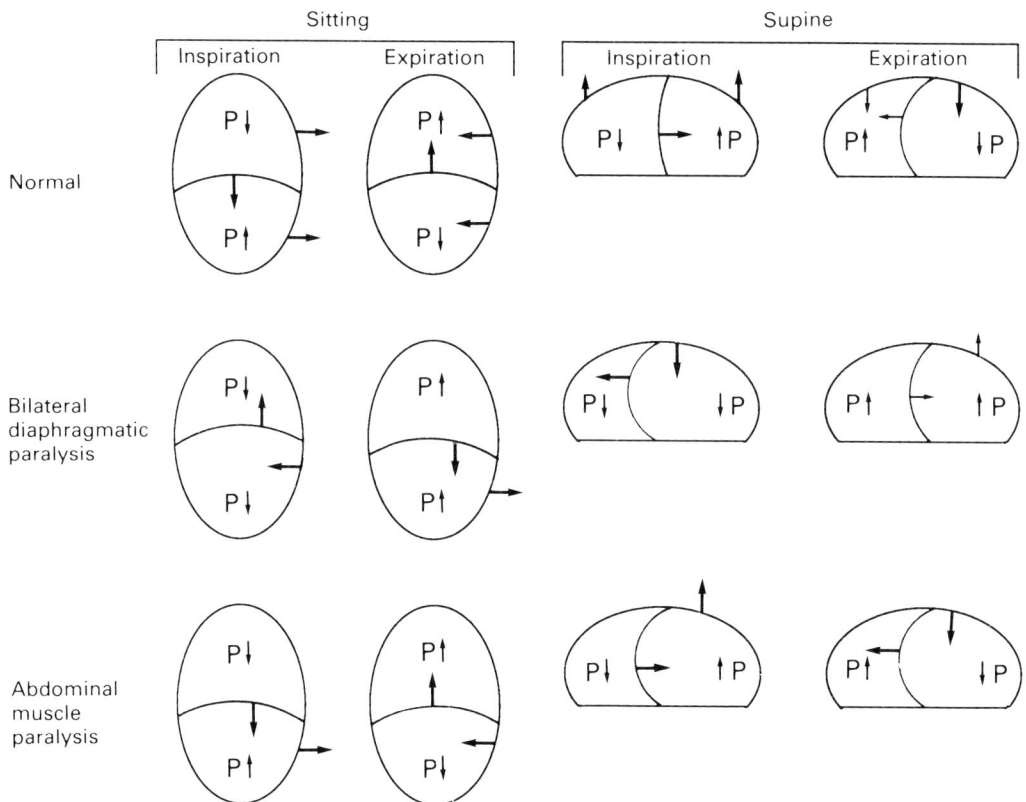

Fig. 7.2. *Pressure and volume changes during respiration with normal muscles, bilateral diaphragmatic paralysis and abdominal muscle paralysis. In the sitting position, the upper compartment represents the rib cage and the lower compartment the abdomen. In the supine position, the left compartment represents the rib cage and the right side the abdomen. The magnitude of the change in volume and pressure (P) is represented by the size of the arrows.*

which presents in a similar way [2585], and the hyperventilation following a sleep apnoea.

Platypnoea is the opposite of orthopnoea and usually indicates either abdominal muscle weakness in the presence of normal diaphragmatic function or severe pulmonary hypertension (Fig. 7.2). Platypnoea with abdominal muscle weakness is seen particularly in quadriplegia, but also in poliomyelitis [1174] and with large anterior abdominal wall hernias [521]. In the upright position diaphragmatic contraction expands the abdomen, but at the end of expiration the diaphragm is in a low and inefficient position. In the supine position, gravity limits the inspiratory abdominal expansion and the weight of the abdominal contents returns the diaphragm to a higher level at the end of expiration. In pulmonary hypertension, the ventilation/perfusion matching at the apices of the lungs improves and the pulmonary artery pressure falls in the supine position [66]. Some patients adopt a prone position, crouching on all four limbs.

INADEQUATE COUGH

Cough is a protective mechanism that prevents the retention of sputum and the inhalation of pharyngeal material into the lungs. Cough is initiated by the mechanical or chemical stimulation of receptors, particularly those in and around the larynx, in the trachea and in the large bronchi [1535]. The threshold of the receptors appears to be lower at the small lung volumes that are seen in many neuromuscular and skeletal disorders. Afferent impulses travel via the 9th and 10th cranial nerves to the nucleus tractus solitarius in the medulla.

Cough can also be purely voluntary. It is a complex act that requires a deep inspiration, glottic closure and subsequent forceful expiration as the glottis opens [1839]. The peak expiratory flow rate may be as high as 5–6.5 l/sec. The clearance of secretions is aided by the reduction of the diameter of the airway during coughing because of compression by the high intrathoracic pressure [1712]. This may be as high as 100 cmH$_2$O [2710]. The kinetic energy is proportional to the square of the velocity so that if, for instance, the area of the trachea is decreased to one-sixth of normal, the linear velocity of the air flow is about 28 000 cm/sec (85% of the speed of sound) [2710]. Dynamic compression and effective clearance of secretions can be extended to the smaller airways by the technique of huffing (p. 281).

An inadequate cough is common, particularly in the neuromuscular disorders, because of:

Damage to sensory fibres

The cough receptors can be inactivated by, for instance, local anaesthetics but more importantly the sensory fibres can be interrupted by lesions of the vagus nerve above the junction of the superior laryngeal nerve (e.g. basal meningitis, tumours, trauma) or medullary disorders such as syringobulbia.

Central nervous system depression

Depression of the level of consciousness from any cause impairs the cough reflex.

Inadequate inspiration

A deep inspiration is needed for the expiratory muscles to be able to generate a high pressure when the glottis opens. The cough may, therefore, be ineffective if there is inspiratory muscle weakness or a reduced chest wall compliance. A $P_{I_{max}}$ of about 30 cmH$_2$O and a VC two to three times the V_T during quiet breathing are usually needed for an adequate cough [1243].

Failure of glottic closure

It is impossible to generate a high intrathoracic pressure if the glottis is unable to provide a tight seal. The explosive quality of the cough is lost and clearance of secretions is impaired. The efficiency of cough is diminished in the presence of a tracheostomy or an endotracheal tube because there is no effective glottis [1074].

Expiratory muscle weakness

The intrathoracic pressure may be inadequate not only because of a failure to take a deep inspiration but also because of expiratory muscle weakness, particularly weakness of the abdominal muscles. The maximal expiratory flow rate only falls if the intrapleural pressure is reduced to about 30% normal [104] and, as long as the maximal expiratory pressure (PE_{max}) is greater than about 20–40 cmH$_2$O, the cough may remain effective [709, 3307].

Impaired sputum clearance

Secretions within the lung may not be expectorated adequately if their viscosity or elasticity is abnormal, if ciliary function is impaired or if the bronchi are occluded.

An inadequate cough leads to an accumulation of bronchial secretions and a failure to prevent pharyngeal material from entering the trachea through the larynx. This tendency is exacerbated if swallowing is also impaired. The inhaled secretions increase the air flow resistance and aspiration pneumonia may result.

The physiotherapy techniques for aiding expectoration are described in Chapter 23. Rehydration, bronchodilators and raising the level of consciousness are indicated in selected cases. Teflon injection into a paralysed vocal cord is less effective in preventing aspiration than it is in improving the voice [683]. Assistance with coughing using a tank ventilator (p. 240) and other mechanical appliances, such as the cofflator [41, 146(b)] and a cough chamber [184], have been shown to be of some value, but are rarely used.

DIFFICULTY IN SWALLOWING

Swallowing, like cough, is a protective reflex whereby pharyngeal material is passed into the oesophagus rather than entering the trachea or being expectorated. Food entering the mouth is chewed and is pushed into the pharynx by the action of the tongue. The soft palate reflexly seals off the nasopharynx and the glottis closes. The cricopharyngeal sphincter opens as the other pharyngeal constrictors contract and the food bolus enters the oesophagus where it initiates peristaltic waves that carry it into the stomach. Swallowing is coordinated particularly in the nucleus ambiguus in the medulla. Respiration is inhibited during swallowing. If the swallow occurs in inspiration, the following expiration is shortened. If it occurs during expiration, this phase is prolonged [2317].

Abnormalities of swallowing are common in neuromuscular disorders that are associated with ventilatory failure [992, 1739, 2335, 2579]. Depression of the level of consciousness predisposes to aspiration of pharyngeal material into the lungs and, even in normal subjects, aspiration is frequent during sleep [1511].

Any of the stages of swallowing may be abnormal. There may be a failure to form or propel the bolus into the pharynx, the pharyngeal motility may be reduced leading to stasis, the velopharyngeal sphincter may be incompetent resulting in nasal regurgitation, the cricopharyngeal sphincter may fail to relax and oesophageal peristalsis may be weak [697, 812, 2397, 2925]. These abnormalities are seen particularly with disorders of the brain stem or of the higher control of the bulbar muscles, such as in Parkinson's disease, multiple sclerosis, pseudobulbar palsy, brain stem strokes or tumours, poliomyelitis, motor neuron disease, idiopathic polyradiculoneuritis, myasthenia gravis and primary muscle disorders, particularly dystrophia myotonica and polymyositis.

The most important respiratory consequence of difficulty in swallowing is the inhalation of pharyngeal material into the trachea and bronchi. This increases the air flow resistance and predisposes to aspiration pneumonia. It is important to treat the cause of the swallowing defect if possible. A diet of a suitable consistency and swallowing with the neck extended may be helpful [2925]. Other trick movements may be required but surgery should be considered if aspiration continues. Dilatation of the criocopharyngeal sphincter is rarely helpful but cricopharyngeal myotomy is often effective if failure of the criocopharyngeal muscle to open is the cause of the swallowing difficulty [862, 1611, 1620, 1838, 2362]. Feeding by a nasogastric tube or gastrostomy may be valuable, but saliva and fluids refluxing from the stomach into the oesophagus can still be aspirated. A cuffed tracheostomy tube is more effective in preventing aspiration and in mild cases the cuff can be deflated between meals. If these measures fail, laryngeal surgery should be considered [683, 1694, 2205]. This entails the loss of the normal voice but is effective in preventing aspiration. Laryngeal stenting is of little value but a total laryngectomy, although irreversible, is effective. Alternative procedures such as laryngeal closure and laryngeal diversion by, for instance, anastomosing the distal trachea to the oesophagus and forming a tracheostomy with the proximal trachea are both effective and can be reversed if necessary.

STRIDOR AND WHEEZE

Stridor due to neurological disease usually indicates that the abductor muscles of the vocal cords are selectively weakened. This is a feature of bilateral lesions of the vagus nerve below the origin of the superior laryngeal nerve or of lesions of the recurrent laryngeal nerves. With more proximal nerve lesions the adductors are also paralysed and although there is a severe motor and sensory laryngeal defect, aspiration rather than stridor develops. Stridor may be improved surgically by cordectomy, arytenoidectomy, extralaryngeal cord displacement such as lateralization of the arytenoids, or re-innervation procedures [683].

Wheezing may be due to inhalation of a foreign body because of difficulty in swallowing or a poor cough. Asthma may be more common in neuromuscular and skeletal disorders than in a normal population, partly because of the small size of the airways associated with the small lung volumes but also because atopy is common in conditions such as neurofibromatosis and Marfan's syndrome, which are associated with scoliosis [2901].

Chapter 8
Physical Signs

Careful observation of the patient can reveal valuable clues to the cause and severity of ventilatory failure. The classical physical signs of lung disease are well described but the signs of chest wall disorders and respiratory muscle weakness are often overlooked. It is also important to search for signs outside the chest: abnormal neurological features may indicate the underlying cause of the respiratory muscle weakness; pigmented patches suggest neurofibromatosis as the cause of scoliosis; etc. Malnutrition and many of the systemic diseases, such as thyrotoxicosis, may show valuable physical signs that point to the physiological cause of respiratory failure.

In this chapter, the signs of lung disease will only be mentioned briefly and emphasis will be placed on the features that throw light on disorders of respiratory control, respiratory muscle action and chest wall movement.

RESPIRATORY CONTROL

Disorders of respiration during sleep are usually detected by non-invasive monitoring techniques (Chapter 9), but observation of the patient by a trained observer provides a valuable corroboration of the validity of the events that are documented. The presence, frequency and duration of apnoeas should be noted and those features suggesting upper airway obstruction should be recorded. Snoring and snorting (p. 79) should be listened for.

The adequacy of voluntary respiratory control is hard to assess clinically with any precision. Disorders of speech and an inability to obey respiratory commands such as 'hold your breath' or 'take a deep breath' may be apparent.

The ability to breathe at a set rate or to take a breath of a given volume may be impaired. Cheyne-Stokes respiration may appear if the medullary respiratory centres are released from the inhibitory influence of the cerebral cortex (p. 56).

The automatic control of respiration determines T_I/T_{TOT}, V_T/T_I and to a lesser extent the respiratory frequency. The normal responses of each of these indices to hypoxia and hypercapnia may be reduced or absent if this control system is damaged. A diminished respiratory drive should also be suspected if the accessory muscles of respiration are not recruited when the blood gases become abnormal or if there is pulmonary disease. A variety of specific respiratory dysrhythmias, such as central neurogenic hypoventilation and apneustic breathing, may appear (Chapter 5). The frequency and tidal volume may be very irregular since respiration depends on voluntary control, which varies from moment to moment.

RESPIRATORY MOVEMENTS

It is conventional to observe and to measure the chest expansion, but much less attention is normally paid to abdominal movement during respiration. The movements of the rib cage and abdomen should be viewed together. Normally, the whole rib cage and abdomen expand and contract almost synchronously, but dissociation of movements may be apparent. The sternum and upper rib cage often continue to move together due to the action of the accessory and intercostal muscles: the abdomen and the part of the lower rib cage that is exposed to abdominal pressure also move as a unit. Dissociation of these two components and other disorganized patterns of respiratory movements are frequently seen.

Abnormal respiratory movements may be the result of respiratory muscle weakness, obesity, skeletal disorders and abnormalities of the lungs and pleura if they alter the regional ventilation. Obesity adds a load to both the rib cage and abdomen, but skeletal deformities influence particularly the movement of the rib cage.

SKELETAL DISORDERS

The most important skeletal disorders that should be recognized are:

PECTUS EXCAVATUM AND PECTUS CARINATUM

These abnormalities are apparent on inspection, and details are discussed in Chapter 16.

RIB ABNORMALITIES

Congenital rib abnormalities are rarely apparent clinically, but occasionally an abnormal rib may be prominent if it grows more than the adjacent ribs. The characteristic appearances of rickets are described on p. 190. Trauma to the chest may result in a flail segment, which moves paradoxically with respiration. This may also be seen following surgery to the ribs, such as thoracoplasty.

ANKYLOSING SPONDYLITIS

Rib cage movement is greatly diminished or even absent and inspiration occurs largely by abdominal expansion.

SCOLIOSIS

The scoliosis should be confirmed to be structural by asking the patient to touch his toes. Postural curves disappear with this manoeuvre. There may be specific features that reveal the cause of the scoliosis, such as Marfan's syndrome or neurofibromatosis. Congenital abnormalities and any associated muscle weakness should be sought. It is important to note the level of the scoliosis, whether there is a single curve or a secondary compensatory curve, the side to which the curve is convex and the extent of the posterior rib hump. It is difficult to analyse the movement of the ribs in scoliosis because of the distortion of the costovertebral joints. Rib cage expansion may be predominantly lateral or anterior, or achieved by extension of the spine. Expansion often takes place obliquely because of the rotation of the spine and there may be paradoxical movement of parts of the rib cage. The accessory muscles of respiration are often used during tidal breathing but abdominal expansion may be more prominent than rib cage expansion.

KYPHOSIS

The level and extent of the kyphosis should be noted and the ability to elevate the ribs assessed.

RESPIRATORY MUSCLE FUNCTION

The physiological actions of the respiratory muscles have been described in Chapter 2, and the effects of weakness of each of the main muscle groups in Chapter 15. Careful examination of the respiratory movements should enable the action of each of the major muscle groups to be assessed. Muscle weakness cannot be distinguished from muscle fatigue on clinical grounds unless it can be shown that weakness develops during the performance of a respiratory activity.

GENERALIZED RESPIRATORY MUSCLE WEAKNESS

Criteria for assessing the severity of weakness of limb muscles, such as the MRC scale [2109], are available but weakness of the respiratory muscles except for the sternomastoids can only be assessed indirectly. It may be apparent from the distress associated with breathing and the inability to speak except in short sentences. Signs of hypoxia or hypercapnia may also be present if respiratory muscle weakness is severe. Milder degrees of generalized respiratory muscle weakness lead to a sequence of changes in respiration.

Rapid shallow breathing

Observation of the respiratory frequency is much neglected and recordings in hospital records frequently bear no relationship to the true respiratory rate [1735]. A rate of 24 breaths/min, or greater, is quite specific for respiratory disorders [1235], of which respiratory muscle weakness is an important example. The ratio T_I/T_E increases as the respiratory frequency rises. This increase in the duty cycle of the inspiratory muscles predisposes to inspiratory muscle fatigue and raises the oxygen cost of respiration. The V_T falls as the respiratory frequency increases, and although this diminishes the work of inspiration during each breath, it increases the V_D/V_T ratio and reduces alveolar ventilation. The small V_T may also lead to closure of the basal airways and ventilation/perfusion mismatching. The mean inspiratory flow rate usually remains constant or may fall despite the reduction in T_I.

Recruitment of accessory muscles

Recruitment of the accessory respiratory muscles is a normal compensation for an increase in air flow resistance or a reduction in the compliance of the lungs or chest wall. These muscles are also brought into action when the ventilation increases during exercise, or if the respiratory muscles are weak or fatigued. Contraction of the sternomastoids may be both seen and felt. The muscles of the shoulder girdle are employed especially when the subject sits or leans forwards with the arms fixed on a supporting surface. Contraction of the abdominal muscles during expiration may decrease the end

expiratory volume below the FRC so that the onset of inspiration can occur through elastic recoil without the need for inspiratory muscle contraction. If the thorax is asymmetrical due, for instance, to scoliosis or thoracoplasty, accessory muscles are recruited earlier and to a greater extent on the less compliant side of the thorax.

Respiratory alternans

Respiratory alternans is characteristic of respiratory muscle weakness or fatigue. The diaphragm or the intercostal and accessory muscles contract on alternate breaths. Each muscle group therefore relaxes alternately so that some recovery from fatigue can take place. A similar pattern may be seen in normal neonates but in some infants the intercostal muscles do not contract and short apnoeas are seen between the diaphragmatic contractions [1942]. Respiratory alternans can be recognized by the alternate expansion and paradoxical movement of the abdomen or rib cage because of failure to activate the intercostal and accessory muscles or diaphragm [597, 2718].

Respiratory muscle incoordination

Several patterns of respiratory movement have been thought to indicate a failure to coordinate the action of the respiratory muscles. The abdomen may expand before the rib cage [1483]. This may be due to relaxation of abdominal muscles that were contracted during expiration, or to a loss of the synchronized contraction of the diaphragm, intercostal and accessory muscles. Relaxation of previously contracted abdominal muscles may also cause paradoxical inspiratory movement of the sternum [1130]. The lower rib cage can move paradoxically late in inspiration [1483] either because of inefficient diaphragmatic contraction or as a result of extension of the spine [2881]. During acute respiratory failure other forms of respiratory muscle incoordination are seen, so that some respiratory muscles may be acting in an expiratory fashion while others are still effecting inspiration [81,

113, 2515, 2881]. The tidal volume improves when coordinated activity of the inspiratory muscles returns [833].

DIAPHRAGMATIC FUNCTION

Contraction of the diaphragm is not usually visible and its function has to be assessed indirectly. Occasionally, however, the peeling off of the diaphragm from the parietal pleura is visible through the chest wall as a ripple that moves with the phases of respiration (Litten's sign). This is rarely apparent unless the intercostal muscles are atrophied, as in, for instance, poliomyelitis [706]. Diaphragmatic contraction can be inferred from the protrusion of the abdomen only if the abdominal muscles do not contract [1125]. Normally, the lower rib cage is also exposed to intra-abdominal pressure and expands with the abdomen. However, if the diaphragm is low and flat, as a result of hyperinflation of the lungs, its contraction draws the lower rib cage inwards. This paradoxical movement was first analysed by Hoover in a series of papers [1464–1467]. Other signs of hyperinflation of the lungs should be sought to confirm this interpretation of the rib cage movement.

Unilateral weakness of the diaphragm is difficult to detect clinically. Occasionally weakness of other muscles with nuclei in C3–C5 seg-

ments may suggest that the phrenic nerve nucleus or its roots are damaged (Table 8.1). Unilateral weakness can be detected by percussing the lower part of the lung during inspiration and expiration. The level of dullness rises paradoxically during inspiration on the paralysed side. The normal inspiratory outward movement of the abdomen may be reduced or absent [1914] on the side of the diaphragmatic paralysis, and expansion of the lower chest may lag behind the normal expansion of the other side. These signs imply that respiratory pressure changes are not conducted uniformly throughout the abdomen [2007]. These subtle physical signs are, however, often absent because of compensation by other muscles.

Bilateral diaphragmatic paralysis is readily recognizable. Profound orthopnoea is present and the patient may only be able to lie flat for a few seconds. This contrasts with pulmonary oedema where orthopnoea develops much more slowly. If diaphragmatic weakness is less severe and the patient can lie flat for a period of observation, the abdomen is seen to move paradoxically inwards as the diaphragm ascends during inspiration [735, 1423]. The negative intrapleural pressure is transmitted across the flaccid diaphragm to the abdominal contents. Paradoxical inward movement of the abdomen is also seen if the abdominal muscles contract during inspiration, even if the diaphragm is

Table 8.1. *Non-respiratory muscles whose spinal cord representation overlaps that of the diaphragm*

Spinal nerve roots	Muscles	Movements tested
C45	Rhomboids	Fixation of scapula while pushing arm backwards
C56	Clavicular part of pectoralis major	Forward movement of elevated arm
	Infraspinatus	External rotation of arm
	Supraspinatus	Initiation of abduction of arm
	Deltoid	Abduction of horizontal arm
	Biceps and brachialis	Flexion of elbow with forearm supinated
	Brachioradialis	Flexion of elbow with forearm semiprone
C567	Serratus anterior	Fixation of scapula while pushing forward with arm
	Teres major	Adduction of elevated arm

normal. This can be distinguished by palpation
of the abdominal muscles. Bilateral diaphragmatic paralysis is accompanied by compensatory
recruitment of accessory muscles.

INTERCOSTAL MUSCLE FUNCTION

The intercostal muscles stabilize the rib cage
when the diaphragm and other inspiratory
muscles lower the intrapleural pressure.
Paralysis may, therefore, be detected by observing an indrawing of the intercostal spaces (Fig.
8.1.). On palpation, the intercostal spaces remain flaccid during inspiration. The thorax fails
to expand and paradoxical movement may be
apparent. This is normal in young children, in
whom the chest wall is extremely compliant,
and is most readily seen during REM sleep when
intercostal muscle activity is reduced [2222].

ACCESSORY MUSCLE FUNCTION

The scalene, sternomastoid and trapezius
muscles are easily observed and palpated [3153].

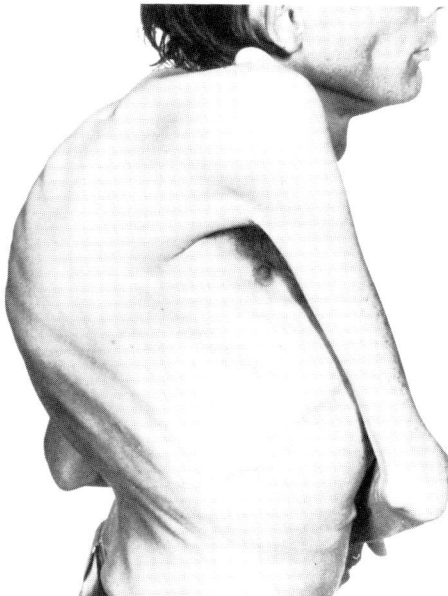

Fig. 8.1. *Severe intercostal muscle wasting following
poliomyelitis.*

The scalene muscles are normally active in quiet
respiration but the other muscles are only
employed in the presence of air flow obstruction,
a decreased lung or chest wall compliance, or
when ventilation is increased, for instance,
during exercise. Their activity during quiet
breathing indicates an abnormality of respiratory mechanics or weakness of other respiratory
muscles, particularly the diaphragm [706].
Hypertrophy of the sternomastoid due to
chronic use can be detected, and its atrophy is
characteristic of dystrophia myotonica.

ABDOMINAL MUSCLE FUNCTION

Abdominal muscle contraction can be most
easily detected by palpation. Their activity during expiration may compensate for diaphragmatic weakness by elevating the diaphragm and
decreasing the end expiratory volume to less
than the FRC.
  Weakness of the abdominal muscles increases
the compliance of the abdomen and, in the upright position, abdominal expansion during inspiration is greater than normal. The abdominal
pressure remains low and the diaphragm
shortens excessively and becomes less efficient.
In the supine position, the weight of the abdominal contents pushes the diaphragm into a
higher position at the end of expiration and the
respiratory movements appear more normal.
Weakness of the rectus abdominis muscle can
be detected by palpating the muscle and observing any movement of the umbilicus when the
patient flexes his neck against resistance while
lying flat.

UPPER AIRWAY MUSCLE FUNCTION

Normal upper airway muscle function ensures
that the airway remains patent during inspiration and slows the rate of expiration during quiet
breathing. Snoring is due to rapid opening and
closing of the upper airway, and in obstructive
sleep apnoeas the airway remains closed during
several inspiratory efforts. Indrawing of the rib
cage accompanies expansion of the abdomen as

the diaphragm descends, as long as the occluded airway prevents any flow of air in or out of the lungs. Weakness or incoordination of the upper airway muscles may also impair the cough and lead to difficulty in swallowing (Chapter 7). The patient should be asked to cough and its adequacy carefully assessed. Swallowing, particularly of liquids, should be observed and any nasal regurgitation, aspiration of fluids into the lungs or sounds indicating pooling of fluid in the pharynx should be noted. Disorders of the innervation of the larynx may cause stridor, voice changes or predispose to aspiration. Direct or indirect laryngoscopy may be required and a thorough neurological examination is necessary to search for the cause of the vocal cord palsy.

Chapter 9
Physiological Investigations

This chapter contains a brief description of the physiological tests that are of most value in assessing ventilatory control, the respiratory muscles and movements of the chest wall. No attempt is made to describe the investigations that are employed to assess lung disease or to provide a detailed plan of the sequence of investigations that may be needed. The investigations have, however, been grouped according to the aspect of the respiratory pump that they test. Sufficient detail is given to provide an understanding of the principles of the investigations and some of their limitations.

RESPIRATION DURING SLEEP

Abnormalities of respiration may only be present during sleep, and investigation during wakefulness may be unrewarding. Several methods of monitoring are often employed simultaneously (polysomnography) (Table 9.1), but they may disturb sleep. The completeness of the study has to be balanced against loss of information due to disruption of the sleep structure. The monitoring equipment should, therefore, be tailored to the questions that are asked of the sleep study. Monitoring of the blood

Table 9.1. *Methods of monitoring respiration during sleep*

Physiological index	Method
Sleep stage	EEG, EOG, EMG
Blood gases	Transcutaneous P_{CO_2} and P_{O_2} monitors Oximeters for Sa_{O_2}
Pattern of ventilation	Pneumotachograph and face mask End tidal CO_2 monitoring Tracheal microphone Thermistor
Tidal volume, rib cage and abdominal movements	Strain gauge Impedance pneumography Magnetometer coils Inductance plethysmography
Site of upper airway obstruction	Fibre-optic endoscopy
Diaphragmatic activity and recognition of type of apnoea	Diaphragmatic EMG Oesophageal and gastric pressures
Cardiac dysrhythmias	ECG monitoring
Hypertension	Automatic sphygmomanometer
Gastro-oesophageal reflux	Oesophageal pH monitor

gases, perhaps with EEG recording to establish that sleep has occurred, is sufficient if the question is whether or not hypoxia or hypercapnia occurs during sleep. More complex equipment to monitor expansion of the rib cage and abdomen is required if accurate analysis of the types of sleep apnoea is needed. An electrocardiographic recording must be added to the blood gas monitoring if nocturnal cardiac dysrhythmias are suspected. These are only some examples of the combinations of equipment that may be needed. The monitoring of the patient should, wherever possible, be supplemented by direct observation by a trained observer. This ensures that the monitoring equipment is functioning correctly and that any faults are promptly discovered. It may also prevent important misinterpretations of artefacts due, for instance, to movement of the patient.

Interpretation of sleep studies is therefore complex and the data from each type of monitor and from direct observation should be carefully correlated to obtain an overall picture of respiration during sleep. Computer analysis of the data is valuable, although clinically significant abnormalities are often apparent from visual inspection of the record (Fig. 9.1).

Interpretation of the observations also requires a knowledge of the factors that alter the sleep structure. The most important of these are:

Unfamiliarity with the equipment

Unfamiliarity with the equipment and the place where the sleep recording is carried out are responsible for the changes in sleep pattern that are frequently observed during the first night of monitoring [30]. The sleep latency time (time before the onset of sleep) is prolonged, the time spent in stage 1 NREM sleep is increased and the time in stage 4 NREM and REM sleep is lessened. The total sleep time is shortened and awakenings are more frequent. If the sleep abnormality is gross it may overshadow these changes, but in milder cases it may not be apparent or may be underestimated, particularly if the abnormalities are present only in stages 3 and 4 NREM and REM sleep. A second night's study may be required.

Sleep studies are usually continued for the whole night, but they can be terminated once the relevant abnormalities have been satisfactorily demonstrated. Sleep studies during the day (nap studies) may be useful, but REM sleep is less likely than at night and false negative results are common.

Drugs

Sedative drugs alter the relative durations of the sleep stages and thereby affect respiration during sleep. They may also decrease respiratory

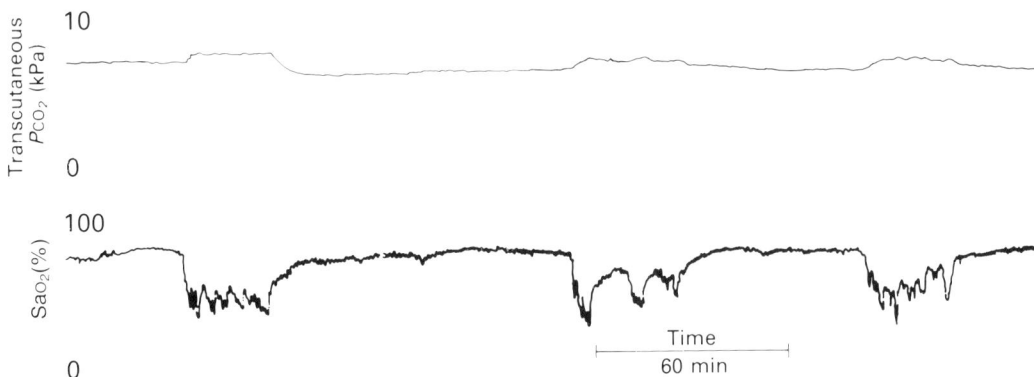

Fig. 9.1. Continuous tracing of transcutaneous P_{CO_2} and oxygen saturation during sleep showing periods of hypoventilation.

muscle tone and respiratory drive. In general, drugs that diminish REM sleep do so only temporarily and REM sleep increases abruptly when they are stopped.

Age

The sleep structure changes with age (p. 34) and this alters the frequency of respiratory abnormalities that are sleep-stage specific.

The most important indices of sleep and respiration that are commonly monitored are:

Sleep stage

Respiration varies with the stage of sleep and it is therefore important to document that sleep has occurred and for how long, and the duration of each sleep stage. An EEG recording is essential, but additional information may be obtained from an electro-oculogram (EOG) and an EMG, usually submental. The EEG criteria for each stage of sleep are described in Chapter 3. The EOG enables rapid eye movements to be detected and the EMG electrode identifies periods when muscle tone is decreased. In combination, these recordings accurately delineate NREM and REM sleep and the tonic and phasic periods of REM sleep. The standard distribution of electrodes of EEG and EOG recordings interferes with sleep, and a simplified system such as that comprising two EEG, an interocular EOG and a single submental EMG electrode is well tolerated and usually sufficient.

Arterial blood gases

This is the most important measurement of respiration during sleep. Abnormalities of the ventilatory pattern are usually of little clinical significance if the P_{O_2} and P_{CO_2} remain normal throughout sleep.

The arterial P_{O_2} and P_{CO_2} can be determined directly by analysis of arterial blood samples. This has the disadvantage that sampling is only intermittent and that it awakens the subject and thereby disturbs sleep. An alternative is to inter-mittently sample arterial blood from an indwelling cannula, but this method does not provide a continuous estimation of the blood gases. The end tidal P_{CO_2} can be determined if an endotracheal tube is in place, or with a tight-fitting face mask, but the latter alters the respiratory pattern.

These methods have been largely superseded by non-invasive techniques for measuring arterial blood gases [2320]. Both the P_{O_2} and P_{CO_2} can be determined transcutaneously [1510, 2012]. The skin is heated to a pre-set temperature of about 43°C, which dilates the cutaneous blood vessels. This not only increases the blood flow to the skin so that it is 'arterialized' but it also ensures that blood flow is almost constant. The temperature rise shifts the oxyhaemoglobin dissociation curve to the right, alters the resistance of the skin to oxygen permeation and increases the oxygen uptake and CO_2 production of the skin. The transcutaneous blood gas tensions are therefore slightly different to the arterial tensions. Conversion formulae are available but there is wide variation between subjects, and individual calibration of the transcutaneous and arterial gas tensions is advisable [2320].

The transcutaneous monitors are sufficiently accurate for clinical purposes but they respond slowly and may not detect short apnoeas. Oxygen saturation monitors react more rapidly. They have a time constant of as little as 3 sec [821, 2579]. They estimate the percentage of oxyhaemoglobin spectrophotometrically. The Hewlett-Packard HP 47201A senses eight wavelengths of light but the newer pulse oximeters, such as the Biox III and Nellcor N, use only two wavelengths. There is no difference in accuracy between these models [2579, 2619, 3204], but a bradycardia delays the response of the pulse oximeters [1107]. Their readings are within 4% of the arterial oxygen saturation estimated directly from arterial blood, as long as the saturation is above 60% [821]. Below this level the Hewlett-Packard model gives falsely low readings and the Biox III model gives falsely high readings [532]. The Hewlett-Packard oximeter readings are altered by skin pigmentation and hyperbilirubinaemia, and carboxy- and methaemoglobin affect both types of oximeter.

Nocturnal hypoxic dips and periods of hypercapnia can be detected by simple inspection of a chart recording of the data obtained. A gradual fall in oxygen saturation, followed by a rapid rise, is characteristic of obstructive sleep apnoeas. The pattern of hypoxic dips has also been used to identify the stage of sleep. Small, irregular variations in oxygen saturation occur during wakefulness, whereas slower variations appear in NREM sleep, together with sinusoidal desaturations during apnoeas. In REM sleep the desaturations are less uniform and more severe [956].

Various statistical indices of oxygen saturation, Po_2 and Pco_2 have proved useful in analysing the blood gas abnormalities during sleep. These indices include the lowest oxygen saturation observed during either NREM or REM sleep, the number of dips of a certain percentage saturation (or kPa) to within a given range of oxygen saturation (such as 70–80%), the mean duration spent with an oxygen saturation within a given range or below or above a given range of saturation [2967], the highest Pco_2 during any sleep stage, or the duration of the Pco_2 above a certain level during any sleep stage. Computer sampling of the sleep recordings may enable these figures to be obtained with only a slight error, except for single events such as the lowest oxygen saturation or the longest apnoea, which may be missed by the sampling technique [3054].

Pattern of ventilation

The frequency of respiration, the respiratory rhythm and the presence of apnoeas can be recorded. Pneumotachographs are accurate but are normally mounted in a face mask which alters the respiratory pattern. They measure tidal volume more accurately than the methods described below. Continuous recording of the expired CO_2 concentration through a nasal cannula detects each respiration by the variation in CO_2 concentration. Errors may result if expira-

tion is purely through the mouth rather than the nose.

The sounds generated in the large airways during breathing can be recorded by a microphone placed over the trachea [694]. This method has proved reasonably satisfactory but noises due to movements and snoring may cause artefacts. An alternative is to fix a thermally sensitive resistor (thermistor) to the nose or mouth, or both. The expired air warms the thermistor and increases its resistance. The resistance changes are electrically processed into a form that can be recorded or displayed. This method is also subject to artefacts, and the thermistor may be displaced during sleep so that false negative results are obtained.

Tidal volume, rib cage and abdominal movement

The tidal volume may be estimated using a pneumotachograph (see above), but assessment of the relative movements of the rib cage and abdomen requires more complex equipment. This is needed to recognize apnoeas and hypopnoeas and for discriminating between central, mixed and obstructive apnoeas. The total number of apnoeas and hypopnoeas of each type can be recorded during each night's sleep or per hour and the longest apnoea, the frequency of apnoeas and the mean duration of each apnoea can be calculated.

The most commonly used methods are:

STRAIN GAUGES

These consist of an electrical conductor, such as mercury, sealed within an elastic tube that surrounds the rib cage or abdomen, or both. The current passing through the conductor varies inversely with its length, so that the resistance increases with inspiration and falls with expiration. These strain gauges have been widely used in the past but are only reliable over a narrow range of tidal volumes and have been largely superseded by newer methods.

IMPEDANCE PNEUMOGRAPHY

The impedance of the thorax changes as its volume alters, but it also varies with the proportions of air, blood and other liquids in the thorax. Circulatory changes may, therefore, be wrongly interpreted as changes in volume. It is usual to measure only one diameter during impedance pneumography, so an accurate assessment of both abdominal and rib cage movements may not be possible. Impedance pneumography may, nevertheless, be useful as an apnoea detector and for monitoring respiratory frequency.

MAGNETOMETERS

In this method a magnetic field is generated by an exciter coil, which is usually placed posteriorly. The voltage detected by an anterior receiver coil is inversely proportional to the cube of the distance between the coils. Magnetometer coils are normally placed on both the chest and abdomen, and respiratory movements that change the distance between them can be detected. Calibration is usually achieved by an isovolumetric manoeuvre. The volume changes of both chest and abdomen can be reasonably accurately measured from their anteroposterior diameter changes, at least in normal subjects [1124, 2102].

INDUCTANCE PLETHYSMOGRAPHY

The electrical inductance of a body is its opposition to a change in the flow of current. This is analogous in mechanical terms to inertia. Inductance transducers, such as the Respitrace system, are placed around both the chest and abdomen [2320]. The changes in cross-sectional area during respiration alter the inductance. This method only samples a small volume of the chest and abdomen, but the results correlate within about 10% with the tidal volumes measured spirometrically [1510, 2732]. Calibration is usually achieved by a simultaneous equation method during two breaths in different positions, an isovolume manoeuvre, or a least-squares or multiple linear regression method [524, 3067]. Calibration may be difficult, particularly if the chest wall is deformed or the patient's position alters during the recording, but accurate measurements can be made throughout the range of the VC.

Cardiac dysrhythmias and hypertension

Nocturnal hypoxia may cause cardiac dysrhythmias. These can be detected readily by continuous ECG recording. Physiological bradycardias occur during REM sleep as part of the increase in parasympathetic activity, but bradycardias are also a feature of sleep apnoeas.

The systemic blood pressure can be recorded automatically at regular intervals and usually rises during hypoxic episodes. Pulmonary artery pressure and cardiac output estimation require a right heart catheter. This is usually only employed for research purposes.

Other observations

The site of any upper airway obstruction may be visualized by introducing a fibre-optic endoscope into the upper respiratory tract and observing the pharyngeal and laryngeal movements. This procedure is surprisingly well tolerated.

Oesophageal and gastric pressures may also be recorded to distinguish central from obstructive sleep apnoeas. Diaphragmatic EMGs can be recorded from oesophageal electrodes (p. 108) and measurement of oesophageal pH may be useful if it is suspected that gastro-oesophageal reflux is the cause of the changes in respiratory pattern.

CONTROL OF VENTILATION

The contributions of the voluntary and automatic components of ventilatory control cannot be completely separated by most of the tests of respiratory drive (Fig. 9.2). The overall respiratory drive to the diaphragm has been assessed

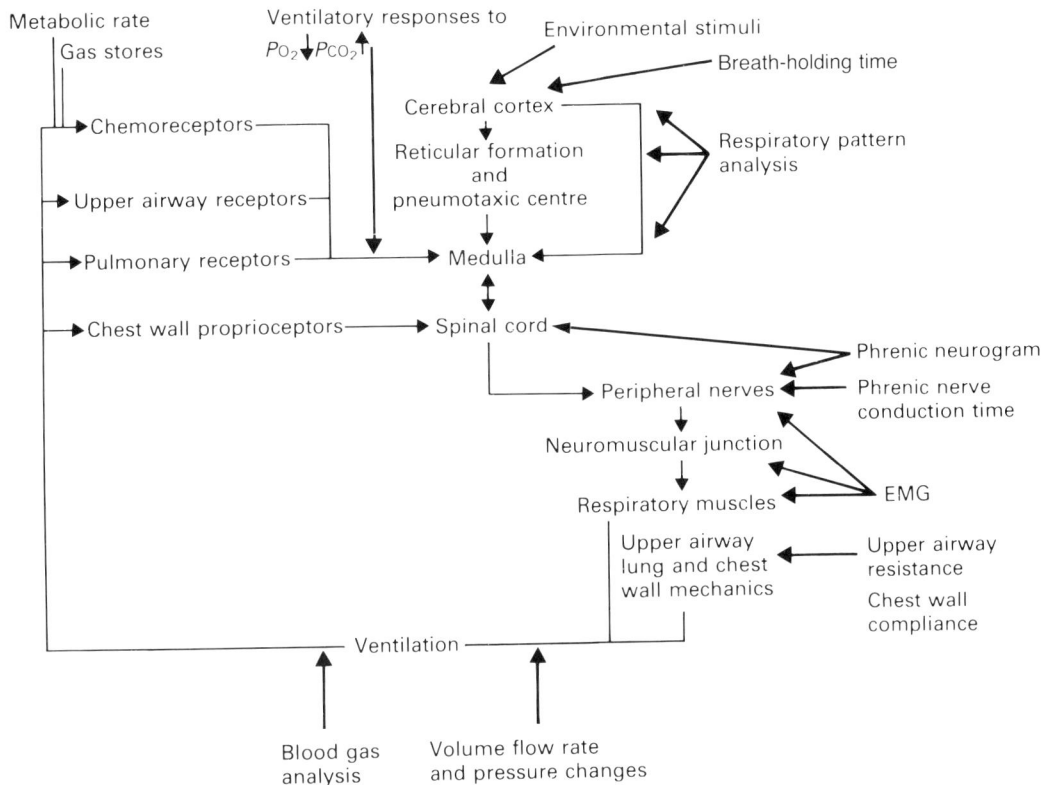

Fig. 9.2. *Diagrammatic representation of the aspects of the respiratory control system that are evaluated by individual tests (indicated by thick lines with arrows).*

experimentally by phrenic nerve recordings (phrenic neurogram). This has the advantage that it is not directly influenced by abnormalities of the neuromuscular junction, respiratory muscles or respiratory mechanics but it only samples the output to one respiratory muscle, the diaphragm. In cats, both the peak and the mean phrenic nerve activity are proportional to the peak inspiratory pressure measured by mouth occlusion [906].

Voluntary control

RESPIRATORY PATTERNS

The recognition of Cheyne-Stokes respiration by clinical observation or by the techniques described above may indicate a defect in the voluntary control of ventilation. An inability to

match the tidal volume or respiratory frequency to preset targets suggests a respiratory dyspraxia (p. 52). Other indices such as T_I, T_E, T_I/T_{TOT} and V_T/T_I have not yet been adequately studied, but may provide valuable insight into the voluntary control of ventilation.

BREATH-HOLDING TIME

The estimation of the breath-holding time is a useful but underused test of voluntary control and of reflex respiratory drives. The sensation of discomfort and breathlessness during breath-holding arises in the respiratory muscles, particularly the diaphragm. The breath-holding time is prolonged if the respiratory muscle contraction can be eliminated [1157], for instance, by curarization [481, 483]. Spinal or epidural anaesthesia to a level of T_I has no effect [899]

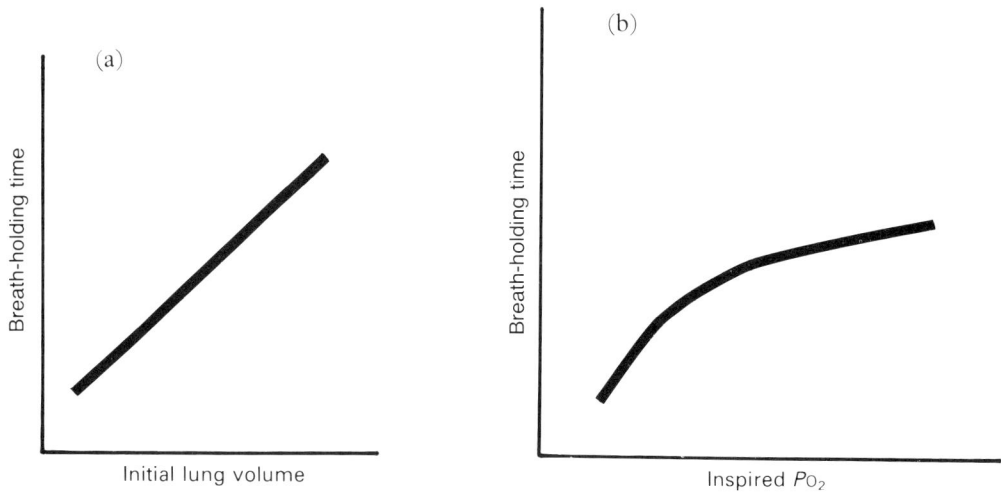

Fig. 9.3. *Relationship of breath-holding time to (a) initial lung volume and (b) inspired* P_{O_2}.

but phrenic nerve block prolongs the breath-holding time [2318]. The sensation of breathlessness probably relates to impulses arising in the muscle spindles or possibly the tendon organs, and can be relieved by a single breath even if this is of a hypoxic or hypercapnic gas mixture [1024].

The breath-holding time varies with the lung volume and blood gases (Figs 9.3 and 9.4). It is more prolonged at high lung volumes [2195] so that at TLC it is normally about 80 sec, at FRC about 30 sec and at RV about 20 sec [2195]. During breath-holding, the volume of gas in the lungs falls since carbon dioxide production is less than oxygen uptake and the gas is compressed by the increasing tension in the respiratory muscles. Breath-holding time is inversely related to the degree of hypercapnia and hypoxia [2195] but the effects of these gases are interrelated [975].

Breath-holding time is prolonged by blocking the vagus nerve [1311, 1315], which implies that afferent impulses originating in the lungs, presumably from stretch receptors, are responsible for increasing the stimulation of the respiratory muscles. The inspiratory movements can be voluntarily inhibited, initially, but then irregular

contractions appear that increase in strength and frequency until the breaking point is reached [33].

The breath-holding time, therefore, reflects the activity of respiratory reflexes and the ability to voluntarily inhibit diaphragmatic contractions. It is prolonged in disorders of the carotid body and in central alveolar hypoventilation, but is reduced to less than 20 sec in functional cardiovascular disorders [1715] and in functional hyperventilation.

Automatic control

RESPIRATORY PATTERNS

The specific patterns of ventilation associated with disorders of the pons and medulla are described in Chapter 5. The equipment used for investigating respiration during sleep may be employed to document these respiratory rhythms.

VENTILATORY DRIVE

The adequacy of automatic respiratory control can be assessed by challenging it with hypoxia,

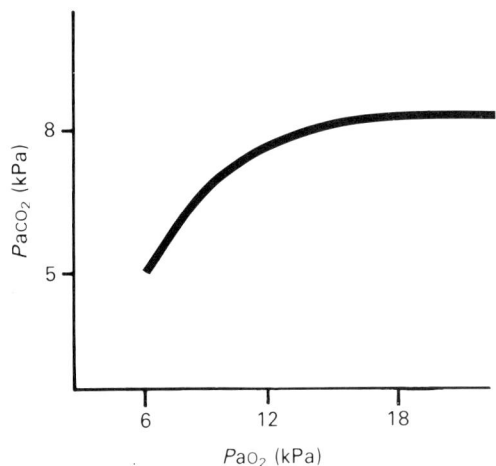

Fig. 9.4. *Relationship of Pa_{CO_2} to Pa_{O_2} at the breaking point of breath-holding in subjects breathing hypoxic and hypercapnic gas mixtures.*

hypercapnia or a mechanical load, and observing the ventilation, tidal volume, frequency, V_T/T_I, T_I, T_E and $P_{0.1}$ [2156].

Hypercapnia

The hypercapnic drive is usually assessed by increasing the concentration of the inspired CO_2 and measuring the ventilatory response. This can be carried out as a steady-state test where a constant level of arterial CO_2 is achieved [2580] or, more commonly, simply and quickly by the rebreathing technique [2577]. The CO_2 stimulus is usually taken as the end tidal P_{CO_2} and the ventilatory response is measured over a period of 15 or 30 sec, or computed as an instantaneous minute volume. The test is carried out under hyperoxic conditions to prevent hypoxia altering the response.

The ventilatory response to a rising P_{CO_2} is linear (Fig. 1.5) and can be described both in terms of its slope (sensitivity) and the intercept on the x-axis (threshold). The results from the steady-state and rebreathing tests are similar, except that the response line is shifted to the right during the rebreathing test by about 1.0 kPa. This difference may be due to the smaller chemoreceptor–arterial P_{CO_2} gradient during

the rebreathing test, in which equilibrium is not attained but in which there is a constant rate of change of P_{CO_2} as opposed to a constant P_{CO_2}.

An abnormal response may be due not only to a reduced chemoreceptor drive but to an abnormality of respiratory mechanics [1251] or respiratory muscle weakness, either of which may limit the ventilatory response. Measurement of the mouth occlusion pressure (see below), which is less dependent on respiratory mechanics, may help to resolve any doubt. A disproportionately low ventilatory response compared to the $P_{0.1}$ suggests that the respiratory mechanics rather than the respiratory drive is abnormal.

Hypoxia

The hypoxic drive is less easy than the hypercapnic drive to test because it is dangerous to induce severe hypoxia and it may be difficult to separate the influence of hypercapnia from that of hypoxia. An indirect measurement of the hypoxic sensitivity can be derived from the ventilatory responses to CO_2 at different inspired oxygen concentrations. The hypoxic drive can also be assessed by rebreathing air or by inspiring a hypoxic gas mixture, but it is essential that the inspired P_{CO_2} is kept constant. These tests are usually carried out by the rebreathing technique [2578], but a steady-state test requires less time for equilibrium than when testing with hypercapnia since the body stores of oxygen are small and the response time of the carotid body chemoreceptors is shorter than the central CO_2 receptors.

The alveolar P_{O_2} may be taken as the P_{O_2} stimulating the chemoreceptors, but the oxygen saturation measured by an oximeter is more commonly used. Ventilation increases hyperbolically as the P_{O_2} falls, but it is linearly related to the oxygen saturation [2578]. Hypoxia itself may cause brain stem depression and diminish the ventilatory response, but this is less likely to occur with the shorter rebreathing test than in the steady-state test [1768].

The quick response of the carotid body receptors has been utilized in observing transient responses to changes in arterial P_{O_2}. Substitution of pure oxygen for air in hypoxic subjects will diminish the ventilation within a few breaths, and a similar technique but using a hypoxic mixture can be used for normal subjects.

Mechanical loading

The ventilatory response to mechanically loading the respiratory system relies on reflexes arising from mechanoreceptors in the chest wall and lungs [543]. It is essential that the blood gases are kept constant since either the hypoxic or hypercapnic drives may modify the response.

The addition of elastic or resistive loads is usually examined during a steady-state test. An elastic load can be achieved by strapping the chest wall or by breathing from a rigid airtight container. A resistive load can be added by breathing through a narrow orifice or by inserting a fine wire mesh into the airway. This may cause hypoventilation if the respiratory muscle strength is reduced or the chest wall mechanics

are abnormal. The changes in ventilation, respiratory frequency, tidal volume and T_I and T_E are recorded. Abnormal responses may reflect disorders of the medullary respiratory centres, cervical cord [2294], peripheral nerves or respiratory muscles.

MOUTH OCCLUSION PRESSURES

The force developed by the inspiratory muscles can be estimated from the mouth pressure generated while the airway is transiently occluded early in inspiration. The occlusion is too brief for the patient to react to it or for any reflex such as the Hering-Breuer reflex to influence ventilation. The maximal rate of change of pressure [2089] or the pressure 0.15 or, more commonly, 0.1 sec after the initiation of inspiration ($P_{0.15}$, $P_{0.1}$) can be measured. This method may be used while breathing air or during other investigations, such as tests of hypercapnia or hypoxia.

It has been proposed that the mouth occlusion pressure is a measure of the intensity of the respiratory drive [3319]. It is measured when

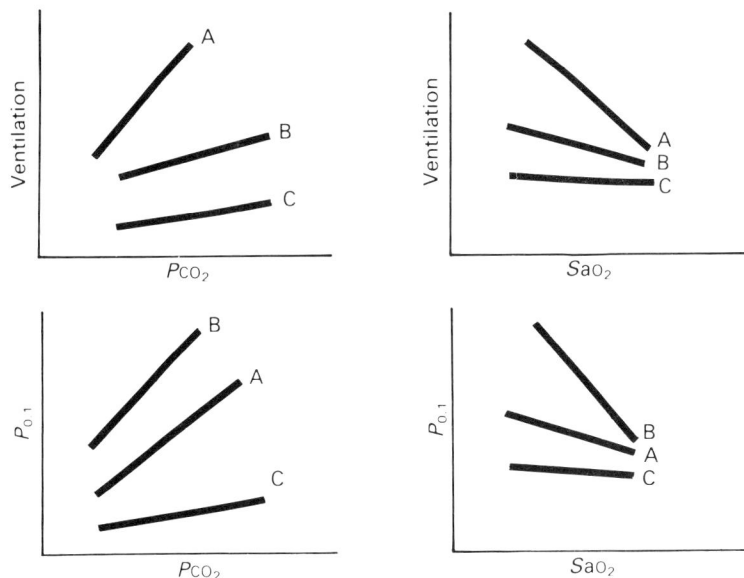

Fig. 9.5. *Ventilatory and mouth occlusion pressure responses to hypercapnia and hypoxia in normal subjects (A), chest wall disorders (B) and central alveolar hypoventilation (C).*

the airway is occluded and is, therefore, independent of air flow resistance. It does, however, depend on the strength of the respiratory muscles [1131] and the mechanics of the chest wall, especially the lung volume [909]. Normal subjects undergoing a rebreathing test progressively lower their end expiratory volume [1232] and, conversely, patients who are hyperinflated increase their end expiratory volume. In both situations, the force generated by the diaphragm alters so that the mouth occlusion pressure changes independently of the intensity of the respiratory drive. The mouth occlusion pressure is, therefore, more a measure of the isometric inspiratory muscle force than of the respiratory drive. It has been used to detect muscle fatigue [468] and may be useful in assessing the contribution of abnormal respiratory mechanics to observed changes in ventilatory drive (Fig. 9.5).

PERIPHERAL NERVE FUNCTION

Disorders of the peripheral nerves supplying the respiratory muscles impair the results of the tests of their function. Only the phrenic nerve is, however, readily accessible for investigation. The phrenic nerve conduction time can be estimated by stimulating the phrenic nerve in the neck and recording the diaphragmatic EMG. The method of locating the 'motor point' of the phrenic nerve was established during the early studies of diaphragmatic pacing (p. 270). Stimulation is usually achieved transcutaneously [2888], but needle stimulation has also been recommended [2010].

The precise distance between the point of stimulation and the diaphragm is uncertain, so that only a conduction time rather than a conduction velocity can be estimated. Autopsy studies of fresh human phrenic nerves suggested that the conduction velocity was about 78 m/sec [1398]. In adults, the phrenic nerve conduction time is usually 7–9 msec [2010, 2295, 2887], with an upper limit of normal of about 9.75 msec [2060]. In children, the conduction time varies from 2.7 to 7.8 msec [406], reflecting both the shorter length of the phrenic nerve and probably the slower conduction velocity in the narrower axons.

CHEST WALL MOVEMENTS

The study of the properties of the chest wall cannot be separated from that of the respiratory muscles, which provide the energy for the respiratory movements and whose activity partly determines the compliance of the chest wall. The movement of individual parts of the chest wall can be estimated by methods such as optical contour mapping [772] (Fig. 9.6), and the overall expansion of the rib cage and abdomen can be assessed by the techniques described above.

The compliance of the chest wall is difficult to measure. Relaxation against an occluded airway at different inspired lung volumes, continuous pressure breathing against a weighted spirometer [932] and periodic interruption of a relaxed expiration from the TLC [1440] have all been used. Each of these techniques requires an oesophageal pressure measurement so that the pressure gradient across the chest wall can be estimated. The results are not repeatable because of the difficulty in ensuring complete relaxation of the inspiratory muscles; EMG recordings may be required to validate the measurements. Periodic interruption of a relaxed expiration from the TLC is probably the least unsatisfactory method.

RESPIRATORY MUSCLE FUNCTION

The force developed by the respiratory muscles reflects not only the properties of the muscles themselves but also the respiratory drive, peripheral nerve and neuromuscular junction function and the mechanical properties of the chest wall and lungs. Each of these components may influence the results of most of the tests of respiratory muscle function. Those tests that require voluntary contraction of the respiratory muscles also suffer from the disadvantage that the degree of motivation may vary. Electrical

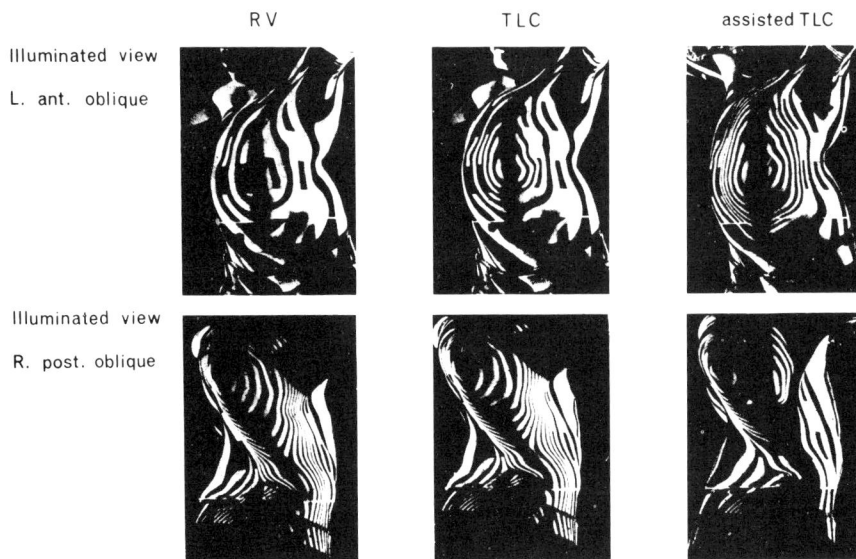

Fig. 9.6. *Optical contour mapping of chest wall movements in a patient with scoliosis. The increase in the number of contour lines anteriorly shows that this region of the chest expands most. Right-hand figures show the chest position during assisted ventilation, which achieves a volume greater than the normal TLC. Reproduced, with permission, from Denison D. Br. J. Dis. Chest, 1982;* **76:** *23.*

stimulation of peripheral nerves with a supra-maximal current overcomes this problem but only a single nerve, the phrenic nerve, is readily accessible for stimulation. Activity of muscles other than the diaphragm cannot be tested in this way unless they are stimulated directly. Electrical activation of the peripheral nerves provides a standardized stimulus to the muscles but this is unphysiological and its relevance to the coordinated function of the respiratory muscles is doubtful. The results of both voluntary and electrical stimulation also depend on the length of the muscles, which can be only indirectly and approximately assessed from the lung volume (p. 18). Changes in the length of the muscles may significantly alter the values obtained and falsely indicate an increase or reduction in muscle strength or endurance.

Strength

INSPIRATORY AND EXPIRATORY MUSCLES

The strength of the inspiratory and expiratory muscles is more difficult to assess clinically than most other muscles. Subjective assessments and grading of the maximal voluntary force using scales such as that recommended by the MRC [2109] are of little value. The only respiratory muscle whose force can be measured directly is the sternomastoid [895, 2239]. The force of the other muscles can only be inferred from changes in volume, flow rate or pressures within the thorax and abdomen.

Volume

Simple tests such as blowing out a match 7.5–15.0 cm from the lips through the wide open mouth correlate with objective changes in volume such as the forced expiratory volume in 1 sec (FEV_1) and the MVV [2363, 2994], but have been superseded largely by more precise tests. The VC is the single most useful volume measurement, since it requires both maximal inspiratory and expiratory efforts. It can be measured simply with a dry spirometer or roughly estimated clinically, since counting to ten at a rate of 2 digits/sec requires an expiratory volume

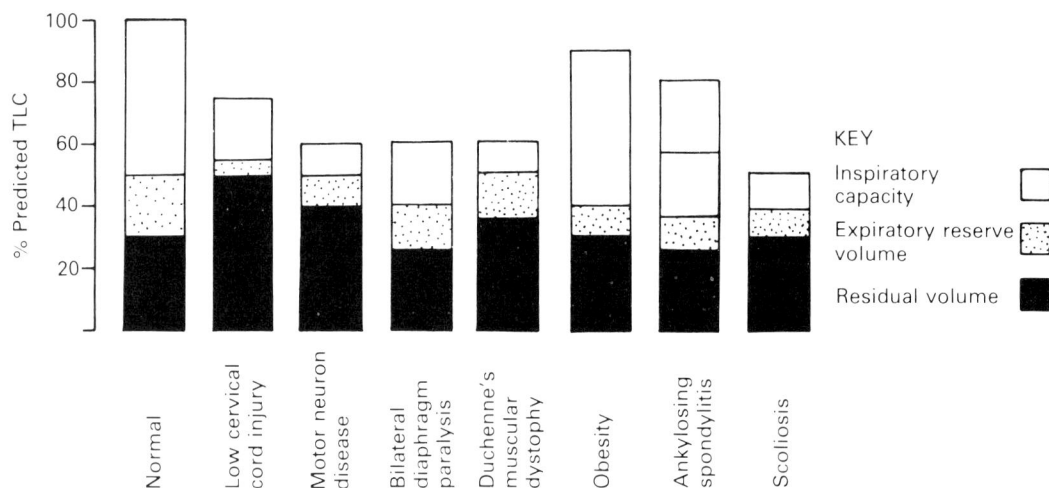

Fig. 9.7. *Bar chart to show lung volumes in normal subjects and some neuromuscular and skeletal disorders.*

of about 1 litre [1367, 3254]. The VC is independent of automatic respiratory control but requires a maximum voluntary effort. It is a good estimate of the respiratory muscle strength and chest wall compliance in the absence of lung disease, although it may be lowered by a secondary fall in lung compliance due to a small lung volume or an inability to take a deep breath.

Changes in the TLC, FRC and RV (Fig. 9.7) are less easily estimated. They require either a body plethysmograph, a gas dilution technique (usually helium) or calculations from chest X-rays. The body plethysmograph measures the amount of compressible gas in the thorax and abdomen, whereas the dilution techniques measure only the volume of accessible gas in the lungs. Both of these methods are, therefore, liable to errors.

The MVV is usually measured over a period of 12 or 15 sec, either at a respiratory frequency chosen by the patient or at a fixed frequency. Normal values vary with the age, height and FEV_1 [264, 1258, 1831]. This test requires motivation and an ability to coordinate rapid respiratory movements, which may be lost in neurological disorders. It is more dependent on

inspiratory than expiratory muscle function, since expiration is largely passive. The MVV falls as PI_{max} is reduced, but it is not a sensitive indicator of respiratory muscle weakness [1831]. The test period of 12 or 15 sec is too short to reveal muscle fatigue, unless this is gross.

Flow rates

The maximal flow rates during inspiration depend on the properties of the respiratory muscles, the compliance of the chest wall and lungs and the air flow resistance. The maximal inspiratory flow rates can be used as a measure of respiratory muscle strength if the respiratory mechanics are normal.

Muscle strength is only estimated by maximal expiratory flow rates over the upper 25% of the VC, since the airways are dynamically compressed at lower lung volumes. The maximal rates of air flow are then limited by the dimensions of the airways and by the elastic recoil of the lungs rather than by muscular effort. The peak expiratory flow rates (PEFR) and FEV_1 provide simple measures of maximal expiratory flow rates.

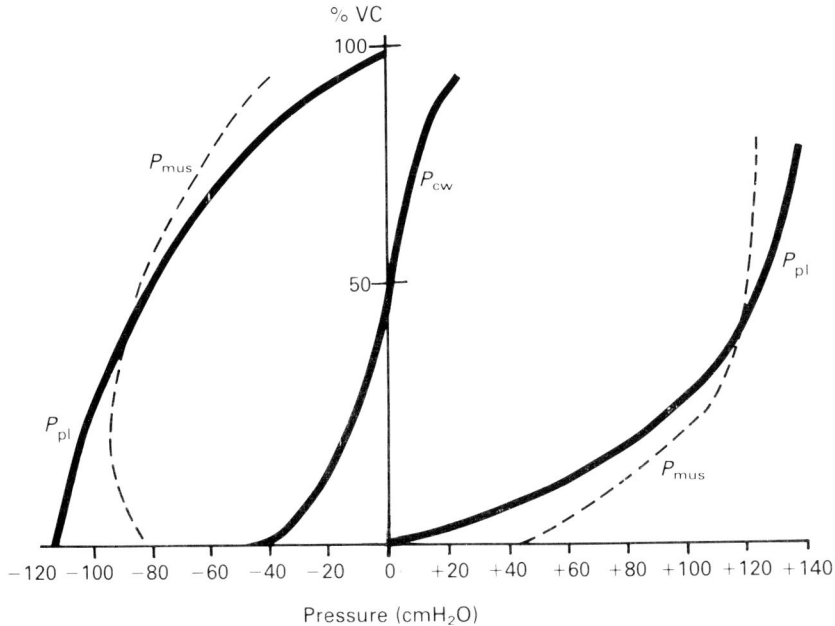

Fig. 9.8. *Volume–pressure diagram to demonstrate contributions of chest wall recoil pressure* (P_{cw}) *and muscle contraction* (P_{mus}) *to pleural pressure* (P_{pl}).

Pressure

Maximal inspiratory and expiratory pressures (P_{Imax} *and* P_{Emax}). The maximal pressures obtainable during inspiration and expiration have been measured in the oesophagus or even nasally [2633], but are most conveniently estimated at the mouth. The P_{Imax} or P_{Emax} that can be sustained for more than 1 sec is recorded. A small leak is introduced into the system to ensure that the muscles of the chest wall rather than those of the upper airway are used. A maximal effort is necessary but it may not be possible to measure the maximal pressures of air leaks around the mouthpiece because the muscles of the lips or cheeks are weak.

The P_{Imax} is greatest at RV and the P_{Emax} at TLC [2549]. The pressures are normally measured at these volumes but P_{Imax} can also be assessed at FRC [2884]. The maximal pressure recordings reflect not only the tension developed by the respiratory muscles but also the elastic recoil pressure of the lungs and chest wall. This varies with lung volume but is usually only a small component (Fig. 9.8).

The maximal pressures correlate in normal subjects with age, height, weight and general muscular strength [311, 2633, 3351], and normal values are available both for adolescents and adults [2990]. The P_{Emax} is greater than the P_{Imax} and the values for women are about two-thirds those of men [311].

DIAPHRAGM

Bilateral diaphragmatic weakness can be suspected clinically from the observation of paradoxical movement of the abdomen and rib cage [735, 1423], which can be demonstrated using the techniques described on p. 95. Ultrasound examination enables the diaphragm to be located even in the presence of a pleural effusion, its thickness to be assessed, and it can show whether movement is normal or paradoxical. It is particularly valuable in infants, to monitor the recovery from diaphragmatic paralysis [70]. The limitations of radiological techniques of assessing diaphragmatic function have become well recognized [735, 1929]. Diaphragmatic paralysis may be suspected from the presence of an elevated hemidiaphragm or both halves of the diaphragm on the chest radiograph, but these appearances may be due to many other causes. Mediastinal shift demonstrated by fluoroscopy is an unreliable sign and paradoxical movement may be due to contraction during inspiration of the abdominal muscles rather than to diaphragmatic weakness [52]. If bilateral diaphragmatic paralysis is suspected, it is essential that the patient is examined in the supine position with a weight on the abdomen, and that screening takes place during sniffing as well as deep breathing. These precautions prevent abdominal muscle contraction during expiration from mimicking diaphragmatic activity. The abdominal muscles can decrease the end expiratory volume below the FRC so that inspiration occurs when the abdominal muscles relax through the elastic recoil of the lungs and chest wall, and in the upright position by the effect of gravity on the abdominal contents as well.

A fall in the VC in the supine position is characteristic of diaphragmatic weakness and is most marked if this is severe and bilateral (p. 162). Diaphragmatic strength can also be estimated from the transdiaphragmatic pressure. This is more complex to measure than the

maximal mouth pressures because a pressure transducer has to be swallowed so that recordings can be made both in the stomach and in the oesophagus. The pressure gradient across the diaphragm, generated by its contraction, can then be recorded (Fig. 9.9). The transdiaphragmatic pressure is normally zero at end expiration (FRC).

There is considerable intersubject variation of the transdiaphragmatic pressure during most respiratory manoeuvres [748, 1118]. The transdiaphragmatic pressure during quiet breathing, at TLC after a slow inspiration from the FRC, and during maximal inspiratory efforts against an obstructed airway at various lung volumes are each subject to wide variation. The transdiaphragmatic pressure can be recorded during inspiration when the abdomen is protruded, in order to minimize abdominal muscle contraction [1118], or more usually during sniffing [2161, 2162]. Sniffing is a simple and easily repeated action that provides reliable results both in normal subjects and in those with diaphragmatic weakness [2150].

The transdiaphragmatic pressure can also be measured when diaphragmatic contraction is initiated by electrical stimulation of the phrenic nerve rather than by voluntary contraction. A single supramaximal current may be used to cause a diaphragmatic twitch. The pressure across the diaphragm correlates with the transdiaphragmatic pressure during sniffing [2147] but even when bilateral supramaximal twitches are induced, the transdiaphragmatic pressure is only about 20% of the maximal pressure [226]. The phrenic nerve can alternatively be stimulated at different frequencies to obtain a frequency–pressure curve that approximates to a frequency–force curve for the diaphragm [127, 2238, 2240].

ACCESSORY MUSCLES

The force generated by the sternomastoid muscles can be measured directly during electrical stimulation of the muscle [2239, 2240]. The significance of the observed changes is uncertain

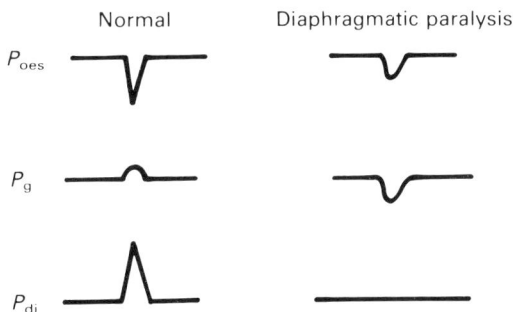

Fig. 9.9. *Effect of diaphragmatic paralysis on oesophageal, gastric and transdiaphragmatic pressures during inspiration, showing inability to generate a transdiaphragmatic pressure.*

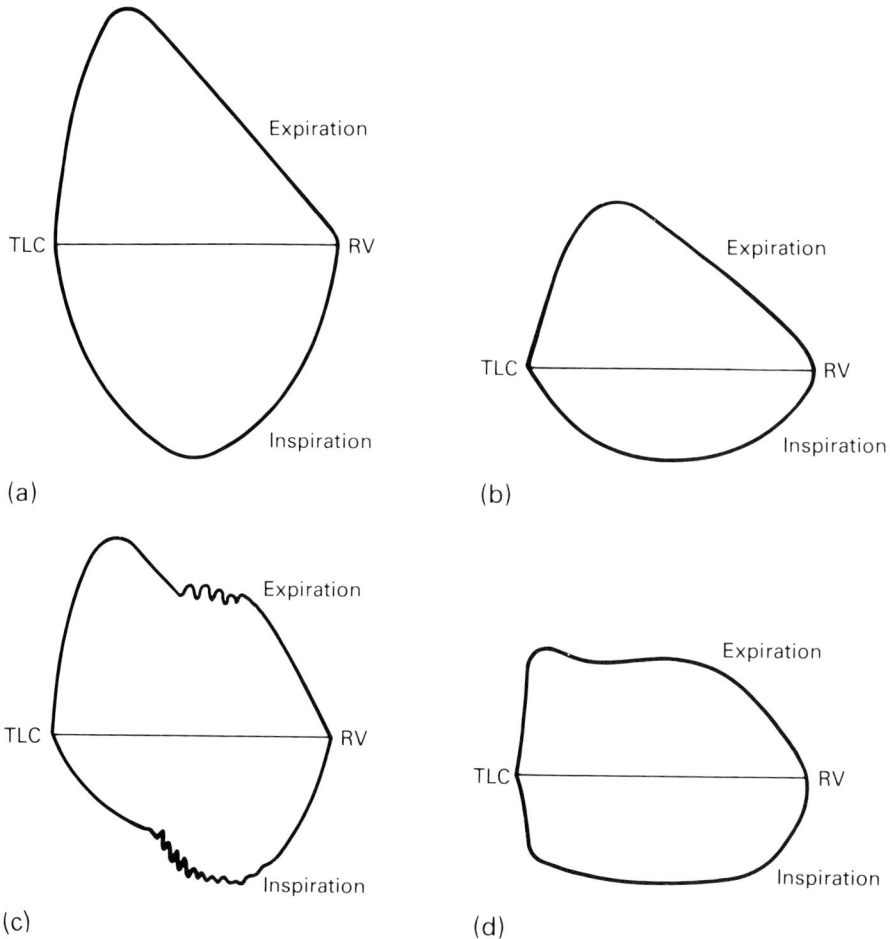

Fig. 9.10. *Flow volume loops in (a) normal subject, (b) respiratory muscle weakness, (c) upper airway oscillation, and (d) fixed upper airway obstruction.*

since sternomastoid function may change independently of the more important respiratory muscles such as the diaphragm.

UPPER AIRWAY MUSCLES

The dimensions of the upper airway can be assessed radiographically, particularly by cephalometry, computerized tomography scans and cinefluoroscopy, as well as by acoustic reflectance (p. 67). Upper airway endoscopy and rhinometry may also give valuable information. The peak nasal inspiratory flow rate is a measure of the air flow resistance in each nostril. Flow volume loops are also sensitive tests of upper airway obstruction or respiratory muscle weakness, both of which reduce the peak inspiratory flow rate [647, 954, 2166, 3238] (Fig. 9.10). Fluttering of the expiratory, and occasionally the inspiratory, loop is common (p. 115).

Endurance

The ability to sustain a force is the endurance of a muscle, and this implies that its diagnosis requires at least two serial measurements. The reduction in force after an interval may be due to muscle fatigue, but this can only be implicated if other factors such as motivation, the mechanical efficiency and the length of the muscle remain constant. Fatigue appears when the force developed reaches a critical fraction of the maximal force and is, therefore, dependent on the strength of the muscle. The tests described above may, as a consequence, give an indication of the likelihood of fatigue appearing, but there are other more direct investigations.

FAILURE TO SUSTAIN VOLUME

Respiratory muscle fatigue can be demonstrated by showing that a given ventilation cannot be sustained. This is usually carried out by assessing the maximal ventilation that can be maintained for a period of time, such as 15 min, under isocapnic conditions (maximal sustainable ventilatory capacity, MSVC). This is usually 50–70% of the 15-sec MVV in normal subjects (Fig. 9.11). This tests both the inspiratory and expiratory muscles, but its value is lessened if lung rather than respiratory muscle disease limits the maximal ventilation. The maximal inspiratory resistance that can be tolerated for a given time, or the duration for which a submaximal ventilation can be maintained, are alternative indicators of endurance and can be shown to fall when muscle fatigue develops.

FAILURE TO SUSTAIN PRESSURE

Muscle fatigue can be demonstrated in a similar way by estimating the maximal inspiratory pressure that can be maintained during each breath for a given period of, for instance, 10 min [2308]. This tests only the inspiratory muscles. The ability to sustain a $P_{0.1}$ in the face of a resistive load may also be used to demonstrate fatigue [468].

Diaphragmatic fatigue may be shown by changes in transdiaphragmatic pressure during sniffing or electrical stimulation of the phrenic nerve. Fatigue shifts the frequency–transdiaphragmatic pressure curve to the right. The loss of force may be more marked at either high- or low-frequency stimulation, indicating high- or low-frequency fatigue, respectively [127, 2238]. Low-frequency fatigue can also be demonstrated by electrical stimulation of the sternomastoid [2239].

SLOWER RELAXATION RATE

The rate of relaxation following a muscle contraction is slower in the presence of muscle fatigue. The mechanism underlying changes in the relaxation rate are uncertain but may involve alterations in adenosine triphosphate utilization [3331, 3334]. Relaxation occurs in two phases. The initial relaxation occurs rapidly but is

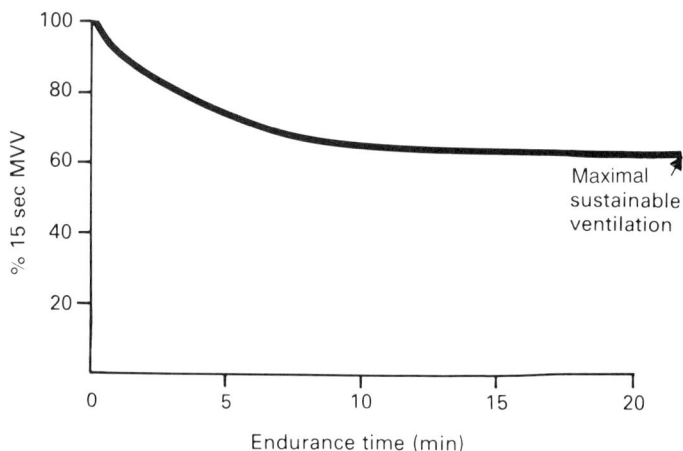

Fig. 9.11. *Decline in maximal ventilation that can be sustained as its duration increases. There is little change after about 15 min and this value, which is about* 60% *of the 15-sec* MVV, *is the maximal sustainable ventilatory capacity* (MSVC).

dependent on the peak pressure, such as trans-diaphragmatic pressure, that has been achieved. Relaxation of type 2 fibres is about twice as fast as type 1 fibres [3333] and selective recruitment of these muscle fibres when high pressures are attained is responsible for the more rapid initial relaxation. The second phase of relaxation occurs exponentially and independently of the peak pressure. Both the maximal relaxation rate and the time constant of the exponential phase can be used as measures of the relaxation properties of the muscle.

A slow relaxation rate is not specific to muscle fatigue since it is also seen if the muscle is ischaemic or shortened excessively. It can be assessed during measurements of PI_{max} or trans-diaphragmatic pressure, either during sniffing [925] or phrenic nerve stimulation [129]. A fall in the relaxation rate usually accompanies changes in PI_{max} and transdiaphragmatic pressure [129, 1882], but is no more sensitive than these observations in detecting muscle fatigue.

ELECTROMYOGRAPHIC CHANGES

The electrical activity recorded from a muscle depends on the action potential of each muscle fibre, the firing frequencies of the motor neurons, the number of motor neurons that are recruited and the distance and conduction properties of the tissues between the muscle and the electrode. The signal obtained can be amplified, filtered, rectified, integrated and recorded. Electromyograms can be obtained from most of the respiratory muscles using surface or needle electrodes, and from the diaphragm with an oesophageal electrode as well. The surface dia-phragmatic EMG may be difficult to obtain and to interpret because of interference from inter-costal and other chest wall muscles. Lack of EMG activity does not necessarily imply relaxa-tion of the muscle, since the electrode may be incorrectly placed.

All of the EMG techniques have the disadvan-tage that they sample only a limited amount of each muscle but it has been shown that for the diaphragm, the amplitude of the EMG reflects the activity in the phrenic nerve [1945]. The amplitude of the EMG does not correlate precisely with the force developed because this depends on other factors such as the length and mechanical efficiency of the muscle, but in certain circumstances it is related to the trans-diaphragmatic pressure [34, 1233] or peak in-spiratory pressure [906].

A variety of indices can be derived from the EMG, such as the peak amplitude or the total electrical activity per breath, although this depends on the duration of the breath as well as on the intensity of the muscle activity. Differ-ent wavelengths of the EMG can be analysed separately [1604]. This 'spectral analysis' has been particularly useful in assessing muscle fatigue. An overall fall in frequency and an increase in amplitude has been recognized for many years to occur during muscle fatigue [590] and spectral analysis has shown that this is due both to an increase in low-frequency activity and a decrease in high-frequency activity [228, 1604]. A fall in the high–low ratio of more than about 20% is usually considered significant [454, 597]. This is detectable before any mechanical consequence of fatigue appears, such as a fall in PI_{max}, transdiaphragmatic pressure or spiro-metry [228, 1261, 2236, 3352]. Determination of the centroid frequency may be even more sensitive [2914].

The EMG features of muscle fatigue differ from the other observations described above in that they do not imply a failure to sustain a force, which is the definition of fatigue. They are better regarded as indicating that the muscle is performing fatiguing work rather than that fatigue has occurred. The EMGs of the respira-tory muscles may also be useful in showing whether individual muscles are active during different respiratory manoeuvres. They may, in addition, indicate the nature of the process caus-ing weakness of the respiratory muscles, al-though an open needle or conchotome muscle biopsy is frequently needed [890, 892].

Part 3
Disorders Causing Ventilatory Failure

Chapter 10
Disorders of Voluntary Control of Respiration

INTRODUCTION

The ability to adapt ventilation to changes in the environment may be lost if the voluntary control system is damaged by disease. The consequences of this may be less prominent than if the automatic control of respiration is deranged, since hypoventilation does not occur either during wakefulness or sleep. Other neurological problems, such as dysphagia, which accompany the loss of voluntary ventilatory control, may be clinically more important.

The loss of voluntary control allows reflex influences on ventilation to become pre-eminent; dysrhythmias such as Cheyne-Stokes respiration, post-hyperventilation apnoea and an abnormally regular respiratory rate (Chapter 5) appear. Voluntary control of ventilation may also be disturbed in functional hyperventilation (hyperventilation syndrome, hysterical hyperventilation), of which periodic or continuous hypocapnia is the main feature. This will not be considered further.

INDIVIDUAL DISORDERS

The many disorders of voluntary ventilation have been the subject of remarkably little attention, although there are a few reviews of the subject [2490, 2491, 2496]. The most important of these conditions are:

Epilepsy

Status epilepticus has a recognized mortality, but it is less widely realized that sudden death may occur in epileptic subjects between obvious fits [1434]. Fits without prominent tonic or clonic activity may be fatal and death may even occur when no motor abnormality is apparent. Changes in cardiac or respiratory reflexes have been held responsible [1434], but the most likely cause is prolonged apnoea due to inhibition of respiratory muscle activity. Breathing ceases during the tonic phase of generalized epileptic fits, with the chest in an inspiratory position, but during 'flaccid' epileptic apnoeas the lung volume is approximately at FRC.

These epileptic apnoeas are characteristic of temporal lobe epilepsy [1550, 2285]. Electrical stimulation of the temporal cortex and limbic system may also cause apnoeas [435, 1602, 3015, 3324], probably by increasing the cortical inhibition of the brain stem respiratory centres [1550]. In one case, infarction of the cingulate gyrus and part of the frontal cortex led to an epileptic apnoea that may have been due to damage to a respiratory stimulating area of the cerebral cortex rather than to stimulation of the neighbouring inhibitory temporal lobe cortex [2724].

Hemiplegia

Analysis of the effects of hemiplegia on ventilation has been hindered by the problem of separately assessing the movements of the two halves of the thorax and abdomen. The wide variety of techniques used has prevented precise comparison of the results of the different studies. The movements of the two sides of the rib cage are symmetrical when ventilation increases 'reflexly', such as while rebreathing gas containing carbon dioxide, and during coughing [216, 1010]. However, during voluntary ventilatory manoeuvres, the diaphragm excursion [1318, 2663] and the expansion of the chest wall on the side of the hemiplegia are diminished [216, 1010, 1549, 1719, 1732, 2979]. Electromyogram activity of the respiratory muscles is also less on the side of the paralysis [746]. The severity of the hemiparesis determines the degree of asymmetrical movement [1732], and paradoxical movement of the chest wall may even be apparent during inspiration [1058]. Paradoxical movement ceases when spasticity of the intercostal muscles appears. This may improve ventilation but is offset by the increase in oxygen consumption during exercise, such as walking, which is due to spasticity of the limbs [190].

These observations can be explained by bilateral representation of the respiratory muscles in the cerebral cortex and decussation of most, but not all, of the descending fibres. Some voluntary activity, therefore, remains on the hemiplegic side. There is considerable individual variation in the amount of residual activity [1732]. In general, movement of the upper chest is more impaired than movement of the lower chest [1010] and corresponding changes in EMG activity have been observed [746]. This suggests that fewer fibres controlling diaphragmatic movement decussate than fibres that supply the intercostal and accessory muscles.

The voluntary manoeuvres that are necessary for the measurement of lung volumes are affected by these abnormalities. A restrictive defect with a diminished TLC, FRC and VC but normal forced expiratory ratio is seen if the hemiplegia is severe [1058]. Both $P_{I_{max}}$ and $P_{E_{max}}$ are decreased [1058, 3343].

Stroke

Strokes are a common cause of hemiplegia, but in addition to the abnormalities discussed in the previous section there may also be changes in the respiratory rhythm. The cortical inhibition of the medullary response to hypercapnia may be lost so that the arterial P_{CO_2} falls; hypoxia

is uncommon [123]. Although these changes have been related to damage to the cerebral hemispheres [1703] or to brain stem lesions [1804, 2765], there is probably no clearcut relationship between the site of the damage to the corticobulbar fibres and the P_{CO_2} [123]. However, if the cerebral damage is bilateral, a wide range of respiratory patterns may be seen. Cheyne-Stokes respiration and Cheyne-Stokes variant carry a better prognosis than most of the other dysrhythmias, especially persistent tachypnoea which has a very poor prognosis [1845, 1846, 2723].

Trauma and other severe illnesses

The changes in respiratory rhythm following head injuries are similar to those following a stroke. The localizing value of these respiratory rhythms after an acute injury is much less than with chronic neurological conditions but they do offer a guide to prognosis. This is poor if there is sustained tachypnoea greater than 25 breaths/min, particularly if the P_{CO_2} is less than 4 kPa, the temperature is greater than 39°C, and extensor rigidity is present [2333, 3221]. Irregular respirations are seen, particularly with medullary but also with pontine lesions, but none of the other respiratory patterns can be correlated with the site of damage [2333].

The prognosis is also poor in critically ill patients in intensive-care units in whom the P_{CO_2} is low [2098]. In coma due to a variety of causes, an increase in regularity of the respiratory rate irrespective of the rate itself is a valuable sign of deepening coma and a worsening prognosis [1855]. A rise in the respiratory rate in this situation often indicates a pulmonary rather than a neurological complication [1855]. A wide variety of other respiratory rhythms may be seen, of which Cheyne-Stokes respiration has the best prognosis [993].

Encephalitis

Acute encephalitis commonly causes changes in the respiratory rhythm, such as Cheyne-Stokes

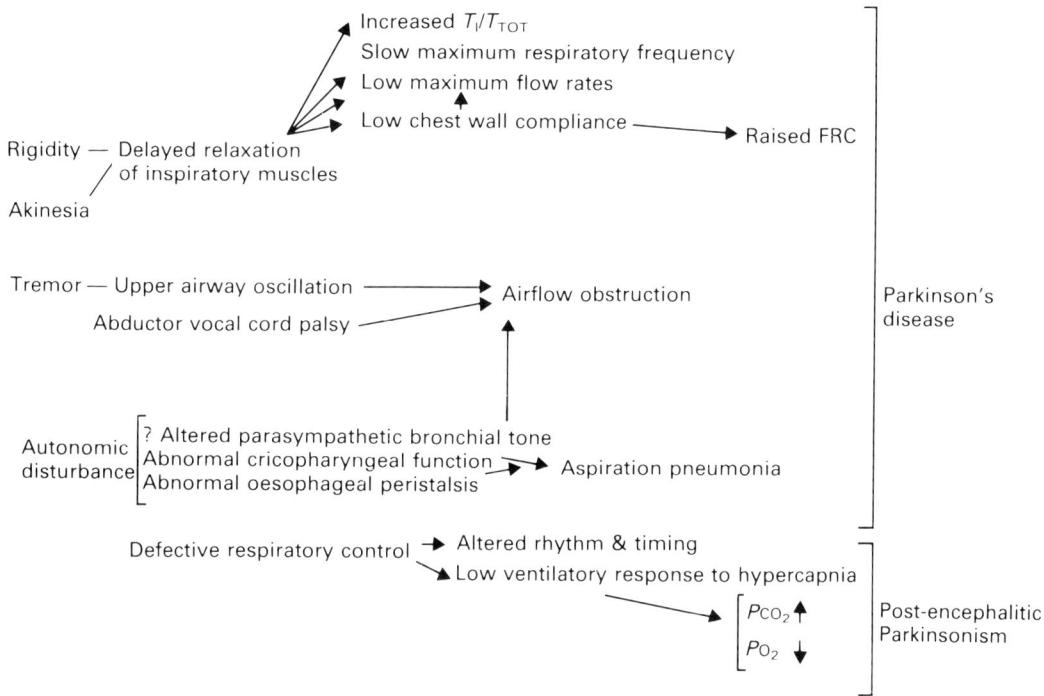

Fig. 10.1. *Flow chart to show effects of Parkinsonism on respiration.*

respiration, as the intracranial pressure rises and the level of consciousness falls. More direct effects on the automatic control of respiration are also well recognized in brain stem encephalitis (p. 121).

Multiple sclerosis

The degeneration of axons in multiple sclerosis is characteristically patchy, but widespread. The corticobulbar and corticospinal tracts are frequently affected. Respiratory failure and even death are commonly due to aspiration pneumonia caused by a poor cough [1308, 1974]. Clinically significant respiratory muscle weakness is unusual, probably because of the bilateral representation within the cerebral cortex. It may, nevertheless, occur in severe multiple sclerosis with quadriplegia [1308] and, occasionally, upper motor neuron weakness of

both halves of the diaphragm is the predominant feature [640, 2640]. This may cause severe intermittent hypoxia during sleep [2640].

Loss of voluntary control of respiration varies considerably in degree. It is seen both in severe multiple sclerosis [2325] and as an isolated abnormality [734], presumably due to damage to the corticospinal pathways in the medulla or high cervical cord.

Parkinsonism (Fig. 10.1)

Parkinsonism is characterized by tremor, cogwheel rigidity and akinesia, which can directly affect the function of the respiratory muscles. Parkinsonism is, however, often only one feature of more widespread neurological damage that may also influence ventilation. For this reason, the individual causes of Parkinsonism are considered separately below.

PARKINSON'S DISEASE

Breathlessness is common in Parkinson's disease but is usually unrelated to its severity [2153]. Depression is frequent and probably contributes to the respiratory symptoms.

The disordered extrapyramidal control of respiratory movements is manifested by activity of the inspiratory muscles which persists into expiration [765, 2449]. Rib cage movement is diminished [1418]. Abdominal muscle EMG activity is also detectable during inspiration [765]. This abnormal activity is less marked in the diaphragm than other inspiratory muscles. These observations suggest that postural control of the respiratory muscles other than the diaphragm overrides their respiratory function so that the respiratory periodicity becomes blurred. Changes in the extrapyramidal control of posture are a more likely explanation than an alteration of the function of the brain stem respiratory centres. The ventilatory response to hypercapnia is normal [1418, 2424] or even increased [960], and the blood gases while awake are also usually normal [1523, 2153, 2287, 2342, 3179]. Obstructive and central sleep apnoeas may be present but desaturation during sleep is uncommon in Parkinson's disease [96, 716, 1353]. The respiratory frequency during sleep is often abnormally regular [2023].

Impairment of voluntary control of V_T and respiratory frequency, and a shortened breath-holding time have been observed [2336] but it is not clear from this report whether these changes were seen in idiopathic Parkinson's disease or post-encephalitic Parkinsonism.

The duration of inspiration is prolonged so that T_I/T_{TOT} is increased [1523]. The resting respiratory rate is often greater than normal and V_T diminished [1523], possibly because of reflexes from chest wall receptors reacting to an increase in muscle tone. This increase in tone and the loss of the normal phasic activity of the inspiratory and expiratory muscles probably underly the respiratory function abnormalities that have been interpreted as being due to air flow obstruction. The ability to generate a rapid air flow is impaired and the respiratory frequency cannot be increased to normal levels [2274, 3179]. The maximal panting rate is diminished [94] and the MVV is less than anticipated from the VC [1418, 1902, 2336, 3179]. Muscle fatigue has been postulated to explain the low MVV but there is no direct evidence for this [93].

The characteristic changes in lung volumes are that the TLC increases slightly [2342] but less so than the RV [2287]. The VC falls slightly and the FRC is slightly increased [2342]. Both the peak inspiratory and expiratory flow rates are low [2287] but the forced expiratory ratio is normal [93]. The chest wall compliance is low [2342], presumably because of the increase in muscle tone, and this leads to the raised FRC. The lung compliance is, however, normal [2342]. The rise in the RV is partially explained by the low chest wall compliance and partly by the fall in P_{Emax} [2336]. Muscular rigidity is probably also the cause of the kyphosis and mild thoracic scoliosis, which is common in Parkinson's disease. The scoliosis is convex to the side of the initial symptoms [870, 2066] and is particularly marked if the Parkinsonism is unilateral.

Most of these changes are reversible with treatment of the Parkinson's disease, although stereotactic surgery did not reliably increase the VC or MVV [1902, 2818, 2918]. Treatment has been recorded as increasing the VC [2111, 2424] and the MVV [2336], and shortening T_I [1523], although these changes may not be seen with low doses of L-dopa [203]. The response of the Parkinson's disease to drug therapy can be monitored usefully by simple serial measures of respiratory function, such as the PEFR and FEV_1 or FVC [1808, 2274].

The direct effects of Parkinson's disease on the respiratory muscles can explain most of the physiological findings. However, many patients are, or have been, tobacco smokers and may have coexistent air flow obstruction [2342]. An increase in parasympathetic tone to the bronchial smooth muscle has also been postulated [2287] but there is no direct evidence for this.

Obstruction of the upper airway is, however, occasionally seen. Flow volume loops have shown rapid oscillations during both inspiration and expiration [2813, 3210, 3239] (Fig. 9.10). Fibre-optic examination has confirmed that the glottis and supraglottic structures adduct and abduct rhythmically at 4–8 Hz. This tremor of the upper airway has the same frequency as that of the limb muscles. Fluttering of the flow volume loop is not specific to Parkinsonism since it is also seen with other neurological disorders [3237, 3238], following burns [1348, 1349], with organic obstruction of the upper airway [3235] in subjects with obstructive sleep apnoeas, and in otherwise normal subjects [3236]. The importance of tremor of the chest wall muscles is uncertain and fluoroscopy has shown no evidence for tremor of the diaphragm [1418, 2336, 2663, 3239, 3240].

Air flow obstruction may also be due to bilateral paralysis of the laryngeal abductor muscles [1452], caused by degeneration in the nucleus ambiguus. Stridor may initially be intermittent, but gradually becomes more persistent and may be extremely loud and present both during wakefulness and sleep [2576, 3223]. It should be distinguished from the bovine cough and hoarse voice that may occasionally be the presenting feature of Parkinsonism and which responds to drug treatment [240]. Dysphagia is often associated with stridor [2486]. It is usually due to a failure of the cricopharyngeal sphincter to open as the food bolus passes into the oesophagus, or to its early closure [2396]. There may also be difficulty in chewing, and abnormalities of oesophageal peristalsis [2437]. Aspiration pneumonia may result [1894, 2152, 2424] and, before the advent of effective drug treatment, this was a common cause of death. Dysphagia, like stridor, may respond partially to L-dopa but cricopharyngeal myotomy may, nevertheless, be required [2396].

POST-ENCEPHALITIC PARKINSONISM

Encephalitis lethargica occurred in widespread epidemics, particularly between 1915 and 1927 and subsequently as sporadic cases. The pathological changes are more widespread than in idiopathic Parkinson's disease [1246, 1477] and disturbances of respiration are more common. A large number of respiratory dysrhythmias appear during the acute illness [1477]. Paroxysmal twitches of the diaphragm and other respiratory muscles, asymmetrical movement of the two halves of the diaphragm and even dissociation of the rates of the two hemidiaphragms may be seen [876]. Rapid respiratory rates of up to 100 breaths/min have been recorded. They can be both episodic or continuous and persist during sleep [3200] and are occasionally associated with severe respiratory failure [187].

After the acute illness a wide variety of respiratory rhythms have been observed [876, 3200, 3201]. These are not related to the severity of the Parkinsonism and probably reflect neurological damage outside the extrapyramidal system. Rapid respiratory rates are more common than bradypnoeas, but these can occasionally be so prolonged as to cause a fatal respiratory arrest. Cheyne-Stokes respiration, apneusis, breath-holding, sighing, yawning, noisy forced expirations, and inversions of the inspiratory/expiratory duration have been observed. Abnormalities of more complex respiratory acts, such as yawning, coughing, hiccoughing and sniffing, are frequent. Difficulty in articulation, such as inappropriate variation in speech and rhythm of the speech, are common [577] and often persistent [1250].

The prognosis of these abnormalities is variable [3201]. They frequently persist for many years. A slightly raised resting respiratory frequency with an inability to alter it, for instance, when asked to hold the breath is common [1671]. The tidal volume is more constant during quiet breathing than in normal subjects and voluntary control over it is impaired [1671, 2336]. The response to exercise is unusual in that both the V_T and the respiratory frequency increase initially [1671]. L-Dopa may precipitate rather than relieve abnormalities of the more complex respiratory acts [2740] and can cause involuntary glottic closure [1343].

These findings are only partially explained by an abnormality of voluntary respiratory control, possibly due to an alteration in extrapyramidal function. There is evidence that the automatic control of respiration is impaired in some cases. The ventilatory response to hypercapnia is diminished [1418, 3077], oxygen desaturation may occur during sleep [1353] and central alveolar hypoventilation many years after the acute illness is well recognized [894, 1087, 3077]. The changes in diaphragm contraction, such as the appearance of an immobile diaphragm and asynchronous contraction of the two halves of the diaphragm may reflect disorganization of the DRG or its connections.

OTHER CAUSES OF PARKINSONISM

Parkinsonism is a feature of several conditions that cause widespread neurological abnormalities. These include multiple system atrophy and taurine deficiency, which is a familial condition in which severe respiratory failure occurs with an impaired ventilatory response to hypercapnia [2444, 2542]. As in multiple system atrophy, the respiratory complications due to degeneration of the medullary respiratory centres are usually more prominent than those of the Parkinsonism itself.

Chorea and athetosis

The respiratory muscles share in the abnormal tone and movements of chorea and athetosis [405]. There have been no detailed studies, but irregular diaphragmatic movements [2663] and asynchronous movement of the two hemidiaphragms [405] have been documented. These abnormalities probably reflect widespread brain damage, which disorganizes both the postural and ventilatory control of the respiratory muscles.

Pseudobulbar palsy

Pseudobulbar palsy is due to bilateral damage to the corticobulbar tracts. Swallowing and speech are affected as well as respiration. Inappropriate behavioural respiratory acts, such as excessive laughing and crying, are common and result from loss of cortical inhibition. This also underlies the increased ventilatory response to hypercapnia, although the response to hypoxia is normal [1419, 2493]. Cheyne-Stokes respiration and post-hyperventilation apnoea are common.

Cerebellar disorders

Physiological studies of the cerebellum have suggested that it may have an important role in controlling ventilation (p. 7), but cerebellar disorders have not been studied adequately in man. The MVV appears to be decreased to a greater extent than the VC [1472], probably because of an inability to perform rapid respiratory movements.

Pontine lesions

The corticobulbar and corticospinal fibres may be damaged by bilateral lesions of the ventral pons. If this is extensive, quadriplegia with paralysis of the lower cranial nerves results. The patient is conscious and this condition has been termed the 'locked-in' syndrome. Voluntary control over ventilation is lost. The respiratory pattern is usually completely regular [2330] with very little breath-to-breath variation in V_T/T_I [2297]. Cheyne-Stokes respiration, which cannot be modified by voluntary effort, may appear [2496].

Medullary disorders

Lesions in the medulla that selectively damage the corticospinal respiratory pathways are rare. They may be seen in multiple sclerosis (p. 113). There is one report of infarction of the medullary pyramids due to syphilitic arteritis [2137]. Ventilation was adequate to maintain life for several weeks but the respiratory rate was regular, in keeping with a disorder of voluntary respiratory control.

Spinal cord lesions

Involvement of the voluntary respiratory pathways in the spinal cord is particularly important if this is above the level of the phrenic nerve nucleus. Selective damage by disease is very rare at this level of the cervical cord, but can occur with multiple sclerosis (p. 113). Surgical interruption of the corticospinal tracts has been carried out for Parkinson's disease [2362]. Unilateral section did not cause any respiratory problems, but simultaneous bilateral operations were occasionally associated with cyanosis and pneumonia.

Chapter 11
Disorders of Automatic Control of Respiration

The automatic control of respiration is closely integrated with the voluntary control (Chapter 1). If the latter is damaged, changes in the automatic control of respiration are seen. These include Cheyne-Stokes respiration and post-hyperventilation apnoea, which appear when the medullary respiratory centres are released from inhibition by the cerebral cortex. Damage to the automatic control of respiration itself may impair the ventilatory response to hypoxia and hypercapnia, and disturb the respiratory rhythm. During wakefulness, respiration is irregular if the metabolic control is abolished, and the respiratory rhythm is determined predominantly by the cerebral cortex. Other well-defined respiratory rhythms, such as apneusis and central neurogenic hyperventilation, are seen with lesions at specific sites (Chapter 5). Hypoventilation may be present during wakefulness but it is a characteristic of damage to the automatic respiratory control that the blood gases can be temporarily returned to normal by voluntary hyperventilation. Tests of voluntary functions, such as the FEV_1, FVC and PEFR, are normal and the lung volumes are normal.

The commonest but, until recently, little-recognized consequence of a failure of the automatic control of respiration is hypoventilation during sleep. Several of the physiological changes in breathing during sleep (Chapter 3) are modified if the automatic control of respiration is damaged. Respiration is particularly dependent on automatic control during NREM sleep and if it fails prolonged central sleep apnoeas appear (Chapter 6). Hypercapnia and hypoxia normally cause arousal, but the thresholds for this response are often abnormal in disorders of automatic respiratory control, so that even severe hypoventilation may not waken the subject.

The tone of all the respiratory muscles except for the diaphragm is diminished in REM sleep so that the FRC falls and ventilation/perfusion mismatching worsens. Respiration becomes more dependent on the diaphragm, and severe hypoxia will develop if this is weak. The importance of changes in upper airway resistance is uncertain but obstructive sleep apnoeas are common, particularly if there are anatomical abnormalities that narrow the upper airway. Each of these mechanisms can cause profound hypoxia and lead to long-term complications, such as polycythaemia, pulmonary hypertension and right heart failure.

INDIVIDUAL DISORDERS

The normal functioning of the automatic control of respiration can be interrupted at various anatomical sites. The most important of these are:

Carotid body

The carotid bodies contain the chemoreceptors responsible for hypoxic control of ventilation and, to a lesser extent, the hypercapnic respiratory drive (Chapter 1). They hypertrophy in response to chronic hypoxia [1790, 1791]. As a consequence, their weight correlates with the weight of the right ventricle [887, 1391], which also increases in chronic hypoxia.

Paraganglionomas are associated with hypoxia, whether this is caused by disease or by altitude [1268, 1390]. The carotid bodies also hypertrophy in the presence of systemic hypertension, even in the absence of lung disease [887, 1391–1393]. This raises the possibility that they are also baroreceptors or that hypertension is related to chronic hypoxia (p. 51).

Hypertrophy of the carotid bodies may, therefore, indicate chronic hypoxia or hypertension, but conversely dysfunction of the carotid bodies may be the cause of hypoxia. This is difficult to diagnose and is, therefore, possibly wrongly, thought to be rare. It should be suspected if the ventilatory response to hypoxia is diminished out of proportion to the ventilatory response to hypercapnia and if there is no other pulmonary, neurological or chest wall disorder. An identical picture can be produced by disorders of the carotid sinus nerve, for example by surgery or possibly in familial dysautonomia, or even by disturbances of the respiratory centres and their pathways within the medulla.

The occurrence of diminished hypoxic ventilatory responses in several members of a family [1486, 2206] may be due to abnormalities of carotid body function. Some patients with central alveolar hypoventilation have absent or very diminished ventilatory responses to hypoxia [955, 2689, 3312], possibly because of non-functioning carotid bodies. This may also be the cause of some fatalities in the sudden infant-death syndrome in which histological changes in the carotid bodies are common [608, 2269]. Carotid body dysfunction may also predispose to ventilatory depression by sedative drugs [208].

Most of the data concerning carotid body abnormalities in man have, however, been obtained from subjects who underwent carotid body resection as treatment for asthma, particularly in the 1940s and 1950s. This was one of a variety of operations on the autonomic nervous system that were popular at that time, including resection of the posterior pulmonary plexus, stellate ganglion block, cervical and thoracic sympathectomy, and vagotomy [7, 222, 315, 1704]. The benefits claimed for these operations [2276, 2844, 3357] were never objectively substantiated and were little different from the results of sham operations [2065, 3368]. More recently, carotid body function has been studied following carotid endarterectomy. In this operation, the nerve to the carotid sinus as well as that to the carotid body is often damaged [3356], in contrast to carotid body resection in which the carotid sinus nerve is not affected. Carotid endarterectomy is, therefore, accompanied by temporary loss of postural control over blood pressure and longer lasting hypertension, in addition to impairment of hypoxic ventilatory responses [1460, 3247].

Unilateral resection of a carotid body has far less effect on respiratory control than bilateral resection. The ventilatory response to hypoxia is about 50% normal [1463] and the arterial P_{CO_2} rises only slightly [3105]. In contrast, after bilateral resection there is very little increase in ventilation in response to breathing hypoxic gas mixtures [231, 360, 529, 1460, 1463, 1958, 1960, 3357]. Injection of lignocaine around the 9th and 10th nerves has similar effects [1314]. The virtual abolition of the hypoxic response after bilateral carotid body resection indicates that in man the aortic bodies contribute very little to the ventilatory response to hypoxia. However, a slight response to hypoxia may be seen in the presence of hypercapnia [3123]. This may originate in the aortic bodies or from the neuroma-like regeneration that has been described after section of the carotid sinus nerve [2192].

The carotid bodies also contribute to the increase in ventilation in response to hypercapnia. The ventilatory response to hypercapnia after carotid body resection is slightly diminished [1460, 1958]. The arterial P_{CO_2} remains normal at rest, although it may rise slightly during exercise [1462, 1958, 3263].

Breathlessness on exertion is uncommon after bilateral carotid body resection, and this may be one reason why it was initially thought to be beneficial in asthma [529, 721]. The breath-holding time is prolonged [898], which may be hazardous during, for instance, underwater swimming when severe hypoxia can develop [529, 721]. The prolongation of the breath-holding time is greatest in hypoxic conditions [721, 3308], but an increase is also detectable during hyperoxia [721] and when breathing air [1315]. The normal bradycardia during breath-holding is not seen, revealing the influence of the carotid bodies on cardiac as well as respiratory control [711, 1266].

The pattern of respiration in normal subjects at sea level at rest is not altered by carotid body denervation [1315]. However, oscillations in the arterial P_{O_2} and P_{CO_2} have an important influence on ventilation [907] and, at least in dogs, transient increases in P_{CO_2} after carotid body denervation shorten the next expiration [358] and a single deep breath prolongs the next expiration [359]. Further studies of these transient changes in ventilation in carotid body disorders are required.

During sleep the carotid bodies normally increase ventilation in response to hypoxia and cause arousal when hypoxia develops. Arousal in response to hypoxia only occurs if the carotid bodies are functioning [3094] and is independent of the ventilatory response to hypoxia. Carotid body denervation does not influence arousal during sleep from other causes, such as laryngeal stimulation [360]. Carotid body dysfunction may therefore be important in the failure to terminate sleep apnoeas and to awaken during periods of nocturnal hypoxia. In one reported case, obstructive apnoeas were severe enough to cause marked ventilatory failure [2406(b)]. The hormonal responses to hypoxia, such as an increase in antidiuretic hormone and corticosteriod levels in the blood, are also mediated by the carotid bodies [2548].

Hypothalamus

Hypothalamic and pituitary lesions are surprisingly rarely associated with disorders of ventilation. Alteration of the control of the body temperature will modify respiration but the somnolence of hypothalamic and pituitary disorders is only rarely due to alveolar hypoventilation [406, 614, 998, 2230]. In most of these cases the hypoventilation may have been secondary to the obesity rather than to any defect in automatic control of respiration. Biochemical abnormalities of hypothalamic and pituitary function, such as impaired prolactin secretion, are not associated with significant oxygen desaturation during sleep [95, 1729].

Midbrain

The experimentally induced changes in ventilation (p. 7) have not been observed with midbrain lesions in man. This region does, however, contain important areas of the reticular formation as well as the corticobulbar and corticospinal fibres whose interruption would be expected to modify respiration.

Pons and medulla

The most important lesions that impair the automatic control of respiration are those within the pons and medulla. These contain the respiratory centres as well as much of the reticular formation. Several characteristic respiratory rhythms are seen (Chapter 5) and nocturnal hypoventilation is an important complication. Lesions within the pons and medulla are frequently associated with dysfunction of the bulbar muscles, leading to complications such as aspiration pneumonia and stridor.

Several metabolic disorders and pathological conditions within the pons and medulla may influence the automatic control of respiration (Table 4.1). These include:

HAEMORRHAGE

Haemorrhages within the medulla or pons are often fatal but if the patient survives, apnoeas and a variety of other abnormal respiratory rhythms such as gasping, grunting, tachypnoea or a short-cycle type of Cheyne-Stokes respiration may be seen [1623, 3037].

INFARCTION

Automatic respiratory control is only impaired by infarction in the medulla if this is bilateral or if it interrupts the descending fibres from the medullary respiratory centres where they decussate in the region of the obex. Survival after bilateral infarction is rare. The voluntary control of respiration is preserved, but respiratory arrests occur during sleep. These may require mechanical ventilation. Autopsy examination has confirmed either bilateral medullary infarction [784] or damage in the region of decussation of descending fibres from the medullary respiratory centres [1872].

The lateral medullary syndrome, due to infarction in the territory of the posterior inferior cerebellar artery, may occasionally be associated with somnolence and hypoventilation [1505]. Obstructive rather than central apnoeas occur and are probably due to the palatal, pharyngeal and vocal cord paralysis causing obstruction of the upper airway [536].

TRAUMA

Head injuries may interrupt the automatic respiratory control pathways, as well as those serving voluntary respiratory control (p. 112). A wide range of respiratory dysrhythmias may be seen either as a direct result of the injury or indirectly through damage to the cerebral vasculature or a rise in the intracranial pressure. The picture may be complicated by other factors such as drug overdosage, alcohol, aspiration pneumonia, chest trauma and occasionally fat embolism or neurogenic pulmonary oedema. Central alveolar hypoventilation is an occasional long-term complication [103, 1139].

NEUROSURGERY

The respiratory consequences of neurosurgery are dealt with in standard textbooks and their physiological consequences have been reviewed [1052(a)]. The effects on respiration reflect not only the surgery and the underlying condition but also complications, such as haematoma and oedema, which increase the intracranial pressure. Cheyne-Stokes respiration is usually associated with supratentorial surgery. Posterior fossa surgery may lead to a variety of respiratory patterns, including apneusis [1437, 1745, 1750, 3072]. Stridor due to vocal cord palsy, difficulty with swallowing leading to aspiration pneumonia and a temporary failure of automatic respiratory control causing sleep apnoeas are well recognized.

TUMOURS

The respiratory consequences of brain stem tumours depend largely on their situation, the rise of intracranial pressure and their effects on the cerebral circulation. Clearcut alterations in the automatic control of respiration are rarely seen. Hypercapnia, which improved with radiotherapy, has been documented [1491] and central neurogenic hyperventilation has been recorded [1805].

ENCEPHALITIS

The effects of encephalitis on the voluntary control of respiration have been described previously (p. 112). Any of the complications discussed in the introduction to this chapter may be seen if the brain stem is involved and automatic respiratory control is impaired.

Rabies encephalitis is unusual in that spasms of the pharynx, larynx and inspiratory muscles, including the diaphragm, may occur even during minor stimulation such as attempting to drink [565]. Spasms of all the inspiratory muscles may cause a prolonged cessation of breathing [3260]. These features are probably due to brain stem encephalitis. Less commonly, a flaccid paralysis develops and leads to respiratory failure [3121] and aspiration pneumonia. Early tracheostomy and intensive-care support is required [695, 1154, 1380].

Late respiratory complications of encephalitis are also recognized. The ventilatory responses to hypoxia and hypercapnia may be diminished [652, 703, 3312]. Central alveolar hypoventilation may develop many years after encephalitis lethargica [894, 1087, 3077] (p. 116), Western equine encephalitis [603, 3312] and probably

other types of viral encephalitis [652, 703, 1596].
Central alveolar hypoventilation following encephalitis may present in childhood [2704].

POLIOMYELITIS

Important disorders of the automatic control of
respiration are a feature of acute poliomyelitis
and are also seen as late complications of this
infection. They are described in Chapter 12.

SYPHILIS

Central alveolar hypoventilation has been
documented in syphilis [2687, 2689] but its
mechanism is obscure. The ventilatory response
to hypoxia is diminished in tabes dorsalis, possibly because of a sensory neuropathy of the 9th
cranial nerve that interrupts afferent impulses
from the carotid body [673]. Sleep apnoeas may
be severe enough to cause nocturnal fits [1778].
Infarction of the medullary pyramids due to
syphilitic arteritis has also been reported [2137]
(p. 116).

MULTIPLE SCLEROSIS

Alterations in the automatic control of respiration, as well as in voluntary control of respiration, are recognized but are uncommon. The
ventilatory response to hypoxia [2640] and to
hypercapnia [640, 1731, 2640, 3229] are usually
normal and the $P_{0.1}$ during hypercapnia is also
normal [3229]. Respiratory dysrhythmias such
as a persistent hiccough [345] may occasionally
be seen. Respiratory arrest during sleep is rare
but has been correlated with autopsy demonst-
ration of demyelination in the medulla, particularly around the obex in the region where the
descending fibres from the medullary respiratory centres decussate [345]. Bilateral diaphragmatic weakness may also cause severe nocturnal
hypoxia without any primary defect of respiratory control, since in REM sleep respiration is
almost totally dependent on normal diaphragmatic function.

MOTOR NEURON DISEASE

Defects in the automatic control of respiration
are rare in motor neuron disease (p. 136), but
there is one case report in which this may have
been present [2140].

SYRINGOBULBIA

Syringobulbia is closely allied to syringomyelia
(p. 135). The fissure-like clefts that extend into
the brain stem can interrupt the corticobulbar
and corticospinal fibres. This may have been
the cause of the single report of cyanotic attacks
occurring during wakefulness in a three-month-
old child in whom a neurenteric cyst had rup-
tured causing a syringobulbia [573].

Involvement of the nucleus ambiguus in the
medulla is more common [43, 1347]. The two
halves of this nucleus are close to each other
and both may be damaged by the syrinx. This
leads to a flaccid paralysis, particularly of the
abductor muscles of the vocal cords so that the
cords adduct. Severe air flow obstruction with
stridor results [43, 2564, 2836, 3342] and this
may cause sudden death unless tracheostomy is
performed. Obstructive sleep apnoeas also occur
and may be severe enough to cause nocturnal
pulmonary hypertension [1347]. They may be
relieved by a nasopharyngeal airway or nasal
CPAP, suggesting that impairment of
pharyngeal innervation as well as a vocal cord
palsy may be important [1347, 3226].
Pharyngeal and palatal weakness and failure of
the cricopharyngeus to relax may also cause recurrent aspiration pneumonias [2328, 2564].

Extension of the syrinx into the brain stem
may penetrate the respiratory centres or their
efferent pathways. Central alveolar hypoventilation has been reported [1139, 2689] and central
sleep apnoeas have been documented in a patient
in whom autopsy examination subsequently
showed the syrinx reaching the nucleus tractus
solitarius [850]. Cardiovascular reflexes may be
deranged; postural hypotension is the commonest complication [2328].

AUTONOMIC DISORDERS

Acquired autonomic disorders, e.g. due to diabetes, are common, but the rarer familial and idiopathic conditions also have important respiratory complications. Familial dysautonomia (Riley-Day syndrome) presents early in life with motor abnormalities, particularly of the parasympathetic system and a sensory neuropathy [2623, 2624]. Scoliosis is common [1408] but is usually of little respiratory significance. Multiple system atrophy includes the Shy-Drager syndrome, olivopontocerebellar atrophy and striatonigral degeneration. In these conditions, neuronal degeneration is widespread but most marked in the basal ganglia, cerebellum and inferior olives. Control of the sympathetic nervous system is defective and is manifested by postural hypotension and other abnormal cardiovascular reflexes [561]. The brain stem respiratory centres share in the widespread degeneration.

The voluntary control of ventilation appears to be completely normal in these disorders. The ability to reproduce a breath of a given tidal volume is maintained [2023] and the initial increase in ventilation on exercise is unimpaired [900]. However, abnormalities of automatic respiratory control are detectable in each of the types of autonomic disorder. In familial dysautonomia, the ventilatory response to hypercapnia is diminished but there is conflicting evidence concerning the response to hypoxia [878, 880, 977]. The breath-holding time is prolonged. Breath-holding spells may lead to unconsciousness in children [2623] and drowning, presumably due to hypoxic cardiac dysrhythmias, has been reported [977]. In multiple system atrophy both hypoxic and hypercapnic ventilatory drives are normal [1924], but in diabetes the response to hypercapnia is diminished [1461], although hypoxic control appears to be normal [467]. In acquired dysautonomias associated with amyloidosis [900] and tabes dorsalis [673], the ventilatory response to hypoxia is decreased.

These abnormalities of automatic control of respiration probably lead to central alveolar hypoventilation in some cases [1031]. Sleep apnoeas may be central [18, 561, 1031, 1065, 1276, 2586] but may be predominantly obstructive [398, 1276, 1303, 1854]. Reflex responses to gastro-oesophageal reflux may be responsible for some of these apnoeas [1276], and vocal cord palsy (see below) may contribute to obstructive apnoeas. Sleep apnoeas occur particularly in NREM sleep [561, 1295] and, in multiple system atrophy, are more frequent when the patient is erect rather than supine [563]. They are often an early feature, and may be useful in predicting the progression of autonomic dysfunction [2023]. The nocturnal desaturation may be severe enough to raise the pulmonary artery pressure through a direct effect of hypoxia on the pulmonary microcirculation. In multiple system atrophy, hypoxia is not associated with systemic hypertension because the autonomic vasoconstrictor reflexes are defective [1303, 1854].

The derangements of the automatic control of respiration are also responsible for several abnormal respiratory rhythms. These include cluster respirations [1924] and apneusis [171], which appear during wakefulness as well as sleep.

Bilateral paralysis of the abductor muscles of the vocal cords occurs in multiple system atrophy, but not in the other causes of autonomic neuropathy. Parkinsonism is also frequent in multiple system atrophy, but neither sleep apnoeas nor vocal cord paralysis correlate with the presence of Parkinsonian features [1137, 2023, 3340]. The vocal cord palsy causes stridor, which may be very loud and intermittent but can occur at night as well as during the day. Voice abnormalities are frequent [1343]. Sleep apnoeas are common in the presence of a vocal cord palsy [18, 1651], and fatal respiratory arrest during sleep may occur [3340]. Histological examination of the posterior cricoarytenoid muscles, which are the sole abductors of the vocal cords, has shown changes indicating denervation [170]. This has been confirmed by surface laryngeal EMGs [1137]. The abductor paralysis is, therefore, probably due to degeneration of the nucleus ambiguus. Lateralization of the vocal cords [1651] or a tracheostomy may be required [1132, 1540].

CENTRAL ALVEOLAR HYPOVENTILATION

The concept of central alveolar hypoventilation and its relationship to sleep apnoeas has been discussed in Chapter 6. In this chapter, its aetiology and the physiological and clinical features are described.

Aetiology

The cardinal feature of central alveolar hypoventilation is that the ventilatory responses to hypercapnia or hypoxia, or both, are diminished or absent. This suggests an abnormality in the medulla or possibly the upper cervical cord or carotid bodies. Abnormalities of the brain stem auditory-evoked potentials have been recorded both in infants [212] and in adults [1934]. However, in most of the reported cases of both congenital and adult onset of central alveolar hypoventilation, no cause has been apparent either clinically or on histological examination of the brain [648, 1052(b), 1833, 2391(b), 2395(b), 3048]. This has led to the supposition that the defect may be at a subcellular level or even that cells with a specific neurotransmitter, such as 5HT, might be deficient [1325, 3048]. In one report a urinary thiamine pyrophosphate inhibitor was present [1937]. In other cases, slight abnormalities in the brain stem, such as a deficiency of the number of neurons in the region of the medullary respiratory centres, have been detected both in infants [1922] and in adults [103, 1031, 2267]. An increased number of capillaries has been noted [2267, 2852], which may be relevant to the increased blood flow to the brain stem that has been reported in patients with sleep apnoeas [2138].

Central alveolar hypoventilation in infants may occur with other congenital abnormalities, such as absence of the external arcuate nucleus [1014] (which has embryological connections with the region of the medullary carbon dioxide receptors), ptosis and dysconjugate gaze [1922], hypotonia [773, 1922] and Hirschsprung's disease [1294, 1325, 3048]. It can rarely be the presenting feature of an astrocytoma [1645] or result from previous encephalitis [2704] or Reye's syndrome [2357]. In older children there may be an association with hypothalamic disease [998, 2230] or autonomic disorders [1031].

Previous encephalitis or poliomyelitis are the most frequently recognized causes of central alveolar hypoventilation in adults, but its appearance may be delayed for many years after the acute episode. Early reports associated central alveolar hypoventilation with a variety of other conditions, but in many cases little evidence was provided to support the diagnosis. The proposed associated conditions are syringomyelia [1139, 2689], severe hypoglycaemia [2689], head injury [103, 1139], mental retardation [2689], syphilis [2687, 2689], brain stem cysts [1139], gliomas [1491], strokes [1143], cyanotic heart disease [1499] and taurine deficiency [2444, 2542]. Correction of the underlying disorder may improve the central alveolar hypoventilation [1491, 1499].

Physiological features

A diminished or even absent ventilatory response to hypercapnia can be demonstrated in most patients with both the congenital [195, 1004, 1521, 2867, 3289] and adult [36, 213, 1227, 1596, 1723, 2566, 2999, 3312] forms of central alveolar hypoventilation (see Fig. 9.5).

A slight but temporary increase in ventilation may be seen, possibly due to activity of the carbon dioxide receptors in the carotid bodies [1004]. In some infants [195, 3289] and adults [1014, 1087], ventilation is diminished by inhalation of pure oxygen, indicating that the hypoxic chemoreceptor influence on ventilation is still present. The ventilatory response to hypoxia may even be normal [2283] but is often diminished [955, 2689, 3312] (Fig. 9.5).

The nature and exact site of the defect in automatic respiratory control, therefore, probably differs from subject to subject and this may be why it has proved difficult to equate central alveolar hypoventilation with any single form of sleep apnoea.

Hypoventilation due to these abnormal ventilatory responses is most apparent during sleep, particularly NREM sleep [195, 1325, 1428]. The ventilatory response to hypercapnia is less during NREM sleep than in either REM sleep or wakefulness [1004]. Sleep apnoeas are more frequent during NREM sleep [648, 1294, 1325] and both central and obstructive apnoeas may be seen [536, 1141, 1428, 1645]. Other respiratory patterns, such as irregular breathing [432, 1326, 2281, 2360, 2787], shallow but regular respirations [193, 2404], bradypnoea [224] and very infrequent sighs or deep breaths [2281] have been recognized.

The automatic control of respiration is severely deranged in central alveolar hypoventilation, but voluntary control is invariably retained [997]. Voluntary hyperventilation is able to return the arterial blood gases virtually to normal [1227, 2999, 3190], and this has been used as a diagnostic test. The breath-holding time is greatly prolonged [603, 2566], even to over 200 sec [1515]. The ventilatory response to exercise is variable. It is usually less than normal [1515, 2566] but may be sufficient to prevent a further deterioration in the arterial blood gases [2687]. Cyanosis may, however, appear on exertion [432, 2614] and the P_{CO_2} may rise [1087] (Fig. 11.1).

Clinical features

Central alveolar hypoventilation is usually diagnosed either in infancy or between the ages of twenty and fifty. In each age group, the presenting features are remarkably stereotyped and largely reflect the consequences of the ventilatory failure itself.

In infants, usually boys, periods of apnoea or cyanosis may be noticed often within a few hours of birth, but occasionally not for several months.

They may occur during feeding or chest infections [648] and hypoxic fits are common [1014, 3379]. Anti-epileptic drugs make these more frequent because of their respiratory sedative action [1014]. Occasionally, however, epilepsy may be due to the underlying disease, such as a glioma, which is also responsible for hypoventilation [1645]. Recurrent chest infections, which may even lead to bronchiectasis, can be a problem and may be related to oesophageal motilty disorders [648]. Right heart failure develops after a few months, due to pulmonary hypertension secondary to chronic hypoxia. The prognosis without ventilatory assistance is poor, and death usually occurs during sleep.

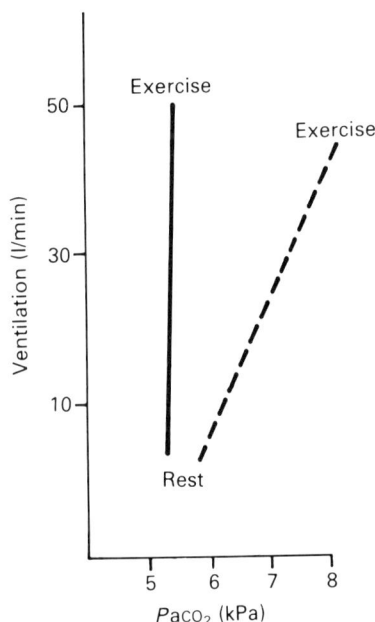

Fig. 11.1. *Ventilatory responses to exercise in normal subjects (continuous line) and central alveolar hypoventilation (broken line). In the latter, the increase in ventilation is insufficient to maintain a normal P_{CO_2}.*

In adults, breathlessness even during exertion is uncommon [2025, 3072], presumably because the defective medullary respiratory centres do not generate enough impulses to drive the respiratory muscles or stimulate the cerebral cortex sufficiently. Symptoms due to the blood gas abnormalities are prominent and may present for several years before medical attention is sought. Somnolence during the day [1515, 1955], early morning headache [445], inability to concentrate, failure of memory, personality change, decrease in libido and frequent episodes of waking at night are common. Carbon dioxide retention may be severe enough for papilloedema to be seen [2978], and central cyanosis, particularly during sleep and on exertion, is frequent.

Right heart failure often develops [193, 2025] and the ECG may show right atrial and right ventricular hypertrophy. The pulmonary artery pressure may be normal [1311] but, in severe cases, it is raised [432, 603, 998, 1035, 1052(b), 1515, 1833, 3190] and increases abnormally rapidly during exercise [603]. Pulmonary hypertension also worsens during episodes of hypoxia [1428], which may be associated with cardiac dysrhythmias [1280, 2969].

Polycythaemia is less common than might be expected from the duration of the symptoms, but it can be severe [571] and may even be confused with polycythaemia rubra vera [2293]. Relief of hypoxia lessens the polycythaemia [3093].

The prognosis of central alveolar hypoventilation in adults is uncertain. If it follows a specific illness, such as encephalitis or acute poliomyelitis, gradual improvement may be seen [3312], but only rarely does this occur in idiopathic cases [1326, 2360]. Even in these, there may be no change in the ventilatory response to hypercapnia [2360]. Death usually occurs at night, presumably because of a cardiac dysrhythmia induced by hypoxia.

HYPOTHYROIDISM

It has long been recognized that some patients in myxoedema coma have a high P_{CO_2}, even allowing for the difficulties in blood gas analysis at low body temperatures [810, 2309, 2331, 3409]. Hypercapnia probably contributes to, but is not the only cause of, the coma. In less-severely hypothyroid subjects, a slow respiratory frequency while awake [810, 2331] and central apnoeas during sleep [2001, 2174] have been documented. Both the central apnoeas and hypercapnia while awake appear to be related to the diminished ventilatory responses to hypercapnia [2081, 2174, 3409] and hypoxia [2174, 3409]. It is uncertain whether these changes in ventilatory drive are purely secondary to the low metabolic rate or are due to a specific effect of hypothyroidism. Treatment with thyroxine lessens the frequency of the apnoeas and improves daytime somnolence [2174].

METABOLIC ALKALOSIS

The ventilatory response to carbon dioxide is reduced in the presence of a metabolic alkalosis. The CSF bicarbonate concentration adapts slowly because the blood–brain barrier is impermeable to bicarbonate and equilibration takes place only by diffusion of carbon dioxide. Nevertheless, ventilation is reduced by a metabolic alkalosis, whatever its cause [2498]. Cheyne-Stokes respiration may be seen and central apnoeas occur, particularly in NREM sleep. Their frequency can be reduced by correction of the alkalosis with, for instance, acetazolamide, but obstructive apnoeas may develop [1517, 2876, 2909].

SEDATIVE DRUGS AND ALCOHOL

Sedative drugs and alcohol have several important effects on ventilation [67, 1300, 1421, 2665]. They reduce the level of consciousness, impair voluntary respiratory control, lessen the ventilatory response to hypoxia and hypercapnia, and may reduce the tone of the upper airway and chest wall muscles. These effects are discussed on p. 68. The most important of the sedative drugs are opiates, benzodiazepines, barbiturates and general anaesthetic agents.

Spinal cord

The descending fibres leaving the medullary respiratory centres enter the spinal cord and can be interrupted selectively by disease or trauma. The most important cause is high cervical cordotomy (p. 128), since the fibres leading to the phrenic nerve nuclei are unaffected by lesions below the level of C3–C5.

Chapter 12
Disorders of the Spinal Cord

The spinal cord contains the descending pathways that serve both voluntary and automatic control of respiration and converge on the motor neurons in the nuclei of the peripheral nerves. Afferent impulses from many types of receptor enter the spinal cord and initiate intra- and intersegmental reflexes (Chapter 1). Disorders of the spinal cord may interfere with the functioning of one or more of these components of respiratory control. Spinal cord lesions are particularly important at or above the level of the phrenic nerve nuclei (C3–C5), since lesions at lower levels will not interfere with the functioning of the diaphragm.

Interruption of automatic pathways in the spinal cord leads to similar physiological and clinical consequences to those seen with medullary disease. Abnormalities of bulbar function are absent but autonomic changes and damage to other spinal cord tracts may be seen. If the normal inhibitory influences on the motor neurons are abolished, the respiratory muscles become spastic and intermittent increases in muscle tone (spasms) may be prominent. Damage to the α motor neurons weakens the respiratory muscles. The consequences of this are described in Chapter 15.

INDIVIDUAL DISORDERS

The most important individual disorders of the spinal cord that affect ventilation are:

Cervical cordotomy

Cervical cordotomy is carried out with the aim of interrupting fibres in the anterolateral spinothalamic tract and thereby alleviating pain. Cordotomy was first performed in 1912 [3019] and for many years an open surgical approach was used. With the introduction of percutaneous cordotomy in the 1960s [1026, 1401, 2248, 2249], the indications for cordotomy widened. Both methods are equally effective and pain relief is prolonged and worthwhile in over 40% of patients with severe non-malignant pain [1548, 1794].

The anterolateral spinothalamic tract is closely related to the descending fibres from the medullary respiratory centres [1026, 1438] (Fig. 12.1). Respiratory complications of cordotomy are common and it may even be impossible to achieve pain relief without injuring the respiratory pathways [236]. Although the automatic control of respiration is deranged by cordotomy,

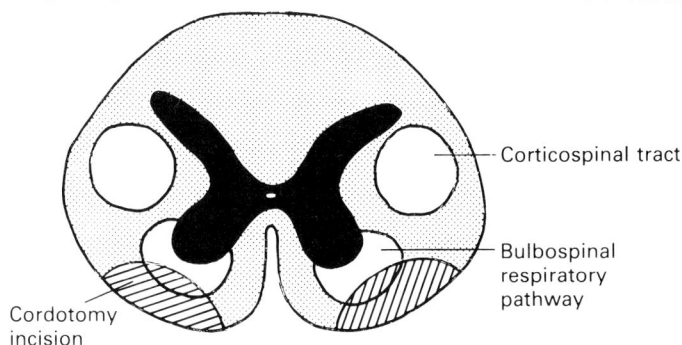

Fig. 12.1. *Site of spinal cord lesion after cordotomy.*

the corticospinal tracts are not affected. They run separately, more dorsally; unilateral paralysis of the respiratory muscles can occur without a hemiparesis, which would be expected if the corticospinal tracts were damaged [2279]. It has been postulated that afferent pathways to the medullary respiratory centres are interrupted by cordotomy [1748, 1782], but there is no direct evidence for this.

The fibres from the brain stem respiratory centres are damaged, particularly if lesions are created within the spinal cord more than 3 mm from its margin [236, 1438] and just lateral to the exit of the ventral root [2279]. Weakness of the respiratory muscles appears on the same side as the cordotomy [1026, 2279]. Diaphragmatic paralysis is seen if the most anterior fibres are damaged [1438]. Inspiratory and expiratory fibres are, however, not completely separable [237].

Unilateral cordotomy hardly affects voluntary respiratory manoeuvres such as the FVC, MVV and PI_{max} and PE_{max} [2709, 3146]. Nevertheless, intra-operative recordings have shown that immediately after a unilateral high cervical cordotomy the ipsilateral intercostal EMG amplitude is diminished and the tidal volume of the ipsilateral lung falls [2279]. Temporary diaphragmatic paralysis on the side of the cordotomy is common [2352] and has been demonstrated by fluoroscopy [1438]. The tidal volume and minute ventilation fall and the respiratory frequency rises both during and for a short while after surgery [236, 1438, 1782, 2709]. Sleep apnoeas are rarely seen [1782], since the respiratory muscles are represented bilaterally in the medullary respiratory centres. Those patients who do develop respiratory complications usually have pre-existing lung disease [3146]. This is often a bronchial carcinoma in the contralateral lung. Post-operatively, a combination of the diseased lung with impaired respiratory muscle function on the side of the cordotomy may cause respiratory failure.

Complications are much more frequent following bilateral cordotomy. Disturbance of bladder and bowel function [1548], hypotension [236, 1753], confusion and hypersomnolence [1755] may appear in addition to the respiratory complications. The latter were not originally considered to be frequent [3060, 3316] but lesions at C4 and higher segments are now recognized to be particularly liable to cause respiratory problems [1026]. The patient may feel unable to breathe deeply enough [1753] but the breath-holding time is not prolonged [1782], presumably because fibres from the medullary centres to the cerebral cortex are still intact, in contrast to those entering the spinal cord.

The changes in tidal volume and respiratory frequency described with unilateral cordotomy are seen [236, 2709] together with a fall in VC [1782, 3146]. However, the most important abnormalities appear during sleep. Sleep apnoeas are frequent, particularly during the first post-operative week, and may be fatal [1025, 1044, 1753, 2249, 2434, 2709, 2861, 3146]. They usually persist for only a few nights, but occasionally may be present for several weeks [554, 1753, 3146] or even longer [1755, 2507]. The ventilatory response to hypercapnia is decreased [1746, 1753] and there is some evidence that this finding can predict which patients will develop sleep apnoeas [2709]. Sleep apnoeas and changes in VC and ventilatory response to hypercapnia are also seen after other types of anterior spinal surgery in the upper cervical cord [976, 1746, 1754].

The risk of respiratory complications with bilateral cordotomy is greatest if the cordotomies are performed simultaneously [236]. If bilateral cordotomy is required, the second operation should be carried out at least several weeks after the first procedure and lower in the cervical cord [2430, 3293]. Respiratory depressants should be avoided post-operatively, since they exacerbate sleep apnoeas. Aminophylline may be of benefit [554] but mechanical ventilation may be required for a few nights post-operatively [2861, 3146].

Trauma and other causes of quadriplegia

A wide variety of spinal cord lesions can lead to quadriplegia, with its serious respiratory

consequences. These include vascular abnormalities, tumours, developmental abnormalities, transverse myelitis, infarction and
trauma. The respiratory complications depend
to a certain extent on the rate of progression of
the condition, but more importantly on the exact
level of the lesion in the spinal cord and its
degree of completeness. The most important
consideration is whether or not the diaphragm
is paralysed because of damage to C3–C5 segments. Several of the accessory muscles of respiration are also supplied from the cervical cord.
Lesions lower in the spinal cord may paralyse
the intercostal muscles that are innervated by
T1–T12, the abdominal muscles supplied by
T7–L1, or the muscles of the pelvic floor that
are supplied by L1–S2.

The respiratory consequences of trauma to
the spinal cord have been studied much more
thoroughly than the other conditions that lead
to quadriplegia. The remainder of this section
will, therefore, deal with the features seen following trauma, although many aspects are common to all the causes of quadriplegia.

Trauma to the spinal cord differs from the
other conditions in that its onset is usually instantaneous. Following spinal cord injury,
'spinal shock' persists for several weeks and is
manifested by hypotonicity. The early mortality
from respiratory complications is high, unless
skilled medical care is given [1563]. Respiratory
problems remain an important cause of death
in the first few months after the injury [2567]
and subsequently [225], although other complications such as renal failure become increasingly
prominent [2340]. If the spinal cord injury occurs before the adolescent growth spurt,
scoliosis frequently develops. Bracing of the
spine at an early stage may slow its progression,
but spinal fusion may be needed [414].

HIGH CERVICAL CORD INJURY

A traumatic complete transverse lesion of the
spinal cord, at the level of C4 or above, usually
causes sudden death unless immediate resuscitation is possible [508]. The only residual func-

tioning respiratory muscles are the sternomastoid and the trapezius, supplied by the 11th
cranial nerve. These are usually unable to maintain sufficient ventilation to support life for long
[3033]. Contraction of these muscles without
any diaphragmatic or intercostal activity elevates the ribs but decreases the lateral diameter
of the lower rib cage [714, 752]. Immediate
IPPV is required and most patients who survive
will require long-term ventilatory support unless function at C4 level returns.

During the stage of spinal shock, tracheal
stimulation, particularly the suction of secretions, may induce severe bradycardia or even
asystole [1563, 2086, 2413]. The mechanism of
this is uncertain but it appears to be due to lack
of compensatory sympathetic reflexes in the presence of hypoxia [711]. This complication can
be treated by atropine and oxygen administration [1032, 2086]. Autonomic dysreflexia may
also cause neurogenic pulmonary oedema, presumably because of increased sympathetic induced vasoconstriction leading to acute hypertension. This may appear spontaneously [2504]
or with minor stimulation, such as traction on
a urinary catheter [1661].

LOW CERVICAL CORD INJURY (Fig. 12.2)

When the lesion in the cervical cord is below
C4–C5, diaphragmatic and cervical accessory
muscle activity is retained but the intercostal
and abdominal muscles are paralysed. The contribution of abdominal expansion to VT and VC
is increased to over 50% [156, 1055, 1056, 1170,
2218]. There is considerable variation between
individuals in the relative expansion of the rib
cage and abdomen [2217, 2218], due largely to
differences in the rib cage and abdominal compliances. The compliance of the abdominal wall
is difficult to measure but it appears to be increased in quadriplegics [223, 258, 930, 1169,
1170]. Although the abdominal muscles may be
spastic, they become atrophied and, on balance,
the abdominal wall is more compliant.

The compliance of the rib cage is less than

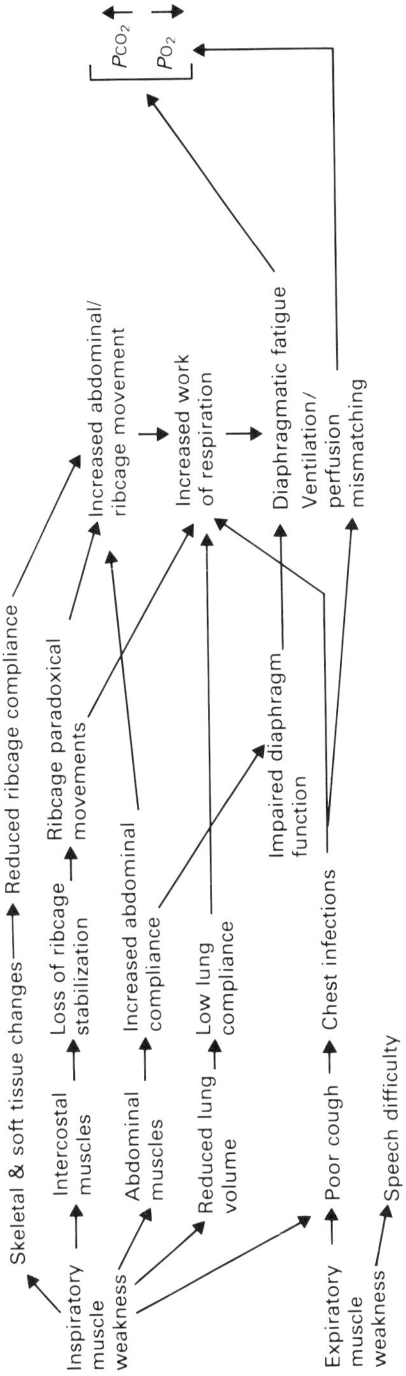

Fig. 12.2. Flow chart to show the effects of low cervical quadriplegia on ventilation.

normal [223, 930], possibly because of spasticity of the intercostal muscles but more probably because of secondary changes in the soft tissues and joints of the rib cage associated with the limited range of respiratory movements. Expansion of the rib cage is limited by the lack of intercostal muscle activity, as well as the decrease in compliance [2223, 2224]. It may even move paradoxically during inspiration, when the diaphragm generates a negative intrathoracic pressure because of loss of the stabilizing effect of intercostal muscle contraction. Paradoxical movement is more marked over the upper rib cage [753, 3213], particularly at low lung volumes when the diaphragmatic fibres are almost parallel to the rib cage and their contraction elevates the lower ribs [714, 753, 2234]. The paradoxical movement and diminished compliance of the rib cage contribute to the increased oxygen consumption during respiration [258, 259, 2926].

The lack of intercostal muscle activity correlates with the fall in lung compliance and FRC [753], probably because of closure of small airways at low lung volumes. There is, however, considerable variation in the extent of intercostal and accessory muscle activity [753, 929]. Much of this represents a stretch reflex rather than true rhythmic respiratory activity. The stretch reflex of the inspiratory intercostal muscles is induced when they are lengthened by paradoxical movement of the rib cage [1309, 2927, 2929]. The stretch reflex should be distinguished from generalized spasms of the intercostal muscles that occasionally occur, inhibiting diaphragmatic activity and causing breathlessness [2929]. Diaphragmatic spasms also occur, particularly in C5 lesions where the innervation of the diaphragm is only partially separated from supraspinal control [2930].

The activity of the intercostal muscles and diaphragm changes during the months after spinal cord injury. Paradoxical movement of the rib cage, which may be obvious initially [1841], improves with time [2218], probably because of both the fall in chest wall compliance and the development of intercostal muscle spasticity.

Diaphragmatic function may return [2474], particularly if the level of the spinal cord lesion falls [144, 2015]. The EMG activity of the diaphragm soon after the injury can be used to predict the degree of eventual recovery of respiratory function [1865]. The VC may increase considerably [144, 507, 1841] and the P_{O_2} may improve [1168].

Postural differences in the VC are prominent in cervical cord lesions if the diaphragm is spared. The VC is maximal in the supine or head-down position [470, 714, 1018, 1317, 2234], in contrast to the postural change with diaphragmatic paralysis (p. 162). In low cervical cord injuries, the excursion of the diaphragm is greater in the supine or head-down position than while sitting, because the weight of the abdominal contents pushes the diaphragm into the thorax during expiration and decreases the residual volume [931]. In the sitting position, the diaphragm remains low during expiration, lessening the ability to take a deep inspiration. Paradoxical movement of the lower rib cage is also minimized in the supine position, because the diaphragm is higher [2234] (see above).

Fatigue of the diaphragm is readily induced in low cervical cord injuries. The causes of this are complex. The work of respiration is increased because of the decreased rib cage compliance and paradoxical rib cage movement. The position of the diaphragm at the beginning of inspiration varies with the posture of the patient (see above) and may not be optimal for its contraction. The diaphragm is also virtually the only inspiratory muscle. This limits the range of muscles that can be recruited when the work of breathing increases or when diaphragmatic fatigue is developing.

Fatigue of the diaphragm may be an important factor in determining whether respiratory failure develops during acute illnesses, such as chest infections. It can be demonstrated readily when an inspiratory resistance is applied [1262, 1263]. Endurance training can improve the EMG features of fatigue and increase the $P_{I_{max}}$ [1262–1264]. Diaphragmatic fatigue is, however, not a feature of the uncomplicated stable state and the MVV is not diminished out of proportion to the VC [259, 1057, 3059(a)].

All the main expiratory muscles are paralysed in cervical cord lesions. Only relatively weak expiratory muscles, such as the clavicular portion of pectoralis major, remain active [750]. Expiration is largely passive and is due to the combination of gravity, elastic recoil of the lungs and, at high lung volumes, elastic recoil of the chest wall as well. The PE_{max} is greatly reduced and is more abnormal than PI_{max} [1055, 2015]. The PEFR, which is effort dependent, is more markedly diminished than the maximal expiratory flow rates at 50% or 25% of the VC, which depend on elastic recoil [1055]. The expiratory reserve volume is very limited [3059(a)] and the inability to exhale fully increases the RV [1053, 3059(a)]. Air flow obstruction does not contribute to this [1057, 1718].

Weakness of the expiratory muscles is largely responsible for the diminished VC seen in cervical cord lesions (Fig. 12.3), but the low TLC also contributes to this [1017, 1055, 1057] (see Fig. 9.7). The TLC is determined by the extent of inspiratory muscle paralysis and the compliance of the chest wall and lungs. Variable

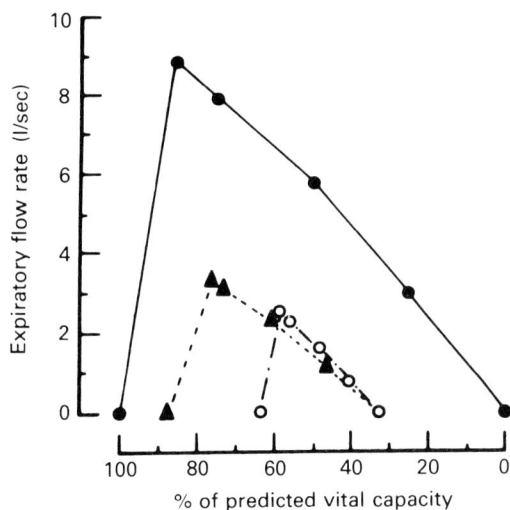

Fig. 12.3. *Expiratory flow rates related to percentage predicted vital capacity in quadriplegia:* (●) *predicted values,* (○) *first week after injury,* (▲) *five months after injury.*

estimates of the lung compliance have been obtained [1055, 1317, 2002, 3059(a)]. This reflects the variation in intercostal muscle activity, which determines the expansion of the underlying lung [753], and the ability to sigh or take deep breaths. The VC is usually between 50% and 70% of the predicted value in complete lesions of the lower cervical cord [259, 1018, 1404, 1718, 2002, 2234, 3059(a)].

Weakness of the expiratory muscles also affects both speech and cough. The voice is usually soft, with little variation in the stress on different words and an inability to articulate long sentences [836]. The volume of air expired during a cough is normal but the peak flow rate and peak oesophageal pressure during coughing are diminished [2234, 2911]. The efficiency of cough is not affected by changes in posture, despite the alterations in VC [1692]. The cough depends more on elastic recoil than on the expiratory muscle activity so that the ability to inspire to a high lung volume is important. The risk of chest infections is determined by the adequacy of the cough and also on the ability to sigh or take deep breaths. Quadriplegic patients who sigh frequently have fewer chest infections than those who cannot sigh [2002]. Frog breathing [2002] and IPPB [1692], which have the same mechanical effect as sighing, can also prevent chest infections. A deep breath not only increases the power of the cough but prevents airway closure and sputum retention. Isotopic techniques have shown that there is little ventilation to the bases of the lungs if there is an inability to sigh [156].

Chest infections are a common and important complication of quadriplegia [2928] and occasionally acute sputum retention presents with loss of consciousness due to acute hypoxia, which simulates a pulmonary embolus. The chest X-ray may be normal but ventilation as well as perfusion is impaired in the affected part of the lung [762].

The arterial blood gases of quadriplegics are remarkably normal despite the extensive respiratory muscle paralysis. This, rather than any abnormality of respiratory control, probably causes the low ventilatory response to CO_2 [2832]. The P_{CO_2} may occasionally be slightly raised [259] but is more often below normal [1057, 1718, 2002, 3059(a)]. The low P_{CO_2} may be the consequence of afferent impulses from lung receptors stimulated by the small lung volumes, or of abnormal reflexes from the respiratory muscles. The arterial oxygen saturation is usually near normal in the stable state after cervical cord injury [1057, 1718, 3059(a)], but hypoxia is present immediately after the injury [1841]. This is due to a variety of factors, including retained secretions, an inability to sigh and suboptimal ventilation/perfusion matching due to defective autonomic control of the pulmonary circulation and airway calibre. Desaturation during sleep is uncommon, except in older subjects or if the diaphragm is weak [393]. The sleep pattern is also abnormal in quadriplegics, in that there is abnormally little REM and stage 3 and 4 NREM sleep [19].

Injuries to the low cervical cord prevent afferent impulses from the chest wall muscles, other than the diaphragm, from reaching the central nervous system. Impulses from the lungs and from receptors in the upper airways are uninterrupted. The ability to detect added loads to respiration may be partially preserved [142, 796], although this varies considerably from patient to patient [143, 2002]. There is no feedback from the muscles of the chest wall to the central nervous system of the tension generated or movement, and this impairs the ability to adapt the pattern of ventilation to changing loads [173, 174, 1205, 1643].

THORACIC AND LUMBAR CORD INJURY

The degree of impairment of ventilation in thoracic cord injuries depends on the level of the spinal cord lesion. The changes in lung volumes and in the FVC and FEV_1 are less marked with low than with upper thoracic cord lesions [1053, 1404, 2354]. Paradoxical movement of the upper rib cage does not occur if only the lower intercostal muscles are paralysed. The VC, MVV, blood gases and ventilation during exercise are usually normal following lumbar spinal cord injuries [1404], but the cough may be impaired because of abdominal muscle weakness [1951].

Friedreich's ataxia

Friedreich's ataxia is the commonest of the spinocerebellar degenerative disorders, although it may be difficult to distinguish from the rarer forms. It involves not only the spinocerebellar tracts but also the dorsal columns and the corticospinal pathways (Fig. 12.4).

It usually becomes apparent in childhood but initially there may be no detectable respiratory or cardiac changes. The first respiratory abnormality is a mild restrictive defect with a normal forced expiratory ratio [441, 3154]. This restrictive defect worsens in adolescence [653] as the neurological deficit deteriorates. The MVV is diminished more than the single breath tests of respiratory function, such as FEV_1 and FVC. This implies that either muscle fatigue develops during the test, or more likely, that coordination of rapid respiratory movements is impaired as in other cerebellar disorders [3155].

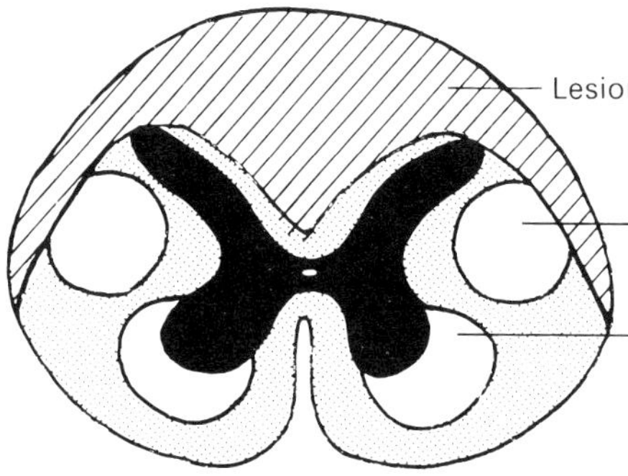

Lesion in Friedreich's ataxia

Corticospinal tract

Bulbospinal respiratory pathway

Fig. 12.4. *Site of spinal cord lesion in Friedreich's ataxia.*

There is no evidence for any abnormality of control of ventilation [220]. The arterial P_{CO_2} is usually normal and the mild hypoxia that is common is due to suboptimal ventilation/perfusion matching [441]. The oxyhaemoglobin dissociation curve is normal [440].

The development of a restrictive defect is usually due to a progressively worsening scoliosis rather than to muscular weakness. The scoliosis almost always develops within a few years of the first features of Friedreich's ataxia becoming apparent [1105, 3154] and is most severe if the condition appears at an early age [1105, 1788]. The primary curve is usually thoracic and convex to the right [61, 1105]. The spine remains well balanced, unlike Duchenne's muscular dystrophy, and pelvic obliquity is uncommon. The scoliosis frequently worsens rapidly after the ability to walk is lost [61, 653] and progresses throughout life, particularly if it is of early onset [460, 1788]. The angle of scoliosis, which may be severe, is not closely related to the severity of the neuromuscular disorder [1395]. It is important to provide support for the spine at an early stage in both ambulant and wheelchair-bound patients. Spinal fusion may prevent a deterioration in lung function. Pectus excavatum may also be present [1395] but has little effect on respiratory function.

Cardiac complications are so common in Friedreich's ataxia as to be an important diagnostic feature separating this condition from the other spinocerebellar degenerations [189, 1203]. The characteristic abnormality is hypertrophy of the left ventricle, which is either concentric or most marked in the interventricular septum [1203, 3118, 3211, 3284]. It has been considered to be similar to hypertrophic obstructive cardiomyopathy (HOCM) but is probably distinct from this condition [3118, 3284]. Extensive fibrosis, with degeneration and hypertrophy of cardiac muscle fibres, develops [654, 1415, 3155, 3211]. Narrowing of the small coronary arteries may also be seen [1415], and contributes to the angina that is frequently present in older patients [1414].

Symptoms of heart disease are often absent [1354] but a systolic murmur [12, 654, 1354, 2438] and a 3rd or 4th heart sound [654] are common. The ECG is usually abnormal but shows non-specific features, particularly left and right ventricular hypertrophy and T-wave changes [12, 1354, 2438, 3155]. The echocardiogram is more sensitive than the ECG in detecting ventricular hypertrophy. Abnormal relaxation of the ventricles, as well as of contraction, has been demonstrated [3118]. The echocardiographic abnormalities may precede the clinical appearance of cardiac disease [12] by many years, although cardiac disease is occasionally the presenting feature [249, 3155].

The severity of the cardiomyopathy is not related to the severity of the neuromuscular disorder [654, 1354], and cardiac failure is often absent even in patients who have longstanding disease. It commonly appears only in the last few months of life [1414] and often deteriorates suddenly because of a dysrhythmia, which is usually atrial fibrillation or a supraventricular tachycardia [653, 1414, 2438].

Syringomyelia

Syringomyelia most commonly involves the cervical and upper thoracic spinal cord, leading to loss of pain and temperature sensation with preservation of light touch, position and vibration sense. Damage to the corticospinal tracts causes upper motor neuron signs in the legs. Lower motor neuron signs develop in the upper limbs (Fig. 12.5). The diaphragm is innervated by C3–C5 and diaphragm weakness might be anticipated to be common. This complication is surprisingly rarely recognized but can cause respiratory failure [204] and may have contributed to the few recorded cases of central alveolar hypoventilation [1139, 2689]. Intercostal muscle atrophy has also been recorded [204, 2836].

Scoliosis, which occurs in about 50% of patients [1489, 3270], is probably due to weakness of the trunk muscles. The level of the spinal curvature correlates with the site of the lower motor neuron lesion [3270]. A double curve

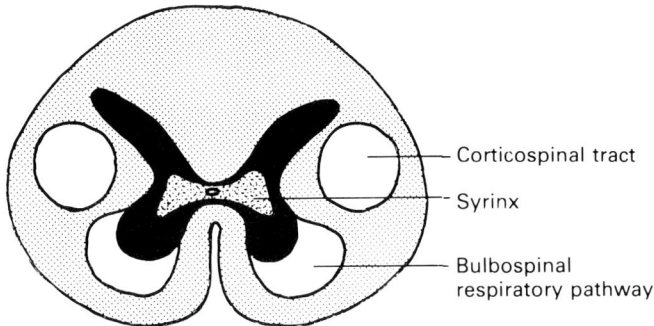

- Corticospinal tract
- Syrinx
- Bulbospinal respiratory pathway

Fig. 12.5. *Site of spinal cord lesion in syringomyelia.*

similar to that seen in idiopathic scoliosis is common [999]. Scoliosis is particularly severe if the syrinx develops before the adolescent growth spurt is completed [1489], and a progressive scoliosis may even be the presenting feature of syringomyelia [160, 2550].

Syringomyelia is commonly associated with myelomeningocoele and abnormalities at the foramen magnum such as basilar impression, Klippel-Feil syndrome or the Arnold-Chiari malformation [1927]. In the latter condition, the cerebellar tonsils herniate through the foramen magnum and this may lead to respiratory consequences additional to those due to the syrinx itself.

Stridor may develop in the Arnold-Chiari malformation but by a different mechanism to that seen in syringobulbia (p. 122). It has been postulated that medullary infarcts or haemorrhages are the cause [2219, 2398] but it is more likely that it is secondary to a raised intracranial pressure [1752]. Stridor usually appears in early infancy rather than at birth and improves when the posterior fossa is decompressed [1698, 2910]. It is probably due to stretching or compression of the vagus nerve, particularly its posterior rootlets which supply the recurrent laryngeal nerve [331, 1225]. Stridor is often associated with other lower cranial nerve palsies, which are probably caused by a similar mechanism. The function of the vocal cords returns more rapidly if the raised intracranial pressure is relieved promptly [331], but in other cases a tracheostomy may be necessary [2728]. Aspiration pneumonia may also be a problem, particularly if laryngeal sensation is absent or if

oesophageal motility or cricopharyngeal function is disturbed [294].

Chronic hypoventilation may develop with the Arnold-Chiari malformation [478]. A diminished ventilatory response, particularly to hypoxia but also to hypercapnia, has been demonstrated [339]. The carotid bodies or medulla may be damaged but it is more likely that the 9th cranial nerve is stretched or compressed in a similar manner to the 10th nerve palsy, which causes stridor. Central sleep apnoeas can be largely abolished by surgical treatment of the deformity [165].

Neurosurgical procedures for syringomyelia and syringobulbia are occasionally followed by sudden death [3341]. This may be due to cardiac dysrhythmias but is more commonly related to derangement of automatic respiratory control [2250, 2422]. Irregular respirations and gasping may be seen post-operatively [1745] and obstructive sleep apnoeas due to post-operative vocal cord paresis are also recognized [18]. This may necessitate a tracheostomy. Careful post-operative monitoring is required to detect these potentially serious complications.

Motor neuron disease (Amyotrophic lateral sclerosis, progressive muscular atrophy, progressive bulbar palsy)

This progressive degenerative disease involves the corticobulbar and corticospinal tracts, as well as the lower motor neurons in the brain stem and spinal cord (Fig. 12.6). Weakness of the muscles of the hand and other limb muscles usually appears first, but eventually this spreads

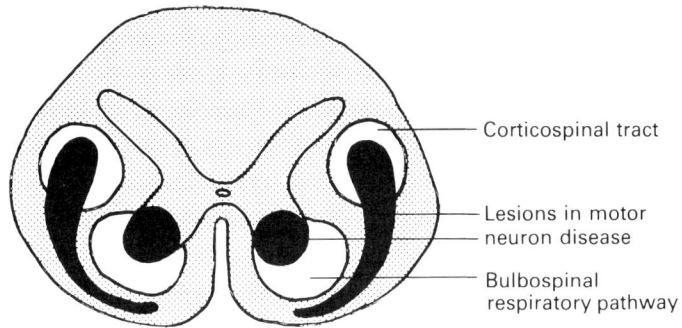

Fig. 12.6. *Site of spinal cord lesion in motor neuron disease.*

to most muscle groups. The respiratory muscles are not spared and bulbar involvement is common. The prognosis in motor neuron disease is poor [1834], particularly if there is bulbar involvement [2253, 2275]. Chest infections, due to aspiration, and respiratory failure are the most common causes of death [948].

Weakness of the limb muscles is usually marked before respiratory muscle weakness becomes clinically apparent. Respiratory impairment is insidious and respiratory failure is a feature of the later stages of the disease [2164, 2952]. The expiratory muscles are weaker than the inspiratory muscles, as judged by changes in PI_{max} and PE_{max} [1743, 1744, 2798], PEFR

[1743] and transdiaphragmatic pressure [1744].

The expiratory muscle weakness largely determines the changes in lung volume (see Fig. 9.7). The fall in VC is closely related to the increase in RV [948, 2855]. Close examination of expiratory flow volume loops has confirmed that the RV is determined by expiratory muscle weakness rather than airway closure, in most patients [1743]. In contrast, the inspiratory muscles are usually strong enough to attain a normal TLC [2798] and to enable sighs and occasional deep breaths, which prevent small airway closure. Lung compliance [2798] and FRC [948, 1743] are, therefore, normal. Serial lung function tests are of some value in predict-

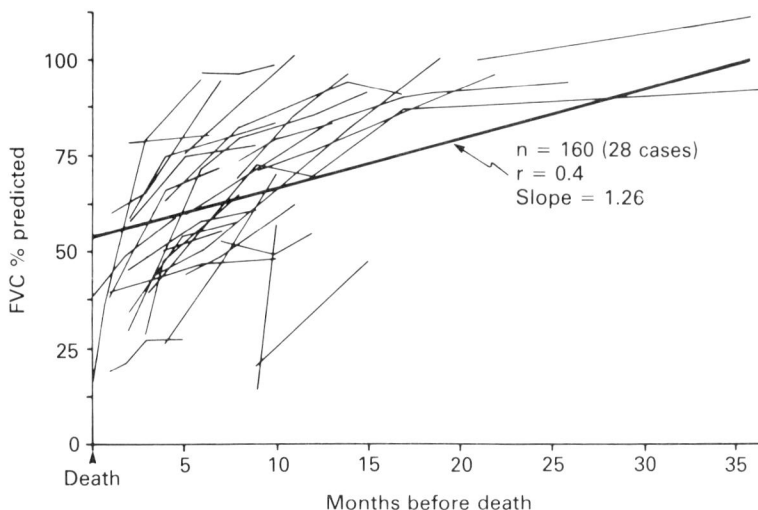

Fig. 12.7. *Serial measurements of vital capacity in motor neuron disease, showing the rapid decline during the months before death. Reproduced, with permission, from* Arch. Neurol. *1979;* **36***: 78. Copyright 1979, American Medical Association.*

ing the prognosis in motor neuron disease. The $P_{I_{max}}$, $P_{E_{max}}$, lung volumes and spirometry appear to be the most useful indices [2275]. A prolonged stable phase is common but a rapid fall in VC usually heralds a very poor prognosis [948, 2134, 2512] (Fig. 12.7).

Weakness of the expiratory muscles reduces the effectiveness of the cough and predisposes to chest infections. This tendency is increased if there is a bulbar or pseudobulbar palsy; 25% of patients present with dysarthria or dysphagia and these features almost inevitably appear eventually [498, 1994]. Aspiration pneumonia is a constant hazard that may cause respiratory failure and is a common cause of death. Dysphagia and aspiration pneumonias frequently prove difficult to treat but surgical procedures, particularly cricopharyngeal myotomy, should be considered [1838, 1994].

Flow volume loops have also shown a pattern in which air flow slows rapidly early in expiration. This can be abolished by insertion of an oral airway, inferring that the obstruction is in the pharynx [367]. Incoordination of the pharyngeal muscles is the most likely explanation, but this has not been observed or recorded directly. Upper airway obstruction may also be due to vocal cord palsy [39, 498, 2763]. Flaccid paralysis of the vocal cords due to degeneration in the nucleus ambiguus is usual, but occasionally spasticity with bilateral cord adduction is seen.

In a few subjects, inspiratory muscle weakness is severe and presents with respiratory failure [64, 1030, 1051, 1427, 2406(a), 2421, 3158]. This may be acute and severe enough to require mechanical ventilation. The diagnosis of motor neuron disease may not initially be apparent but muscle wasting and fasciculation are usually present. In almost all the reported cases, orthopnoea has been a prominent feature [715, 1260, 2167, 2312, 3395], indicating that bilateral diaphragmatic weakness is present. This has been confirmed in one case by the finding of a low transdiaphragmatic pressure [64, 1319]. Autopsy examination has revealed degeneration in the ventromedial region of the anterior horn of

C3–C5, corresponding to the site of the lower motor neurons of the phrenic nerve [1051, 2406(a)]. These patients have a relatively good prognosis, providing that adequate long-term ventilatory support is provided and that bulbar weakness is not present. Temporary spontaneous improvement may even be seen.

Ventilatory failure in the absence of bilateral diaphragmatic weakness is a late complication. The P_{CO_2} remains normal until muscle weakness is extensive [2512], but it may rise preterminally to high levels [963, 2855]. Once significant hypoxaemia has developed, the progression of the disease is usually too rapid for polycythaemia or right heart failure to develop. Pulmonary hypertension may, however, be present and become rapidly more severe on exertion [2855].

The distribution of the degeneration within the central nervous system makes it unlikely that the automatic as opposed to the voluntary respiratory pathways would be involved. Sleep apnoeas are uncommon [2184] but, in a single case, moderately severe carbon dioxide retention with hypersomnia in the presence of normal spirometry raised the possibility of an abnormality of automatic respiratory control [2140]. Hypoxic episodes, particularly during REM sleep, would be expected in the presence of bilateral diaphragmatic paralysis (p. 77), but this does not imply any abnormality of ventilatory control.

Spinal muscular atrophy

Spinal muscular atrophy is an autosomal recessively inherited condition in which the lower motor neurons progressively degenerate [2426]. The bulbar and proximal muscles of the limbs, particularly the lower limbs, are worst affected. The severity of spinal muscular atrophy ranges from rapidly progressing weakness and hypotonia, which is fatal in infancy or early childhood (Werdnig-Hoffman disease), to a slowly developing illness with a moderately good prognosis (Kugelberg-Welander disease).

Death usually occurs from respiratory complications in the rapidly progressive form of the disease [1355, 2834]. Feeding difficulties are prominent and aspiration pneumonia is common [455, 2427]. The diaphragm is relatively spared [455] but in rare cases, possibly due to a genetic variant [2031], it is weak and this leads to respiratory failure. The diaphragmatic paralysis may be either unilateral [2258] or bilateral [2123], and at autopsy it is largely membraneous with only a few muscle fibres [2123]. The prognosis is poor, even with mechanical ventilation and plication of the diaphragm.

Respiratory complications are less prominent in the more benign forms of spinal muscular atrophy. The intercostal muscles become weak but diaphragmatic paralysis is uncommon [735, 1423]. Weakness of the bulbar muscles contributes to respiratory infections and abdominal muscle weakness lessens the effectiveness of the cough [2834]. Asymmetrical weakness of the trunk muscles commonly leads to a severe and progressive scoliosis, which is usually a single thoracolumbar curve [238, 2615, 2834]. Spinal fusion may be required to maintain a satisfactory posture and to prevent a deterioration in respiratory function [817, 2615, 2834].

Poliomyelitis (Fig. 12.8)

ACUTE POLIOMYELITIS

Infection with the poliomyelitis virus causes an acute febrile illness, with mainly upper respiratory symptoms in children and gastrointestinal symptoms in adults. It may progress to cause paralysis, which is of the lower motor neuron type (Fig. 12.9). The clinical picture varies according to which cranial and spinal nerve nuclei are damaged. The frequency of paralysis was recorded as between 30 and 80% in different epidemics [1798, 1819, 2974], although many of the milder cases probably remained unrecognized. About one-third of those paralysed required ventilatory support [1342, 1817]. Paralysis is often asymmetrical, and milder and less extensive in children than in adults [3282].

Acute poliomyelitis is now rare in the developed countries [223], although the ease of travel and antigenic evolution of the virus, which enables it to be pathogenic even in immunized subjects [2471], suggest that it may become more common again. Before the introduction of effective immunization in the 1950s, it was responsible for widespread epidemics.

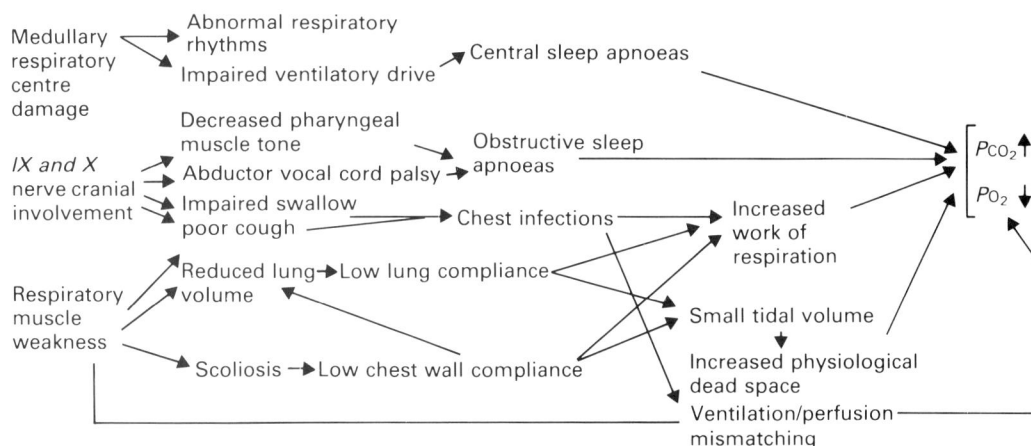

Fig. 12.8. *Flow chart to show the effects of poliomyelitis on ventilation.*

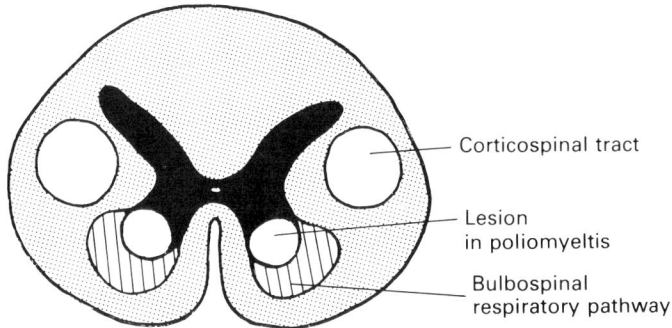

Fig. 12.9. *Site of spinal cord lesion in poliomyelitis.*

Several occurred in Great Britain during the 1950s, and in the USA it has been estimated that between 1949 and 1953, 18.5–37.2 per 100 000 were infected [568]. Particularly severe epidemics broke out in Scandinavia between 1952 and 1954. In Copenhagen in 1952, 2241 confirmed cases of poliomyelitis were admitted to the Blegdam Hospital, of which 1250 were paralysed and 345 required respiratory support [1819]. In that year, 58 per 100 000 of the population of Denmark developed paralytic poliomyelitis [568]. This epidemic spread to Sweden and, in 1953, 953 patients were admitted to hospital in Stockholm alone [3085].

Most of the information concerning the respiratory effects of acute poliomyelitis is derived from epidemics such as these, with the result that modern investigative techniques have been applied only to small numbers of patients. The careful observations made when poliomyelitis was common have, however, enabled various patterns of respiratory involvement to be recognized.

Respiratory muscle weakness

Respiratory muscle paralysis can occur rapidly, so that within a few hours the patient is completely dependent on a ventilator [2824]. However, all degrees of severity of respiratory muscle involvement are seen, and in mild and moderately severely affected subjects the weakness may be patchy and asymmetrical. There appears to be no particular predilection for the diaphragm, although this can be paralysed.

The weakness of the respiratory muscles causes a restrictive defect. The fall in VC [401, 1961] is a valuable indicator of the severity of respiratory muscle involvement. The weakness of the respiratory muscles lowers both PI_{max} and PE_{max} [401] and prevents full inflation and deflation of the lungs. The TLC is therefore diminished and the RV is increased [973, 1342, 1961, 3218]. In most studies the FRC was found to be normal [29, 973], although in one report it was abnormally low and the RV was normal [946]. The MVV is decreased to a greater extent than the VC, suggesting that the endurance of the respiratory muscles is lessened [1961].

The VC is also affected by changes in the lung and chest wall compliance. The lung compliance falls [637, 974], probably because of small airway closure as a result of the inability to take deep breaths: it can be increased temporarily by deep breathing [970]. The chest wall compliance is also diminished [974], perhaps because of changes in the soft tissues and joints of the chest wall secondary to the restricted range of tidal respiratory movements. The fall in compliance of the lungs and chest wall together is considerable [29], and correlates with the fall in VC [401, 548].

Bulbar involvement

Bulbar involvement is one of the most important complications of poliomyelitis, and the prognosis without treatment is much worse than in the pure spinal type of infection (p. 318). Involvement of the higher cranial nerves, such as the facial nerve, has virtually no respiratory consequences and does not adversely affect the prognosis [2973, 3085].

Impairment of the cough reflex and difficulty with swallowing are common. Aspiration of secretions into the tracheobronchial tree predisposes to acute bronchitis and pneumonia, and may obstruct the airway, increasing the work of the already weakened respiratory muscles.

Bulbar poliomyelitis also occasionally causes paralysis of the abductor muscles of the larynx due to involvement of the nucleus ambiguus. The vocal cord paralysis may be unilateral [971], or bilateral when the flaccid cords lie almost in the midline during inspiration but are blown apart on expiration. Bilateral paralysis is present in < 10% of patients with bulbar palsy [1904]. It can cause aspiration pneumonia stridor and severe obstruction of the airway, which may require a tracheostomy [905, 1904, 2528]. A unilateral abductor cord paralysis usually causes a weak cough but no air flow obstruction [2528].

The medullary centres controlling the heart and circulation are often involved in bulbar poliomyelitis [159, 1424]. Hypertension is occasionally seen [246] and may be due partly to hypoxia [651]. More commonly, hypotension develops and may be severe enough to cause shock [1424, 2502]. Changes in vasomotor tone are at least partially responsible but myocarditis, due directly to the poliomyelitis virus, or dysfunction of the heart secondary to severe hypoxia, may contribute. The pulmonary artery pressure may rise [1342] and pulmonary oedema may develop.

Respiratory centre abnormalities

Involvement of the medullary respiratory centres is almost invariably associated with other features of bulbar infection. Difficulty in swallowing and abnormalities of temperature control and blood pressure are common [922]. Histological studies have shown degenerative changes in the medulla that are most marked ventrolaterally [159, 415, 987, 2499, 2808].

Failure of the respiratory centres may not appear until a few days after the onset of respiratory muscle weakness. It usually presents with changes in the rhythm of respiration. The earliest abnormalities are sleep apnoeas [2499], but in more severe cases apnoeas appear during wakefulness as well [415, 1904, 1988, 2499]. The apnoeas can be terminated by ordering the patient to breathe [1904, 2787]. Other abnormal respiratory rhythms, such as slow [2787] or irregular [415, 1904, 2787] respirations or clusters of breaths [2787], may be seen. The ventilatory response to hypercapnia is diminished [2499] but breathlessness is not a feature and the VC may be completely normal.

The diagnosis of respiratory centre failure in acute poliomyelitis may be difficult if respiratory muscle weakness is also present. Both may cause a deteriorating level of consciousness and other symptoms, such as headaches, if hypercapnia and hypoxia are severe. Abnormalities in respiratory rhythm are, however, not seen with pure respiratory muscle weakness except during REM sleep with bilateral diaphragmatic paralysis, and they suggest involvement of the respiratory centres.

LATE CONSEQUENCES OF POLIOMYELITIS

Most subjects who have suffered from paralytic poliomyelitis are left with some degree of disability. Weakness of the legs is more common than weakness of the arms, and it has been estimated that in 1958 over 250 000 subjects in the USA were partially disabled because of poliomyelitis [1798]. Psychological problems are common, disruption of the family structure is frequent and full-time employment is often difficult to obtain [44, 1369, 1453]. Physical problems, such as recurrent urinary tract infections and calculi, frequently develop [330, 379, 1369, 2452, 2686, 2966].

Respiratory muscle weakness

Recovery of muscle strength from the acute poliomyelitis infection is unpredictable but may continue for up to two years. It tends to be less complete if the acute infection is contracted as an adult [1453]. The weakest muscles during the acute illness recover least [2452]. It has also become apparent that muscle weakness can begin to progress faster than would be expected through the normal processes of ageing, many years after the acute infection. The mechanism of this 'post-poliomyelitis amyotrophy' is still uncertain but is probably related to loss of a critical number of the few remaining motor neurons [1823, 2095].

The return of respiratory muscle strength after the acute infection is shown by improvement in the VC, $P_{\mathrm{I_{max}}}$ and $P_{\mathrm{E_{max}}}$ and by an increasing independence from mechanical ventilatory support [356]. However, the strength of the paraspinal and other trunk muscles is often asymmetrical and a scoliosis develops. This is severe in about 10% of those who require mechanical ventilation during their acute illness [2452]. A double structural curve in the thoracic and lumbar spine or a long 'C'-shaped curve is common [2094]. The scoliosis progresses at a constant rate until the onset of puberty and then at a faster but still constant rate [210]. The VC fails to increase at a normal rate if the angle of scoliosis is greater than 30° at puberty, particularly if there is also paralysis of the intercostal muscles and deformity of the ribs [1555].

The detailed effects of scoliosis on respiratory function are discussed in Chapter 16. It appears to be less important than the respiratory muscle weakness in determining the compliance of the

respiratory system [1605]. In adults, the VC falls at almost 2% per year in those with ventilatory failure [146(b)], but the relative contributions of a worsening of respiratory muscle weakness, progression of the scoliosis and of soft tissue and joint changes are uncertain. Erosion of the upper margins of the ribs, particularly the posterior 2nd and 3rd ribs, also occurs but is probably of no functional significance [263].

Bulbar involvement

Bulbar function may continue to improve after the acute illness for up to two years [1620]. Recovery may be complete but in many cases a complex combination of abnormalities persists. These include palatal weakness, weakness of the pharyngeal constrictors and failure of the cricopharyngeus muscle to relax during swallowing [348]. Swallowing may be helped by trick movements of the head and neck, but the risk of aspiration pneumonias persists. If the cricopharyngeus is the main problem, cricopharyngeal myotomy may be of considerable benefit [334, 1620, 1964].

Respiratory centre abnormalities

The respiratory centres may also only partially recover after acute poliomyelitis. The ventilatory response to hypercapnia is often diminished [1907, 2499, 2999], although ventilation during hypoxia and exercise may be normal

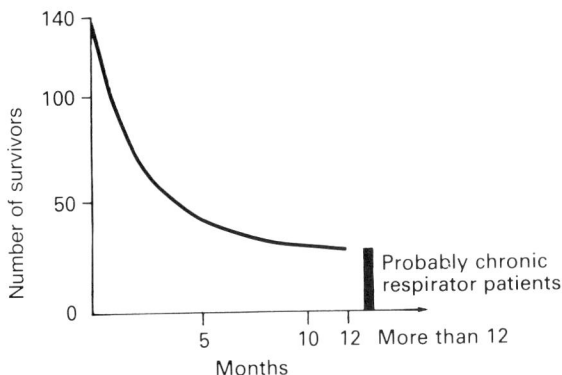

Fig. **12.10.** *Number of survivors of acute poliomyelitis with respiratory failure who required mechanical ventilation following the 1952 Copenhagen epidemic. Fifty-six additional patients developed respiratory failure, but survived without mechanical ventilation. Reproduced, with permission, from Lassen H.C.A., ed.* Management of life-threatening poliomyelitis Copenhagen 1952–56 with a survey of autopsy findings in 115 cases. *Churchill Livingstone: Edinburgh 1956.*

[2999]. The impaired response to hypercapnia is, in some cases, predominantly due to respiratory muscle weakness rather than to respiratory centre dysfunction. The $P_{0.1}$, which is less dependent on these mechanical factors, may be normal, despite a reduced ventilatory response to hypercapnia [2429]. Persisting abnormalities of the respiratory centres are only seen if the acute illness caused a bulbar palsy [1428, 2499].

Respiratory failure

The gradual improvement in respiratory muscle strength and bulbar and respiratory centre function lead to increasing independence from any mechanical ventilatory support required during the acute poliomyelitis infection. For instance, in the 1952 Copenhagen epidemic, of the 345 patients who initially required assisted ventilation, only 60 did so at three months, 32 at eight months, 29 at one year and 25 (7%) of these required long-term ventilation (Fig. 12.10). Recovery was least complete in those with the worst paralysis during the acute illness and the longest interval before any recovery was apparent [1819].

Long-term follow-up studies have shown that about 10–30% of patients initially requiring mechanical ventilation still needed this [25, 28, 44, 731, 780, 1819, 2288, 2452]. In one report, as many as 67% of patients required some form of respiratory assistance, but the details were not specified [1369]. Many of these subjects will have required continual ventilatory support since their acute infection, but some develop respiratory failure after many years of adequate respiratory function [45].

The late appearance of respiratory failure is usually multifactorial. Both respiratory muscle weakness and abnormal respiratory centre function have been implicated [2787, 2999] but in some cases other factors such as a severe scoliosis [1803] and diminished compliance of the respiratory system [1605] may have been important. Respiratory failure may, of course, be precipitated by intercurrent illnesses, sedation,

including alcohol, or an increase in weight, but it often develops insidiously, with somnolence as the predominant symptom [1296, 1336, 1803, 3132]. Hypoxia and hypercapnia are more marked at night than during the day and the pattern of breathing during sleep is irregular [1428, 2499, 3198]. Central sleep apnoeas are common [1296, 1428]. Obstructive and mixed apnoeas also occur [1296] but if they predominate, a search for an anatomical cause such as a vocal cord paralysis is indicated [1618].

Respiratory failure is often chronic and severe, and pulmonary hypertension due to hypoxia is well recognized [996, 1013, 1341, 1428, 1920, 3198]. It is particularly marked during nocturnal hypoxic episodes [1296, 1428], and leads to right ventricular hypertrophy [330, 549, 1429, 2592] and right ventricular failure [1341, 1413, 1429, 3030]. Polycythaemia also occurs [549, 1441] and, occasionally, left ventricular failure confined to the side of the chest with the greater respiratory muscle weakness may develop [1329]. This may be the result of local hypoxic vasoconstriction secondary to inadequate ventilation on the side of the respiratory muscle weakness.

Tetanus

Tetanus is due to the liberation of the exotoxin tetanospasmin by *Clostridium tetani*. Tetanospasmin increases both somatic and sympathetic reflex excitability. The autonomic effects include hypertension and hypotension, tachycardias, excessive sweating and increased salivation. Rigidity of skeletal muscles and intermittent spasms are characteristic. In severe infections, the period between the first symptom and the first muscle spasm is short and the spasms, once they develop, are more frequent.

The first symptom is usually trismus, with or without dysphagia, due to incoordination of the bulbar muscles. Mild hypoxia is common [1717]. Nursing in a quiet environment together with sedative drugs such as diazepam or chlorpromazine is often sufficient, although, rarely, these drugs may lead to hypoventilation.

Once spasms occur, the prognosis is worse and more intensive treatment is required. Laryngeal spasms cause stridor and occasionally acute airway obstruction and death through hypoxia. Spasms of the chest wall muscles splint the thorax and prevent inspiration. Severe hypoxia may develop if these follow in rapid succession. Less commonly, the brain stem is involved and prolonged apnoeas are seen. The inability to swallow the excessive saliva not only obstructs the upper airway but may lead to aspiration pneumonia. Occasionally, diffuse lung shadowing resembling adult respiratory distress syndrome develops [539].

These complications require curarization and IPPV [885, 2415, 2971]. Mechanical ventilation is often needed for about ten days but full recovery of respiratory muscle power may be delayed for weeks or months.

Stiff-man syndrome

In this uncommon condition, there is a gradual onset of generalized muscle rigidity with superimposed episodic exacerbations or spasms, which may be extremely painful [380, 1195, 2198]. The increase in muscle tone appears to be due to release of inhibition of the lower motor neurons. All the respiratory muscles may be affected and spasms of the diaphragm are seen [2356]. The rigid muscles give rise to difficulty in breathing, which may be described as a tightness in the chest [2198, 3087], and to a weak voice. A restrictive defect develops [1195], but this can be reversed by muscle relaxants such as diazepam [1475]. The muscle rigidity decreases during sleep and there are no reports of nocturnal respiratory failure.

Chapter 13
Disorders of the Peripheral Nerves

Many of the disorders of peripheral nerves affect the distal parts of the limbs preferentially and do not have any respiratory consequences. Some are less selective and can occasionally cause respiratory failure, and a few have a predilection for the nerves supplying the respiratory muscles. The physiological effects of respiratory muscle weakness due to peripheral nerve damage are identical to those of the primary respiratory muscle disorders that are described in Chapter 15.

INDIVIDUAL DISORDERS

The most important peripheral nerve disorders with respiratory complications are:

Acute idiopathic polyneuropathy (Landry-Guillain-Barre syndrome)

Acute idiopathic polyneuropathy frequently follows a recognizable event, such as an infection, although in some cases no such cause may be found. The characteristic histological appearance is of a lymphocytic infiltration of the nerve roots caused by a cell-mediated hypersensitivity to myelin [2997]. The motor functions of the peripheral nerves are disturbed more than the sensory functions.

The distribution of the peripheral nerve damage varies considerably. It is uncertain how frequently the respiratory muscles are involved, partly because of different criteria used for the diagnosis in different studies, and partly because mild weakness often passes unnoticed. Respiratory problems severe enough to require assisted ventilation are seen in 15–30% of patients who are admitted to hospital [831, 1090, 1992, 2209, 2997]. Respiratory failure may even be the presenting feature [2814]. Any of the respiratory muscles, including the diaphragm, may be affected [1388, 2814]. The phrenic nerve conduction time is usually prolonged [2060], especially if the illness is severe [1215].

Respiratory complications were at one time the most common cause of death. The mortality has been greatly decreased over the last thirty years by improvements in the management of respiratory complications, particularly respiratory failure, sputum retention and pneumonia [1388, 2487, 2571, 2997, 3107]. The consequences of prolonged immobilization, such as pulmonary embolus [2555], still arise but as the mortality from respiratory problems has fallen the relative importance of cardiovascular complications has increased [722, 3192]. Autonomic disorders of the heart rate, such as a fixed tachycardia, postural hypotension and hypertension, are common but are not related to the severity of the muscle weakness [3192].

Weakness of the respiratory muscles may progress rapidly and become severe. Assessment of respiratory muscle strength is most simply carried out by recording serial VC measurements. A fall to around one litre (or about 25% of the predicted value or < 15 ml/kg body weight) usually indicates that mechanical ventilation will be required [1416, 2209, 2305]. If the VC is falling rapidly, mechanical ventilation should be instituted before these levels are reached. Estimation of $P_{I_{max}}$ and $P_{E_{max}}$ may also be useful. The PEFR has been recommended as a measure of respiratory muscle strength [2079] but is not reliable. Prolongation of the phrenic nerve conduction time is a sensitive indicator of impending ventilatory failure, but this technique is not widely available [1215].

IPPV is usually preferable to negative pressure ventilation [1090, 2571] since bulbar function is so often compromised [1226]. There is a risk of aspiration pneumonia unless the airway is protected, particularly if the cough is also weakened through involvement of the expiratory muscles. A bilateral abductor palsy of the vocal cords, which can be detected by examination of flow volume loops, may also develop [1388, 2690]. The widespread use of a cuffed endotracheal tube has reduced the mortality, although occasional patients can be managed with a negative pressure ventilator if their bulbar function is normal [1801].

Recovery may be rapid, in which case tracheostomy is not needed [215, 2303], but commonly ventilation is required for several weeks [1222]. It is uncertain whether the duration of ventilation is related to the age of the subject [1222, 1977, 2209]. On rare occasions, recovery may be delayed for many months [3107] but may then occur remarkably quickly [1711, 3318]. Extubation is usually possible when the VC approaches about 50% of the predicted value [1673].

Complete recovery is usual but is not invariable. It is less complete if there is a long delay between the time of greatest muscle weakness and the start of any improvement [875, 1711, 1926]. A residual respiratory disability is infrequent [1416], although in almost 50% of patients the spirometric values remain below normal [2013]. The improvement in the phrenic nerve conduction time also lags behind the clinical improvement [1215].

Miller-Fisher syndrome

The Miller-Fisher syndrome is an acute inflammatory polyneuropathy [2464] that has many similarities to acute idiopathic polyneuropathy. It is characterized by the presence of an external ophthalmoplegia with ataxia and areflexia. The VC can fall rapidly because of respiratory muscles weakness [319, 1921, 2464], and

apnoeas may appear [46]. IPPV is required for these complications.

Spontaneous improvement is usually seen within a few days, but in severe cases it may be delayed for several months and plasmapheresis may be required [1921].

Neuralgic amyotrophy (cryptogenic brachial plexopathy)

Neuralgic amyotrophy typically presents with sudden onset of shoulder pain followed by weakness of the shoulder muscles [1095]. This may follow a viral infection [3187] but can appear without any antecedent illness. It has many similarities to post-immunization neuropathy. Both appear to be the result of an allergic reaction that causes patchy demyelination in the brachial plexus and neighbouring nerves. If the diaphragm is paralysed it is usually on the side of the shoulder pain [1095], but occasionally it is bilateral [40, 491, 1224, 3187]. A vocal cord palsy may also develop [3378].

Recovery usually occurs within a few weeks but, although this may be clinically complete [783], EMG and physiological abnormalities may persist [1224].

Post-immunization neuropathy

Immunization with non-human serum can cause a wide variety of neurological complications due to hypersensitivity reactions. Encephalitis, meningitis, myelitis, polyneuritis and mononeuritis have all been described [2160]. They are particularly common with tetanus and diphtheria antitoxin but toxoids against these and other infections can cause similar problems, especially with booster injections [1455, 2509, 2545].

The initial manifestations may be urticaria and features of serum sickness but these are usually followed after a few days by the neurological features [873, 1190, 2976]. The inflammation frequently affects the brachial plexus but diaphragmatic paralysis also occurs [1045, 1985, 2976, 3381]. This is usually limited to the side of the immunization but occasionally is bilateral [191, 621, 1985] and rarely may be associated with a vocal cord palsy [1045, 2654].

Recovery usually occurs within a few weeks but may occasionally be delayed for over a year [621, 2976]. This is particularly likely if there is a long interval between the injection and the development of the neuropathy [1455].

Herpes zoster

This common condition affects particularly the dorsal root ganglia and causes sensory symptoms, but occasionally motor changes are detectable. These are usually attributed to infection spreading to the spinal cord or even to the anterior roots [3017, 3142] but muscle weakness can occur with lesions confined to the dorsal roots [2280].

Muscle weakness is by far the most common motor disorder but myoclonus, which responds to clonazepam, has also been recorded. Myoclonus of the abdominal muscles causes breathlessness and staccato speech, due to the repetitive interruption of expiration. The flow volume loop shows an expiratory flutter [2411] (Fig. 9.10).

Paralysis of any of the respiratory muscles may follow Herpes zoster but this is rarely recognized unless the diaphragm is involved. Weakness of, for instance, one or a few adjacent intercostal muscles would be unlikely to cause any symptoms or readily detectable physical signs. Diaphragmatic paralysis occurs when C3–C5 roots are involved. This is uncommon and in two large series it was observed in only 2.4% and 9.7% of patients with Herpes zoster [1389, 1468].

Diaphragm paralysis is always unilateral and, therefore, rarely symptomatic. The diagnosis is suggested by the finding of a high hemidiaphragm on the chest radiograph, especially if a previously normal radiograph is available. The rash of Herpes zoster precedes the muscle paralysis in about 75% of cases [3142], but if it is absent the diagnosis is unlikely to be made [869]. Some cases of 'cryptogenic peripheral neuropathy' may be due to Herpes zoster

infections without a rash. Serial estimation of antibody levels is required to confirm the diagnosis.

The prognosis for diaphragmatic paralysis in Herpes zoster is variable. There is usually little recovery [82, 403, 869, 1335], although partial return of function may be observed, usually over a period of months [778, 2408, 3017].

'Cryptogenic peripheral neuropathy'

The cause of phrenic nerve palsy often remains uncertain [827, 1893, 2627, 3381], even if it is bilateral [1030, 1459, 3023]. About 75% of cases occur in men and there is occasionally a vocal cord palsy as well [1038, 2475]. The diaphragm paralysis is usually asymptomatic if it is unilateral, but presents with sudden onset of breathlessness if it is bilateral [1459]. There is usually little recovery but some function may return after about one year [827, 2475, 3023].

In many of these cases it is likely that a phrenic neuritis is responsible for the diaphragm weakness. The EMG features consistent with a phrenic neuritis have been demonstrated [3023] and a more widespread peripheral neuropathy may subsequently become apparent, particularly if the diaphragmatic paralysis is bilateral [333, 791, 1178]. Diaphragmatic weakness may accompany or follow a febrile illness that may be due to a viral infection causing a mononeuritis of the phrenic nerve. A similar immunological reaction may be responsible for bilateral diaphragmatic paralysis seen as a non-metastatic manifestation of malignancy [3151]. This should be distinguished from Hedblom's syndrome [1575], which is probably not a discrete entity but is said to cause a transient diaphragmatic weakness, with evidence of myositis.

Diaphragmatic paralysis is occasionally associated with pneumonia or pleurisy and occurs on the same side as the infection [658, 1038]. It is usually transient but the mechanism is uncertain. A toxic phrenic neuritis has been proposed but there is no evidence for this and it is more likely to be due to reflex inhibition of phrenic nerve activity. A similar diaphragmatic paralysis is occasionally seen with asthma [2696].

Diphtheria

Infection with *Corynebacterium diphtheriae*, once common in developed countries, is now rare. Respiratory complications may occur in several ways. The throat infection leads to the formation of a membrane, which may extend to the nasopharynx and larynx and obstruct the airway. This can be severe enough to require endotracheal intubation or tracheostomy [802, 3156]. This complication occurs early in the course of the infection, before the later problems due to the exotoxin liberated by the organism. This exotoxin not only causes a cardiomyopathy [2270] but also a segmental demyelination affecting motor fibres in particular. The cranial nerves, particularly the 9th and 10th, are the first to be involved [2753]. The resulting bulbar palsy usually appears one or two weeks after the onset of the infection and may require endotracheal intubation [1306]. Between the fifth and seventh week from the onset of the throat infection, the neuropathy may become more widespread and paralysis of some or even all of the respiratory muscles appears [1987, 2063]. Diaphragmatic paralysis has long been realized to be a serious complication [50, 2197, 2412] but is seen in less than 3% of infections [1197, 2197]. Intercostal muscle paralysis is also recognized [3350].

The paralysis of the respiratory muscles recovers completely over a few weeks or months, providing adequate ventilatory support can be given initially. Tank [1197, 3173], cuirass [2108] and positive abdominal pressure ventilators [1657, 2029, 2030] have proved successful in the past, but IPPV is preferable if bulbar palsy is present.

Porphyria

Axonal degeneration of the motor peripheral nerve fibres is common in the hepatic porphyrias, especially in acute intermittent porphyria. Porphyric exacerbations may lead to extensive paralysis and even to a flaccid quadriparesis. The respiratory muscles are not spared and respiratory failure may develop suddenly [3002]. Mechanical ventilatory support is often required [1422] and recovery may only be partial. The brain stem respiratory centres can also be damaged by cerebrovascular complications of porphyria. This causes respiratory dysrhythmias, such as central neurogenic hyperventilation [162], and may contribute to hypoventilation.

Trauma

The phrenic nerve may be damaged by trauma at any point from the spinal cord to the diaphragm. Diaphragmatic function is permanently lost if the nerve is completely interrupted, although re-suturing of the cut ends may lead to some return of activity [2130]. Anastomosis of the phrenic nerve to the facial nerve has also been performed with some success [1356].

Phrenic nerve function often returns if the damage is less severe. Improvement may occur within a few weeks but more commonly it takes six to eighteen months. The interval before the function returns is determined by its severity and the site of the injury. The axons within the phrenic nerve remyelinate at a rate of about 1 mm per day. The phrenic nerve is approximately 40–45 cm long in adults, so that with a proximal injury recovery would be expected between twelve and eighteen months.

The phrenic nerve is commonly damaged with trauma to the neck or in the region of the clavicle. Both blunt and penetrating injuries can lead to loss of function. Surgical procedures in the neck [2213, 3021] and thorax may be responsible. Phrenic nerve avulsion and similar procedures were widely used to treat pulmonary tuberculosis before chemotherapy became available (p. 192). Surgery may damage the nerve directly or by injury to the vasa nervorum. The low temperatures required for cold cardioplegia during cardiac surgery may lead to post-operative phrenic nerve paralysis [1970, 2061], particularly on the left, but occasionally bilaterally [528, 1716]. The degree of recovery varies with the extent of the injury. The phrenic nerve is not damaged by laparotomy but post-operative incoordination of the diaphragm is common [2517]. It may even appear paralysed, probably due to inhibition by visceral reflexes initiated by, for instance, gut distension [1967, 2941].

Neonatal diaphragmatic paralysis may be caused by cardiac or thoracic surgery or by birth trauma. Surgical damage to the phrenic nerve requires positive pressure ventilatory support and consideration of diaphragm plication [1245, 2106, 2857]. Birth trauma is commoner in males and is usually associated with a difficult delivery, often a breech or requiring forceps, and with brachial plexus injuries, Horner's syndrome or a sternomastoid haematoma [13, 74, 301, 518, 1245, 2610, 2972]. The injury is usually on the right side but may be bilateral [47]. It usually presents within 24 h of birth and the diagnosis can be confirmed by fluoroscopy. Mild cases are probably common and the diaphragmatic weakness is often transient; full recovery usually occurs within about three months of birth [74, 2610, 2972].

These traumatic causes of diaphragmatic paralysis in the neonate should be distinguished from primary disorders of muscle, such as dystrophia myotonica and congenital eventration of the diaphragm. In this condition the muscular region of the diaphragm is replaced by fibrous tissue. It is commoner in males and in the left hemidiaphragm [2627] but is occasionally bilateral and may be associated with other congenital or chromosomal abnormalities [3304]. Diaphragmatic agenesis is rare [2332, 3177].

Compression and malignant infiltration

Any of the nerves supplying the respiratory muscles may be damaged by compression or malignant infiltration. The most important example is phrenic nerve involvement by a bronchial carcinoma.

Charcot-Marie-Tooth disease

This inherited chronic demyelinating disorder of peripheral nerves and their roots initially affects the distal limb muscles. Respiratory complications are uncommon and occur late in the natural history. Diaphragmatic weakness, which is usually bilateral, is probably due to phrenic nerve involvement since there is no response to phrenic nerve stimulation [527, 1813]. The respiratory muscle weakness may be severe enough to cause ventilatory failure [527, 604]. A scoliosis may appear in any part of the thoracic or lumbar spine [704] and contribute to the restrictive defect. It is, however, usually mild and is only apparent in around 10% of subjects [1408].

Chapter 14
Disorders of the Neuromuscular Junction

The output from the central nervous system is transmitted to the muscle fibres across the neuromuscular junction. A defect at this site is therefore manifested as muscle weakness, but an important feature is that the muscle is readily fatiguable. The implications of respiratory muscle fatigue are discussed in Chapter 2 and the consequences of respiratory muscle weakness in Chapter 15.

INDIVIDUAL DISORDERS

Disorders of the neuromuscular junction are less common than those of the central nervous system, the peripheral nerves or muscle fibres. The most important are:

Myasthenia gravis

The characteristic feature of myasthenia gravis is the fatiguability of skeletal muscle due to circulating antibodies against the acetylcholine receptors on the post-synaptic membrane. Myasthenia gravis can present in several forms.

NEONATAL MYASTHENIA GRAVIS

This occurs only in children of myasthenic mothers. It is unusual in the first few hours of life because anticholinesterase drugs cross the placenta from the maternal circulation and protect the child. Myasthenia usually appears within 48 h of birth and may last for up to six weeks. It affects about 12% of children born to myasthenic mothers [2277] and is probably due to antibodies that cross the placenta from the mother [859].

The usual presentation is with feeding difficulties but respiratory problems, at least partly due to aspiration of pharyngeal secretions, are also common. Anticholinesterase treatment is effective.

INFANTILE (CONGENITAL) MYASTHENIA GRAVIS

This rare condition develops within the first two years of life. It tends to run a benign course but can occasionally be severe [2344]. Cyanosis and apnoea [2011], and dysphagia with aspiration into the tracheobronchial tree, may occur [627]. Anticholinesterase treatment is effective.

JUVENILE MYASTHENIA GRAVIS

This condition is similar to adult myasthenia gravis except that it arises before the age of twenty years. It may not represent a distinct entity and appears to have a similar autoimmune basis to adult myasthenia. Respiratory problems similar to those of adult myasthenia gravis occur in about 40% of patients [965] and occasionally may appear suddenly [1895].

ADULT MYASTHENIA GRAVIS

Weakness in adult myasthenia gravis is usually first apparent in muscles supplied by the cranial nerves, but the respiratory muscles are also commonly affected. The muscles are fatiguable and respiratory muscle weakness is therefore episodic. It may be precipitated by, for instance, undue exertion, infection, surgery and labour [115, 968, 2350, 2698, 2699]. Deterioration after surgery is particularly likely if the myasthenia is longstanding, if the dose of anticholinesterases is high, if there is chronic respiratory disease or if the pre-operative VC is less than about 3.0 l [1228].

The pattern of involvement of skeletal muscles varies considerably. Weakness of the bulbar musculature may be the predominant feature and lead to aspiration of secretions into the tracheobronchial tree [115]. Occasionally, a bilateral abductor vocal cord palsy is present and causes stridor [2179]. This may appear after prolonged phonation [1048], cause an intermittent cough and respiratory obstruction [2819], or even be the presenting feature of myasthenia [616, 1022].

More commonly, the muscles of the chest wall are involved. Both inspiratory and expiratory muscles become weak, but the latter are usually disproportionately affected [2631]. Diaphragm weakness is usually mild [2148]. A restrictive defect appears [744, 2631], the FEV_1 is reduced and the diminution in maximal voluntary ventilation is proportional to the fall in the FEV_1 [2631]. Air flow obstruction is not a feature and the compliance of the lungs is normal [744]. Further studies of the fatiguability of the respiratory muscles are required.

It is important to distinguish respiratory muscle weakness from other complications of myasthenia gravis. Interstitial pulmonary fibrosis is well recognized [1991] and since collagen diseases such as systemic lupus erythematosus (SLE), scleroderma and polymyositis [732] also occasionally occur with myasthenia, the respiratory complications of these conditions must be considered (see Chapter 15). Myocarditis leading to abnormal left ventricular function [111] and conduction defects with dysrhythmias, such as sinus bradycardia, atrial fibrillation and ventricular ectopics, are also well recognized in myasthenia gravis [1123].

Treatment with anticholinesterases reverses the changes in respiratory function and increases the outward recoil of the chest wall, presumably by altering the chest wall muscle tone [743, 744, 2033, 2632]. However, overdosage with these drugs can produce exactly the same pattern of respiratory muscle weakness as is seen in patients who are untreated. Respiratory failure may be precipitated acutely by edrophonium when this is used to distinguish between a myasthenic and a cholinergic crisis, and facilities for intubation should be available. Bronchospasm due to the muscarinic-like action of these drugs may also occur.

While anticholinesterase drugs are the mainstay of treatment of myasthenia gravis, in more severe cases respiratory muscle weakness may require high-dose steroid treatment with or without the use of immunosuppressant drugs such as azathioprine. Paradoxically, steroids may sometimes induce respiratory muscle weakness of sufficient severity to require ventilation [968]. Plasmapheresis is also effective in severely affected patients [718, 719, 1113, 1221]. This should be repeated over several days to remove a sufficient quantity of circulating antibody against the acetylcholine receptor. A marked increase in respiratory muscle strength may be seen and, while this can occur rapidly [1113], improvement may be delayed if weakness has been severe and protracted before treatment [718] (Fig. 14.1).

Plasmapheresis may also be used to improve respiratory function before thymectomy [768]. This frequently reduces the muscle weakness [2806] but was at one time associated with a high mortality [2399]. This was largely due to an inability to cough or swallow adequately or to maintain an adequate level of ventilation postoperatively. These respiratory complications were greatly reduced by the introduction of routine post-operative tracheostomy and positive pressure ventilation combined with a decrease in anticholinesterase treatment [2387]. More recently it has been shown that most patients can be quickly weaned from IPPV [2954] and that it is possible to predict which patients will develop respiratory complications after a trans-sternal incision so that tracheostomy can be performed selectively. Post-operative ventilation may be needed if the pre-operative VC is less than about 2 l. Other less-impor-

(a)

(b)

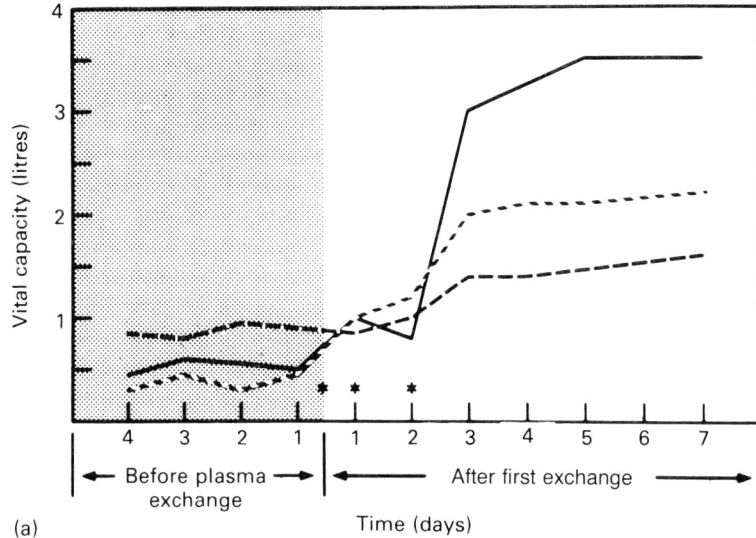

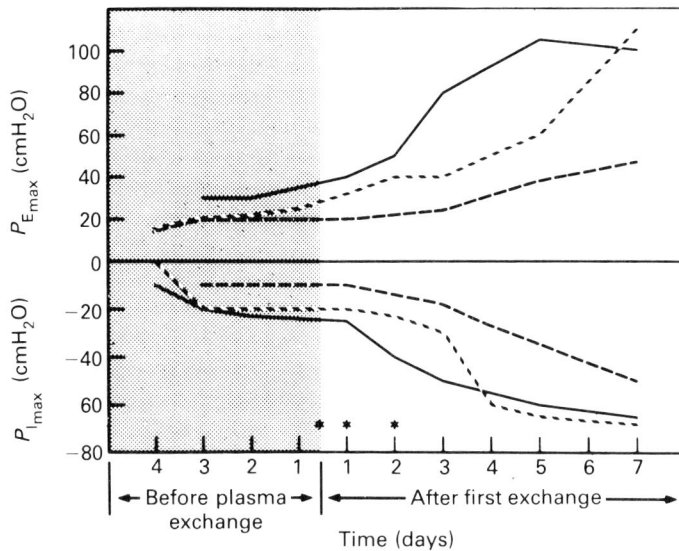

Fig. 14.1. *Effects of plasmapheresis in myasthenia gravis in three patients: (a) improvement in vital capacity, (b) improvement in $P_{I_{max}}$ and $P_{E_{max}}$. Reproduced, with permission, from Gracey D.R. et al. Mayo Clin. Proc. 1982; 57: 742–6.*

tant predictive features appear to be the duration of the myasthenia, the pre-operative anticholinesterase dosage, the presence of respiratory disease and possibly the presence of bulbar dysfunction and the finding of a thymoma at surgery [1219, 1871, 1923]. Post-operative ventilatory support is needed less frequently with a trans-cervical than with the more usual transsternal approach [902].

If ventilation is required for more than 24–28

h, it is usually needed for a prolonged period. A tracheostomy should be carried out at the time of the thymectomy in high-risk patients [1923]. Assessment of when to extubate the patient may be difficult, and regular estimation of PI_{max} and PE_{max} and VC is of value. A PI_{max} of > 20–30 cmH$_2$O and a PE_{max} of > 40 cmH$_2$O, together with a VC of > 15 ml/kg body weight and an adequate cough, usually indicate that weaning will be successful [768, 902, 3391].

Thymectomy is a frequent indication for mechanical ventilation in myasthenia gravis, but this may also be required for both myasthenic and cholinergic crises. Endotracheal intubation and IPPV is usually the treatment of choice because of the presence of bulbar weakness and the risk of aspiration. The prognosis of patients requiring mechanical ventilation was, at one time, poor [115, 2698] but has improved considerably with intensive treatment of the myasthenia and modern methods of intensive-care support [968, 1218]. The long-term prognosis of patients who have required mechanical ventilation does, however, vary according to the precipitating factor responsible for the ventilatory failure. The prognosis is better if this is due to a cholinergic crisis, pregnancy or thymectomy, but worse in older subjects with no detectable cause for their exacerbation [115, 968].

Mechanical ventilation is usually required only as a temporary measure. Chronic hypoventilation is rare [559, 968] and is usually due to bilateral diaphragmatic weakness [735]. Long-term ventilatory support may be required.

Lambert-Eaton syndrome

This syndrome is usually associated with a small-cell carcinoma of the bronchus. This causes antibodies to be produced, which decrease the presynaptic release of acetylcholine. Although the Lambert-Eaton syndrome has some similarities to myasthenia gravis, the cranial nerves are less frequently and the proximal muscles more commonly affected. Weakness of the respiratory muscles may develop rapidly, particularly after muscle-relaxant drugs, and IPPV may be required [1223]. Treatment with guanidine may be of some benefit, but promising results have been reported with immunosuppressant treatment and plasmapheresis [1223].

Botulism

Botulism is caused by the exotoxin of *Clostridium botulinum* and is usually acquired by eating contaminated meat. The exotoxin decreases the presynaptic release of acetylcholine and leads to an extreme degree of muscle fatiguability. Within 12–36 h the muscles supplied by the cranial nerves become weak. Severe paralysis of the respiratory muscles is a frequent finding. The VC may improve temporarily with edrophonium [2563], demonstrating that the weakness is due to severe muscle fatigue. Intermittent positive pressure ventilation is usually required and recovery, although slow, is normally complete.

Tick paralysis

This condition occurs particularly in the USA, Canada, Australia and Africa, and is due to a toxin liberated by pregnant female ticks of various species. The toxin interferes with the presynaptic liberation of acetylcholine and also diminishes the post-synaptic receptor sensitivity [1200]. The ticks become attached to the skin, usually of the head and neck, and inject the toxin in their saliva.

Tick paralysis is commoner in children than in adults. After a mild febrile illness, a rapidly developing, often ascending, paralysis of skeletal muscles occurs. This may spread to the bulbar and respiratory muscles [2820] and IPPV may be required. It improves rapidly when the tick is removed from the skin [760].

Drugs

A variety of drugs can hinder transmission across the neuromuscular junction. This may lead to the persistence of ventilatory depression post-operatively or the unmasking or worsening of myasthenia gravis [100]. Presynaptic acetylcholine release is impaired by drugs such as chloroquine and lincomycin, post-synaptic inhibition by procainamide, tetracycline and polymyxins, and a combination of both actions by aminoglycosides, phenytoin, chlorproma-zine, lithium and propranolol. Penicillamine acts post-synaptically by causing antibodies to be formed against the acetylcholine receptor, thus mimicking myasthenia gravis.

Organophosphate chemicals are long-lasting anticholinesterases and in toxic doses can cause severe respiratory muscle weakness.

Chapter 15
Disorders of the Respiratory Muscles

The ability of the respiratory muscles to ventilate the lungs adequately depends both on the contractile properties of the muscles and on the mechanical properties of the chest wall and lungs (Chapter 2). While the contractility of the respiratory muscles is influenced by many physiological factors, there are also a large number of disorders in which the muscle contractility is pathologically diminished. The respiratory complications of these are commoner than is usually recognized [389]. Respiratory failure may appear in adult life but also neonatally [3242] or during infancy and childhood [918], particularly with the congenital myopathies. Respiratory failure often progresses slowly but can appear suddenly, particularly if there is an intercurrent illness such as a chest infection. Respiratory failure is usually closely related to the degree of respiratory muscle weakness but occasionally occurs with only mild impairment of muscle function. In such cases an impaired respiratory drive may be responsible [224, 497, 2626, 3292]. An increase in the central drive to the muscles is required to generate a given force if the muscles are weak [1260]. This compensation is impaired if the respiratory drive is defective and, as a result, muscle weakness becomes apparent at an early stage.

Many of the disorders of respiratory muscles run a protracted course and lead to chronic hypoxic pulmonary hypertension. Initially, pulmonary hypertension may only be present during episodes of hypoxia during sleep, but in more severe cases it is continuous. Hypoxia is largely due to alveolar hypoventilation but suboptimal ventilation/perfusion matching is often important, particularly if the diaphragm is weak or if there is associated lung disease. The latter

should be carefully distinguished from hypoventilation due to respiratory muscle weakness.

Scoliosis is common in many of the disorders of the respiratory muscles, particularly Duchenne's and limb girdle muscular dystrophies. It is also a prominent feature in respiratory muscle weakness caused by neurological conditions such as quadriplegia, poliomyelitis, Friedreich's ataxia, syringomyelia, spinal muscular atrophy and familial dysautonomia [999, 1408, 2428, 2871, 2915]. In general, scoliosis is uncommon if the axial muscles remain strong. It is, however, an early feature of some conditions, such as Friedreich's ataxia, and it often progresses rapidly during the adolescent growth spurt and may continue to worsen even after growth is complete. Scoliosis in neuromuscular disorders usually affects a considerable length of the spine and is more commonly convex to the right than would be expected from the distribution of the muscle weakness [2428]. Unlike congenital scoliosis, the spine often remains flexible. Respiratory function in neuromuscular disorders often worsens when a scoliosis develops. This is discussed in Chapter 16.

PHYSIOLOGICAL EFFECTS

The physiological consequences of respiratory muscle weakness depend largely on which muscles are affected:

Generalized respiratory muscle weakness
(Fig. 15.1)

This causes a restrictive defect with a small VC, due to both a reduction in the TLC and an

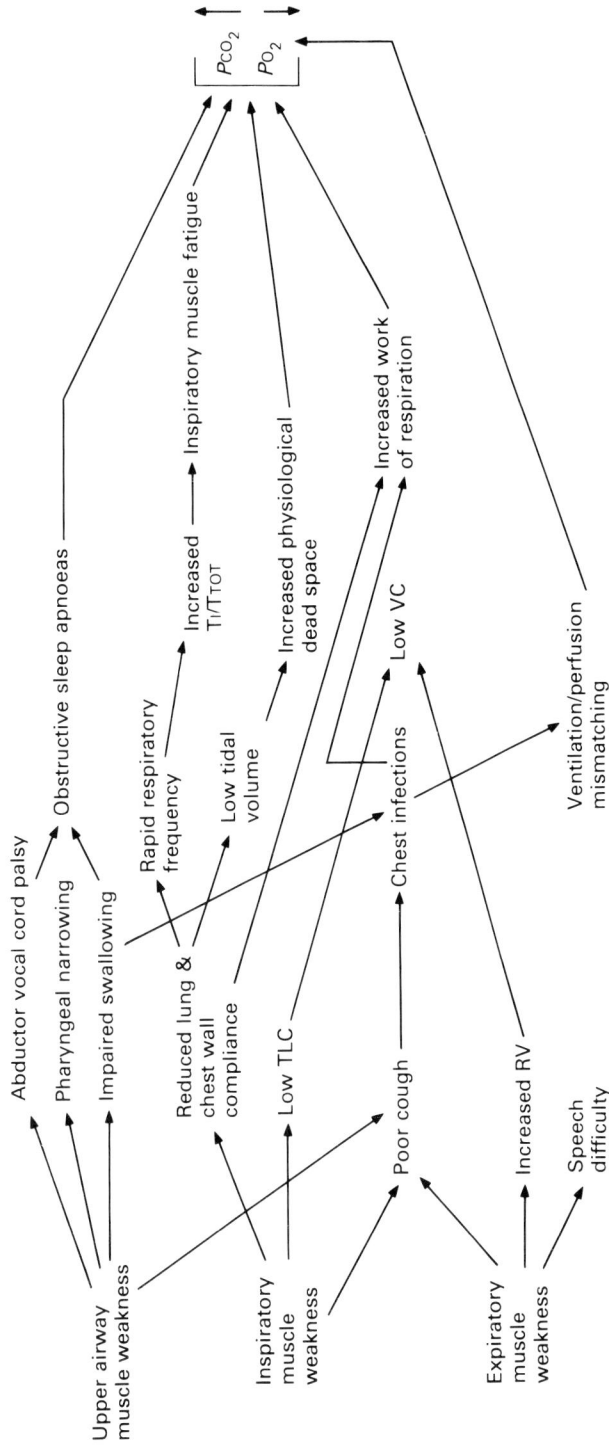

Fig. 15.1. *Flow chart to show effects of respiratory muscle weakness on ventilation.*

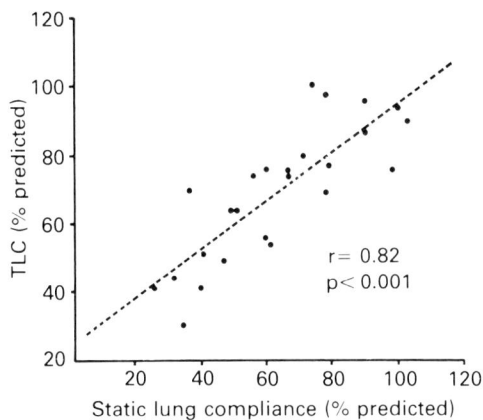

Fig. 15.2. *Relationship between total lung capacity (% predicted) and static lung compliance (% predicted) in patients with respiratory muscle weakness. Reproduced, with permission, from De Troyer A. et al. Thorax 1980; 35: 603– 10.*

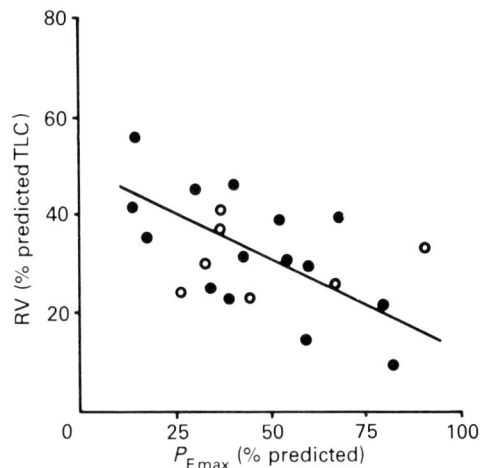

Fig. 15.4. *Relationship of residual volume (expressed as % predicted TLC) to P_{Emax} (% predicted) in patients with myopathies (●; regression line) and myopathies with chronic lung disease (○). Reproduced, with permission, from Braun N.M.T. et al. Thorax 1983; 38: 616–23.*

increase in the RV. The TLC falls because of the weakness of the inspiratory muscles and the reduction in pulmonary [747] and chest wall [932] compliance (Fig. 15.2). The lung compliance is diminished largely because of basal airway closure at small lung volumes, which leads to collapse of distal lung units [745, 1122] (Fig. 15.3). This tendency is exacerbated by an inability to sigh or take deep breaths and often

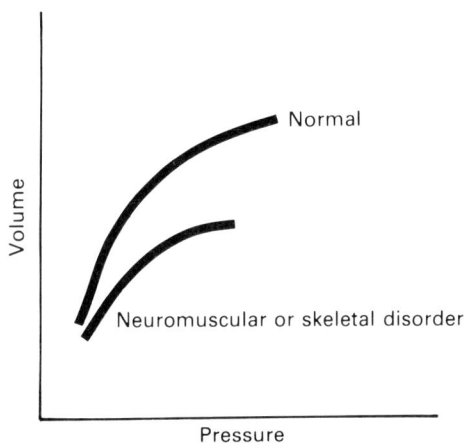

Fig. 15.3. *Volume–pressure curve of lungs of normal subjects and in neuromuscular or skeletal disorders, showing lower compliance and maximum recoil pressure in the latter.*

by a poor cough that leads to sputum retention and areas of lung collapse. The reduction in chest wall compliance may be related to changes in respiratory muscle tone or, in some cases, to mechanical inefficiency of inspiration because of paradoxical movement of the chest wall. Changes in the soft tissues and joints of the rib cage are probably also important. The increase in the RV is less than might be expected from the degree of expiratory muscle weakness because of the increased elastic recoil of the lungs associated with low compliance [742, 745, 1648] (Fig. 15.4).

The changes in the FRC are variable. The reduction in lung compliance and increased elastic recoil of the chest wall tend to lower the FRC but these effects may be obscured by changes in inspiratory and expiratory muscle tone. The MVV is diminished in proportion to the VC [745, 1075, 1648]. Maximal inspiratory and peak expiratory flow rates, which depend on respiratory muscle strength, are reduced.

The fall in the VC is an important feature of respiratory muscles weakness but changes in the P_{Imax} and P_{Emax} precede any change in the lung volumes [312, 389, 766, 1253]. The trans-dia-

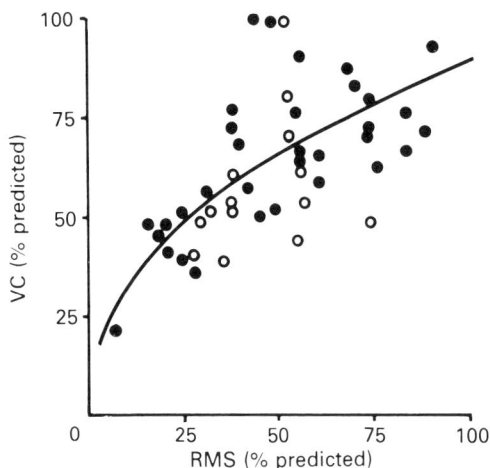

Fig. 15.5. *Relationship between vital capacity (% predicted) and the mean of PI_{max} and PE_{max} (% predicted RMS) in patients with myopathies ($\bullet$; regression line) and myopathies with chronic lung disease ($\circ$). Reproduced, with permission, from Braun N.M.T. et al. Thorax 1983; **38**: 616–23.*

phragmatic pressure is also diminished if the diaphragm is weak. The relationship between PI_{max} and PE_{max} and the VC is curvilinear [389, 392] (Fig. 15.5). The VC falls more than would be expected from the change in maximal pressures alone because of the reduced lung and chest wall compliance.

The combination of respiratory muscle weakness and a low lung and chest wall compliance leads to an increase in respiratory frequency and a decrease in VT [1122, 1367]. As a result the dead space to tidal volume ratio increases and alveolar ventilation falls. As the respiratory frequency rises, TE falls more than TI, with the result that the inspiratory muscle duty cycle ($TI/TTOT$) increases. The mean inspiratory flow rate may not increase because of the muscle weakness but the work of respiration is greater than normal. These factors all contribute to the appearance of respiratory muscle fatigue which, although it has rarely been documented in disorders of respiratory muscles, is probably a major factor in the development of both acute and chronic respiratory failure. Temporary increases in air flow resistance or decreases in compliance due to acute illnesses may precipitate

respiratory muscle fatigue and require intensive treatment.

In the absence of an acute illness, however, hypercapnia is usually a late feature of respiratory muscle weakness. It may appear during wakefulness if the VC falls below about 55% predicted, or if the PI_{max} and PE_{max} are below about 30% predicted [389, 392] (Fig. 15.6). It appears at an earlier stage during sleep than during wakefulness. Hypoventilation may be the result of a fall in VT, which increases the physiological dead space, obstructive apnoeas due to loss of tone in the upper airway muscles, or central apnoeas, especially if the diaphragm is weak or if there is an abnormality of the automatic respiratory drive. The fall in the PO_2 may be out of proportion to the rise in the PCO_2 because of suboptimal matching of ventilation and perfusion. This occurs particularly at the bases of the lungs at low lung volumes during REM sleep when muscle tone is reduced.

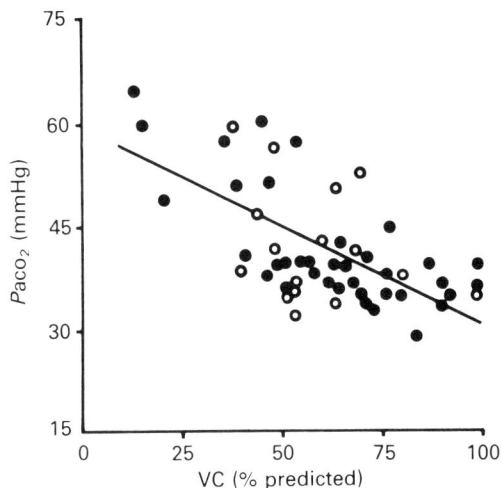

Fig. 15.6. *Relationship between $PaCO_2$ (mmHg) and vital capacity (% predicted) in patients with myopathies ($\bullet$ regression line) and myopathies with chronic lung disease ($\circ$). Reproduced, with permission, from Braun N.M.T. et al. Thorax 1983; **38**: 616–23.*

Selective respiratory muscle weakness

DIAPHRAGMATIC WEAKNESS

The physiological effects of diaphragmatic paralysis are influenced by the presence of pulmonary or chest wall disease, the severity of the paralysis and the age of the subject. The most important distinction, however, is whether the diaphragmatic paralysis is unilateral or bilateral.

Unilateral

Adults. Unilateral weakness of the diaphragm is most commonly due to one of the conditions described in Chapter 13, which damage the phrenic nerve. It is also a feature particularly of poliomyelitis and dystrophia myotonica. During inspiration the diaphragm normally descends, but if it is paralysed it moves upwards (paradoxically) into the thorax. The intrathoracic pressure during inspiration is less than the intra-abdominal pressure because of the action of the intercostal and accessory muscles, and this draws the diaphragm upwards. This paradoxical movement decreases the V_T and the mechanical efficiency of breathing. In the supine position, the weight of the abdominal contents pushes the paralysed diaphragm further into the thorax and decreases the FRC. The abdominal contents splint the diaphragm in an expiratory position so that it moves relatively little, even though it is paralysed. With the subject lying on one side, the lowermost half of the diaphragm behaves in this way if it is paralysed, while if the paralysed hemidiaphragm is uppermost it moves paradoxically [2667].

The maximal inspiratory pressure and transdiaphragmatic pressure are reduced in hemidiaphragmatic paralysis, particularly if the lungs are also abnormal [1812, 1914]. The impairment of inspiratory muscle strength is partially compensated for by recruitment of intercostal, accessory and abdominal muscles, and shortness of breath is unusual unless there is pulmonary disease. Exercise tolerance appears to be unimpaired [2520].

Most of the early data on the effects of unilateral diaphragmatic paralysis on the VC were gained from subjects with tuberculosis who underwent phrenic nerve crush or avulsion. These

studies were complicated by the presence of parenchymal lung disease, which was usually worse on the side of the phrenic nerve interruption. The findings are discussed on p. 192. More recent studies in patients without lung disease have shown a fall of 20–25% in the VC when upright [97, 98, 580, 1212, 2618, 3120, 3286], although in one study [944] little change was observed. A further fall of about 15% occurs when the subject lies supine [580, 1212], whereas normally the postural fall in the VC is less than about 10% [62, 316]. The FEV_1 and MVV decrease in proportion to the fall in the VC [97, 3120]. The TLC and FRC also diminish to a similar extent to the VC when sitting [874, 2618] and fall further when supine [580]. The RV is unchanged [874], since expiratory muscle strength is largely preserved (Fig. 9.7).

The distribution of ventilation and perfusion in the lungs has been studied by bronchospirometry and by isotopic techniques (Fig. 15.7). Ventilation is slightly diminished on the side of the diaphragmatic paralysis when the subject is sitting [874, 3120, 3286]. Both ventilation and perfusion are most affected at the base of the lung [97, 3286] and the ^{133}Xe washout time is prolonged [874, 2618]. In the supine position, ventilation is further diminished on the side of the diaphragm paralysis [3120]. When lying on one side with the paralysed hemidiaphragm lower-most, the ventilation is diminished and perfusion is increased to the lower lung. This shunt of blood is responsible for significant hypoxaemia. If the paralysed side is uppermost, both the ventilation and perfusion are decreased on the abnormal side [97]. Pulmonary angiography has not shown any significant anatomical changes in the pulmonary vasculature [3120] but at bronchography the bronchi to the lower lobes appear kinked, particularly when lying on the side of the paralysed hemidiaphragm [97].

The oxygen uptake measured by bronchospirometry is disproportionately decreased on the side of the hemidiaphragmatic paralysis [3214]. This presumably reflects mismatching of ventilation and perfusion and is related to the

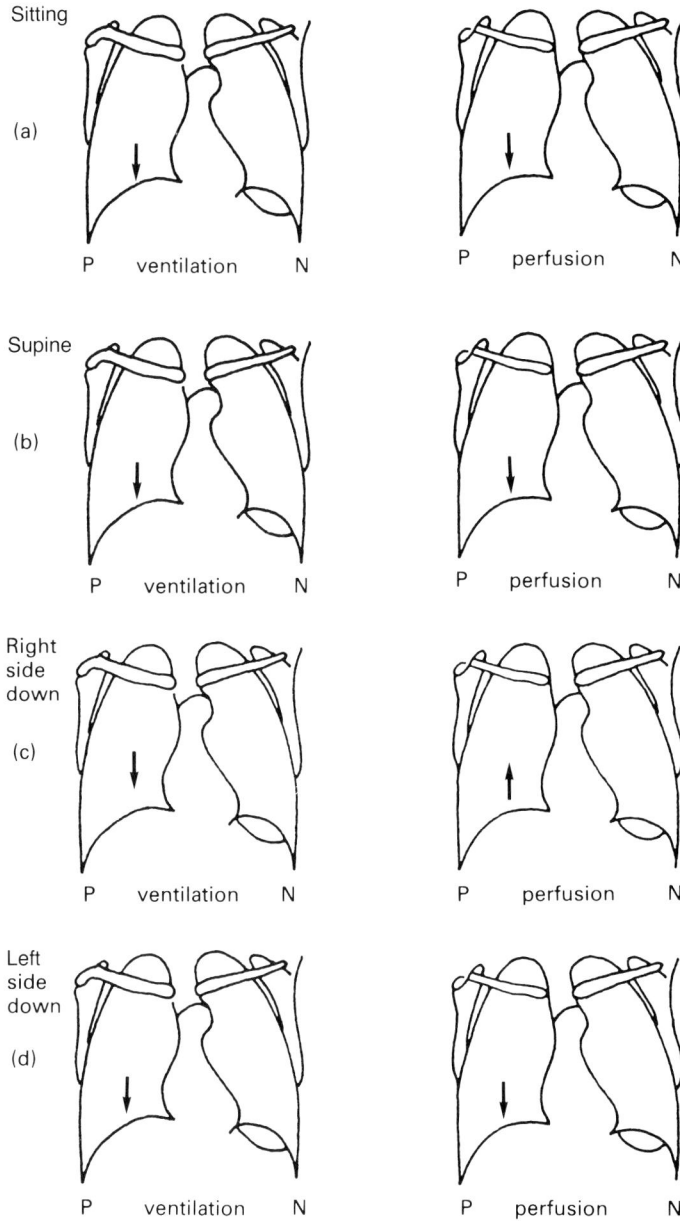

Fig. 15.7. *Changes in ventilation and perfusion with unilateral diaphragmatic paralysis in the sitting (a), supine (b), and right (c) and left (d) side down positions. P=paralysed hemidiaphragm; N=normal hemidiaphragm.*

hypoxaemia, which usually is not present when sitting [97, 580, 1985]. Hypercapnia does not appear in any position during wakefulness or during sleep [580, 1985]. The respiratory drive is normal: the $P_{0.1}$ in response to hypercapnia is even increased, probably because of reflex compensation for the hemidiaphragmatic paralysis [874].

Diaphragmatic plication for hemidiaphragmatic paralysis is rarely required if the lungs are normal because the respiratory symptoms and physiological deficit are mild. Non-respiratory symptoms occasionally require surgery [1547, 558, 2017]. Breathlessness may be troublesome if the diaphragmatic paralysis is associated with pulmonary disease, and in this situation plication may be beneficial. Breathlessness [1816, 2017, 3374], VC [1816, 2056, 3374], FRC and P_{O_2} all improve and the lung volumes are less abnormal in the supine position [3374]. Occasionally plication fails and replacement of the diaphragm by synthetic material such as Marlex mesh is required [355]. Some return of function has also been reported following anastomosis of the phrenic to the facial nerve [1356].

Infants. The causes of diaphragmatic weakness in infancy have been discussed on p. 149. The consequences of unilateral diaphragmatic paralysis in adults, although detectable, are often clinically unimportant. In infants, however, weakness of the diaphragm has a much more marked impact on respiration and usually causes ventilatory failure. There are several physiological features in the newborn that contribute to this. The sternum and ribs are more horizontal than later in life and consequently the range of rib cage expansion is limited if the diaphragm is paralysed [2106]. Secondly, the rib cage of neonates is more compliant than that of adults [2222]. During REM sleep, the intercostal and accessory muscle tone diminishes so that the rib cage is less stable. The negative intrapleural pressure generated by diaphragmatic contraction can cause paradoxical movement of the rib cage. This impairs the efficiency of diaphragmatic function and contributes significantly to respiratory failure if the diaphragm is weak [429, 2251]. Thirdly, the respiratory rate of neonates is faster than later in life and the T_E in particular is shortened. The duty cycle of the inspiratory muscles is, therefore, increased and this predisposes to inspiratory muscle fatigue [2252]. The diaphragm of neonates fatigues more quickly than that of adults [1942, 2251] as there are relatively more type 2 muscle fibres, which are susceptible to fatigue [428, 886, 1634, 1635]. Electromyogram

evidence for diaphragm fatigue, particularly a decrease in the high/low frequency ratio, has been observed [2251], even in certain physiological circumstances such as REM sleep.

Ventilatory support or diaphragmatic plication is usually required under the age of about three years [1245, 1970]. The choice and timing of treatment depends on the probability of recovery from the condition that caused the phrenic nerve damage or diaphragmatic paralysis. If the outlook is good it is preferable to support ventilation either by endotracheal intubation with IPPV or by CPAP [1333, 1970, 2668]. These methods of positive pressure ventilation stabilize the diaphragm and prevent its paradoxical upward movement during inspiration.

Surgical plication lowers the diaphragm and increases the lung volumes. It probably prevents basal airway collapse and increases the compliance of the lungs [2825]. The diaphragm becomes fixed [1245, 2056] but there is no increase in transdiaphragmatic pressure after plication and any improvement is purely due to the increase in lung volumes and to prevention of paradoxical movement rather than to return of active contraction [2825]. Bilateral plication for bilateral diaphragmatic paralysis in infants is of little value, presumably because neither of the hemidiaphragms can contract [2830]. Plication does not appear to prevent a return of function at a later date if there is recovery from the cause of the paralysis [2830].

Plication in infants and young children is a safe, effective form of treatment and may allow weaning from ventilatory support [301, 567, 1573, 2830]. It is generally reserved for those patients who still require ventilatory support after a period of observation of about three months or who still have difficulty with breathing.

Bilateral

Adults. Bilateral diaphragmatic weakness may be seen in almost any of the disorders that affect

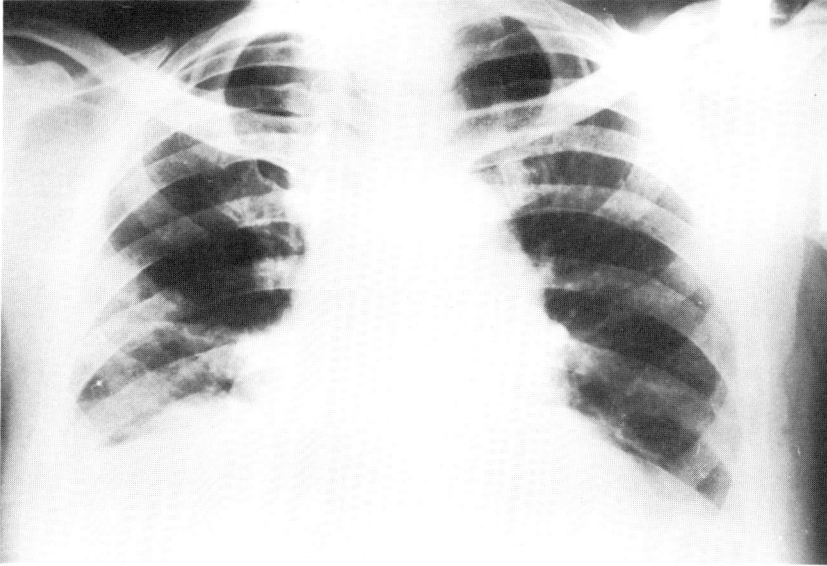

Fig. 15.8. *Chest radiograph showing elevation of diaphragm and basal lung collapse, particularly on the right, due to bilateral diaphragmatic paralysis.*

the respiratory muscles, but it is particularly a feature of acid maltase deficiency and SLE. Severe weakness is also seen in high cervical cord lesions, poliomyelitis, motor neuron disease, acute idiopathic polyneuropathy, and cryptogenic peripheral neuropathy, which may occasionally be familial [2200].

The physiological abnormalities seen with bilateral diaphragmatic paralysis in adults are much more marked than with hemidiaphragmatic paralysis. The fall in intrathoracic pressure during inspiration leads to paradoxical movement of the diaphragm (Fig. 15.8). The pressure changes are transmitted across the flaccid diaphragm so that the abdominal pressure falls during inspiration and the anterior abdominal wall moves paradoxically. This may not be apparent while sitting or standing if contraction of the abdominal muscles during expiration raises the abdominal pressure and elevates the diaphragm so that the end expiratory volume is less than the FRC. The lungs inflate without diaphragmatic activity when the abdominal muscles relax during inspiration, because of the outward elastic recoil of the chest wall [1742, 1929].

The maximal transdiaphragmatic pressure is grossly diminished and may even be zero [735] with bilateral diaphragmatic weakness. The diaphragm is the main inspiratory muscle and, consequently, PI_{max} is also greatly reduced. Exercise tolerance is much more markedly diminished in bilateral than in unilateral diaphragmatic paralysis [2520]. The maximal inspiratory flow rates are low but PE_{max} is well preserved [1985].

The VC in the sitting position is about 50% predicted [735, 2776, 3023] but it may fall by a further 50% when supine [735]. Proportionately smaller changes are seen with lesser degrees of diaphragm weakness [2150]. The influence of the supine position on the VC is greater with bilateral than with unilateral diaphragmatic weakness since the weight of the abdominal contents pushes both halves of the diaphragm into the thorax. The loss of inspiratory capacity is greater than would be expected from the degree of diaphragm weakness because of a reduction in lung compliance [1120, 2300] (see Fig. 9.7).

The distribution of ventilation and perfusion is also influenced by position (Fig. 15.9). While

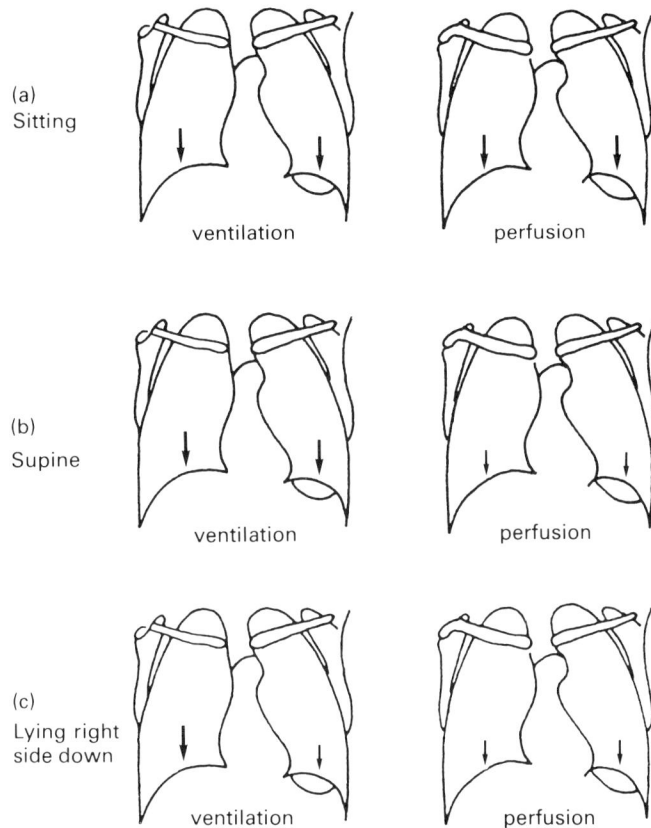

(a)
Sitting

ventilation   perfusion

(b)
Supine

ventilation   perfusion

(c)
Lying right
side down

ventilation   perfusion

Fig. 15.9. *Changes in ventilation and perfusion with bilateral diaphragmatic paralysis in the sitting (a), supine (b) and right side down (c) positions. The size of the arrows indicates the degree of change.*

sitting, there is a slight loss of basal ventilation and of the normal gradient of perfusion from the apex to the bases of the lungs [73]. In the supine position, the ventilation is even more diminished at the bases [73] and the A–a oxygen gradient increases so that the P_{O_2} falls [1490] and P_{CO_2} may rise [1930]. When lying on one side the perfusion is greater to the lower lung, as in normal subjects, but the ventilation is more diminished in the dependent lung [73, 1930, 1931]. The shunt of unoxygenated blood through the lungs may be considerable.

These postural changes are partly responsible for the hypoxia that has been observed during sleep. The fall in P_{O_2} during sleep is related to the transdiaphragmatic pressure and to the degree of hypoxia during wakefulness [736]. Changes in respiratory pattern and muscle tone also contribute to the blood gas abnormalities.

A rapid respiratory rate with small V_T [1490] and short T_I is characteristic of bilateral diaphragmatic paralysis. This pattern may be initiated by afferent impulses from receptors in the lungs that respond to the small lung volumes [2298, 2300, 2959]. In dogs, vagotomy returns this respiratory pattern to normal [2322]. Rapid, shallow breathing increases the dead space so that at any given minute ventilation the alveolar ventilation is lessened. During REM sleep, intercostal and accessory muscle activity is abolished and if the diaphragm is paralysed, respiratory muscle activity may cease. This mimics a central sleep apnoea, although there is no abnormality of central control of respiration. Hypercapnia frequently develops during sleep [735, 2300], although it is less common during wakefulness.

Infants. The respiratory effects of bilateral diaphragmatic paralysis in infants are similar to those of unilateral diaphragm paralysis, but more severe. Ventilatory failure is invariable and mechanical ventilatory support is required.

INTERCOSTAL AND ACCESSORY MUSCLES

Paralysis of the cervical accessory muscles impairs the ability to elevate the upper rib cage and sternum. Intercostal muscle paralysis also limits rib cage movement but, in addition, their stabilizing effect on the rib cage is lost. The negative intrapleural pressure generated by diaphragmatic contraction, therefore, causes paradoxical movement of the rib cage during inspiration. The VC and MVV are both decreased.

ABDOMINAL MUSCLES

Weakness of the abdominal muscles influences both inspiration and expiration. If the muscle tone of the abdomen is reduced, the compliance of the abdomen increases. Contraction of the diaphragm will, therefore, increase the abdominal expansion relative to that of the rib cage in the supine position. The weight of the abdominal contents ensures that the diaphragm is elevated during expiration. However, while sitting or standing, the return of the diaphragm to a normal end-expiratory level is prevented by the gravitational effects on the abdominal contents. The diaphragmatic fibres are, therefore, too short to contract effectively during inspiration [1174].

The abdominal muscles normally contribute to expiration at high minute volumes and their paralysis diminishes the $P_{E_{max}}$, PEFR and VC and increases the RV. The effectiveness of cough is diminished, particularly while sitting or standing [707].

UPPER AIRWAY MUSCLES

Upper airway muscle weakness may lead to upper airway obstruction (Chapter 6), impairment of cough, difficulty in swallowing and stridor (Chapter 7).

INDIVIDUAL DISORDERS

The classification of the large numbers of disorders that affect primarily the muscles rather than the neuromuscular junction, peripheral nerves or spinal cord is difficult. It rests not only on the clinical pattern of muscle involvement and the genetic basis of the disorders, but on EMG and muscle biopsy findings [3257]. Some of these conditions are associated with respiratory problems that may be severe, whereas in other disorders respiratory complications are virtually unknown. In this chapter, only those muscle disorders with respiratory consequences are considered.

Muscular dystrophies

The classification of these diseases is in a state of flux but the feature common to all of them is that they are progressive genetically-determined degenerative myopathies [1086]. They can be grouped according to their genetic inheritance.

X-LINKED

Duchenne's muscular dystrophy (progressive muscular dystrophy)

This is the commonest of the muscular dystrophies and usually becomes apparent by the age of five. It almost exclusively affects boys but when it is seen in girls it is usually milder and inherited in an autosomal recessive way. The muscle weakness initially involves the proximal limb muscles and is steadily progressive. The ability to walk is commonly lost between the ages of eight and twelve and death usually occurs in the second or third decades. Respiratory muscle weakness is almost invariable, and causes most of the respiratory complications. These are responsible for over 75% of deaths in Duchenne's muscular dystrophy [1134, 1531, 3233].

Lung volumes. Breathlessness on exertion is uncommon in young children with Duchenne's muscular dystrophy and it rarely develops later because of the steady decrease in the amount of physical exertion that is possible.. The abnormalities in respiratory function are mild before the age at which the ability to walk is lost. The growth of the thorax proceeds almost normally and there is little loss of respiratory muscle strength [1785]. The lung volumes are, there-

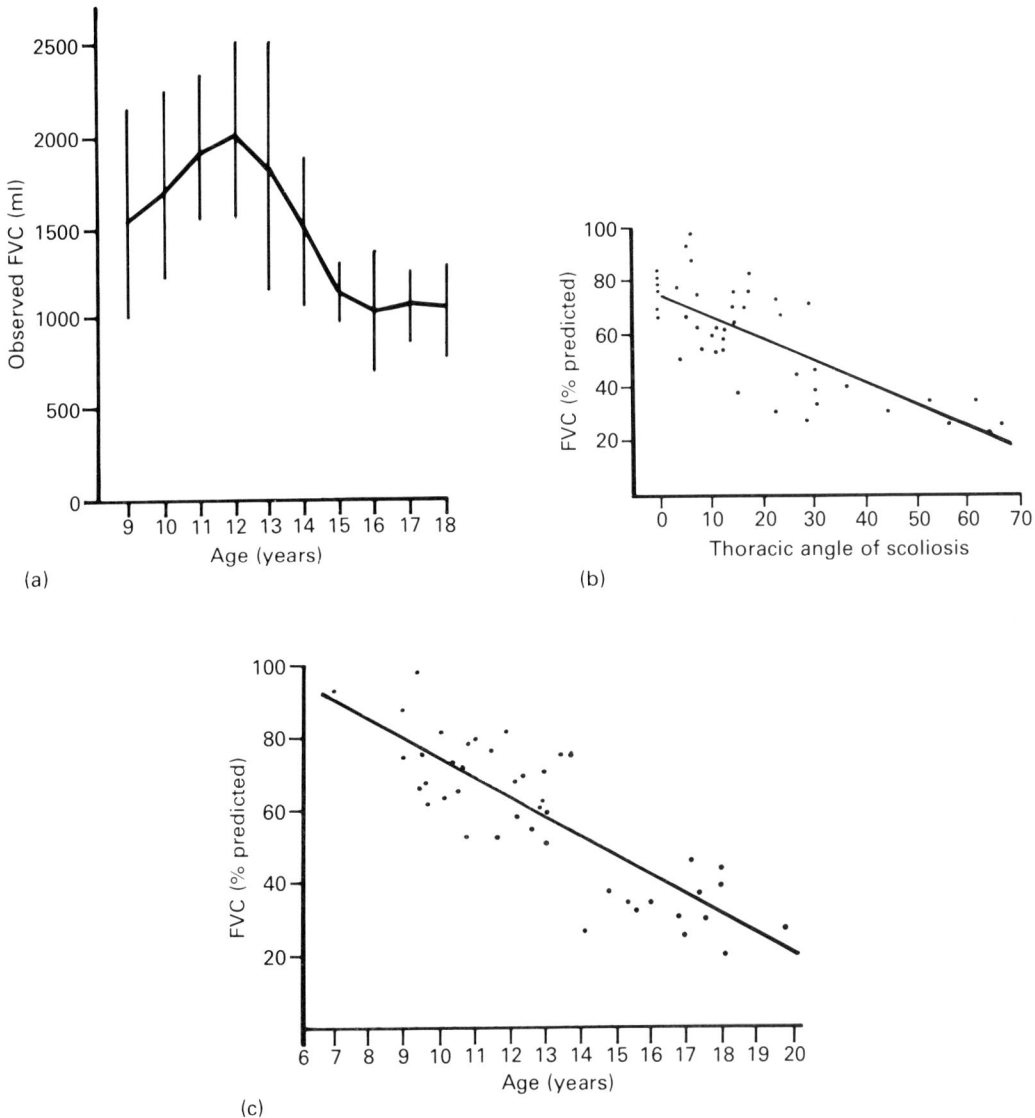

Fig. 15.10. *Duchenne's muscular dystrophy: (a) relationship of forced vital capacity to age, (b) relationship of forced vital capacity (% predicted) to angle of scoliosis, (c) relationship of forced vital capacity (% predicted) to age. Reproduced, with permission, from* J. Pediatr. Orthoped. *1983;* 3: *349–50.*

fore, well preserved but at about the stage when walking becomes impossible the VC begins to fall (see Fig. 15.10). This is partly due to the development of a scoliosis (see below) and partly to the loss of respiratory muscle strength. The PI_{max} and PE_{max} begin to decrease [1531, 1785, 3233] and a restrictive defect is apparent [1537, 2745, 2754]. A raised RV [1949, 3233] is followed by a fall in the TLC [3233] (Fig. 9.7). The FRC remains normal [1345, 1949]. The increase in RV and decrease in TLC and VC correlate with the loss of respiratory muscle strength [1531]. Air flow obstruction is not a feature of Duchenne's muscular dystrophy [442, 1345], and lung compliance when corrected for the small lung volumes is also virtually normal [1345].

The VC reaches its peak around the age of 10–12 years [147, 2617] and then falls steadily. This peak VC gives the best estimate of the life span of the individual patient [2616, 2617]. The fall in VC is linearly related to age [1566] (Fig. 15.11).

Respiratory muscle weakness. The inspiratory and expiratory muscles are involved to an equal extent. The PI_{max} and PE_{max} fall in parallel [1531] but, interestingly, the diaphragm is often relatively spared. Only one study [1345] has implied that involvement of the diaphragm is common, and this has not been substantiated. There is no difference between the supine and standing VC [1531] or MVV [3233], which would be expected if bilateral diaphragmatic weakness was present. Orthopnoea is uncommon and this sparing of the diaphragm may explain the delay in the appearance of respiratory failure until the muscular dystrophy is well advanced [2299]. Rib cage expansion is, however, often minimal and weakness of the cervical, accessory and abdominal muscles may be profound. Weakness of the expiratory muscles lessens the effectiveness of coughing. Pneumonias occur particularly in the lower lobes [1134, 3233]. Aspiration may be a contributory factor but pharyngeal and oesophageal function is usually normal [2335]. The inability to cough adequately and

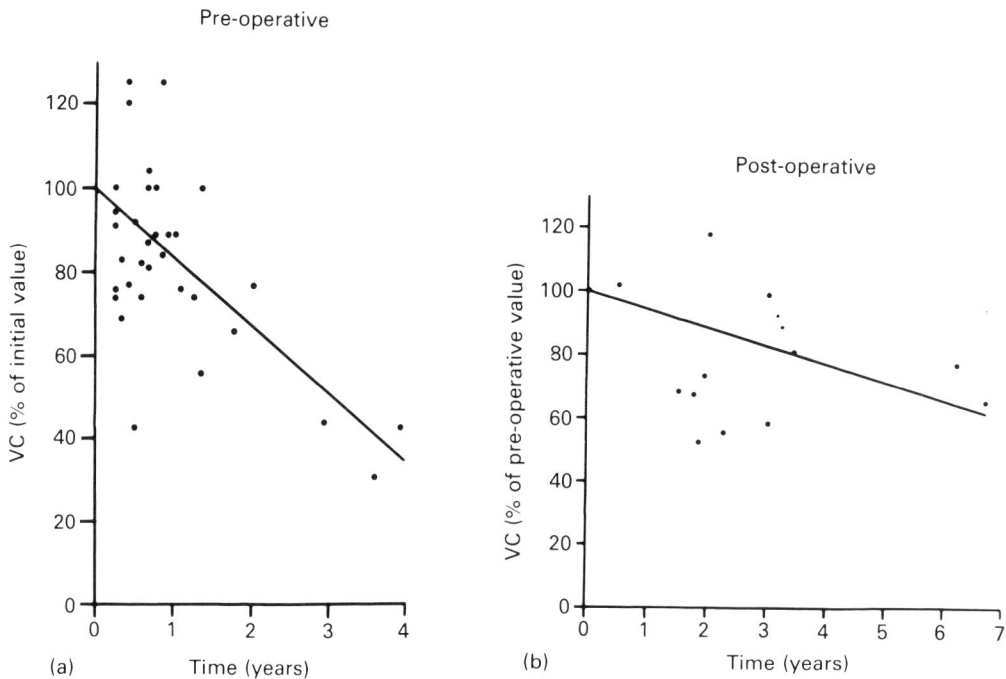

Fig. 15.11. *Deterioration of vital capacity in Duchenne's muscular dystrophy: (a) before spinal fusion, (b) after spinal fusion. Reproduced, with permission, from Jenkins J.G. Crit. Care Med., 1982;* **10**: *647.*

susceptibility to respiratory-depressant drugs renders surgery hazardous [1652].

Ethical problems may arise as to how intensive treatment should be during acute infections. The quality of life before the infection is the most important aspect to bear in mind; even extreme degrees of physical disability may be remarkably well tolerated. Physiotherapy, suction of secretions, prompt intravenous antibiotic treatment, rehydration and even a minitracheostomy may be appropriate. If these measures are taken, the mortality during acute respiratory infections is remarkably low, except in the presence of very advanced disease [3233].

Scoliosis. Respiratory function is also compromised by the development of a scoliosis. This often develops shortly before the ability to walk is lost [2599, 2660] and is almost invariably shortly afterwards [1785]. It appears to be due to generalized weakness of the trunk muscles leading to collapse of the spine rather than to an asymmetrical weakness of the paraspinal and other muscles [2661]. It often progresses rapidly, particularly during the adolescent growth spurt. If the pelvis is level the scoliosis is usually low thoracic, but if there is pelvic obliquity it is usually thoracolumbar or lumbar [3337]. If the lumbar curve is greater than about 35°, progression is inevitable [3277] and may be rapid [1481].

Lumbar curves may cause backache and difficulty in sitting but it is only curves affecting the thoracic spine that have a bearing on respiratory function [1785]. The percentage predicted FVC is linearly related to the angle of thoracic scoliosis (Fig. 15.10). This close association between the angle of thoracic scoliosis and respiratory function is important since the scoliosis is readily treatable by spinal fusion. Following this procedure the VC falls at only about 25% of the pre-operative rate [1566] (Fig. 15.11). Post-operative complications are greater if the VC is less than about 30% predicted at the time of surgery [1566]. A temporary tracheostomy may be required, par-

ticularly if the cough is weak [2752]. Spinal fusion should therefore be considered early, probably once the scoliosis is between 25° and 35° [1116, 1785, 2616, 3115], at which stage the VC is relatively well preserved.

Not all patients, however, develop a scoliosis. In a significant number the spine becomes hyperextended in a stable though stiff position, despite weakness of the extensor muscles [1117, 1345, 1949, 3337]. It is uncertain why this position occurs but in one study it was seen in the oldest surviving patients [3337]. It may help to preserve lung function in a similar manner to spinal fusion, although at the cost of difficulty in obtaining a comfortable sitting position.

Respiratory control. There is no evidence for an abnormality of respiratory drive in Duchenne's muscular dystrophy. The ventilatory response to inhaling 5% CO_2 is normal [1531] and more complex studies measuring respiratory frequency, V_T/T_I and $P_{0.1}$ in addition to minute ventilation have shown virtually normal responses to hypercapnia, hypoxia and hyperoxia [219].

Chronic respiratory failure. Chronic respiratory failure is a well-recognized complication of Duchenne's muscular dystrophy, but it usually appears late in its natural history. Even nocturnal hypoventilation is usually mild and a late complication [2980]. In the earlier stages mild hypoxia may be present [1345, 1537], but this is not invariable [1531]. Hypoxia in the presence of a normal P_{CO_2} is due to suboptimal ventilation/perfusion matching at the bases of the lungs secondary to respiratory muscle weakness. The P_{CO_2} may rise temporarily during chest infections [1949] but this does not necessarily indicate a poor prognosis [3233]. Conversely, once the P_{CO_2} is raised in the absence of a chest infection, the outlook is poor [1531] unless ventilatory assistance is provided.

It is uncertain as to why hypercapnia should appear after a long period of normocapnia in the presence of respiratory muscle weakness. It is possible that V_T falls, increasing the dead space to tidal volume ratio, and the respiratory frequency increases, increasing the T_I/T_{TOT}. This would decrease alveolar ventilation and also, by increasing the duty cycle of the inspiratory muscles, predispose to respiratory muscle fatigue.

Cardiac complications. Cor pulmonale, which is a feature of several chronic muscular disorders, is not apparent in Duchenne's muscular dystrophy. The cardiac complications are dominated by the specific cardiomyopathy associated with this condition. The myocardium shows extensive muscle fibre loss, with replacement by fatty connective tissue [1134, 3061] and multifocal degeneration of conducting tissue [2783]. The posterior wall of the left ventricle is worst affected and in older subjects becomes thin [1167]. Left ventricular function progressively deteriorates [1420, 1498], although in some subjects the cardiac output is increased [3106] and the pulmonary capillary wedge pressure is normal [99]. Pulmonary hypertension is rarely severe [99, 1073, 3061].

A sinus tachycardia and a third or fourth heart sound are common [1420, 2442] but heart failure often appears only pre-terminally and may be precipitated by chest infections [1420]. The heart is usually of normal size, radiographically, until the late stages of the disease. The ECG is normal in almost 50% of patients [2783]. A short PR interval, atrioventricular block, bundle branch block, and other intraventricular conduction defects are all seen [2783]. Characteristically, the ECG shows a tall R wave in V_1 and deep narrow Q waves in lateral chest leads, indicating an electrically non-functioning posterior wall of the left ventricle [1498].

Cardiac dysrhythmias may appear during surgery [591]. Cardiac arrest during or after surgery, possibly due to an abnormal response to succinylcholine, can even be the presenting feature [2841]. Verapamil, a calcium channel blocker widely used for treating cardiac dysrhythmias, may also induce weakness and lead to acute respiratory failure [3394].

Becker's muscular dystrophy

This is much less common than Duchenne's muscular dystrophy. The distribution of the weakness is similar in the two conditions, but the age of onset is later (usually around ten years) and its progression is much slower. The ability to walk, for instance, is not lost until the age of about twenty-five years. Similar respiratory complications to Duchenne's muscular dystrophy might be expected but they appear to be surprisingly mild. There are, however, very few adequate studies, possibly because of the rarity of the condition. In one series, patients with classical Becker's muscular dystrophy had normal spirometry, although a group intermediate between Duchenne's and Becker's muscular dystrophies showed a moderately severe restrictive defect [2617]. Cardiac involvement is probably more common than was initially thought [2442]. The ECG may show changes of left and also of right ventricular hypertrophy [914, 3250].

AUTOSOMAL RECESSIVE

Limb-girdle muscular dystrophy

This is probably a heterogeneous group of conditions and analysis of the respiratory complications is, therefore, difficult. In mild cases, spirometry is normal [2617] or only slightly impaired [2745] but early and fairly selective involvement of the diaphragm may occur [2299]. This may be severe enough to cause nocturnal hypoxia, especially in REM sleep [2959], and for assisted ventilation to be required [2289]. Cardiac abnormalities such as a third and fourth heart sound may be present [2442].

AUTOSOMAL DOMINANT

Facioscapulohumeral muscular dystrophy

This condition is more clearly defined than limb-girdle muscular dystrophy and is often mild, only slowly progressive, and associated with a normal life-span. Respiratory muscle involvement is not a prominent feature [2299, 2617] but, occasionally, the diaphragm may be weak [3365]. Dysphagia and aspiration pneumonias are uncommon [2335] and cardiac involvement is rare [2442].

Dystrophia myotonica (myotonia atrophica, Steinert's disease)

Dystrophia myotonica is characterized by myotonia (failure of muscle relaxation), muscle weakness and atrophy. In addition, a variety of features unrelated to skeletal muscle involvement are common. These include frontal baldness, cataracts and testicular atrophy, and this condition is best regarded as a multisystem disorder [1360].

At one time dystrophia myotonica was thought to be rare before puberty but it is now recognized to occur even in young children [803]. The neonatal form is almost invariably associated with a history of dystrophia myotonica in the mother rather than the father, suggesting that an intra-uterine factor is responsible for its appearance [37, 1361]. Respiratory complications are common and often severe [37, 2943]. Respiratory muscle strength may be insufficient to take the first few breaths after delivery [349] and mechanical ventilation is frequently required [37]. Feeding difficulties leading to aspiration of secretions into the lungs may also be a problem [2537, 2943, 3304]. The diaphragm may be extensively involved [349] but, more commonly, weakness is only diagnosed from the presence of a unilateral, usually right-sided, elevated hemidiaphragm on the chest radiograph [37, 572, 2537, 3304].

Respiratory muscle weakness. In adults, dystrophia myotonica first affects the facial muscles, the sternomastoids and the limb muscles. Weakness of the respiratory muscles can be detected frequently by physiological tests but is often clinically unimportant. A fall in P_{Imax} and P_{Emax} is the earliest observable abnor-

mality [217, 1128, 2854]. The P_{Emax} is reduced more than P_{Imax} [1253, 2854] and this underlies the ineffective cough from which many of these patients suffer. The diaphragm is not usually selectively weakened [2853, 2854] but, occasionally, unilateral elevation of a hemidiaphragm, usually the right side, is seen radiographically [516, 517, 574, 883, 2946] (Fig. 15.12). The elevated hemidiaphragm moves poorly fluoroscopically and may be histologically abnormal, showing the variation in muscle fibre size and central chains of nuclei that are seen in other skeletal muscles [516, 517].

The respiratory muscle weakness leads to a restrictive defect. The VC and TLC fall, often with a slight increase in RV [883, 1664, 1889, 2854]. There is little change in the FRC [2854] and the FEV_1/FVC ratio is normal [1664, 2854].

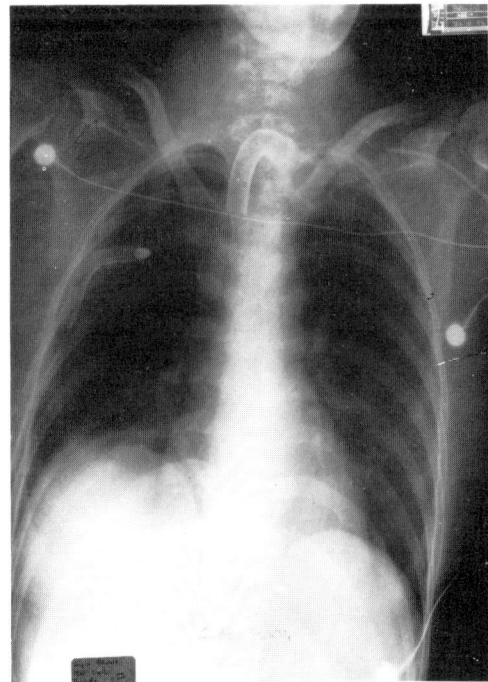

Fig. 15.12. *Chest radiograph of patient with dystrophia myotonica showing elevated right hemidiaphragm and right basal consolidation due to aspiration pneumonia. This precipitated acute ventilatory failure requiring tracheostomy and IPPV, which was complicated by right pneumothorax requiring an intercostal drain.*

Respiratory muscle weakness may also show itself by the development of fatigue at high minute ventilations, such as during exercise. Alternating thoracic and abdominal expansion reflects the inspiratory action of the diaphragm and intercostal muscles during alternate breaths [217].

Myotonia. Myotonia is of less respiratory significance than muscle weakness. It might be anticipated to occur during rapid deep breathing such as in a MVV manoeuvre, but even in this situation it is not prominent. Any reduction in MVV is proportional to the fall in VC [2854] and is, therefore, related to respiratory muscle weakness rather than to myotonia. It has been proposed that the rapid respiratory frequency at rest that has been observed is due to myotonia of the respiratory muscles during inspiration [217]. This could stiffen the chest wall or derange proprioceptive reflex control of respiration, but the evidence is indirect and any abnormality in respiratory rate may well be due to a reduction in lung compliance due to the restrictive defect rather than to myotonia [1121].

Myotonia may, however, be responsible for the unusual jerky movements of the diaphragm that have been noted on fluoroscopy [239, 488, 1663]. Myotonic discharges have been recorded from diaphragmatic EMGs during quiet breathing [2989] but the clinical importance of these movements is uncertain. Myotonia is unlikely to be responsible for the elevation of the diaphragm noted above since prolonged contraction of the diaphragm would lower rather than raise it. Myotonia has been implicated in causing obstructive sleep apnoeas (see below) and can cause problems during general anaesthesia (see below).

Respiratory control and respiratory failure. Respiratory control in dystrophia myotonica has been investigated closely because of the occasional association of severe respiratory failure and hypersomnia. The ventilatory response to hypercapnia [218, 502, 1664, 2853] and probably to hypoxia [502] is subnormal, except in mildly affected subjects [1128]. The ratio V_T/T_I is also less than normal in the presence of hypercapnia or hypoxia [218]. However, these ventilatory responses depend not only on the respiratory drive but also on other factors, such as respiratory muscle strength, air flow resistance and the compliance of the respiratory system. The $P_{0.1}$, which is relatively independent of these other factors, is normal [218]. This suggests that the respiratory drive itself is normal, but that either respiratory muscle weakness or possibly the lung or chest wall compliance limits the ventilatory responses to hypercapnia and hypoxia. This is supported by the finding that the ventilatory response to hypercapnia correlates with the VC and with the maximal mouth pressures [2853].

Despite these findings, which suggest a normal central control of respiration, frequent irregularities of resting tidal breathing have been noted [2853]. Prolonged central [595, 1344, 3225] and obstructive [458, 693, 1281, 1292, 3076, 3225] sleep apnoeas occur, particularly during REM and stages 1 and 2 NREM sleep. Cheyne-Stokes respiration has also been noted [596, 1663]. Fibre-optic endoscopy has shown that the supraglottic mucosa completely occludes the airway during obstructive sleep apnoeas [458]. In one study the frequency of obstructive sleep apnoeas was significantly diminished by phenytoin treatment, suggesting that upper airway myotonia was responsible for the airway occlusion [3076].

These abnormalities in respiratory pattern have been found particularly in patients with respiratory failure while awake [596, 1344, 3076]. Respiratory failure may be severe enough to cause polycythaemia [202, 239] and pulmonary hypertension [202, 595, 1663, 1664, 2637]. The latter may be present both during the day and at night but can worsen dramatically during sleep apnoeas if they are sufficiently prolonged to cause severe hypoxia [595, 1281]. The pulmonary artery pressure may also rise considerably during exercise if desaturation occurs [2637].

Hypersomnia frequently accompanies respiratory failure [458, 1664], but in some patients appears to be unrelated to this [693, 1281, 2456] and improvement in the arterial blood gases may not abolish the hypersomnia [595]. Its association with frequent nocturnal apnoeas and a diminution in the proportion of REM sleep suggests that it is caused by sleep deprivation rather than hypoxaemia [1889].

Chest infections. Chest infections are frequent in patients with dystrophia myotonica [3291]. They are partly due to the ineffective cough related to weakness of the expiratory muscles and larynx, but swallowing abnormalities and aspiration of food and secretions into the lungs is another important factor. Aspiration may go unnoticed by the patient [2536, 2538] but, more commonly, it causes recurrent coughing [1953]. Dysphagia occasionally occurs [2477] and there may be difficulty in chewing due to myotonia of the facial and masticatory muscles [2477].

Observations of swallowing have shown several abnormalities. The clearance of fluid from the pharynx is greatly prolonged [2536, 2538], oesophageal peristalsis is diminished [1376, 1888, 2477, 2538], abnormal cricopharyngeal function is common [1376, 2477] and the vocal cords may fail to adduct completely during swallowing [2538]. The oesophageal abnormalities do not appear to correlate with the FEV_1, VC or MVV [1088]. Both the skeletal and the smooth muscle of the oesophagus may function abnormally [739, 2556]. These changes are part of a widespread disturbance of bowel motility [1888].

Radiographic examination of swallowing with contrast media has clearly demonstrated pulmonary aspiration [2536] and bilateral lower lobe bronchiectasis, presumably a result of long-standing aspiration [2536]. Lung abscesses may develop [3291] and bronchopneumonia is a common cause of death [313, 488].

Infections may also be related to immunological abnormalities. Low immunoglobulin concentrations are common and have even been recommended as a screening test for apparently unaffected relatives of subjects with dystrophia myotonica [2651]. More rarely, thymomas may be present [494, 2243] and may impair immunity [1783], leading to recurrent infections.

General anaesthesia. General anaesthesia may be dangerous in dystrophia myotonica for a variety of reasons [49, 738, 2243]. These patients are very susceptible to respiratory sedatives and any of this group of drugs may cause hypoventilation [2186]. Facilities should always be available for post-operative ventilation [3137]. This enables secretions to be aspirated from the chest as well as maintaining adequate ventilation. Respiration is also depressed in some patients by thiopentone, although others are completely unaffected by this drug [1128, 2568]. The airway may obstruct post-operatively because of weakness of the sternomastoid muscles [3291] and the post-operative course is often complicated by an inability to cough adequately [318].

Non-depolarizing muscle relaxants are well tolerated but succinylcholine frequently induces marked myotonia [2414] and should always be avoided. Succinylcholine is particularly dangerous if the airway has not been secured, but even then myotonia of the respiratory muscles can hinder adequate ventilation [2186]. Myotonia is not prevented by spinal or regional anaesthesia [1630] and may be precipitated post-operatively by shivering due to halothane anaesthesia [2568]. Halothane also induces cardiac dysrhythmias [1629].

Pre-operative evaluation should include a careful clinical assessment of any respiratory muscles weakness and abnormality of swallowing and cough, together with an ECG, spirometry and arterial blood gas analysis.

Cardiac complications. Cardiac involvement only occurs in some families with dystrophia myotonica [1385] and can usually be suspected from the ECG [574, 1714, 2425]. A fourth heart sound is common [2443] but the characteristic feature is damage to the His-Purkinje conducting system and, less commonly, the sinus node [2443]. The sick sinus syndrome [124], atrial flutter, atrial fibrillation [488], bundle branch block [574], intraventricular conduction defects [1721, 2220] and third-degree atrioventricular block are all well recognized. Left ventricular dysfunction and thickening of the left ventricle [2588] is probably more common than has been recognized. The histological changes in cardiac muscle are similar to those in skeletal muscle [988, 1842]. Mitral valve prolapse may be present [1202, 1385, 2220, 3073] but coronary artery disease is unusual and the blood pressure is commonly normal or low [2346, 3018].

Oculopharyngeal muscular dystrophy

This conditions occurs particularly in subjects of French–Canadian descent. It shows similarities to dystrophia myotonica but weakness of ocular and pharyngeal muscles is characteristic. Little is known of the frequency and severity of respiratory muscle weakness but dysphagia and aspiration pneumonias are frequent [2335]. Pharyngeal contractions during swallowing are weak and failure of the cricopharyngeal sphincter to relax completely is common [862]. Cricopharyngeal myotomy may be beneficial.

Myotonia congenita (Thomsen's disease)

This condition may occasionally be inherited recessively rather than dominantly. Its onset is usually in childhood and it progresses slowly. Myotonia and weakness of the limb and facial muscles develop, but very little is known of the respiratory muscle involvement. It one case, EMG features of myotonia of the scalene muscles and diaphragm were associated with breathlessness and tightness of the chest on exertion, which may have been due to myotonia of the respiratory muscles hindering expiration [928].

Congenital myopathies

These disorders typically present neonatally as a floppy infant, or with muscle weakness that appears during childhood and progressively worsens. The term is, therefore, slightly inaccurate since abnormalities may not be present until some time after birth. However, all these conditions have, or are thought to have, a genetic basis and appear early in life. They have been classified according to their biochemical and structural abnormalities.

BIOCHEMICAL ABNORMALITIES

Acid maltase deficiency (Pompe's disease)

There are a large number of biochemical abnormalities causing congenital myopathies but only acid maltase deficiency is recognized to cause respiratory complications. It is one of the glycogen storage diseases. In the typical form of the disease, glycogen accumulates in every tissue of the body. This causes a severe myopathy, with death from respiratory or cardiac complications usually before the age of two [1450, 1900].

A milder form has also been recognized, which presents in adult life without visceral involvement [917, 918, 1488] and in which muscle weakness is both myopathic and due to denervation [1622]. It is in this group of patients that bilateral diaphragmatic weakness is remarkably common [1900, 2134, 3186]. The VC and PI_{max} may be very much reduced [2706]. Diaphragm weakness may occur in the presence of very little weakness of the limb muscles [2956] and respiratory failure may even be the presenting feature [628, 798, 1915, 2706]. Respiratory failure is usually due purely to the muscle weakness [389] but ventilatory drive may be subnormal and contribute to the respiratory failure [224]. Prolonged survival with assisted ventilation has been recorded [781, 1915] but highprotein diets that increase muscle protein synthesis [2965] can lead to significant improvements in respiratory muscle function [2057] (Fig. 15.13).

Organic aciduria

Respiratory problems may also occur in association with the secretion of large amounts of

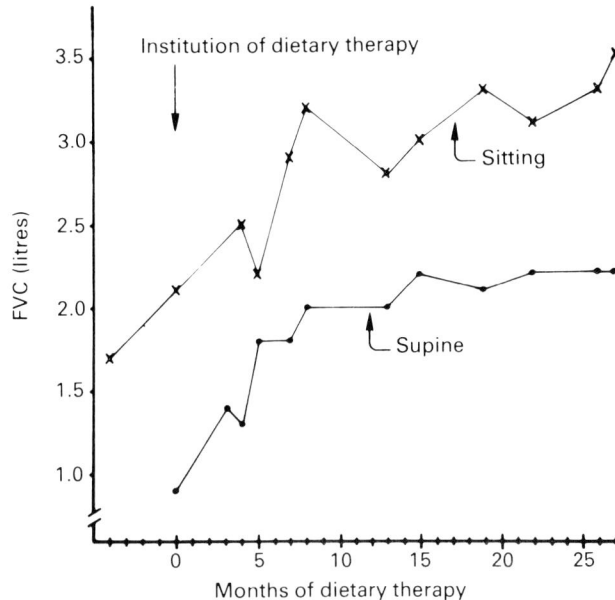

Fig. 15.13. *Improvement in forced vital capacity in a patient with acid maltase deficiency with a high-protein diet. Reproduced, with permission, from Margolis M.L. & Hill A.R. Am. Rev. Respir. Dis. 1986;* **134**: *328–31.*

organic acids in the urine. These conditions are not, strictly speaking, myopathies but they may present neonatally or in infancy with pneumonias, tachypnoeas or stridor [533, 1186, 1637, 3242]. The metabolic acidosis increases ventilation by its effect on the respiratory centres but it also causes hypotonia and respiratory muscle weakness. The organic acidurias are probably heterogeneous but the response to biotin is dramatic in some cases [533, 1637].

STRUCTURAL MYOPATHIES

Degenerative myopathies

The muscular dystrophies fall into this group but have been considered separately earlier in this chapter.

Mitochondrial myopathies

These myopathies may be associated with a variety of other abnormalities, such as lactic acidosis. The abnormal mitochondria impart a 'ragged red' appearance to the muscle fibres. The mitochondrial abnormality is present in every tissue and a cardiomyopathy may develop. Respiratory problems are quite common and hypercapnia, a restrictive defect due to muscle weakness and a diminished ventilatory response to CO_2 have been recorded [847, 1688]. In the Kearns-Sayre syndrome (oculocraniosomatic syndrome), both inspiratory and expiratory muscles may be weak and the ventilatory responses to hypoxia and hypercapnia are reduced [497, 3292].

Nemaline myopathy

This condition is frequently associated with dysmorphic features, such as a high arched palate. Respiratory complications are well recognized. Neonatal hypoventilation may be severe [1979] and aspiration in the neonatal period may lead to pneumonia [1621, 1776, 2862]. In other cases the major feature is a proximal muscle weakness. This may progress slowly during adult life but its severity is very variable. In the more severely affected subjects respiratory infections may be frequent and even fatal [1471, 1487]. Respiratory muscle weakness occasionally causes ventilatory failure [1352, 1973, 2626, 3257] and the

nemaline rods can be demonstrated in the diaphragm and in other respiratory muscles [419,
1352].

Centronuclear (myotubular) myopathy

Neonatal respiratory failure may be the presenting feature of this condition [609, 920]. It appears to be due to respiratory muscle weakness
rather than to aspiration, although this may occasionally be an important factor [2254]. In
some families the neonatal mortality due to respiratory failure may approach 100% [198].
Temporary mechanical respiratory assistance
may be required in milder cases until muscle
strength improves [241], but this may need to
be continued in the long-term [2357].

Reducing body myopathy

This condition may cause the chest wall to become extremely stiff and ventilation to be impaired [3257].

Congenital fibre-type disproportion

Small type 1 muscle fibres are the characteristic
feature of this myopathy. Respiratory muscle
weakness may become severe enough to cause
respiratory failure and require assisted ventilation [1861]. Respiratory infections are
common.

Myositis

Inflammation of the skeletal muscles is a feature
of many conditions, most of which have no respiratory complications. Respiratory complications are, however, important in the
following:

TRICHINIASIS

This infection is acquired by eating under-
cooked meat, usually pork, containing the larvae
of *Trichinella spiralis*. The larvae migrate to
skeletal muscle where they encyst and cause a
diffuse myositis [834], which in severe infections
may affect cardiac muscle [196, 1236]. At the
stage of migration, the larvae may also cause
bronchitis, bronchopneumonia, pulmonary infarction and pleurisy, occasionally with an effusion [2183].

Trichiniasis was at one time very common
and a cause of considerable morbidity. Its prevalence has fallen but occasional outbreaks still
occur. The larvae have a predilection for the
respiratory muscles. The tongue, larynx, intercostal muscles and particularly the diaphragm
are often affected. Myalgia is frequent [353] and,
less commonly, a marked restrictive defect is
seen [2658]. This may be severe enough to cause
ventilatory failure, usually during the fourth to
sixth week of the illness [3040], and to require
IPPV [387]. Spontaneous improvement usually
occurs if ventilation can be supported, but can
be hastened by prednisolone [2658].

POLYMYOSITIS AND DERMATOMYOSITIS

These conditions are characterized by a symmetrical proximal muscle weakness, which in
dermatomyositis is accompanied by cutaneous
changes. Respiratory failure may occur in severe
cases because of generalized weakness of the
respiratory muscles [201, 1558] and, rarely, as
the presenting feature if the diaphragm is selectively involved [332]. This has also been recorded with post-viral myositis [776]. Intermittent positive pressure ventilation is required together with high-dose corticosteroids. This is
effective in increasing respiratory muscle
strength, as indicated by maximal mouth pressures and transdiaphragmatic pressure [2072,
2812(b)], and facilitates weaning from the ventilator [1378].

Respiratory failure may also occur because of
pulmonary infiltrations similar to cryptogenic
fibrosing alveolitis [846, 2488, 2756] or because
of aspiration pneumonia. This carries a poor
prognosis [2110]. The pharyngeal muscles are
often weak, oesophageal peristalsis diminished
[793, 813] and the cough inadequate [1410].
The cricopharyngeal sphincter may fail to relax

during swallowing, although this can be improved by cricopharyngeal myotomy [1611].

These respiratory problems may be complicated by cardiac involvement causing supraventricular and ventricular dysrhythmias, atrioventricular block, cardiac failure, pericarditis, mitral valve prolapse and pulmonary hypertension [336, 1204, 1638, 2581].

SYSTEMIC LUPUS ERYTHEMATOSUS (SLE)

The best-recognized respiratory complications of SLE are interstitial fibrosis, and pleurisy with or without a pleural effusion [1451]. Pulmonary haemorrhage, pulmonary hypertension, chest infections and pulmonary oedema due to renal failure may also appear [2845, 3202]. Myositis is, however, more common than is usually thought and has important respiratory consequences. It affects particularly the proximal muscles [1536, 3196] and is distinct from the steroid myopathy that commonly develops during treatment [2068].

Myositis can weaken both the inspiratory and the expiratory muscles. The $P_{E_{max}}$ may be decreased [1119, 2068] but the most prominent abnormalities are usually diaphragmatic. These were first noticed in the 1950s. It was recognized that the diaphragms were often raised on the plain chest radiograph [1443, 2263, 2924, 3320] and the term 'shrinking lungs' was applied [1443]. Fluoroscopy [2727] and comparison of inspiratory and expiratory films [901] showed that diaphragmatic movement was diminished and in some patients breathlessness was out of proportion to the extent of the lung or pleural disease [3320].

Diaphragm weakness may also be indicated by orthopnoea [1443] and by paradoxical movement of the abdominal wall [1119]. It should be distinguished from the pulmonary and pleural complications of SLE, which cause a restrictive defect with a low carbon monoxide transfer factor [555, 1119, 2068, 2924]. Diaphragm paralysis, however, also lowers the maximum transdiaphragmatic pressure and $P_{I_{max}}$ [1119, 1553, 2068, 3152]. At autopsy

examination, inflammation and fibrosis of the diaphragm has been observed [2727], although the normal response to phrenic nerve stimulation observed in a single patient raises the possibility that a defect in central nervous control of diaphragmatic movements may also be involved [2139].

Respiratory muscle involvement in SLE is not related to other features of the activity of the disease, either serological or clinical [1553, 2068, 2924]. Conversely, there may be no improvement in respiratory muscle strength despite improvement in the other manifestations of SLE [2727]. Steroids do not appear to reverse the radiological diaphragmatic elevation [1443] but there have been no adequate studies of their effect on respiratory muscle weakness. Nebulized salbutamol has been reported to increase the VC in a patient with diaphragmatic weakness without altering air flow obstruction [3152]. This improvement was probably due to its inotropic effect on the diaphragm (p. 300) rather than to any influence on the disease process itself.

SYSTEMIC SCLEROSIS (SCLERODERMA)

The cardiac [1015] and pulmonary complications [3531] of systemic sclerosis are well recognized and are as important as involvement of the limb muscles, skin and joints in limiting the exercise ability [329]. Pulmonary changes are common, often slowly progressive [152, 2821], and may be detected by a fall in carbon monoxide transfer factor before there are any radiographic changes [20]. The commonest complication is interstitial fibrosis but bronchiolectasis, pulmonary vascular disease and possibly pleural involvement also occur [1522, 2393, 2736, 3008], together with aspiration pneumonias if the oesophagus is affected [2032].

Systemic sclerosis might be expected to cause a restrictive defect if the skin over the thorax was extensively involved. In practice this is extremely rare, although it is difficult to separate the effects of skin involvement from that of the underlying intercostal muscles. By analogy with ankylosing spondylitis, fixation of the rib cage alone should be insufficient to cause ventilatory failure. The skin over the whole of the rib cage and abdomen would need to be stiffened to cause this complication. In the few patients who have been tested, the chest wall compliance has been found to be normal [2736] and there are no well-documented cases of ventilatory failure due simply to cutaneous involvement with systemic sclerosis.

Sclerodermatous myopathy is probably more important and has been recognized to be of more than one type [586]. In the commoner form, the muscle biopsy shows no inflammation but there is extensive fibrosis and variation in muscle fibre size. Clinically significant respiratory muscle weakness is uncommon but, occasionally, diaphragm and intercostal muscle weakness can be severe enough to cause ventilatory failure [1522, 2730].

The less common inflammatory form of myopathy, which is indistinguishable histologically from polymyositis, can also cause ventilatory failure. Unlike the more common form, this myopathy may respond to steroids with, for instance, a significant improvement in the PI_{max}, PE_{max} and TLC [537].

A complication of systemic sclerosis that could affect the mechanics of ventilation is rib osteolysis. Notching or loss of bone substance over the superior aspects of the ribs posteriorly is characteristic. It may be bilateral and even lead to complete transection of the rib [2393, 2480]. An identical type of osteolysis is seen in rheumatoid arthritis [63] and poliomyelitis [263]. The mechanism of resorption of the ribs is completely unknown but may be related to vascular changes in the periosteum. The functional importance of rib osteolysis is uncertain but it is unlikely to be great unless it is very extensive.

Metabolic, endocrine and drug-induced myopathies

The most important of the metabolic, endocrine and drug-induced disturbances that cause respiratory problems are:

MALNUTRITION

The effects of malnutrition on respiration are complex. It can cause anaemia and a decrease in immunity as well as biochemical changes within the lungs [2744]. The production of surfactant and lung growth may be impaired [881] and atrophy of the lung parenchyma may be accelerated [118]. The effects of malnutrition are often difficult to separate from those of the disease causing it, particularly during an acute severe illness.

Weight loss in chronic respiratory failure is probably due to a combination of an inadequate diet and a raised metabolic rate [422, 1534, 3345, 3346]. The latter is due to increased work of respiration caused by the abnormal respiratory mechanics and to a raised food-induced thermogenesis [1183]. Weight loss in chronic air flow obstruction has poor prognosis [3220] and often occurs in stages that are related to acute illnesses [3345].

Wasting of the respiratory muscles is closely linked to wasting of the muscle mass of the body as a whole. In malnourished subjects, the diaphragmatic muscle bulk is diminished [105, 108] and the diaphragm muscle fibres show considerable variation in size [107]. Malnutrition causes a selective atrophy of type 2 fibres. Their cross-sectional diameter is decreased so that the cross-sectional proportion of the fatigue-resistant type 1 fibres increases [1647, 2673, 2674].

Respiratory muscle strength is therefore decreased to a greater extent than endurance [1941, 2674]. The contractility of the muscle fibres is probably also reduced because of alterations in intracellular electrolytes or energy substrates [2673]. Loss of strength, indicated by a fall in PI_{max}, is proportional to the loss of body muscle mass [1646] but the force of the muscle at low stimulation frequencies increases [1941]. This is due to the relative increase of type 1 fibres, whose twitches fuse into a tetanic contraction at lower stimulation frequencies than type 2 fibres, and to a slowing of the relaxation rate of the muscle fibres by malnutrition, which also leads to fusion of the individual twitches into a tetanic contraction at lower stimulation frequencies.

Refeeding after a period of malnutrition reverses the atrophic changes in the respiratory muscles [1647], improves contractility [1941] and the PI_{max} [896, 1646, 3347]. Refeeding also increases the metabolic rate and the respiratory drive. The ventilatory response to hypoxia and hypercapnia is reduced in subjects who have been starved [805, 3345], in proportion to the decrease in metabolic rate, but is restored by refeeding [118, 805]. This change is particularly marked with a high-protein diet [117, 1034]. The increase in ventilation may not, however, be beneficial if the ventilatory capacity is limited.

Respiratory failure may also be precipitated if a high-carbohydrate diet is taken. This increases the respiratory quotient so that more CO_2 is produced at any given oxygen consumption [116, 675, 2764]. There is no change in the ventilatory response to hypercapnia [2691] and the PCO_2 may rise. A refeeding diet should, therefore, have a high fat content if there is severe chest wall or pulmonary disease.

Further studies are required to show in which situations these deleterious effects of refeeding are outweighed by an improvement in respiratory muscle endurance, blood gases or prognosis. In many cases the factor limiting the ventilation is a diminished compliance or increased air flow resistance, and any benefits from refeeding are slight.

ELECTROLYTE DISTURBANCES

Specific nutritional deficiencies and electrolyte disturbances may also impair respiratory function. Hypokalaemia from any cause leads to muscle weakness and, if it is severe, to post-exercise rhabdomyolysis [1710]. The respiratory muscles share in this muscle weakness and although it is usually not sufficient to cause respiratory failure by itself, it may be a contributory factor in a variety of situations, such as following surgery. Episodic hypokalaemia is also responsible for one form of periodic

paralysis in which the respiratory muscles are occasionally involved. Hyperkalaemia can also cause periodic paralysis but ventilation is rarely affected.

Phosphate deficiency is seen most frequently in alcoholics, during refeeding after weight loss and with aluminium and magnesium-containing antacids that bind phosphate in the gut [1709]. Chronic respiratory acidosis may cause a phosphaturia. Phosphate deficiency increases the affinity of haemoglobin for oxygen because of the fall in 2, 3-DPG, and may lead to haemolysis. Muscle weakness is often pronounced and may be severe enough to cause acute ventilatory failure [2291]. The transdiaphragmatic pressure during phrenic nerve stimulation falls [128]. Ventilatory failure may be precipitated by glucose, which increases the phosphate uptake by the cells and causes an acute fall in the serum phosphate concentration. Both the transdiaphragmatic pressure [128] and ventilatory failure [2291] improve when phosphate is given.

Magnesium deficiency may occur in alcoholics and during treatment with diuretics, and causes a reversible loss of muscle strength [2898]. Histological changes, including rhabdomyolysis, appear if the deficiency is severe [685]. The maximal inspiratory and expiratory pressures are reduced [2202]. This contrasts with the decrease in respiratory drive and fall in the level of consciousness seen in hypermagnesaemia [966, 1569].

Iron deficiency has been shown in experimental animals to reduce the endurance of muscles in tests involving running ability [979]. This effect is independent of the haemoglobin concentration. The fall in PI_{max} documented in patients with chronic renal failure probably also has a metabolic basis [1185].

ACROMEGALY

The respiratory manifestations of acromegaly are predominantly due to upper airway obstruction (p. 72), but a proximal myopathy is also characteristic of this condition. This can weaken the respiratory muscles and may also predispose to obstructive sleep apnoeas by reducing the tone of the upper airway muscles.

HYPERTHYROIDISM

Muscle weakness is a common feature of thyrotoxicosis [2557]. The proximal muscles are the most commonly affected and a bulbar palsy, which may be acute and cause aspiration pneumonia, is well recognized [877, 1616]. This improves with treatment of the thyrotoxicosis but other associated conditions, such as myasthenia gravis and hypokalaemic periodic paralysis, should be excluded. The PI_{max} and PE_{max} frequently diminish [2149, 3038, 3262] and respiratory muscle weakness probably underlies the restrictive defect that is characteristic of hyperthyroidism. The VC is decreased [3038] largely because of an increase in the RV rather than a fall in the TLC [2609, 3262].

Breathlessness on exertion is a common symptom of thyrotoxicosis but is only partly due to respiratory muscle weakness. The oxygen uptake at any given level of external work is increased so that the maximal oxygen uptake is reached at a lower work rate [1649]. Maximal exercise ventilation is normal [1649] but ventilation is increased during submaximal exercise [1115, 3038]. The respiratory frequency rises rapidly and although this increases the physiological dead space, the P_{CO_2} remains normal [3038]. The control of respiration during exercise is complex and the significance of the raised ventilatory responses to hypercapnia [919, 3412] and hypoxia [3412] is uncertain. Reflexes originating in chest wall proprioceptors may be responsible for the observed changes during exercise.

HYPOTHYROIDISM

There is some evidence for respiratory muscle weakness in hypothyroidism. The MVV is reduced and improves when thyroxine is given [3354]. The PI_{max} also increases with thyroxine [3281]. Respiratory muscle weakness may be due to peripheral nerve damage as well as to a myopathy. The phrenic nerve conduction time may be prolonged and demyelination and fibrosis of the phrenic nerve has been demonstrated at autopsy examination [1339].

CUSHING'S SYNDROME AND CORTICOSTEROID TREATMENT

A proximal myopathy that may affect the respiratory muscles is a common feature of Cushing's syndrome and corticosteroid therapy. The myopathy is part of the catabolic influence of the glucocorticoid hormones. Type 2 muscle fibres selectively atrophy. The myopathy is dose related but is most marked with the fluorinated corticosteroid drugs such as dexamethasone, betamethasone and triamcinolone.

ALCOHOL

The effects of alcohol on muscle function are complex. Excessive intake of alcohol is often associated with malnutrition but it also appears to cause a specific proximal myopathy that is reversible when the alcohol consumption ceases. Bouts of heavy drinking superimposed on chronic excessive alcohol consumption may cause painful, acute muscle weakness associated either with a normal or high serum potassium concentration.

Chapter 16
Obesity and Disorders of the Sternum, Ribs and Spine

Obesity and skeletal disorders of the thorax are an important group of conditions that frequently impair ventilation. In some cases, particularly the neuromuscular diseases causing scoliosis, the respiratory muscles are also weak. These conditions are discussed in Chapter 15, and in this chapter the respiratory consequences of the skeletal disorders themselves are considered. Thickening of the pleura, pleural effusions and pneumothoraces have similar effects on ventilation to many of the skeletal disorders of the thorax, but these are adequately covered in the standard textbooks of respiratory medicine. A variety of abdominal conditions, including pregnancy and ascites, cause a similar restrictive defect [2720].

PHYSIOLOGICAL EFFECTS

Most of these disorders decrease the compliance of the chest wall and the volume of the rib cage [261]. The changes may be slight, for instance, in sternal abnormalities but considerable in severe scoliosis or following thoracoplasty. Characteristically, TLC is decreased, RV decreases or even increases slightly, the RV/TLC ratio increases and the VC is reduced. The fall in TLC is due to the low chest wall compliance, the fall in lung compliance due to the small lung volume and often to impairment of respiratory muscle function. Even in the absence of a primary muscle disorder, the maximal pressures are usually diminished. The distortion of the rib cage puts the respiratory muscles at a mechanical disadvantage. The asymmetrical thorax associated with scoliosis often leads to the inspiratory muscles on one side of the chest being short-ened and on the other side overstretched at the end of expiration so that the strength of contraction is hindered on both sides. Excessive shortening of the diaphragm also appears to be a feature of obesity.

The FRC is usually decreased, but in proportion to the fall in TLC so that the FRC/TLC ratio remains approximately normal. The exception to this is ankylosing spondylitis where the chest wall becomes fixed at its relaxation volume, which is greater than the normal FRC. Air flow obstruction is not a feature of these conditions but the PEFR is reduced if respiratory muscle function is impaired or if there is a severe restrictive defect.

The decrease in lung volume causes the basal airways to close and diminishes the lung compliance. The ventilation and perfusion are imperfectly matched and hypoxia results. The regional ventilation and perfusion are influenced by local variations in intrapleural pressure due to localized deformities of the rib cage or inspiratory muscle weakness. The failure to match ventilation and perfusion diminishes the carbon monoxide transfer factor (unless polycythaemia develops in response to hypoxia) but when corrected for the lung volume, the transfer coefficient is increased. This distinguishes restrictive defects due to chest wall disease from intrapulmonary disease.

The development of the lungs is hindered if the anatomical abnormalities of the rib cage appear at an early age. The development of the lungs appears to be dependent on the mechanical forces generated by the chest wall. The number of alveoli normally increases until the age of about eight years. If the thoracic cavity is small, the adult number of alveoli is not attained. The severity of this hypoplasia of the lungs varies according to the age of onset of the skeletal disorder and its severity. The commonest causes are congenital and infantile idiopathic scoliosis, early onset kyphoses, particularly those due to tuberculosis, and asphyxiating thoracic dystrophy. A similar failure of lung development is recognized with congenital diaphragmatic hernia [1700] and in experimental animals with a variety of disorders, including thoracoplasty, that reduce the volume of the thorax [1898, 1899].

The reduction in chest wall and lung compliance increases the work of respiration. In ankylosing spondylitis and most of the other skeletal disorders, the compliance of the rib cage is disturbed but that of the abdomen remains normal. In contrast, in obesity both the abdominal and rib cage compliance are reduced. The work of breathing in the presence of this elastic load is minimized when the tidal volume is small and the respiratory frequency is rapid (p. 22). This breathing pattern is characteristic of obesity and skeletal disorders of the thorax.

An abnormally rapid respiratory frequency is also adopted when ventilation increases, for instance, during exercise or during the MVV manoeuvre. The dead space to tidal volume ratio is increased and, in order to maintain a normal alveolar ventilation, the ventilation during exercise is greater than normal. This, together with a low maximal exercise ventilation, limits exercise ability. This contrasts with normal subjects whose exercise is limited by circulatory rather than ventilatory factors.

The pattern of small tidal volumes and a rapid respiratory frequency is also observed during sleep and may lead to hypoventilation. Reduction in the respiratory drive and muscle tone decreases the FRC, worsens ventilation/perfusion matching and contributes to hypoxia. Central sleep apnoeas occur during REM sleep and also during NREM sleep if the ventilatory drive is unable to cope with the abnormal mechanics of the chest wall and lungs. Obstructive sleep apnoeas may also be present, possibly because

the upper airway becomes smaller when the FRC falls [1446, 1449]. Adipose tissue in the neck contributes to narrowing of the upper airway in the obese.

The ventilatory drive is usually normal in obesity and skeletal disorders unless chronic hypercapnia has developed. A mildly defective ventilatory drive will become apparent at an early stage since the respiratory muscles require a greater than normal stimulation in order to overcome the impaired respiratory mechanics. It is uncertain what determines whether hypercapnia develops. The small tidal volumes decrease the alveolar ventilation at any given minute ventilation and the rapid respiratory frequency increases the duty cycle of the inspiratory muscles and contributes to respiratory muscle fatigue.

Pulmonary hypertension and right ventricular hypertrophy and failure will develop if hypoxia is severe. Pulmonary hypertension is partly due to the increased pulmonary vascular resistance secondary to hypoxia, but failure of development of the lung, as in congenital scoliosis, or the presence of lung disease may contribute.

INDIVIDUAL DISORDERS

Obesity (Fig. 16.1)

The association of obesity with respiratory problems has long been recognized [1773, 1774, 1826]. Caton in 1889 described respiratory efforts against a closed glottis, which led to recurrent cyanosis [513], and in 1901 Sainton recorded that somnolence that developed with obesity disappeared with loss of weight [2751]. Further cases were documented by Cutting in 1944 [701] and Kerr in 1936 [1655], and in 1937 Spitz [3022] linked obesity with cyanosis and polycythaemia. In the 1950s and early 1960s, awareness of the association between obesity and respiratory and right heart failure grew, and several cases were reported [137, 365, 450, 500, 666, 835, 933, 1129, 1323, 1580, 2136, 2921].

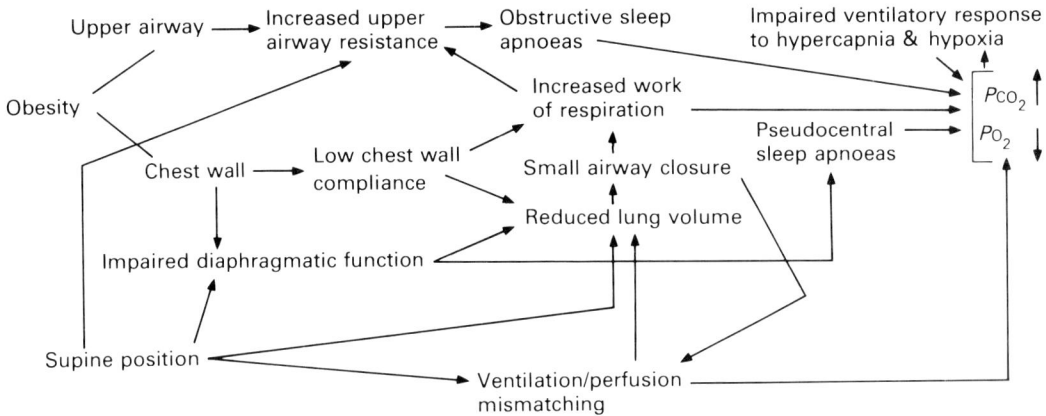

Fig. 16.1. *Flow chart to show the effects of obesity on ventilation.*

Caton in 1889 [513] first drew a comparison between the obese patient and the fat boy in Dickens' 'The Pickwick Papers'. This was reaffirmed by Osler in his book entitled 'The Principles and Practice of Medicine' published in 1907 [2386]. This analogy was revived by Burwell et al. in 1956 who coined the term 'Pickwickian syndrome' to describe the combination of obesity, hypoventilation, somnolence, right heart failure and polycythaemia [450]. Unfortunately, this term is inaccurate since it was not Mr Pickwick himself whom Dickens portrayed as obese and somnolent in 'The Pickwick Papers' but Jo, the fat boy [620, 2467]. This term is, therefore, best avoided and has been replaced largely by the 'obesity hypoventilation syndrome'.

The name 'Pickwickian syndrome' implied that hypoventilation in association with obesity was a discrete entity. It was seen as similar to central alveolar hypoventilation in that no primary lung, heart, neuromuscular or other chest wall disease was present and in that voluntary hyperventilation could improve the blood gases [1323]. The cause of the hypoventilation has, however, been disputed. A large number of physiological abnormalities of respiratory control and mechanics in the obese have been demonstrated [2670, 2874]. Emphasis was initially placed on the direct mechanical effects of the adipose tissue on respiration and later on defects in respiratory control. More recently obstructive sleep apnoeas have been held responsible for the respiratory and cardiac failure but it is likely that these complications are due to an interaction of several physiological changes rather than to any single abnormality. The most important of these are:

SLEEP APNOEAS

Descriptions of obstructive sleep apnoeas are recognizable in several early accounts of the respiratory problems of obesity [513, 835, 933]. Sleep apnoeas were proposed as the cause of oxygen desaturation in the mid-1950s [933, 2921]. Their importance was suggested by the observation that polycythaemia in the obese is associated with only a slight fall in the oxygen saturation during wakefulness [3276]. It was not, however, until 1965 that air flow obstruction during sleep was precisely documented and the idea of pharyngeal occlusion due to loss of muscle tone was proposed [1093, 1094]. These observations were soon confirmed [867, 1284, 1771, 3255], although central and mixed apnoeas were also recognized [562, 1094]. Most of the apnoeas occur during stages 1 and 2 NREM or REM sleep [562, 3141].

The exact site of the obstruction during sleep apnoeas has been investigated extensively. Rhinometry has shown that nasopharyngeal resistance is increased in the obese [76] and rises further in the supine position [77] and during sleep [75]. Pharyngeal obstruction has been confirmed by cinefluoroscopy [3255] and is also suggested by the improvement in sleep apnoeas following the insertion of a nasopharyngeal airway [867, 2942]. Other studies have shown more complex abnormalities. Serial radiographs have revealed that obstruction initially occurs at the level of the soft palate and this is followed by progressive collapse of the airway towards the larynx during the stronger inspiratory efforts later in the apnoea [2548]. Direct observation through the fibre-optic bronchoscope has confirmed that obstruction may take place at the level of the glottis as well as in the pharynx [1759].

The pathogenesis of obstructive apnoeas is described in Chapter 6. In the obese, the accumulation of fat in the neck is thought to lead to narrowing of the pharynx and thereby to predispose to obstructive apnoeas. Computerized tomography scans have not shown fat adjacent to the pharynx but the normal soft tissues are probably displaced inwards by the subcutaneous fat [337, 1350, 3111]. The pharyngeal cross-sectional area correlates with the FRC [1446, 1449]. The FRC is reduced in the obese, particularly in the supine position (see below), and this further increases the risk of obstructive apnoeas. Weight loss reverses these abnormalities, decreases the number of apnoeas and hypopnoeas, and improves nocturnal oxygen saturation [1359].

LUNG VOLUMES (See Fig 9.7)

Obesity causes a restrictive defect due to changes in the chest wall compliance and function of the respiratory muscles (see below). The expiratory reserve volume is most consistently diminished [450, 692, 952, 1323, 2574] and is associated with a low FRC [692, 915] but a normal RV [692, 1323, 3195]. The inspiratory capacity is more nearly normal than the expiratory reserve volume and, consequently, the TLC and VC are only slightly reduced [951, 2574]. The forced expiratory ratio is normal and the MVV falls in parallel with the VC [692, 2670].

These changes in expiratory reserve volume and FRC are particularly marked in the supine position [3195] when the weight of the abdominal contents raises the end expiratory position of the diaphragm. The closing volume is often greater than the FRC [951] so that the small airways close [818]. This causes ventilation/perfusion mismatching [197, 1454], widening of the A–a gradient [1323, 2747] and hypoxaemia [952, 1580]. Hypoxaemia can be relieved by taking a few deep breaths, which open the basal airways [2747], and is proportional to the reduction in expiratory reserve volume [952]. This [560, 915, 2574, 3090, 3224] and the P_{O_2} [560, 952, 3090] both improve if weight is lost.

COMPLIANCE

Obesity not only leads to obstruction of the upper airway but adds a restrictive load to the respiratory system, thus increasing the elastic work of ventilation [2272]. Studies of the total respiratory compliance using the relaxation method have shown that loading the thorax shifts the volume–pressure curve of the respiratory system to the right without altering the compliance, but abdominal loading decreases the compliance [2882]. In obese subjects, fat is present around the rib cage and in the abdomen and the net result is a combination of both of these effects. The chest wall compliance is reduced [2670, 2883], but the static lung compliance is normal [818].

The reduced respiratory system compliance leads to a rapid respiratory frequency with a small tidal volume [1950], particularly in the supine position [2747]. This increases the dead space to tidal volume ratio [1628] and the T_I/T_{TOT} ratio, which predisposes to respiratory muscle fatigue.

The oxygen consumption of respiration is increased by these mechanical abnormalities [951, 1628, 2874, 2883]. The extra weight also raises the oxygen consumption of the body as a whole during exertion [724] and the maximal oxygen consumption, even when corrected for body weight, is diminished [724]. Arterial oxygenation and CO_2 consumption during exercise improve after weight loss [1554].

RESPIRATORY MUSCLE FUNCTION

Both PI_{max} and PE_{max} are reduced in the obese [106]. Severe hypoxia secondary to the obesity may diminish respiratory muscle contractility; in one autopsy report there was extensive infiltration of fat into the diaphragm and intercostal muscles, which may have impaired their function [945]. However, in most cases changes in the length or configuration of the diaphragm because of the fat in the abdomen are more important [1938]. The maximal transdiaphragmatic pressure falls in the supine position [2878] when the diaphragm is elevated by the weight of the abdominal contents. The high position of the diaphragm may overstretch its fibres. This may reduce its function as much as when the diaphragm is excessively shortened if the lungs are hyperinflated (p. 28).

RESPIRATORY DRIVE

The combination of hypoventilation and obesity is associated with a reduced biochemical respiratory drive. If the PCO_2 is normal, the ventilatory response to hypercapnia is retained [692], but once the PCO_2 rises it becomes diminished [1084, 1993, 3411] (Fig. 16.2). The diaphragmatic EMG activity [1944] and $P_{0.1}$ [1940] are also normal in the obese without CO_2 retention, but are reduced in those who hypoventilate. In this situation, weight loss improves the ventilatory response to hypercapnia [450, 3411], but in non-hypoventilating subjects there is no significant change.

The ventilatory responses to hypoxia follow a similar pattern. In hypoventilators the re-

sponse to hypoxia is diminished [1084, 3411] (Fig. 16.2), but it is normal if the PCO_2 is normal [1770]. Neither the ventilatory response to hypoxia or to hypercapnia correlate with the severity of sleep apnoeas [1084].

These findings indicate that it is some other factor and not the obesity itself or its direct consequences, such as a fall in the chest wall compliance or respiratory muscle function, that diminish the hypercapnic and hypoxic drives.

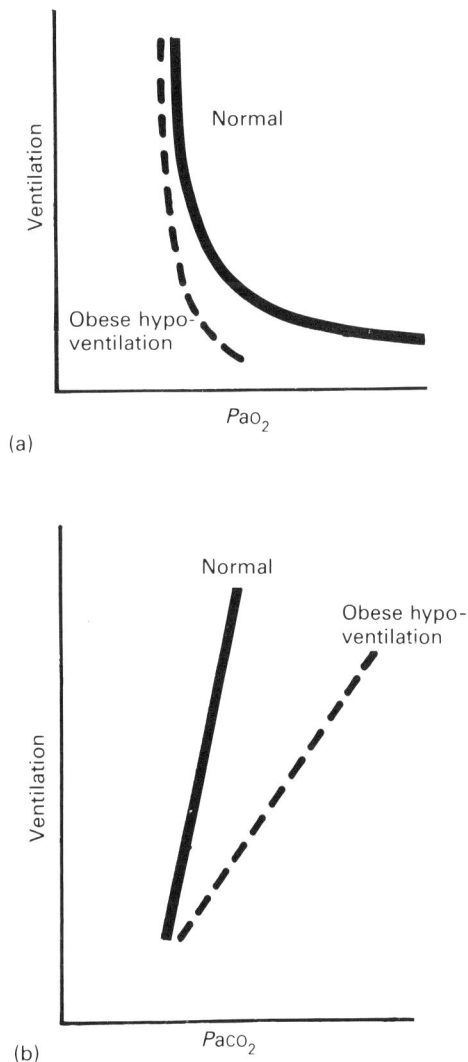

(a)

(b)

Fig. 16.2. *Ventilatory responses of obese hypoventilators and normal subjects to (a) hypoxia and (b) hypercapnia.*

The hypercapnic drive is blunted if prolonged hypoventilation increases the CSF bicarbonate concentration, and the responses to both hypercapnia and hypoxia are lessened by factors such as a direct depressant effect of severe hypoxia and sleep deprivation.

There is no doubt that obesity is related to ventilatory failure and that weight loss improves the blood gases during wakefulness [450, 835, 3090] and lessens somnolence [3141]. In any individual subject there may be a critical weight above which respiratory failure appears. Respiratory failure is commonly equated with the presence of frequent obstructive sleep apnoeas and severe episodes of nocturnal oxygen desaturation. Hypoventilation rarely develops in the absence of frequent obstructive apnoeas [1358, 1585]. It can nevertheless do so [2173] and the relationship between sleep apnoeas and ventilatory failure during wakefulness is not clearcut. Obstructive apnoeas and arousals from sleep may be frequent without any abnormality of the waking blood gases [1305], and there is considerable variation in the frequency of apnoeas and severity of nocturnal hypoxia in those with respiratory failure or somnolence. Close examination has shown no differences in the frequency of obstructive apnoeas in obese subjects with and without hypercapnia while awake [376, 1084] or right heart failure [2829]; improvement in hypercapnia is not always related to changes in the frequency of apnoeas [2560].

These observations indicate that although obstructive sleep apnoeas are almost invariably present if there is ventilatory failure, they alone are not sufficient to cause this. It is likely that there is a further factor that prevents P_{O_2} or P_{CO_2} from returning to normal between the sleep apnoeas. In the obese, the chest wall compliance is not related to the P_{CO_2} [1944], but several of the other physiological abnormalities described above are probably important. Hypercapnia would persist after an apnoea if the normal hyperventilatory reaction to an apnoea is absent or if V_T is reduced. Studies of obese subjects with the Prader–Willi syndrome have identified that a low hypercapnic respiratory drive is a risk factor for respiratory failure independent of obesity [2377]. The low chest wall compliance and impaired diaphragmatic function reduce V_T but increase the respiratory rate, lessening alveolar ventilation and predisposing to respiratory muscle fatigue. Ventilation/perfusion mismatching also contributes to hypoxia, which is common in the supine position in the obese. The depth of oxygen desaturation is greater during sleep in the supine position than in the sitting position [1989]. The FRC is less when supine and, particularly in the presence of air flow obstruction when the closing volume is increased, this would impair matching of ventilation and perfusion [376]. The function of the diaphragm is also reduced in the supine position and this is anticipated to worsen in REM sleep when diaphragmatic tone is lost.

Right heart failure is predominantly due to pulmonary hypertension secondary to hypoxic pulmonary vasoconstriction. It would be anticipated particularly if the severity and duration of hypoxia is severe. Right heart failure has been observed particularly if oxygen desaturation is present during wakefulness [2828] and it is not closely related to the degree of desaturation during sleep alone [2828, 2829]. Hypoxia during wakefulness occurs if there is hypoventilation, or if ventilation/perfusion matching is impaired by any of the factors mentioned above or by coexisting lung disease.

Isolated right ventricular hypertrophy in the absence of left ventricular hypertrophy is very uncommon in the obese [57, 69]. The weight of the heart increases with the degree of obesity [69, 2975], reflecting left rather than right ventricular hypertrophy. Some of this increase in weight is due to fatty infiltration into the heart muscle and an increase in the epicardial fat [69]. The increased blood volume and cardiac output [56, 1824], and hypertension due to reflex hypoxic systemic vasoconstriction, contribute to left ventricular hypertrophy.

Sternal abnormalities

Most of the inflammatory and neoplastic disorders of the sternum have little effect on ventilation unless they cause pain. Fracture of the sternum, particularly traumatic, may form part of an anterior flail segment, which may seriously impede ventilation. This subject is covered in textbooks of thoracic surgery and will not be considered further. Severe congenital defects of the sternum, such as agenesis or a bifid sternum, are rare but may also cause paradoxical movement and require surgery in the neonatal period to stabilize the anterior chest wall [2073]. The two most important developmental abnormalities of the sternum are pectus carinatum and pectus excavatum, but there are a wide variety of protrusion and depression deformities of the sternum, costal cartilages and anterior ribs.

PECTUS CARINATUM (Fig. 16.3)

In pectus carinatum, the sternum protrudes anteriorly and the chest is often narrowed transversely. The deformity may be present at birth but becomes more marked during growth, particularly at puberty. Prominence of the upper sternum is common in ventricular septal defects associated with pulmonary hypertension and a raised pulmonary vascular resistance [726, 727]. Atrial septal defects, however, are associated with a unilateral bulge over the hypertrophied right ventricle but not with pectus carinatum [726].

The cause of pectus carinatum is uncertain. Excessive contraction of the lateral diaphragmatic fibres leading to a narrowing of the chest in the transverse diameter and anterior protrusion of the sternum has been postulated [400, 410]. A more probable cause is excessive growth of the ribs or costal cartilages [1867, 1868, 2655]. If this is asymmetrical, the sternum becomes oblique and the costochondral joints or even the anterior parts of the ribs may protrude anteriorly [1868].

Pectus carinatum is less common than pectus excavatum. Its respiratory consequences have rarely been investigated and are probably of little importance. Chest pain may arise at the insertions of the intercostal muscles anteriorly or

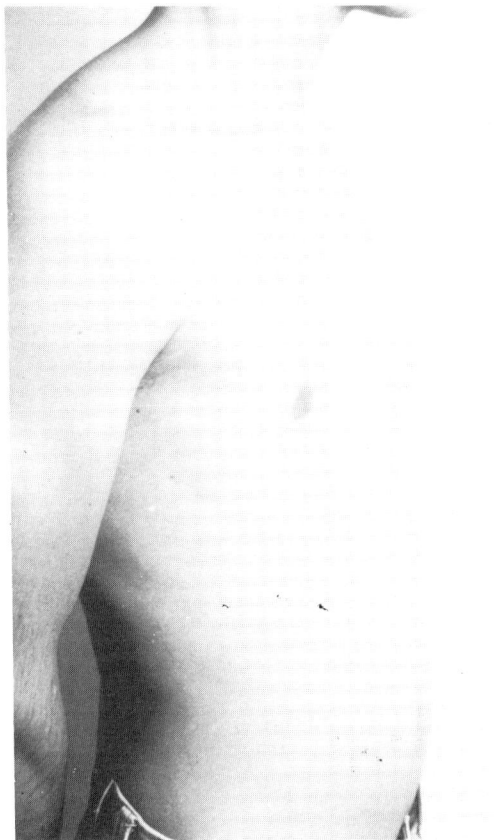

Fig. 16.3. *Asymmetrical pectus carinatum with protrusion of anterior ribs on left.*

in the abnormally–positioned costal cartilages and anterior ribs. The lung volumes and maximal expiratory flow rates appear to be normal [512] and the diaphragm is larger than normal because of the shape of the thorax [1867]. The compliance of the chest wall has not been studied. Surgery is only indicated for cosmetic reasons and does not improve respiratory function or exercise ability [461].

PECTUS EXCAVATUM (Figs 16.4 and 16.5)

Pectus excavatum (funnel chest) is often present soon after birth. It may worsen with growth, particularly at puberty, but can also regress in adult life. It is occasionally familial [1304, 2347, 2749] and may occur in the same individual or in the same family as pectus carinatum [1304,

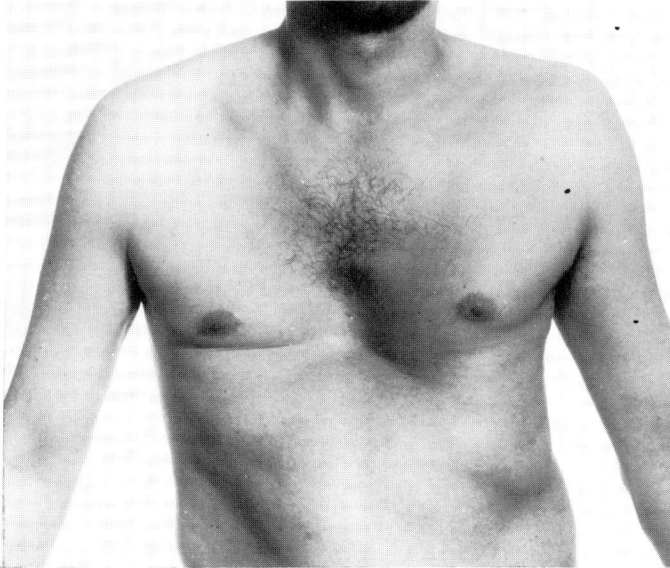

Fig. 16.4. *Pectus excavatum.*

2433, 2749]. It may be associated with the straight back syndrome or with a thoracic kyphosis [1316, 1866, 1911], although these are of little functional significance. Scoliosis and other congenital abnormalities may also be present [1304, 1911].

Overgrowth of the ribs pushing the sternum inwards [2265] or a congenitally short central tendon of the diaphragm [1866, 1868] have been proposed as the cause of pectus excavatum, but they are unlikely [1570, 1571]. An increased inward pull on the sternum by the sternal diaphragmatic fibres or an abnormally compliant chest wall are more probable [409, 557]. Paradoxical movement of the sternum with respiration is seen in neonates in the presence of upper airway obstruction or pneumonia and other conditions that increase the force of diaphragmatic contraction. This is usually transient but if the decreased intrapleural pressure is maintained the sternal depression may become fixed. Upper airway obstruction due to enlarged tonsils or adenoids [949, 1881, 2364], laryngotracheomalacia [677] or bronchomalacia [1156] may be responsible. These precipitating causes may disappear so that later in

life the aetiology of the sternal depression is not apparent.

Pectus excavatum is associated with Marfan's syndrome, Ehlers-Danlos syndrome and hyperflexibility of the joints with hypotonia [1316]. These conditions would suggest that an unusually compliant sternum would predispose to pectus excavatum.

The assessment of the respiratory importance of pectus excavatum has been hindered by difficulties in quantitating the severity of the deformity. Three-dimensional measurements [1495], radiological indices [149, 2693], Moire topography [2822] and even measuring the volume of liquid that can be contained in the deformity [816] have all been recommended. None are entirely satisfactory.

Many patients are asymptomatic but, if the deformity is severe, breathlessness on exertion or a sensation of a precordial pressure may be noticed [943]. Physiological investigations have shown remarkably little respiratory deficit and these symptoms have been thought to be psychological. In most studies the TLC, FRC, RV and VC have been normal or only slightly diminished [512, 983, 1096, 2385, 2508]. The

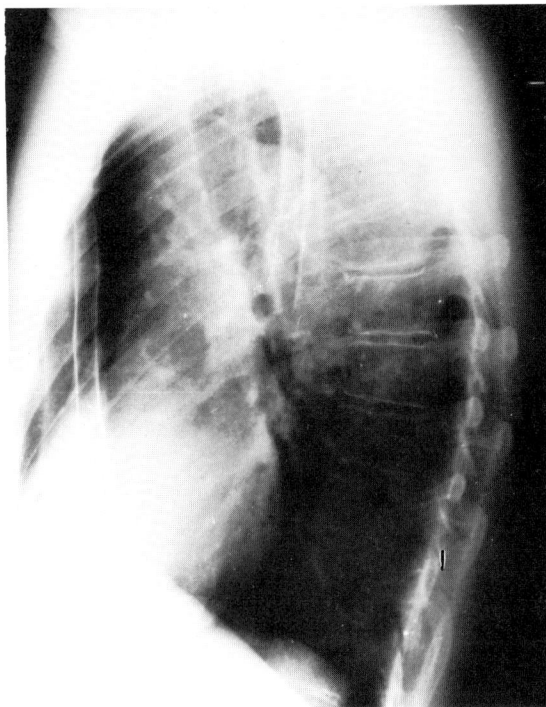

Fig. 16.5. *Lateral chest radiograph showing narrowed anteroposterior diameter of lower thorax at the level of the sternal depression in pectus excavatum.*

MVV [2508, 3273], FEV$_1$/FVC, flow volume loop and lung compliance are all normal [512]. The mild restrictive defect is in keeping with the small volume of the thorax, and is lost by the depression of the sternum. Chest wall mobility both at rest and after exercise is unimpaired [2103] and arterial blood gases at rest [983, 1096, 3273] and on exercise [3273] are also normal.

Pectus excavatum may, however, affect cardiac function. The heart is usually displaced to the left by the sternum, although occasionally it remains under the sternum or is even displaced to the right [410]. The rotation of the displaced heart explains the frequency of right axis deviation on the ECG and the occasional finding of tall P-waves in lead 2 [943, 2082]. Left ventricular function is unimpaired [1972, 2605], although in a single patient a congenital posterior left ventricular diverticulum was associated with pectus excavatum [2708]. Pectus excavatum is also associated with mitral valve prolapse [2045, 2762, 3145].

Right ventricular function, pulmonary artery pressure and cardiac output are normal both at rest and on exertion in the large majority of subjects with pectus excavatum. Radionuclide scans have, however, indicated that although the ventricular function is normal, the volume of both the left and right ventricles increases after surgical repair of the deformity, suggesting that mild compression was present before surgery [2446]. In a few patients, catheter studies have shown evidence of clinically significant cardiac compression. An early diastolic dip and late diastolic plateau in the right ventricular pressures [433, 790, 943, 1096, 1972, 2570, 2657], similar to that seen in constrictive pericarditis, has been recognized. This pattern implies that right ventricular filling is impaired, probably due to compression between the sternum and the spine of the right atrium or, less likely, the superior and inferior vena cavae. Compression of the pulmonary outflow tract, together with its closeness to the anterior chest

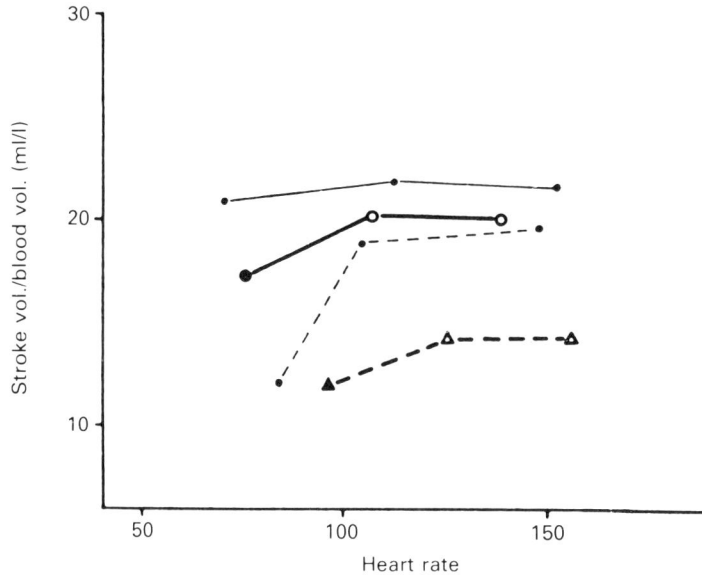

Fig. 16.6. *Relationship of stroke volume to heart rate during exercise in pectus excavatum:* —— *supine;* - - *sitting;* — *normal subjects supine;* - - - *normal subjects sitting. Reproduced, with permission, from Bevegard S.* Acta. Med. Scand. *1962;* **171:** *695–713.*

wall, is probably responsible for the systolic murmur that may be heard, particularly during deep inspiration [790, 1304]. The right pulmonary artery may occasionally be obstructed selectively, since at bronchospirometry the oxygen uptake may be reduced only in the right lung [3120]. Ventilation is normal, which implies that either ventilation/perfusion matching is impaired in the right lung or, more probably, that its perfusion is diminished.

Restriction in right ventricular filling may also occur during exercise, particularly in the sitting position when the heart becomes more caudal and is compressed by the deformity. An inability to increase the cardiac output during exertion while sitting, but not while supine, is characteristic [221, 276, 1096, 3246] (Fig. 16.6), and exercise is limited by circulatory rather than ventilatory factors. The heart rate increases rapidly but the stroke volume does not [276]. In rare instances, the compression of the heart leads to right atrial distension and supraventricular tachycardias [816, 2035] or atrial fibrillation [2570]. In severe cases, dysrhythmias may be precipitated by exertion [2796] or even by standing.

Surgical correction of the pectus excavatum has waxed and waned in popularity since the original operations of Meyer in 1911 and Sauerbruch in 1913 [3246]. Surgery is safe [2433] but appears to have little effect on the mild restrictive defect or exercise ability [410, 461, 983, 1096, 1316, 2385] or on cardiac function during exercise [2446]. However, if the right ventricular filling is impaired, the exercise ability improves following surgery [221] and atrial dysrhythmias due to the deformity are also relieved [816, 2035, 2570]. The systolic murmur may also disappear post-operatively [816, 1802, 1911] and the amplitude of the P-waves decreases [816]. Surgery may also be required for cosmetic reasons, although the result can be disappointing since the scar may be more noticeable than the pectus excavatum [1570, 1571, 2265].

Rib abnormalities

Abnormalities of the ribs are common but they do not usually interfere with respiration unless they cause pain during respiratory movements. The most important are:

Fig. 16.7. *Congenital rib abnormalities with no significant effect on ventilation: (a) bilateral cervical ribs, (b) abnormal joint between the left 1st and 2nd ribs anteriorly, (c) fusion of left 4th and 5th ribs posteriorly.*

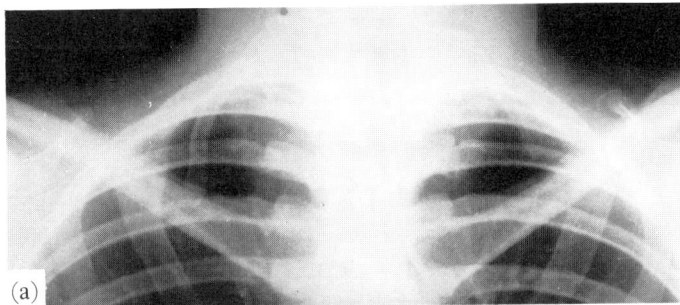

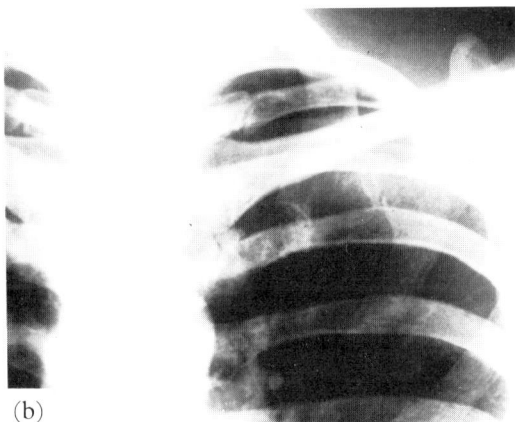

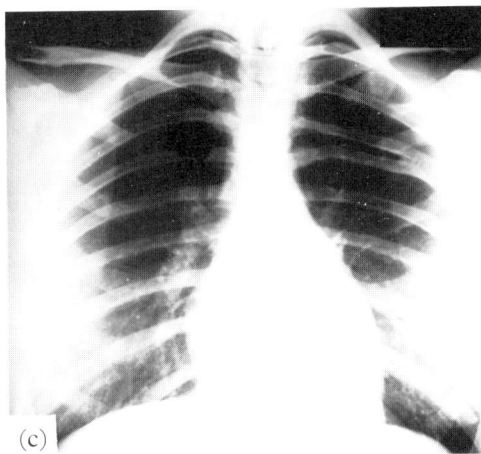

OSTEOMYELITIS, TUMOURS AND EXOSTOSES

These may be conspicuous but unless they are very extensive they rarely impair the expansion of the rib cage. They may, however, directly involve the intercostal muscles and underlying pleura and lung. Chest wall pain may also re-flexly alter intercostal muscle function.

CONGENITAL ABNORMALITIES

The commonest congenital abnormalities are bifid ribs, abnormal intercostal joints or the presence of cervical ribs (Fig. 16.7). Only rarely do they cause any detectable changes in respiratory function. Multiple congenital rib abnormalities may contribute to ventilatory failure if they are in the region of the insertion of the diaphragm (Fig. 16.8) or if the absence of several ribs causes paradoxical chest wall movement.

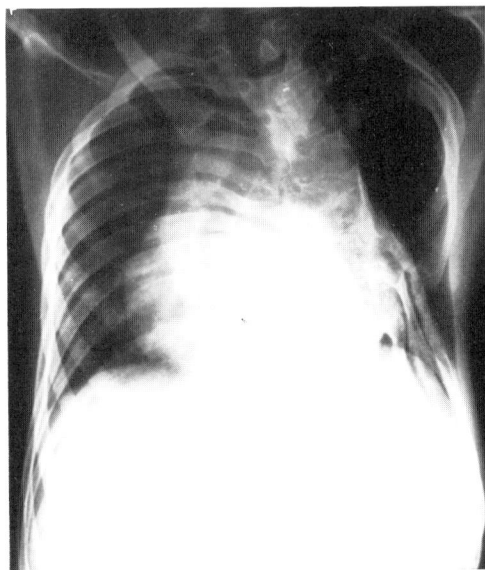

Fig. 16.8. *Multiple congenital left rib abnormalities associated with scoliosis due to congenital abnormalities of mid-thoracic spine.*

GENERALIZED SKELETAL DISORDERS

Generalized bone disorders occasionally affect the ribs sufficiently to impede ventilation. In rickets, deformities such as symmetrical grooves anteriorly along the line of the costochondral joints, Harrison's sulcus at the site of the insertion of the diaphragm, and enlargement of the costochondral junctions (rachitic rosary) are well documented. Their physiological effects have not been adequately studied.

In Klinefelter's syndrome, a restrictive defect is recognized [1508(a), 3222] that may be due to an abnormally compliant chest wall. This could be due to the lack of testosterone, but testosterone replacement does not improve respiratory function [1153]. If respiratory failure occurs it is usually due to obstructive sleep apnoeas secondary to obesity rather than to the chest wall abnormality [809].

Relapsing polychondritis may involve the costochondral joints but the respiratory complications of this condition are predominantly due to changes in the cartilage of the trachea and bronchi [2144].

ASPHYXIATING THORACIC DYSTROPHY
(JEUNE'S DISEASE)

This rare generalized disorder of cartilage is characterized by radiological changes in the pelvis and phalanges and the presence of short limbs. The ribs, which are a type of long bone, are also shortened so that the rib cage becomes narrowed. The abdomen often protrudes and respiratory movements are almost entirely abdominal [982]. The failure of rib growth impairs lung development so that the number of alveolar ducts and alveoli are reduced [982].

Respiratory failure often appears in infancy or childhood [1340, 2343], but in the milder forms it may be delayed or possibly even absent [1737]. Renal failure may develop [2343] in those who do not die of respiratory failure in childhood. The heart is not involved, although it may appear large on the chest radiograph because the rib cage is so small. Attempts at surgical reconstruction of the rib cage and splitting

of the sternum to allow lung growth have been largely unsuccessful [194, 863, 2575].

TRAUMA

Traumatic damage to the rib cage is dealt with in thoracic surgical textbooks and has recently been well reviewed [2720].

THORACOPLASTY AND OTHER SURGICAL TREATMENTS FOR TUBERCULOSIS

The natural history of pulmonary tuberculosis has been completely changed by modern chemotherapy. Streptomycin became available in 1945, PAS in 1946, and isoniazid in 1952. Over the next few years it was shown that long-term treatment with combination chemotherapy could completely arrest the progress of the disease and virtually eliminate the risk of a relapse [684]. Until then, a variety of surgical treatments were employed to treat pulmonary tuberculosis. Resection of parts of several ribs (thoracoplasty) was commonly carried out. This operation is still occasionally required to eliminate persistent air spaces as a result of chronic pulmonary infections and for cosmetic reasons in scoliosis (p. 212).

Thoracoplasty was frequently combined with other surgical procedures in an attempt to arrest the tuberculosis. Its effects are often inseparable from these and from the late results of the tuberculous infection itself. These are, therefore, briefly considered in this section.

Tuberculous infection

Untreated pulmonary tuberculosis may cause extensive necrosis of lung tissue, which leads to a restrictive ventilatory defect. Pleural involvement [2482] and tuberculous osteomyelitis of the spine (p. 200) may also contribute to this. Decortication of the thickened pleura is of some benefit but is less successful than with pleural thickening from other causes [855, 1196]. Air flow obstruction is common following pulmonary tuberculosis [288, 394, 2460, 2462, 2646, 3029, 3398], although early studies did not always take into account the effect of tobacco smoking [2071]. The severity of the air flow obstruction is related to the extent and the duration of the tuberculous infection [288, 289] and is largely irreversible [2462].

Air flow obstruction can result in three ways. First, bronchial stenoses can result from infection of the large airways such as the larynx, trachea and main and segmental bronchi, which occurs particularly with extensive pulmonary tuberculosis [139, 1533, 1595, 2026, 2755]. Secondly, diffuse inflammation of the small airways (endobronchitis), which is also associated with extensive tuberculosis of long duration [1334, 1797, 2453], may lead to more generalized air flow obstruction. Thirdly, lymph node inflammation can involve and obstruct the adjacent bronchi.

If the tuberculosis is untreated, death usually occurs from the infection itself before respiratory or right heart failure appear. Pulmonary hypertension is usually mild, even in extensive disease [3208], and right ventricular hypertrophy is less common in untreated tuberculosis than in many other chronic lung diseases. In a study of 18 000 consecutive autopsies, only 3.7% of subjects dying with pulmonary tuberculosis showed right ventricular hypertrophy [1252] although smaller series showed a higher prevalence [11, 2286]. There are no comparable data for the frequency of hypercapnic respiratory failure, but this is probably uncommon. It may be prevented to a large extent by chemotherapy but, conversely, some patients who would previously have died of their tuberculosis now survive with extensive lung disease and may develop this complication [1568, 1878].

Surgical treatments

The principle of surgical treatment was that if the tuberculous cavities could be closed the infection would be arrested. Various methods of collapsing the lung to close the cavities were devised. The infection was frequently controlled [1029, 1208, 2849] but most of the procedures had deleterious mechanical effects on the rib cage and pleura, which impaired respiratory function. Surgical treatments were often combined either simultaneously or sequentially, so that it is difficult to analyse the consequences of each procedure, particularly if there was also extensive pulmonary or pleural tuberculosis. Most of the data are derived from studies of respiratory function during the weeks and months after surgery, and there is relatively little information on the long-term consequences. The most important of the surgical procedures were:

Scaleniotomy and intercostal neurectomy. These operations were carried out to prevent expansion of the lung, but were found to be ineffective. Intercostal neurectomy diminished the ipsilateral chest wall movement in humans [55] and in dogs [54], and frequently caused a scoliosis convex to the side of the surgery [297]. These effects were not seen with scaleniotomy but upper rib cage expansion was reduced and the VC fell temporarily [55].

Pneumoperitoneum. Introduction of air into the peritoneal cavity elevated both of the hemidiaphragms so that bilateral disease could be treated. Unfortunately, this was often ineffective because the bases of the lungs were preferentially collapsed, whereas the tuberculous infection was usually apical. The FRC and RV fell by about 20%. There was a smaller reduction in the TLC, VC and FEV_1 [1918, 2419, 2912, 3375]. These changes were less marked in the supine than in the erect position [3375]. The air in the peritoneal cavity was absorbed rapidly after treatment was discontinued and no long-term respiratory consequences of pneumoperitoneum are known.

Artificial pneumothorax. Instillation of air extrapleurally (p. 193) or into the pleural cavity was widely used to collapse the lung. The pneumothorax was often maintained for several years by regular injection of air and was occasionally needed bilaterally. The complications of this procedure were mainly pleural. Vascular adhesions between the lungs and the parietal pleura were common and adhesiotomy frequently resulted in a haemothorax. Pleural effusions also led to the pneumothorax being abandoned. Pleural thickening and calcification, which was often gross, resulted from both of these complications (Fig. 16.9).

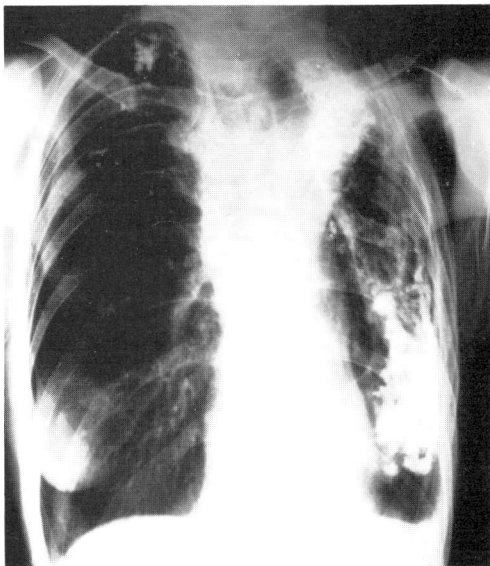

Fig. 16.9. *Chest radiograph showing extensive left pleural calcification following artificial pneumothorax for pulmonary tuberculosis. Calcification within the lung is also visible, particularly at the right apex.*

Extrapleural pneumothoraces hardly altered the VC [60, 1066] but by the technique of bronchospirometry [305, 1552] a fall in the TLC, RV and expiratory reserve volume on the side of the pneumothorax was noted [1067]. An intrapleural pneumothorax caused a restrictive defect, which varied according to the amount of air instilled and the properties of the underlying lung. The VC commonly fell to about two-thirds that predicted, with a lesser fall in the TLC [670]. Bronchospirometry revealed that the major change in the lung volumes was on the side of the pneumothorax but that it also had an effect on the contralateral lung [1067, 2812]. The oxygen uptake was diminished more than the VC and the minute ventilation was least affected [1066, 1072]. This suggests that the pneumothorax impaired the matching of ventilation and perfusion to the collapsed lung. Reduced perfusion has been confirmed isotopically [522].

The recovery of lung function was very variable after the lung had expanded and the pneumothorax treatment had been discontinued [425, 2482]. This probably reflected the degree of pleural thickening that the pneumothorax caused [2208]. Significant improvement may be seen following decortication, even many years after the artificial pneumothorax, as long as the underlying lung remained normal [2453]. This was, however, often damaged by the tuberculous infection. The extent of this correlated with the reduction in the carbon monoxide transfer factor after the pneumothorax treatment had been completed [3189].

Phrenic nerve crush, section and avulsion. Collapse of tuberculous cavities was also achieved by crushing, cutting or avulsion of the phrenic nerve in order to paralyse the diaphragm. This procedure was only carried out unilaterally because of the severe consequences of bilateral diaphragmatic paralysis (Chapter 15). Crushing the nerve was introduced so that diaphragmatic function would recover over a period of months, by which time the tuberculosis would be healed. There is some evidence from long-term studies that recovery of function was complete [2459].

The hemidiaphragm was not always totally paralysed because accessory phrenic nerves commonly join the main phrenic nerve trunk within the thorax below the level of surgery (p. 27). Unless the nerve was completely avulsed, the physiological consequences of phrenic nerve interruption were variable. They also depended upon the presence of pulmonary and particularly pleural disease on the side of the operation [2833]. Extensive pleural adhesions appeared to minimize the change in position of the diaphragm. In general, however, there was a slight fall in the VC [1072, 1912, 2812(a), 3294, 3396] and this could be decreased further by the addition of a pneumoperitoneum [1918, 2913].

Bronchospirometric studies showed that the reduction in lung volumes was more marked on the side of the phrenic nerve surgery. Inspiration was more impaired than expiration so that the TLC and inspiratory capacity were more affected than the RV or expiratory reserve volume [1067, 2913]. The oxygen uptake of the lung on the side of the phrenic nerve surgery was reduced more than the VC [3214], presumably because of mismatching of ventilation and perfusion.

Pulmonary resection. Resection of infected lung was hazardous before the advent of chemotherapy, but was often combined with this in the 1950s until it was realized that drug treatment alone was sufficient. The fall in the FEV_1, VC and MVV was in general proportional to the amount of lung removed [291, 698, 779, 1020, 1799]. The reduction was about 10–15% with a segmentectomy, 15–20% with a lobectomy [1918] and about 30% with a pneumonectomy [668, 698]. The MVV was reduced more than the VC [347]. The changes were often less than expected because the resected lung tissue was abnormal and poorly functioning [287, 304, 364, 2165, 2472]. As a consequence, the oxygen saturation often improved post-operatively [2472] with removal of lung tissue that was responsible for shunting blood through the lungs. Pneumonectomy after an unsuccessful extensive thoracoplasty did not alter the lung volumes or the MVV [1071], but the addition of a thoracoplasty to a pneumonectomy reduced respiratory function [289, 1433, 3140]. Unexpectedly severe deterioration in respiratory function was occasionally seen post-operatively if there were complications such as intrathoracic bleeding, a persistent air space, protracted lung collapse or impaired diaphragmatic movement [2128].

The pulmonary artery pressure remained within normal limits at rest following resection [2126] but rose abnormally rapidly during exercise [447]. Resection of lung tissue reduces the size of the pulmonary microcirculation so that when the cardiac output is increased during exercise fewer vessels can be recruited and the pulmonary vascular resistance rises. Fatal cor pulmonale was a recognized problem of lung resection for tuberculosis [1432]. Late respiratory failure is, however, rare if the function of the contralateral lung is normal but pneumonectomy combined with phrenic nerve interruption may lead to respiratory failure [1085]. The combination of pneumonectomy with a thoracoplasty also appears to increase the risk of late respiratory failure relative to that of a pneumonectomy alone [1482].

Extrapleural pneumolysis. Collapse of tuberculous cavities could be achieved by separating the parietal pleura from the ribs (extrapleural pneumolysis). The most effective technique was mobilization of the apex of the lung, as in Semb's extrafascial apicolysis. The extrapleural space could be filled with air (extrapleural pneumothorax, p. 191), paraffin, muscle grafts, fat or solid foreign bodies (plombs) such as lucite balls (Fig. 16.10), polythene bags or drilled spheres. These operations reduced the VC by only about 10% [787, 1070, 1072, 3349] and did not lead to a scoliosis, pleural thickening or paradoxical movement of the chest wall [3349]. However, migration of the plombs and extrapleural infection were frequent complications [112, 2896].

Thoracoplasty (Fig. 16.11). The removal of varying lengths of the ribs enabled the chest wall to collapse in on the infected lung (Fig. 16.12). The early operations, such as Sauerbruch's paravertebral thoracoplasty, were extensive and as many as eleven ribs were resected. Less radical surgery was found to be equally effective and caused fewer respiratory problems and less chest deformity.

Thoracoplasty was carried out extensively, especially between 1930 and 1955. It has been estimated that between 1951 and 1960 about 30 000 operations were performed in the UK alone [2461]. The mortality of such patients is greater than normal, particularly from cardiac or respiratory failure. These complications are

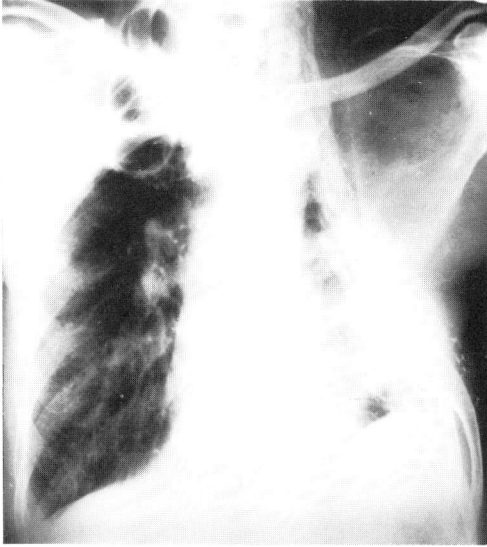

Fig. 16.10. *Chest radiograph showing right apical plombage with lucite spheres and left seven-rib thoracoplasty.*

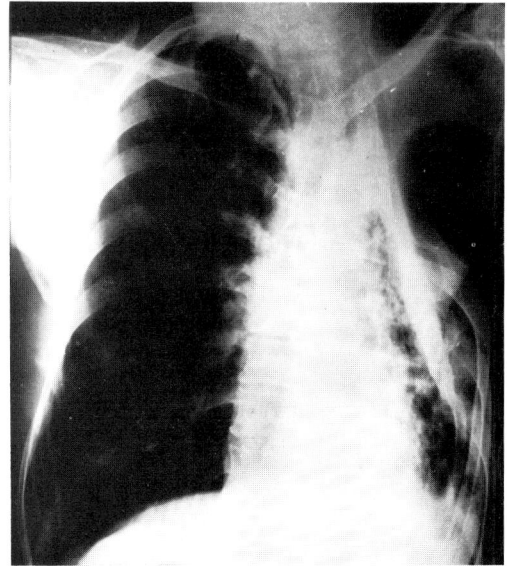

Fig. 16.12. *Chest radiograph showing left seven-rib thoracoplasty with mild upper thoracic scoliosis. Left lung is grossly reduced in volume and shows bronchiectasis due to the tuberculous infection.*

related to the extent of the tuberculosis and to whether or not an artificial pneumothorax was induced on the contralateral side to the thoracoplasty, since this may have lead to pleural thickening or because it indicates extensive tuberculous damage to the underlying lung [2461].

A restrictive defect was recognized as an inevitable consequence of thoracoplasty. The TLC was decreased more than the FRC or RV

[1375, 1614, 1996]. The severity of the restrictive defect is related to the extent of the thoracoplasty [779]. A five-rib thoracoplasty decreased the FEV_1 by about 20% [1799], an eight-rib thoracoplasty by about 35% [1918] and the fall in VC was about 45% with a nine- to eleven-rib thoracoplasty [3396]. In some cases the change

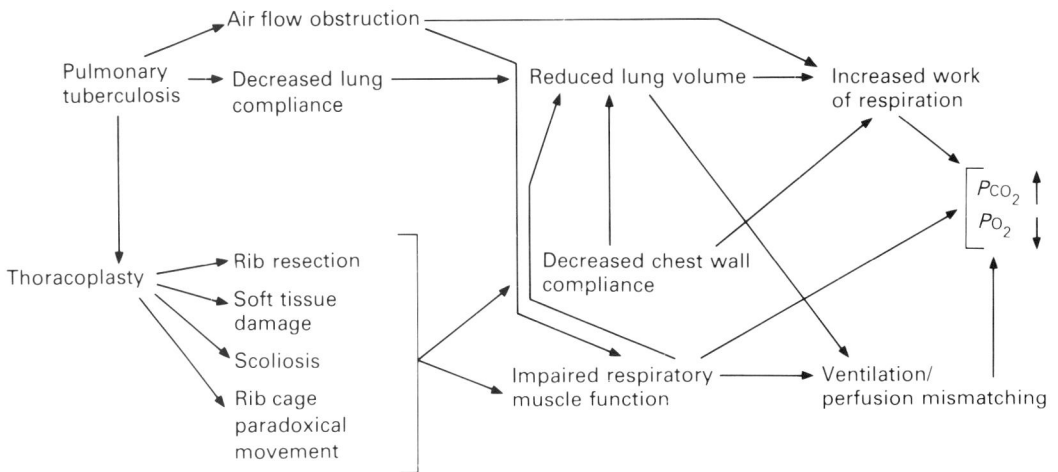

Fig. 16.11. *Flow chart to show effects of thoracoplasty and pulmonary tuberculosis on ventilation.*

in lung volumes was less than expected, presumably because of pre-existing damage to the underlying lung [290]. If the operation was carried out in separate stages, the greatest change in the VC was seen after the first stage, which involved resection of the upper ribs [1912]. The fall in the VC was shown by bronchospirometry to be more than twice as great on the side of the thoracoplasty as on the contralateral side [60]. The ventilation of the lung on the side of the thoracoplasty was reduced less than the oxygen uptake and the VC [1072, 2482].

These observations were made shortly after the surgical procedure; it remains uncertain whether the restrictive defect subsequently changes. The rib cage deformity is permanent but compensatory overinflation of the contralateral lung would be anticipated. Conversely, progressive changes in the soft tissues and joints of the rib cage might decrease the chest wall compliance and worsen the restrictive defect. There are no longitudinal studies of patients who have undergone thoracoplasty and there is conflicting evidence as to whether the interval since the thoracoplasty correlates with the ventilatory function [1482, 3029, 3398].

There are several interrelated causes for the restrictive defect. The resection of the ribs has

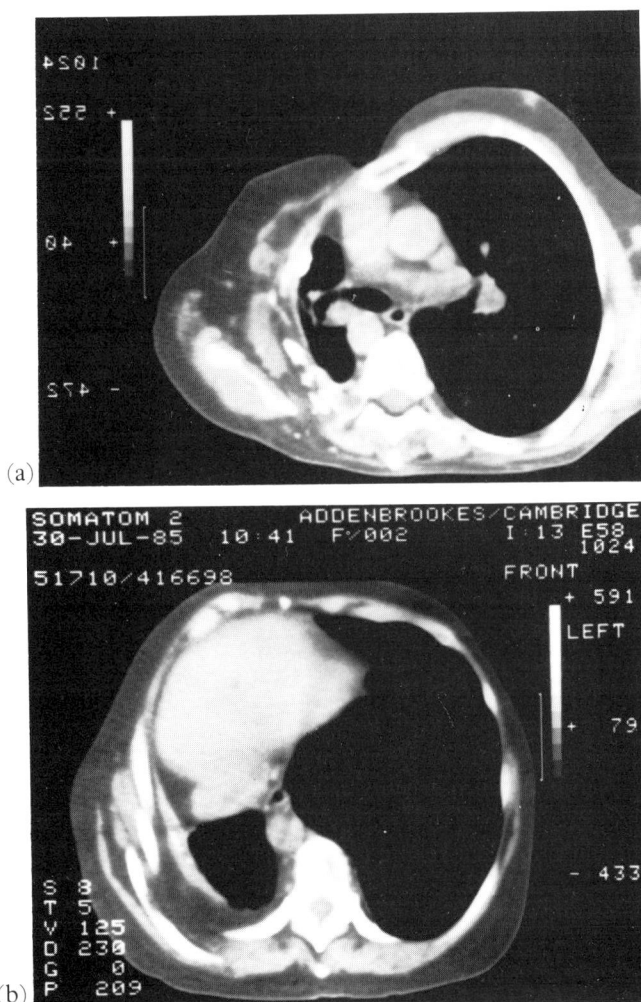

Fig. 16.13. Computerized tomographic scans after thoracoplasty through (a) upper and (b) lower chest, showing rib resection and distortion, ipsilateral pleural thickening and calcification, and the small ipsilateral lung.

the direct effect of drawing in the remaining tissues of the chest wall in the area of the thoracoplasty. The stability of the rib cage is lost and paradoxical movement at the site of the surgery is commonly seen. This is particularly a problem if the anterior parts of the upper ribs are resected. The compliance of the lungs and chest wall are both reduced. Lung compliance falls because of the effects of the tuberculous infection itself and because of the loss of lung volume secondary to the thoracoplasty. Pleural thickening may be marked and can be caused either by the tuberculosis itself, a previous artificial pneumothorax or by the thoracoplasty since this involves dissection close to the pleura [138, 2208] (Fig. 16.13). Thoracoplasty also damages the soft tissues of the rib cage leading to fibrosis. The costovertebral joints may not be damaged at the time of surgery but the small range of movements after the thoracoplasty probably induces changes that decrease the compliance of the chest wall.

This is also reduced by the almost invariable development of a thoracic scoliosis [1905]. The curve is convex to the side of the thoracoplasty, in contrast to the scoliosis due to a tuberculous empyema, which is concave to the affected side [3034]. The curvature often progresses for many years after the thoracoplasty, but about half of the final curvature is apparent within the first week and two-thirds within the first six months [297, 1947]. The angle of curvature is not related to the age of the patient or to whether a pneumonectomy is also carried out, but it does correlate with the number of ribs removed [1947]. About 3° of scoliosis develops per rib resected but the scoliosis is less if there is a long interval between the stages of the thoracoplasty, during which time reossification of the ribs can occur [2526].

The scoliosis is probably due to unequal muscle power on the two sides of the thoracic spine. Several muscle groups are damaged at thoracoplasty. If the transverse processes are removed the paraspinal muscles are disturbed, if the 1st and 2nd ribs are resected the scalene muscles are removed, if the anterior segments of the 2nd, 3rd and 4th ribs are resected the function of the pectoralis minor is altered and when the scapula is freed the upper fibres of the serratus anterior are damaged. The scoliosis becomes particularly severe if the head, neck and tubercle of the rib and the transverse processes of the vertebrae are removed [1516, 1947] or if the anterior segments of the 2nd, 3rd and 4th ribs are resected [2526]. A similar scoliosis also develops if a thoracoplasty is carried out for indications other than tuberculosis [777].

Interference with the function of the respiratory muscles, particularly the inspiratory muscles, also contributes to the restrictive defect. The PI_{max} and maximal transdiaphragmatic pressure are both decreased and the fall in the latter is related to the fall in the VC [2459]. This is reflected in the change in lung volumes in that the TLC is diminished more than the RV, which primarily depends on expiratory muscle strength [1067]. The intercostal and shoulder-girdle muscles are directly damaged by the surgery but the number of ribs resected does not correlate with the PI_{max} [2459]. Distortion of the rib cage may, however, put the inspiratory muscles at a mechanical disadvantage and reduce the pressures that they can develop. The excursion of the diaphragm observed at fluoroscopy is diminished on the side of the thoracoplasty, both at rest [1070, 1382, 1614] and immediately after exertion [1381]. If the thoracoplasty is extensive the contralateral diaphragmatic movement may also be reduced [787, 1614]. Although the exact causes of the dysfunction of the diaphragm are not yet established, this is probably one of the most important complications of thoracoplasty.

The fall in lung and chest wall compliance together with any air flow obstruction (p. 190) increase the work of the inspiratory muscles. Muscle fatigue probably develops in certain circumstances, such as during chest infections or during prolonged or severe exercise. The exercise ability of subjects who have undergone thoracoplasty is less than normal [1614]. Exercise is limited by ventilatory factors rather than by the cardiovascular system as in normal sub-

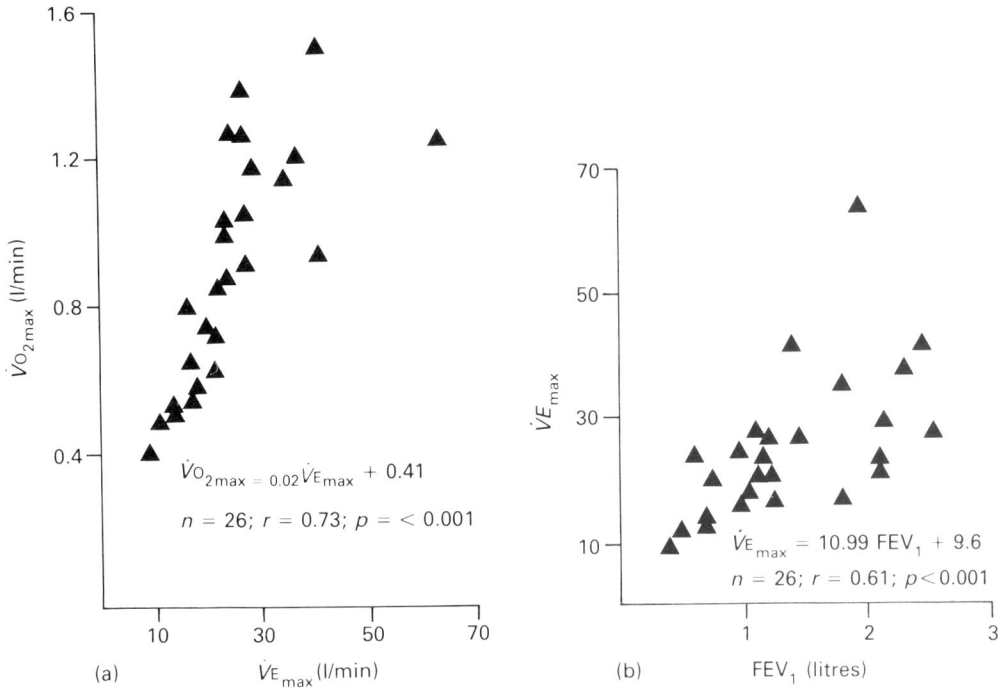

Fig. 16.14. *Exercise responses following thoracoplasty: (a) relationship of $\dot{V}_{O_2\,max}$ to $\dot{V}_{E\,max}$, (b) relationship of $\dot{V}_{E\,max}$ to FEV$_1$.*

jects (Fig. 16.14). The maximal exercise ventilation correlates not only with the FVC and maximal tidal volume, but with the FEV$_1$ and the maximal respiratory frequency. This suggests that although the restrictive defect is important in limiting exercise ventilation, air flow obstruction also contributes to this. There is no correlation between maximal oxygen uptake and the arterial blood gases, angle of scoliosis or the number of ribs resected [2459].

Respiratory failure occasionally occurred immediately after thoracoplasty if the pre-operative lung function was poor [471, 1905]. Most of the deaths in the first few years after the thoracoplasty were due to a relapse of the tuberculosis, but longer-term follow-up has shown that respiratory failure commonly develops [271, 1469, 2038, 2803, 2950, 2951].

Chronic hypoxia is partly due to suboptimal ventilation and perfusion matching [1482, 3029]. The lung on the side of the thoracoplasty may partially be responsible but both its ventilation [2208] and perfusion [787] are considerably reduced and the function of the contralateral lung is relatively more important. Hypoxaemia worsens during sleep since the FRC falls and this leads to basal airway closure and worsening of ventilation/perfusion matching.

Hypoxaemia is also due to alveolar hypoventilation. The degree of hypercapnia is related to the fall in $P_{I\,max}$ and maximal transdiaphragmatic pressure [1678, 1679]. In some patients, hypercapnia persists during the day. This is also related to the $P_{I\,max}$ and maximal transdiaphragmatic pressure (Fig. 16.15). The PEFR and FEV$_1$ correlate with the blood gases [2462], and the extent of pleural thickening bilaterally, particularly on the contralateral side to the thoracoplasty, is related to the P_{CO_2} [2207]. The severity of the scoliosis appears to be unimportant in most cases [2207] but may occasionally be significant [671].

The gradual worsening of these factors may explain the late appearance of respiratory failure

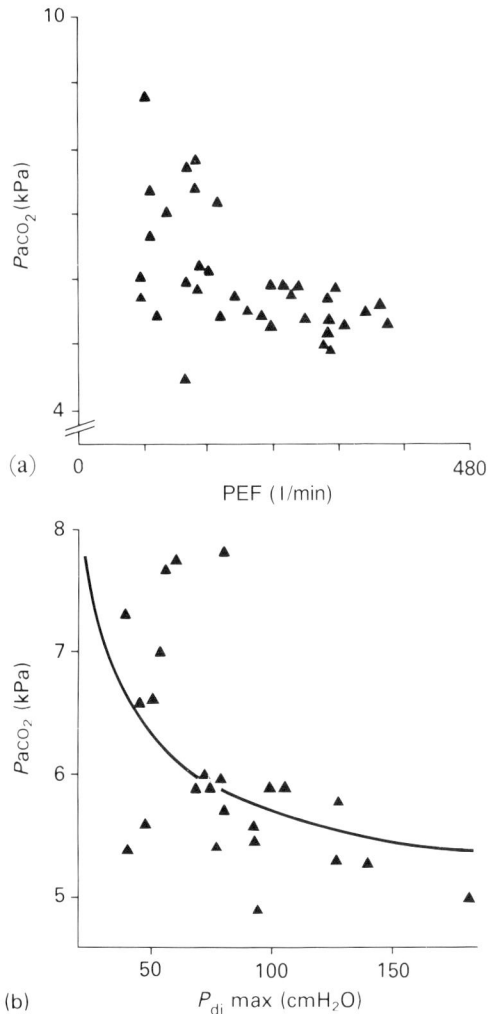

Fig. 16.15. $Pa\text{CO}_2$ following thoracoplasty: (a) relationship to peak expiratory flow rate, (b) relationship to maximum transdiaphragmatic pressure. Reproduced, with permission, from Kinnear et al., unpublished observations, and Phillips et al. Thorax 1987; 42: 348–52.

after thoracoplasty but the normal decrease with age of the respiratory drive, chest wall compliance and inspiratory muscle strength probably contribute. Respiratory failure may worsen rapidly after a long period of stability. An identifiable cause, such as chest infection, is not always present but respiratory muscle fatigue, an increase in respiratory frequency and a fall in tidal volume may determine when this deterioration occurs.

Right heart failure was rarely the cause of death in the first few years after a thoracoplasty unless there was pre-existing chronic bronchitis or emphysema [1068, 1208]. It is, however, a common late complication of thoracoplasty [424, 1082, 2208, 2460, 2461, 3399] and is due to pulmonary hypertension caused by a raised pulmonary vascular resistance [1482]. Pulmonary hypertension may be difficult to recognize from the clinical signs and ECG [2463]. It is probably determined by the extent of the damage to the pulmonary microcirculation by the tuberculous infection and the degree of hypoxia during both sleep and wakefulness.

Spinal disorders

Disorders of the spine may interfere with ventilation by impinging on the spinal cord or peripheral nerves, or by mechanically limiting the expansion of the rib cage. The effects of neurological involvement have been described in Chapters 12 and 13. The most important conditions that have mechanical effects on respiration are:

ANKYLOSING SPONDYLITIS

Ankylosing spondylitis often presents with inflammation of the sacro-iliac joints but this may spread up the spine to affect all the intervertebral and costovertebral joints. The sterno-manubrial, costochondral and chondrosternal joints may also be involved. The inflammation subsides in the later stages of the disease but the joints become ankylosed and the spinal ligaments calcify. The result is a rigid rib cage, little spinal mobility and often a pronounced kyphosis [1373]. Chest pain during sudden movements such as coughing, tightness in the chest and an inability to take a deep breath may be noticed while the inflammation is active [1371, 1372, 1598]. These symptoms originate either in the joints themselves or in the muscles of the chest wall [1470] but become less prominent as the disease advances.

Lung volumes and respiratory muscles (see Fig. 9.7)

The typical changes in lung volume are that the TLC and VC fall slightly and the RV and FRC increase [1033, 1064, 1372, 2121, 3185, 3401]. With the exception of Parkinsonism, the increase in the FRC is unique among chest wall diseases. It results from the rib cage becoming fixed at its own relaxation volume. This is greater than the normal FRC, which is influenced by the inward pull of the elastic recoil of the lungs. The fall in the VC is proportional to the degree of vertebral ankylosis [2121] and fall in chest wall compliance, but is not related to the degree of kyphosis or to the duration of the disease [2885]. Early studies showed that the VC could be increased and RV decreased by radiotherapy [1371, 2694]. Physiotherapy may also be of benefit, particularly in the early stages of the disease [1256, 1593]. Non-steroidal anti-inflammatory drugs increase chest expansion but not the VC [1033].

The ankylosis of the intervertebral, costovertebral and other chest wall joints may severely limit the expansion of the rib cage [1256, 1371, 1591]. The chest wall compliance falls [1372, 2885], although the lung compliance remains normal [1064, 1372, 1598]. The immobility of the rib cage is thought to lead to atrophy of the intercostal muscles [1593], which can cause paradoxical movement of the rib cage during inspiration. The EMG features of muscle fatigue have been demonstrated when the V_T increases [3188], although presumably intercostal muscle contraction is virtually isometric because of the fixation of the rib cage. Both $P_{I_{max}}$ and $P_{E_{max}}$ are diminished [3185].

Diaphragmatic contraction is relatively more important than intercostal and accessory muscle contraction in ankylosing spondylitics than in normal subjects. The diaphragmatic excursion is greater than normal both when assessed fluoroscopically [1383, 2695] and by more sophisticated analysis of abdominal and thoracic movements [1256, 1593]. It largely compensates for the inability to expand the rib cage and minimizes the change in lung volumes [3188].

The MVV is even less abnormal than the VC [1064, 2600, 2694, 2695, 3401], probably because the diaphragm enables an unusually high proportion of the VC to be utilized. The ventilatory responses to exercise are remarkably normal and exercise is usually limited by circulatory factors [911].

It might be expected that since the lung expansion is almost solely due to diaphragmatic contraction, the ventilation to the bases would be greater than normal and that ventilation and perfusion might not be matched. Underventilation of the apices has been reported in one study [3053] but this has not been confirmed [2410]. The physiological dead space and A–a oxygen gradient are both normal [2163, 3185] and the carbon monoxide transfer factor is also normal [578]. These findings indicate that fixation of the rib cage does not cause significant ventilation/perfusion mismatching.

Respiratory failure

Respiratory failure is extremely uncommon in ankylosing spondylitis. The rib cage rigidity alone probably never leads to either respiratory failure or right heart failure, probably because compensation by the diaphragm prevents any major change in lung volumes or the distribution of ventilation. Other causes for respiratory failure should be sought. These include:

Air flow obstruction. Air flow obstruction is not a feature of ankylosing spondylitis [1064] unless there is cricoarytenoid arthritis. This may cause either stridor or respiratory failure [1892, 3363]. It usually occurs in longstanding ankylosing spondylitis and may present with slowly worsening hoarseness of the voice and breathlessness, with stridor as a later manifestation. Tracheobronchial aspiration may develop because of the immobility of the larynx during swallowing [248]. In the early stages, some response to prednisolone may be seen [282] but tracheostomy may be required. This can be technically difficult because of the flexion deformity of the neck, and arytenoidectomy may be necessary.

Pleural thickening and effusion. Respiratory failure may occur in the rare cases of ankylosing spondylitis that are associated with widespread pleural thickening [2707]. Pleural effusions have also been described [1682] but are often transient [2707].

Aspiration pneumonia. Ankylosing spondylitis is occasionally associated with oesophageal motility disorders, which may lead to pulmonary aspiration [2835].

Associated lung diseases. Apical fibrobullous lung disease is well recognized in ankylosing spondylitis and may be complicated by infection with fungi such as *Aspergillus fumigatus* and by saprophytic mycobacteria [1430, 1497, 2707]. There may also be a predisposition to pulmonary tuberculosis [1373, 1430].

Surgery. Respiratory failure may follow surgery, particularly laparotomy in which diaphragmatic function is impaired post-operatively. Thoracotomy is usually well tolerated unless the phrenic nerve is damaged [1371, 3136, 3401].

Cardiac complications

Right heart failure rarely occurs because of the respiratory complications of ankylosing spondylitis, but the heart may be involved in the disease process itself. The aortic valve cusps become shortened and thickened and a subaortic ridge of inflammatory tissue develops. These features are seen particularly in older subjects with more severe disease [3194]. Intraventricular conduction defects, including third-degree atrioventricular block, occur [254] and aortic regurgitation and aortic dilatation are well recognized [445].

KYPHOSIS

Kyphosis of the thoracic spine has many causes but most of these are not associated with any significant changes in respiratory function (Fig. 16.16). The most important exception is tuberculous osteomyelitis of the spine (Pott's disease) (Fig. 16.17). This often spreads to more than one vertebra and causes a very sharp kyphosis (gibbus) with a relatively mild scoliosis. In addition to the kyphosis, the costovertebral joints

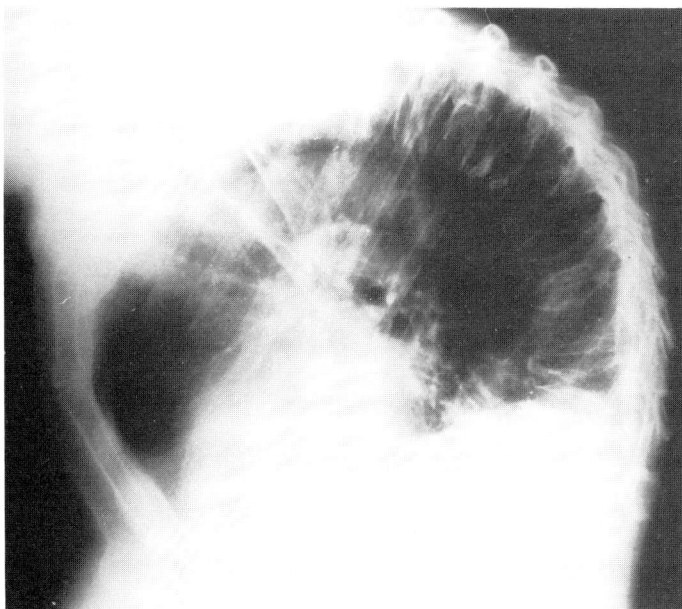

Fig. 16.16. *Lateral radiograph showing marked thoracic kyphosis due to osteoporosis in a sixty-five-year-old female. No respiratory complications.*

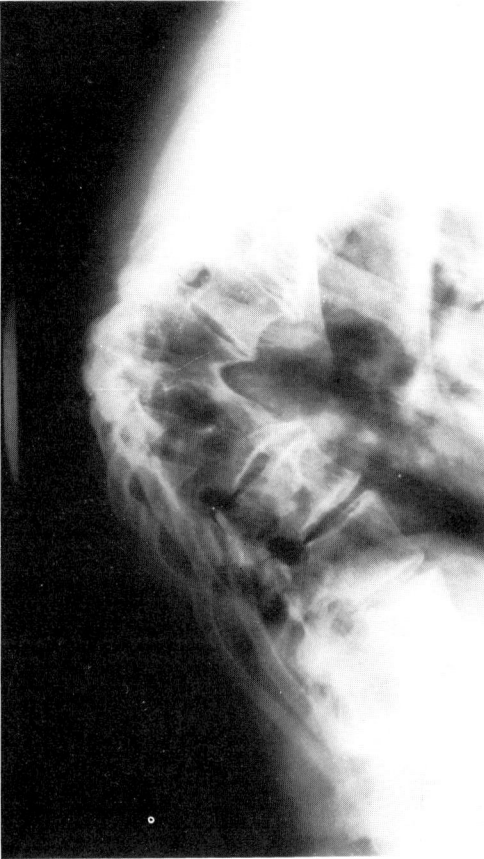

Fig. 16.17. *Lateral radiograph of spine showing sharp mid-thoracic kyphosis noted at age 2 years. Chronic ventilatory failure developed at age 55 years.*

become ankylosed and this limits the expansion of the rib cage. Diaphragmatic contraction is therefore particularly important. Tuberculous osteomyelitis is most common at the thoracolumbar junction but respiratory complications occur most frequently if the infection is higher in the thoracic spine [2345]. A restrictive defect in which the TLC is decreased more than the RV is characteristic [1811, 3386]. This may be improved by surgical treatment [3386].

Ventilatory failure is unusual in tuberculous osteomyelitis. In most of the reported cases the infection was contracted early in childhood and may have prevented the normal development of

the lung. In one carefully studied case the number of alveoli was decreased and the variation in alveolar size was abnormally great [247]. It is uncertain exactly how hypoplasia of the lungs leads to ventilatory failure later in life, but alterations in the chemical drive to respiration acquired early in life may contribute to this complication (p. 8).

Chronic hypercapnia can be severe [397, 1135, 2353, 3198] and exacerbations may be precipitated by, for instance, acute chest infections or asthma [1341]. Pulmonary hypertension [1341] and right heart failure [397, 638, 1341] develop, probably because of the chronic hypoxia and reduced size of the pulmonary vascular bed. Both respiratory and cardiac failure may appear during pregnancy, partly because of the increase in blood volume and partly because the enlarging uterus limits the excursion of the diaphragm [250, 534, 1583, 1730].

Hypertension is occasionally associated with severe kyphosis. Hypoxic vasoconstriction may be responsible but in severe cases there is a marked angulation of the aorta at the level of the kyphosis and this could, like aortic coarctation, cause hypertension [10, 638, 871].

STRAIGHT BACK SYNDROME

In the straight back syndrome, the normal thoracic kyphosis is lost. This may cause a mild restrictive defect [1862, 2917] but the cardiac features are more prominent. The heart and great vessels are compressed between the spine and anterior rib cage in a similar manner to pectus excavatum. A systolic murmur may be heard [717, 2572, 2573, 2856, 2917]. This may reflect compression of the right ventricular outflow tract or pulmonary artery, but mitral valve prolapse is also recognized [1435, 2045, 2762, 3145]. Occasionally, the right ventricular end diastolic pressure is raised [1862] and an early diastolic dip and late diastolic plateau in the right ventricular pressures are seen [1862, 2856]. This implies that right ventricular filling is hindered by compression of the heart or great vessels and this is probably also responsible for vessels and this is probably also responsible for the diminished cardiac output during exercise [2856].

SCOLIOSIS (Fig. 16.18)

Scoliosis is a lateral curvature of the spine that is invariably associated with rotation of the vertebral bodies (Figs 16.19 and 16.20). This leads to a lordosis, which is unstable because its axis is posterior to the vertebral bodies [792, 2642]. There is no kyphosis and the term kyphocoliosis is, therefore, inaccurate.

Scoliosis is a purely descriptive term and it may be caused by a variety of conditions that have little else in common (Table 16.1). This heterogeneity has caused problems in analysing the respiratory effects of scoliosis. The most important distinction is between those conditions with normal and those with abnormal respiratory muscle strength and endurance. The latter have been described in Chapters 12–15, and this chapter deals primarily with the respiratory effects of the skeletal deformity itself rather than muscle weakness.

The severity of the spinal curvature is an important factor determining the respiratory abnormalities, but difficulties in accurately assessing the deformity have hindered analysis of this relationship. A large number of methods have

been proposed for assessing the severity of scoliosis [3175] but the method of Cobb [589] is the most widely used. Its accuracy can be improved by computerization [1565]. Estimation of the degree of rotation of the spine is more complex but techniques using measurement of the rib hump [3056], plain radiographs [2112] and CT scans [3, 4] have been developed. The degree of lordosis can also be assessed from CT scans [3, 5].

If the scoliosis appears before the age of about eight years it may prevent the normal multiplication of alveoli so that the lung fails to develop fully. In congenital scoliosis the spine is also often rigid and there may be multiple rib abnormalities that impair ventilation, particularly if they are in the region of the insertion of the diaphragm (p. 189). In contrast, the scoliosis of neuromuscular disorders is often capable of considerable extension but may worsen when sitting or standing because of the effect of gravity. An exception is the scoliosis of the rigid spine syndrome, which is associated with a variety of myopathies and may lead to ventilatory failure [2505, 3358].

In many of the neuromuscular disorders the scoliosis is long and may affect both the thoracic and the lumbar spine [999]. In other conditions such as neurofibromatosis it may be severe and affect only a short length of the thoracic spine.

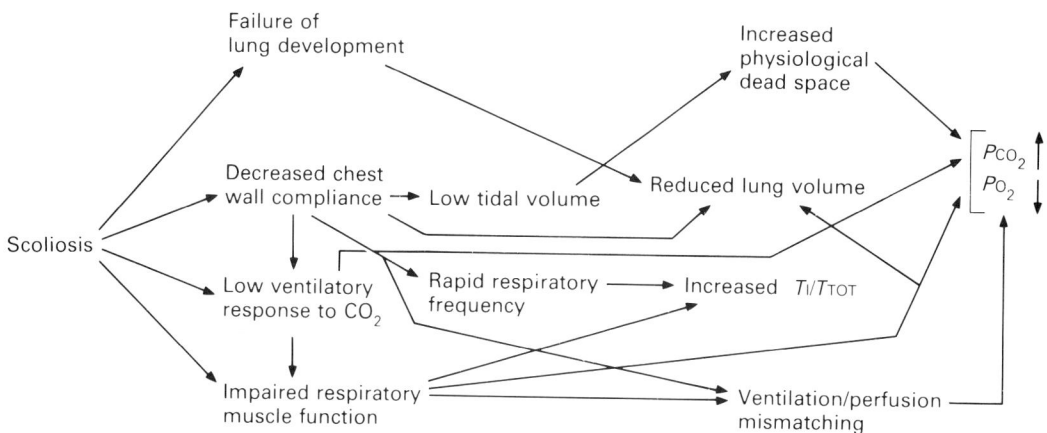

Fig. 16.18. *Flow chart to show effects of scoliosis on ventilation.*

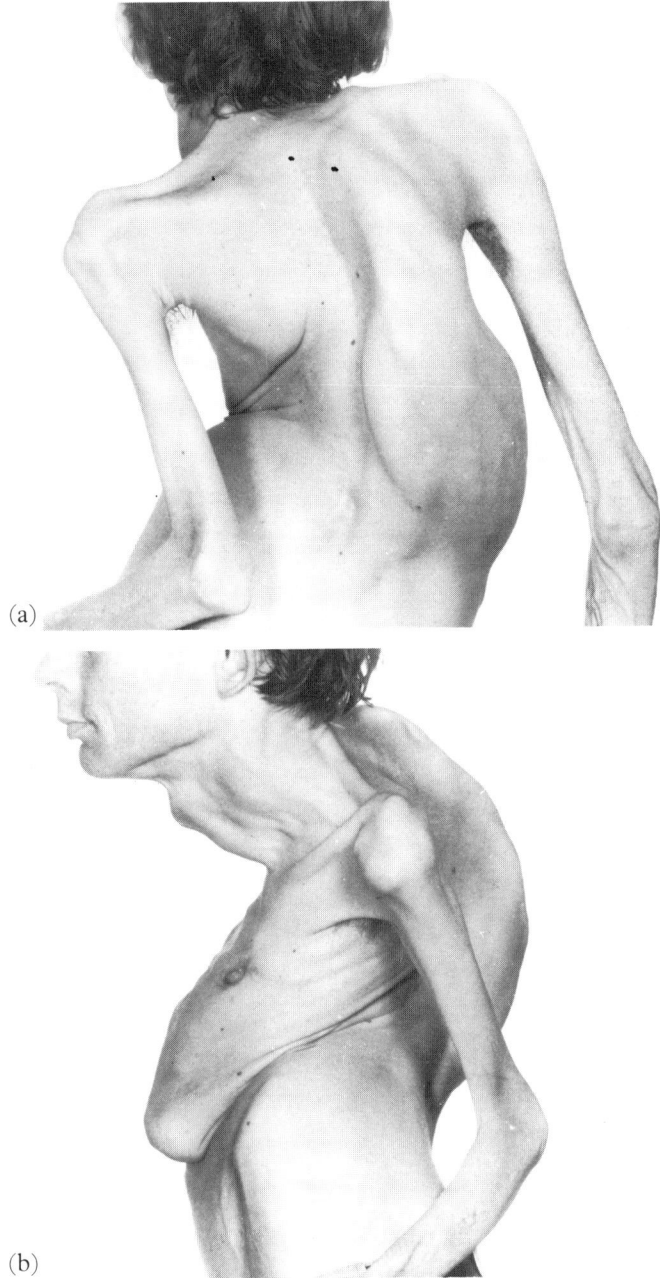

Fig. 16.19. *Severe long thoracic scoliosis following poliomyelitis. (a) Scar from spinal fusion operation is visible. (b) Pronounced rib hump due to rotation of spine is apparent.*

In general, the higher the curve in the thoracic spine, the more marked are the cardiac and respiratory consequences [1000]. Lumbar scolioses have no such sequelae.

Compliance, lung volumes and respiratory muscle function

The combination of a lateral curvature, rotation and lordosis of the thoracic spine greatly alters

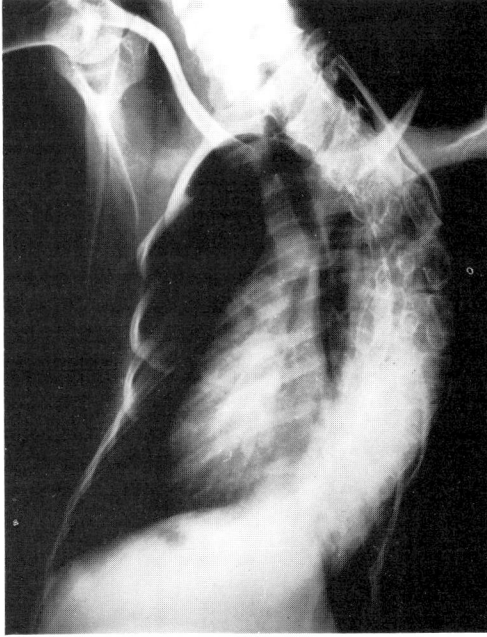

Fig. 16.20. *Chest radiograph showing severe long thoracic scoliosis following poliomyelitis. Left-sided ribs are markedly thinned and lie almost vertically, indicating gross intercostal muscle weakness.*

the configuration of the rib cage (Fig. 16.21). Despite this, the ribs move parallel to the axis of their necks as in normal subjects [1591], although this axis is positioned obliquely. The distortion of the rib cage puts the respiratory muscles at a mechanical disadvantage. The hemithorax on the side of the convexity of the scoliosis tends to be relatively overinflated and that on the concavity underinflated [1588]. This concept is helpful in analysing the mechanics of the rib cage but it has been difficult to develop because of the problems in measuring the relative movements of the two halves of the thorax independently when they are so distorted and the surface markings of each lung are uncertain.

The $P_{I_{max}}$ and $P_{E_{max}}$ are reduced in scoliosis even in the absence of muscle weakness, but even more so if this is present [637, 642, 1588, 1913, 2439]. The $P_{I_{max}}$ and maximal transdiaphragmatic pressure correlate better with the VC than with the angle of scoliosis [642, 1588,

1913], although this may also be important [2439]. This suggests that there are more subtle anatomical changes, such as the degree of rotation or lordosis, that determine the length and mechanical advantage of the respiratory muscles. A fall in the VC when changing from the sitting to the supine position has been noted and this suggests that even in the absence of muscle weakness, diaphragm function is impaired by the scoliosis [2145]. However, at fluoroscopy, diaphragmatic movement appears normal [2934].

The abnormal configuration of the spine and rib cage decreases the compliance of the chest wall [260, 1606], particularly in older subjects [495, 3169]. The compliance of the lungs is also diminished [260, 496, 642]. The dynamic lung compliance can be increased by IPPB, indicating that airway closure during tidal breathing is partly responsible [642]; this is confirmed by the finding that the closing volume is often above the FRC [306, 310].

The deformity of the rib cage and the loss of strength of the respiratory muscles characteristically causes a restrictive defect [260]. It is, however, difficult to assess the normal values for lung function in scoliosis. The spinal curvature shortens the stature so that falsely low predicted values are obtained from measurements of height. There is no ideal way of allowing for this loss of height. Corrections using the length of the tibia [3402, 3403], foot and hand size [153] and radiological methods of assessing the degree of spinal curvature [307, 3217] have been proposed. The most commonly used method is to measure the arm span from which a corrected value for height can be derived, by dividing the span by approximately 1.03 [1409, 1577, 1777, 1906].

The TLC, FRC and VC are diminished but the RV may increase slightly [1046, 1606, 2743] (see Fig. 9.7). In idiopathic scoliosis, the VC correlates best with the angle of scoliosis but this association is also seen with the changes in RV, TLC, FRC and MVV [306, 338, 1046, 1431, 1606, 1779, 1874, 2044, 2053, 2864, 3283, 3299]. This correlation does not hold in

Table 16.1. *Causes of scoliosis*

Non-structural	Structural
Postural	Idiopathic—infantile, adolescent
Sciatic	Osteopathic—congenital, e.g. hemivertebrae
Compensatory	—thoracoplasty
Inflammatory (e.g. perinephric abscess)	Neuromuscular—e.g. syringomyelia, Friedreich's ataxia, poliomyelitis, Duchenne's muscular dystrophy
	Connective tissue disorders—Marfan's syndrome, neurofibromatosis, osteogenesis imperfecta
	Pleuropulmonary—empyema, pneumonectomy, unilateral lung fibrosis

neuromuscular disorders since the changes in lung volumes are due to weakness of the respiratory muscles, particularly the diaphragm, as well as the degree of deformity [1000, 1605, 2529, 3299]. The fall in the VC in congenital scoliosis is related to the angle of scoliosis, but for any degree of deformity the VC is less than that in idiopathic scoliosis [1796, 2392]. This may be due to the rigidity of the spine, congenital hypoplasia of the lungs or congenital rib abnormalities.

These relationships between lung volumes and the angle of scoliosis have been studied more intensively than the other aspects of the spinal deformity, largely because these are difficult to measure. There is, however, some evidence that the degree of lordosis and possibly the degree of rotation of the spine are also important. The changes in the FRC, VC and FEV_1 correlate with the severity of lordosis assessed by CT scans in idiopathic scoliosis and, to a lesser extent, with the degree of rotation [5]. The VC, FRC and MVV are lower when the lordosis is severe [2278, 3359] and the improvement in VC following spinal fusion in such subjects is proportional to the correction of the lordosis [3359].

The age at which these lung volume abnormalities develop depends on the age of onset of the scoliosis. The fall in VC correlates more closely with the angle of scoliosis when this is of early onset than when it is first noticed during adolescence [2247]. In the latter, severe scoliosis

often has less effect on the volume of the lungs. The normal adult number of alveoli may not be attained if the scoliosis develops before the age of about eight years. The total capillary surface area is reduced and the size of the remaining alveoli is more variable than normal [335, 725, 861, 1155, 2359], although there is remarkably little difference in the size of the two lungs as estimated from CT scans [303].

Lung volume measurements are difficult in young children but a decrease in the VC and TLC have been detected in teenagers shortly after the appearance of adolescent idiopathic scoliosis [436, 2053, 2991]. The reduction in the VC and MVV is related to the PI_{max} and PE_{max}, but not to the angle of scoliosis [2991]. In adult life the VC remains stable in subjects with idiopathic scoliosis as long as it is above about 50% of normal, but it may fall if it is less than this [386].

Air flow obstruction occasionally accompanies scoliosis. Bronchography has demonstrated that the bronchi are of variable calibre and that this is probably related to the size of the individual lobes of the lung [499]. It is a clinical impression that asthma is common in scoliosis and atopy is frequently seen in some disorders of connective tissue causing scoliosis, such as neurofibromatosis and Marfan's syndrome [2901]. The small size of the airways enhances the increase in air flow resistance bronchoconstriction occurs.

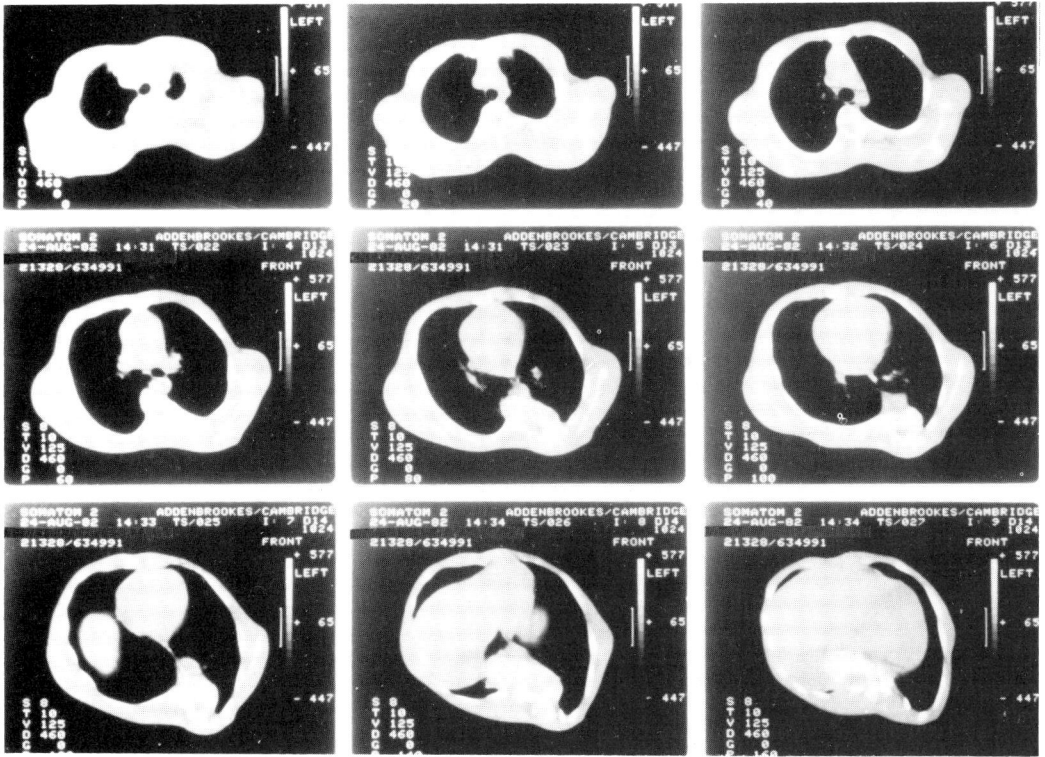

Fig. 16.21. *Computerized tomography scan in scoliosis, showing distortion of lungs and mediastinum.*

Exercise

The limits of exercise tolerance in severe scoliosis are usually set by the respiratory deficit [2902], although in some subjects orthopaedic problems of the legs and spine may be important. The oxygen consumption during walking is increased and this is related to the VC, but not to the angle of scoliosis, the balance of the spine or the presence of pelvic obliquity. This suggests that a factor connected with the VC, probably the compliance of the respiratory system, raises the oxygen consumption as the intensity of the exercise and ventilation increase [1909].

The exercise ability is further limited since not only is the oxygen consumption for any given level of work increased but the maximal oxygen consumption is diminished [2902] (Fig. 16.22). In younger subjects with mild deformities due to adolescent idiopathic scoliosis, the

degree of physical unfitness is more commonly the limiting factor [309, 800, 1321, 1848, 2904]. They show no [1847] or only minor abnormalities of ventilation during exercise [2703, 2992], which are related to the angle of scoliosis [564].

In adults with severe deformities, the maximal exercise ventilation is diminished in proportion to the fall in the FEV_1 [2902]. The ventilation at any given oxygen uptake is greater than normal [800, 2902, 2904] so that the reduced maximal exercise ventilation is reached at a lower oxygen uptake than expected. The tidal volume increases initially during exercise to a maximum and then remains constant while the respiratory frequency rises [2902, 2904]. The maximum tidal volume, although less than normal, is a higher percentage of the VC than in normal subjects [2902]. The oxygen consumption of the respiratory muscles increases

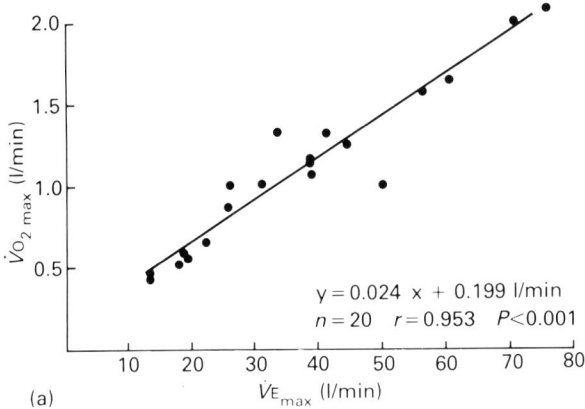

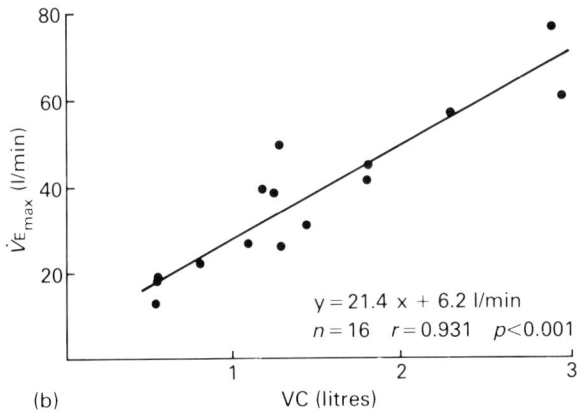

Fig. 16.22. *Exercise responses in scoliosis: (a) relationship between maximum oxygen consumption and maximum exercise ventilation, (b) relationship between maximum exercise ventilation and vital capacity. Reproduced, with permission, from Shneerson J.M. Thorax 1978; 33: 457–63.*

rapidly as V_T rises because of the reduced chest wall and lung compliance [260] and it may account for a significant proportion of the total oxygen consumption. Early reports [2743, 2869, 3182] suggested that the P_{O_2} dropped during exercise, particularly if cor pulmonale was present [260], but subsequent studies have shown no consistent change in P_{O_2} or P_{CO_2} [2120, 2902].

The cardiac output increases normally during exercise [260, 1047] and left ventricular function, as indicated by the pulmonary wedge pressure, is also normal [260, 2120]. Pulmonary artery pressure, however, rises rapidly [1047, 1135, 2119, 2120, 2903] and the rate of increase is linearly related to the oxygen uptake [2903]. It is also inversely proportional to the VC, FRC

and TLC but unrelated to the angle of scoliosis or P_{O_2} and is hardly affected by breathing pure oxygen [2903].

These observations suggest that pulmonary hypertension is due to an increase in the pulmonary vascular resistance. This appears to be due to a limitation in the size of the pulmonary vascular bed, which is related to the size of the lungs. Vascular distension and recruitment of unperfused vessels normally occurs during exertion so that the pulmonary vascular resistance falls. The density of intra-acinar capillaries is normal in scoliosis [725, 861] (Fig. 16.23) but if the lungs are of a size such that the VC is <1–1.5 l these adaptations are insufficient to accommodate the increased cardiac output and pulmonary artery pressure rises [2903].

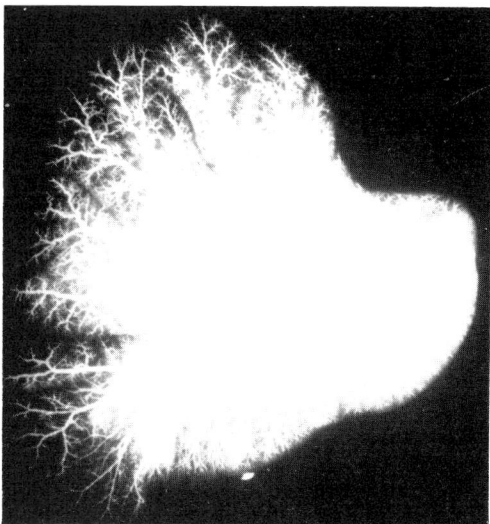

Fig. 16.23. *Post mortem pulmonary angiogram of lung in scoliosis, showing normal pattern of small blood vessels.*

Control of ventilation

The observation that respiration is depressed with sedatives such as morphine [710] raised the possibility that ventilatory control was defective in scoliosis.

The ventilatory responses to both hypoxia [2143, 2992] and hypercapnia in idiopathic scoliosis are usually decreased [1606, 1610, 1792, 2429, 3269], but this is probably secondary to the abnormal mechanics of the chest wall rather than to a primary fault in the respiratory drive. The ventilatory response correlates with the compliance of the respiratory system and the VC and TLC [1606, 1607, 1610]. In idiopathic scoliosis, the $P_{0.1}$ in the presence of hypercapnia is normal since it is less dependent on the mechanical properties of the lungs and chest wall [2795]. The ventilatory response to hypercapnia also improves after spinal fusion [1874, 1875], presumably reflecting the improvement in the compliance and function of the respiratory muscles. The ventilatory drive does, however, decrease in the presence of chronic hypercapnia, probably because of the increase in CSF bicarbonate [260].

Respiratory failure

The earliest abnormality of the blood gases is a fall in the P_{O_2}. This may become apparent soon after the onset of scoliosis [436, 2868, 3269] and is due to mismatching of ventilation and perfusion. The P_{O_2} is related to age, the angle of scoliosis, the VC, the compliance of the respiratory system [1399, 1607, 2117] and to the $P_{I_{max}}$ and maximal transdiaphragmatic pressure [1913].

The distribution of ventilation and perfusion between the two lungs might be expected to be grossly disturbed by the anatomical changes. The initial bronchospirometric study indicated that ventilation was greater on the side of the convexity of the spine [3041], but a subsequent study gave the opposite result [3299]. This latter finding has been confirmed by isotope ventilation scans [1234, 1919, 3300]. Ventilation appears to be least in the region of the maximum convexity of the spine [2843], although this regional difference has not been confirmed [806].

No such difference between the lungs has been detected by isotope studies of perfusion, although a single study using pulmonary angiography has suggested that blood flow is greater on the side of the convexity of the spine [499]. Perfusion in the lungs is largely determined by gravitational forces and normally increases towards the bases of the lungs. This gradient is often absent in scoliosis [806, 2868, 3300, 2843] and may even be reversed [155]. This abnormality of basal perfusion is worse if the angle of scoliosis is severe [310]. It may reflect an increase in pulmonary vascular resistance at the bases of the lungs secondary to the anatomical deformity or to hypoxic vasoconstriction caused by basal airway closure.

Ventilation/perfusion mismatching is responsible not only for hypoxaemia in the absence of hypercapnia but also for a reduction in the carbon monoxide transfer factor. If this is corrected for the lung volume the transfer coefficient is above the normal range [771, 2530, 2920].

Acute ventilatory failure may be precipitated by an intercurrent illness, particularly chest infections or asthma, possibly because respiratory muscle fatigue develops in response to the extra work of respiration. Chronic hypercapnia is common in neuromuscular disorders, which cause scoliosis, but the majority of scoliotics with normal respiratory muscles never develop this complication. Hypercapnia may, nevertheless, occasionally be severe [995, 996] and in idiopathic scoliosis the P_{CO_2} is inversely related to the compliance of the respiratory system [1607]. Hypercapnia in idiopathic scoliosis is uncommon if its onset is after the age of about five years [386]. The cause of this is uncertain but a low chest wall compliance, failure of the lung to develop normally and abnormalities of respiratory drive may all contribute.

Hypoventilation during wakefulness is probably preceded by hypoventilation during sleep, although hypercapnia is usually present in the day as well if nocturnal hypoxia is severe [2145]. Oxygen desaturation is more marked during REM than NREM sleep [1274, 1293, 2143, 2145, 2802] (Fig. 16.24). It is predominantly due to hypoventilation rather than to ventilation/perfusion mismatching since it is paralleled by a rise in P_{CO_2} [2145, 2802]. Central sleep apnoeas are frequent, particularly during REM sleep [2141, 2143], but desaturation may occur without apnoeas, especially in NREM sleep, probably becuse of a fall in V_T and a consequent rise in the physiological dead space [1274, 2145]. The severity of oxygen desaturation during sleep correlates with the oxygen saturation during wakefulness and also with the FEV_1, VC and fall in VC when changing from a sitting to a supine position [2145].

The development of respiratory and right heart failure can be fairly accurately predicted from the age of onset, severity and level of the scoliosis, the presence or absence of muscular weakness or a progressive neurological disease, and the VC [88, 386]. Normal blood gases while awake and asleep usually indicate a good prognosis and, overall, this is better in idiopathic scoliosis than in other types of scoliosis [615, 3283]. Occasional patients survive despite several of these high-risk factors [1047, 2700], al-

though in some cases the scoliosis deteriorates late and was not as severe earlier in life.

The cause of death in most patients with severe scoliosis is of cardiac or respiratory origin [2264, 2313, 2907]. Pneumonia and respiratory failure are particularly common in neuromuscular disorders, whereas cardiac failure is commoner in those without muscular weakness [2907]. Hypoxic dysrhythmias during sleep are probably responsible for many of these deaths [335]. The prognosis after the initial episode of acute respiratory failure precipitated by, for instance, a chest infection is quite good [1891, 2977] but depends on many factors, including the intensity of subsequent supervision and the provision of assisted ventilation.

Cardiovascular complications

Right ventricular failure is well recognized to occur transiently during episodes of acute respiratory failure, but chronic right ventricular failure is a late complication of severe scoliosis [260] and is associated with severe nocturnal hypoxia [2145]. Autopsy series have shown right ventricular hypertrophy in about 75% of subjects with severe scoliosis [148, 1252, 2907].

Right heart failure in spinal deformities has been considered to be a distinct disorder [2900] and has received names such as pulmonocardiac failure [531] and heart failure of the hunchback [1341]. It is, however, completely analogous to right ventricular hypertrophy in chronic lung disease. Left ventricular hypertrophy is also common in scoliosis and may be due to hypertension secondary to chronic hypoxia or to other causes, such as congenital renal or ureteric abnormalities [148].

Right ventricular hypertrophy is due to pulmonary hypertension. This is uncommon in younger subjects with idiopathic scoliosis [2119, 2120, 2636] but is frequent in older subjects with severe scoliosis, particularly when this is congenital or due to a neuromuscular disorder [260, 2810, 2908]. The normal cardiac output and pulmonary wedge pressure [260] indicate that the pulmonary hypertension is due to a

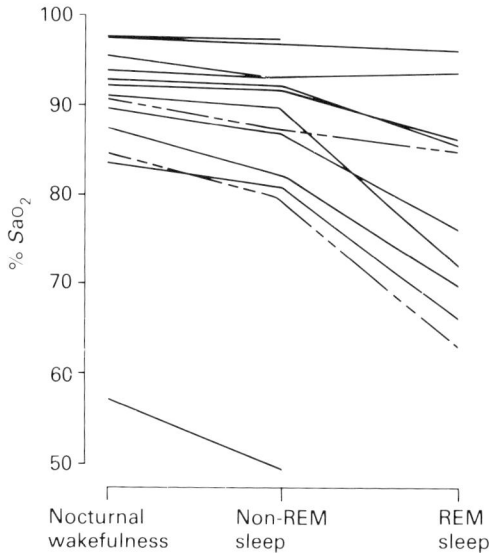

Fig. 16.24. *Changes in mean oxygen saturation during wakefulness, NREM and REM sleep in twelve patients with scoliosis. Reproduced, with permission, from Midgren et al. Br. J. Dis. Chest. 1988. (In press.)*

raised pulmonary vascular resistance. The early idea that the pulmonary vessels were kinked and distorted has not been verified but the pulmonary artery pressure while awake does correlate with the degree of hypoxia [1399, 1920, 2115, 2118, 2908] (Fig. 16.25). Hypoxia causes both pulmonary arterial vasoconstriction and, if prolonged, smooth muscle hypertrophy [1379, 2268, 2591]. Polycythaemia may also contribute to the raised pulmonary vascular resistance. The pulmonary artery pressure rises rapidly during exercise if the lung volumes are reduced (see above), but the size of the lungs does not determine the pulmonary artery pressure at rest [2908] (Fig. 16.26).

The chest deformity frequently makes it difficult to determine the presence or severity of pulmonary hypertension clinically, although this is likely if the pulmonary second sound is louder than the aortic second sound [2908]. The skeletal deformity has remarkably little effect on the interpretation of the ECG [1155] but the QRS axis may be misleading [23, 1512, 3184].

The ECG is insensitive in detecting right atrial or right ventricular hypertrophy but the presence of a tall P-wave is the most useful sign [2908]. A prolonged interval between pulmonary valve closure and tricuspid valve opening is more sensitive [2908] but echocardiography is often difficult because of the distortion of the anterior chest wall.

Congenital heart disease is commoner in scoliosis than in the normal population. It occurs in over 3% of idiopathic scoliotics and 7% of congenital scoliotics [2907]. Conversely, between 2% and 10% of subjects with congenital heart disease have a significant scoliosis [1962, 2582, 3244], although these figures need to be interpreted with care because of the high early mortality of these patients. Idiopathic scoliosis in association with congenital heart disease usually appears between the ages of ten and nineteen, is commoner in girls, and is usually convex to the right [244, 2582, 3244]. A wide variety of congenital heart defects may be seen [244, 2907, 3244]: the most common are cyanotic heart disease, especially Fallot's tetralogy [207, 244, 1590, 1962, 2713, 3317], coarctation of the aorta [2506] and mitral valve prolapse [1435, 2045, 2531, 2762, 3145]. Scoliosis may also coexist with congenital heart defects in certain disorders such as Marfan's syndrome and with a cardiomyopathy in, for instance, Friedreich's ataxia and Duchenne's muscular dystrophy.

Pregnancy

The blood volume normally increases by up to 25% during pregnancy and scoliotics with pre-existing pulmonary hypertension may develop right heart failure. Termination of pregnancy may be required for this reason, as well as to prevent ventilatory failure [242]. Nevertheless, patients with severe ventilatory abnormalities may tolerate pregnancy surprisingly well [2054]. Breathlessness increases because the enlarging uterus elevates the diaphragm and occasionally because of the development of left heart failure. Respiratory failure usually occurs late in pregnancy, but is common if the respiratory muscles are weak [357, 737, 1504, 2314]. Positive or negative pressure ventilation may be required [2314, 2805].

Care should be taken with opiate analgesics during delivery because of the risk of respiratory depression [958]. The pain of labour increases ventilation and can even return a previously elevated P_{CO_2} to normal [1496]. Pelvic abnormalities may be present, particularly if the scoliosis is in the lumbar spine [1730, 2455], but narrowing of the pelvic outlet is uncommon. If this is satisfactory and if the abdominal and diaphragmatic muscle strength is normal, a trial of spontaneous labour is usually indicated. Vaginal delivery is possible in most patients [786, 2919] and this can be hastened by the use of forceps if necessary [851]. The maternal mortality is, nevertheless, increased and in one study was 2.6% with a perinatal mortality of 3.8% [2455].

Pregnancy is, therefore, not without its risks and it may be best to advise against it, especially if the scoliosis is part of a hereditary disease such as a muscular dystrophy with other more

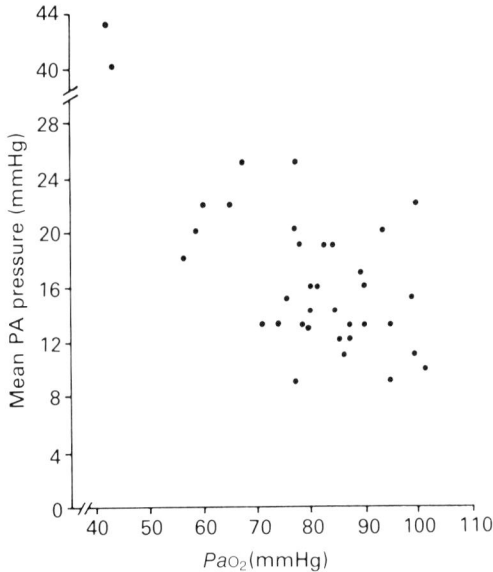

Fig. 16.26. *Relationship between the rate of rise of mean pulmonary artery pressure with oxygen uptake (sPAP/$\dot{V}_{O_2}$) and vital capacity during exercise in scoliosis. Reproduced, with permission, from Shneerson J.M. Thorax 1978; **33**: 747–54.*

serious manifestations, or if the physical capacity or prognosis of one or both parents is limited.

Surgery

The restrictive defect caused by the scoliosis does not, by itself, significantly increase the risk of surgery unless it is severe. Particular care is necessary if the scoliosis is due to a neuromuscular disorder that has caused respiratory muscle weakness or if the blood gases are abnormal [83]. Pulmonary hypertension increases the danger of anaesthesia and of blood loss, and care is needed with sedation post-operatively [1608]. Malignant hyperpyrexia is associated with chest wall deformities and with many of the neuromuscular disorders, and in some myopathies myoglobinuria may occur [1609]. Cardiac dysrhythmias are a feature of some diseases causing scoliosis, such as Duchenne's

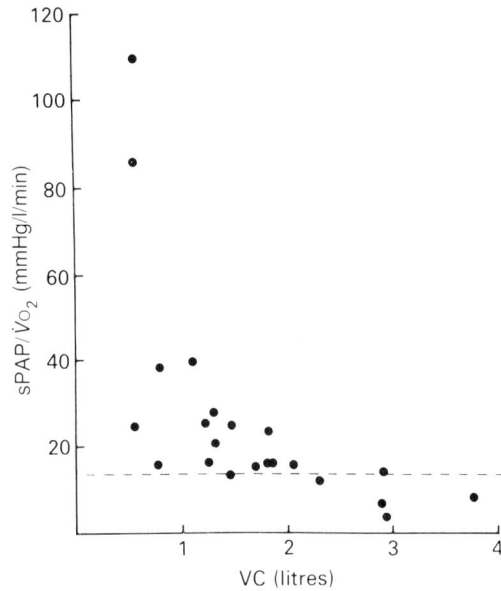

Fig. 16.25. *Relationship between mean pulmonary artery (PA) pressure and P_{aO_2} in scoliosis at rest. Reproduced, with permission, from Shneerson J.M. et al. Thorax 1977; **32**: 700–5.*

muscular dystrophy and Friedreich's ataxia, and cardiac monitoring may be required during surgery. Pre-operative assessment of high risk patients should include blood gas analysis, spirometry, chest X-ray and an ECG.

Orthopaedic treatment

All the methods of external support for the spine have the potential to restrict respiratory movements. The Risser localizer cast, which has been extensively used in the past, decreases the VC and MVV [1270, 2043, 2355]. Even lightweight polypropylene braces lower the VC, especially if the scoliosis is severe and is well corrected by the brace or if the diaphragm is weak [2319]. The Milwaukee brace does not have this disadvantage [1270, 2355, 2859] and oxygen consumption during slow walking is even diminished, presumably because of the mechanically more efficient posture [1908].

Removal of the posterior sections of the ribs, which comprise the rib hump, has been carried out particularly for cosmetic reasons. This 'costectomy' or thoracoplasty does not influence exercise ability [1320] and has only a slight effect on the VC, TLC and MVV [1320, 2055], in contrast to the consequences of thoracoplasty in tuberculosis.

Spinal fusion may be required to prevent progression of the scoliosis, to stabilize the spine (particularly in neuromuscular disorders), for cosmetic purposes, to relieve backache and, in selected cases, to improve cardiac or respiratory function or to prevent its deterioration. Spinal fusion may be carried out by a posterior approach using the Harrington instrumentation, or the Luque method which is particularly suited to neuromuscular disorders, or by an anterior approach as in the Dwyer operation. The compliance of the respiratory system is diminished immediately after surgery and right-to-left shunting through the lungs is considerable [1903]. Careful observation is required in high-risk cases at this stage and IPPV may be required post-operatively.

Realization of the risks of spinal fusion has

led to several trials of physical training programmes in an attempt to improve the pre-operative cardiac and respiratory status. In uncontrolled studies, slight improvements in heart rate, MVV and maximal oxygen uptake have been recorded [308, 309, 1206, 1207, 3057]. These have not been confirmed in the only controlled study of physical training and no changes in the VC or the ventilatory responses during exercise were seen [2906]. General physical training is unlikely to lessen the respiratory complications of spinal fusion in adolescent idiopathic scoliosis, although specific training of the respiratory muscles may be of use in selected patients with severe deformities or possibly those with muscular weakness (Chapter 23).

Most interest has focused on the long-term effects of spinal fusion on respiratory and cardiac function. Many of these operations are carried out in childhood and adolescence and the influence of growth on respiratory function is difficult to separate from that of the spinal fusion. Few studies have taken this into account and none have been controlled since, for ethical reasons, surgery has not been withheld from patients for whom it is indicated.

Most of the data have been collected from patients with adolescent idiopathic scoliosis and remarkably few changes in respiratory function have been found post-operatively. There is a slight improvement in $P_{I_{max}}$ [642] and in the ventilatory response to hypercapnia [1874, 1875], both of which suggest that the mechanics of the chest wall have been improved. However, the VC has not changed in most studies [924, 1406, 2043, 2116, 2868, 2905, 3404], although it may increase slightly [1101, 1102, 1337, 1777, 1874, 1910, 2355] or even decrease [3301]. There is little change in the FEV_1 [1337, 2905] or MVV [2355, 2905, 3301], although a slight improvement may be seen [1102, 1910, 2801]. The TLC remains unchanged [2116, 3404] or increases slightly [1101, 1102, 1910]. Ventilation/perfusion matching does not alter significantly and isotope lung scan appearances are also unchanged [2868]. The arterial P_{O_2} and oxygen saturation may remain the same [1777, 2355,

3301] or improve [1874, 1875, 2868]. The oxygen consumption while walking slowly is less after spinal fusion [1909], probably because of improvement in the mechanical efficiency of walking but possibly because of improvement in the compliance of the respiratory system. A slight improvement in P_{O_2} during exercise has been noted [2868] but there is no significant change in maximum oxygen uptake or maximum exercise ventilation despite a slight improvement in the submaximal ventilatory indices [2823, 2846, 2905].

These rather disappointing results in idiopathic scoliosis may well apply to congenital scoliosis as well but there have been no adequate studies. In one report on patients who had already developed right heart failure due to congenital or infantile idiopathic scoliosis, little improvement was seen after spinal fusion [3122].

In contrast, the benefits of spinal fusion in scoliosis due to muscle weakness can be considerable. The rate of fall of the VC in Duchenne's muscular dystrophy can be slowed considerably (see Fig. 15.11) and the VC has been shown to increase in arthrogryposis after spinal fusion [439]. In scoliosis associated with myelomeningocoele, stabilization of the spine increases the maximal expiratory flow rate and the MVV as well as increasing the FRC [172].

More experience has been gained in poliomyelitis in which an improvement in the VC [1213, 1910], which may be considerable if the scoliosis is high and severe [1270, 1271], has been observed. The P_{O_2} and P_{CO_2} may improve following traction for scoliosis pre-operatively [327] and, in a group of patients in whom right heart failure had already developed, traction followed by spinal fusion increased the VC by 80% and improved the P_{O_2}, P_{CO_2} and, in one subject, the pulmonary artery pressure [3122].

These short-term improvements in neuromuscular disorders are encouraging but there are no studies that indicate whether spinal fusion performed in childhood or adolescence prevents respiratory failure from appearing in adult life. The risk of respiratory failure developing is greatest if the onset of the scoliosis is before the age of five or if there is respiratory muscle weakness. Surgery to prevent respiratory failure should, therefore, be directed towards these groups of patients. It should be designed to improve the mechanics of the chest wall and the function of the respiratory muscles. It is likely that further studies will show that spinal fusion is not necessarily the best procedure to achieve these aims and that surgery to the ribs or even the diaphragm is required.

Part 4
Treatment of Ventilatory Failure

.

Chapter 17
Negative Pressure Ventilation

The principle of negative pressure ventilation is that the pressure around the thorax and abdomen is lowered relative to the mouth pressure. Air is, therefore, drawn into the lungs through the mouth and nose and expiration occurs passively due to elastic recoil of the lungs and chest wall. The subatmospheric pressure around the chest and abdomen is attained by enclosing the trunk in an airtight rigid enclosure. This is connected to a pump that is capable of evacuating air from the space between it and the patient.

There are three main types of negative pressure ventilator or 'body respirator': the cuirass, jacket and tank ventilators (Fig. 17.1). The term cuirass originally signified a breastplate, which was usually used for military purposes. It has come to mean a rigid shell that encloses the whole or part of the chest and abdomen for the purpose of assisting ventilation. In the past, ventilatory equipment that would now be termed a cuirass has been referred to as a jacket respirator. The essential difference between a jacket (wrap or poncho) and a cuirass is that the jacket consists of impervious material supported by a rigid frame around the chest wall, whereas in a cuirass the impervious cover and the rigidity are provided by a single structure, the cuirass shell. When negative pressure is applied within a jacket, the garment collapses onto the rigid frame. Tank ventilators, in contrast to cuirasses and jackets, enclose the whole of the body up to the neck in an airtight chamber that is intermittently evacuated. They have received various synonyms in the past, such as cabinet, chamber, box and body respirators or ventilators, and 'iron lungs'.

The relative merits of these three types of negative pressure ventilator have recently been reviewed [1426, 1683] and are summarized in Table 17.1. They can all be used to provide positive pressure to the thorax and abdomen during expiration, as well as negative pressure during inspiration (p. 241).

CUIRASS VENTILATION

Historical development

The earliest cuirass designs date from the second half of the 19th century. In 1874, von Hauke described a sheet iron cuirass that consisted of an anterior shell. This made contact with the chest wall by pneumatic rubber seals [1384, 3252]. Alexander Graham Bell designed a cuirass in 1882, in which an anterior and a posterior shell were bolted together [3372]. Breuillard developed a cuirass in 1887 [1136], but the first model to be extensively used was the Biomotor designed by Eisenmenger in 1904 [87, 903]. His cuirass comprised a rigid dome that covered the abdomen but only the lower part of the chest. The inspiratory flow rates generated by the Biomotor had a 'physiological waveform' [991] and the inspiratory/expiratory ratio could be varied. Positive pressure could also be applied by inflating a rubber balloon inside the shell.

A variety of respiratory and non-respiratory conditions were treated with the Biomotor [904, 991] but the main stimulus to the development of cuirass ventilation was the large number of patients with respiratory muscle paralysis due to poliomyelitis. In 1918, Steuart devised a box-like cuirass in which the whole trunk but not the limbs was enclosed in a rigid chamber [3050]. This model was only developed after an

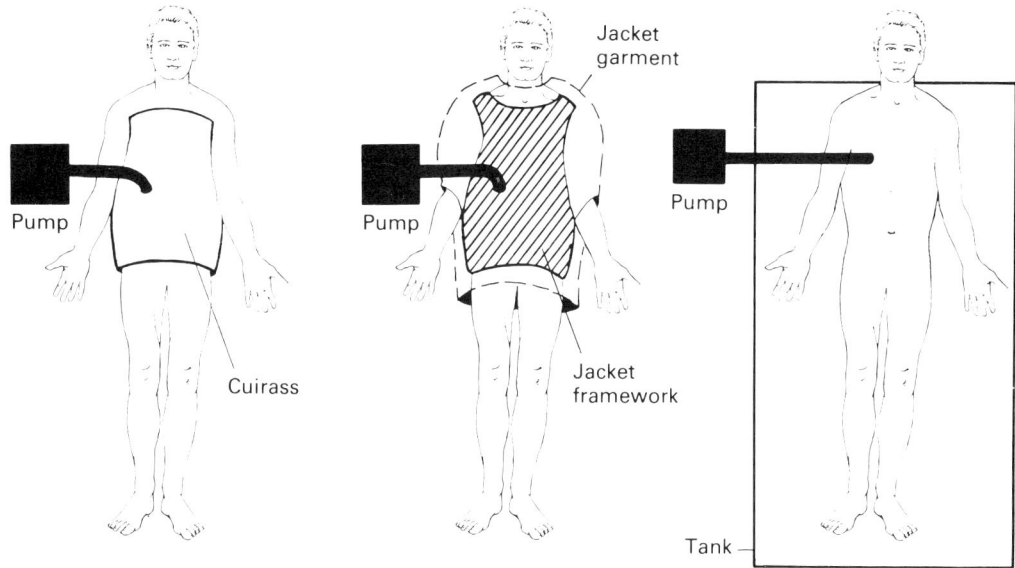

Fig. 17.1. *Diagrammatic representation of cuirass, jacket and tank ventilators. The cuirass provides a rigid and impermeable enclosure around the thorax and abdomen, whereas these two functions are performed separately by the framework and garment of the jacket. The tank is similar in principle to the cuirass, but encloses the whole body up to the neck.*

epidemic of poliomyelitis had finished, and it was never used. During the 1930s, respiratory failure caused by poliomyelitis was treated with Eisenmenger's Biomotor [904], but because of pressure on the sternum it was often poorly tolerated [314].

Several new types of cuirass were subsequently developed until the advent of effective immunization for poliomyelitis, when interest in cuirass development virtually ceased for over twenty years. Criteria for the design and performance of cuirasses were laid down by the USA

Table 17.1. *Comparison of cuirass, jacket and tank ventilators*

Criterion	Cuirass	Jacket	Tank
Size	smallest	intermediate	largest
Portability	portable	portable	immobile
Assistance required	unusual	usual	invariable, except with modern domiciliary designs
Claustrophobia	rare	uncommon	common
Mobility during treatment	little	little	very little
Pressure sores	occasional	uncommon	uncommon, except around neck
Use with tracheostomy	easy	difficult	difficult
Relief of inspiratory muscle activity	least	intermediate	greatest
Tidal volume	least	intermediate	greatest

Council on Physical Medicine in 1947 [659]. These criteria had considerable influence over the acceptance of subsequent designs of cuirass for clinical use. The most important types of cuirass in use from the 1930s until the epidemics of poliomyelitis in developed countries were prevented in the 1950s were:

SAHLIN-STILLE CUIRASS

This cuirass was designed by Sahlin in Scandinavia and the results of its use in providing prolonged ventilatory support were described in 1936 [1001]. The dome of the cuirass was bolted to a table underneath the patient to minimize air leaks and contact with the patient, but the necessity for the patient to be immobile frequently led to pressure sores.

BURSTALL JACKET RESPIRATORY (Fig. 17.2)

This was developed in response to the 1937 poliomyelitis epidemic in Melbourne, but was not available until this epidemic had finished.

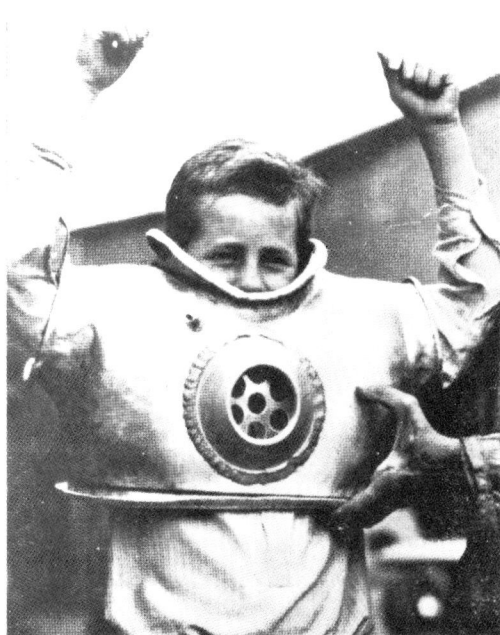

Fig. 17.2. *Burstall 'jacket' respirator. Reproduced, with permission, from Burstall A.F.* Br. Med. J. *1938; 2: 611–12.*

This cuirass was made of one piece of aluminium that enclosed the chest and upper abdomen. It was supplied in three sizes and was fitted by being passed over the patient's head. This procedure took two people about 7 min [449]. It was intended that several cuirasses could be powered simultaneously by a single tank ventilator pump [2129].

LAFFER LEWIS APPARATUS

This cuirass was developed in Australia in 1938, independently of Burstall's cuirass [2108]. It had a longitudinal joint with quick-operating clamps and enclosed most of the abdomen as well as the thorax. It was suitable for use with equipment necessary for splinting the limbs if they were weakened by poliomyelitis.

LONDON COUNTY COUNCIL CUIRASS RESPIRATOR

This was designed by Henderson and was in use in the London County Council's hospitals from 1938 [2108]. It was constructed of aluminium and enclosed the thorax. It consisted of an anterior and posterior shell with airtight joints between them. It could be applied much more easily than the Burstall cuirass and gave greater freedom of arm movement [2129].

TURNER JACKET RESPIRATOR

This aluminium cuirass was designed in 1939 and was similar to the London County Council cuirass [2108].

LIEBLE AND HALL CUIRASS

This was introduced in Toronto for use in poliomyelitis in 1937. It enclosed both the chest and abdomen but was subsequently modified and constructed in plastic by Collins and Drinker in 1939 [649, 1136].

BLANCHARD RESPIRATOR

This cuirass was constructed of plastic and came into use in 1948 [660].

MULLIKIN RESPIRATOR

This was similar to the London County Council cuirass but it was subject to mechanical failures. It was found to be unacceptable for use by the American Council on Physical Medicine in 1949 [663].

CHESTPIRATOR CHEST RESPIRATOR

This American cuirass was capable of applying both positive and negative pressure and was in use from 1949 [661].

MONAGHAN RESPIRATOR

This successful cuirass was designed by Monaghan, the chief engineer at The Children's Hospital, Denver and was mass produced from 1949. The findings of a government survey of 400 000 Americans during the 1930s were used to design six sizes of cuirass [649, 662]. It was constructed of plastic and consisted of an anterior shell with a rubber seal. It was held onto the patient by leather straps.

FAIRCHILD-HUXLEY CHEST RESPIRATOR

This American cuirass was constructed of plastic; models enclosing only the thorax or both the thorax and abdomen were manufactured. It came into use in 1950 [665] and was fitted with feet to prevent the cuirass from compressing the chest wall during inspiration. An alarm was designed to indicate power failure or a drop in pressure within the cuirass.

TECHNICON-HUXLEY CHEST RESPIRATOR

This cuirass was similar to the Fairchild-Huxley chest respirator and was also constructed of plastic. It enclosed both the thorax and the abdomen and was produced in four sizes [2201].

DRAGER CUIRASS

This was similar to the Technicon-Huxley cuirass [2201].

FREIBURG CUIRASS

This cuirass, designed in Scandinavia, was extensively used for treating poliomyelitis after the Second World War.

KIFA RESPIRATOR

This Swedish cuirass consisted of an aluminium anterior shell and had rubber seals. It could be fitted with an alarm bell to signify power failure [1640].

SPIRASHELL CUIRASS RESPIRATOR

This cuirass was developed in the UK in the early 1950s. It was constructed of plastic and fitted with foam rubber seals [2602].

HEMO-DYNE VITAL CAPACITOR

This American cuirass was introduced in 1959 [3373]. It was mainly used experimentally to study the physiological effects of cuirass ventilation [1023, 1114, 3305]; its clinical applications were limited.

Modern cuirass construction and design

The ideal cuirass should not only be an effective ventilator but should be comfortable, light, portable and easy for the patient to wear without requiring help from another person. The development of modern synthetic materials has made it possible to improve on the older designs and to more nearly achieve these properties. Fibreglass [2527] and vitrathene [416] are not only light, rigid and impervious to air but can be readily moulded to form a cuirass that will fit each patient individually. This is particularly important if the thorax is deformed since the cuirasses of standard shape do not give an airtight seal or allow adequate expansion of the whole of the thorax and abdomen. Even in subjects with normal anatomy, individually-made cuirasses are superior to the standard models.

In an attempt to overcome this problem, some of the older types of cuirass were made in different sizes, e.g. Eisenmenger's Biomotor, Sahlin-Stille cuirass, Burstall jacket respirator, Fairchild-Huxley and Technicon-Huxley chest respirators and the Monaghan respirator. Some of these older models are still available. The Huxley cuirass and a cuirass similar to the Monaghan respirator are supplied by Lifecare (available from Thomas Respiratory Systems, 3 Cholmeley Crescent, Highgate, London N6 5EZ) at a cost of about £400. The Emerson Customfit cuirass is available in three sizes from E & G International Inc., 269 Giralda Avenue, Coral Gables, FL 33134, USA (cost approx. £300).

Some suppliers, such as E & G International Inc. and Thomas Respiratory Systems, construct cuirasses for patients with deformed chests from measurements of each patient, but these cuirasses are often uncomfortable and ineffective. The use of poorly-fitting equipment was largely responsible for the unpopularity of cuirass ventilation in the past, but it is now possible to construct efficient and comfortable cuirasses. The most reliable method is to make a cast of the patient's chest and abdomen and to design the cuirass from this. The method used in the Assisted Ventilation Unit at Newmarket General Hospital has proved to be simple and effective [416] (Fig. 17.3). The cost is approximately £100. The cuirass shell is moulded from a plaster-of-Paris cast of the subject's chest and abdomen. It is essential that this cast should accurately represent the contours of the patient and extend down to the pelvis and to the lateral chest and abdominal wall. The plaster cast is built up over areas that are either prominent or likely to expand during inspiration, but not over the sides of the cuirass that will form a seal with the patient's chest and abdomen.

The material from which the cuirass will be made (vitrathene) is rendered malleable by heat so that it can be applied to the cast. When it sets in a rigid form it is removed from the cast, trimmed to fit the patient exactly and the edges covered with soft material such as foam rubber. This is protected from damage by neoprene, which is impervious to air. The cuirass is fitted to the patient at each stage so that adjustments can be made. A Velcro back-strap is useful in minimizing air leaks and a hole is cut in the centre of the cuirass for tubing that connects it to the pump.

It is important to review the functioning of the cuirass periodically, since air leaks may develop if the materials wear or if the patient changes weight. Some leakage of air is inevitable but it can be minimized by using an impervious yet soft edging material that conforms to the contours of the body and the underlying surface.

Pressure areas may develop if the cuirass is applied too tightly. They are particularly common over bony prominences, such as the hips and ribs, in scoliotic subjects. The breasts occasionally become sore through pressure, and compression of the lateral cutaneous nerve may result in meralgia paraesthetica. Care in moulding the cuirass and in applying the foam to the edges should prevent these complications. Backache occasionally develops, probably due to movement of intervertebral and costovertebral joints that have been immobile for a long period.

Cuirass pumps

The negative or subatmospheric pressure within the cuirass is generated by a pump, which evacuates the air. The earliest cuirass pumps were hand pumps, e.g. von Hauke's cuirass [1384], or foot pumps, e.g. Eisenmenger's Biomotor [87, 903], or even relied on steam, e.g. Breuillard's cuirass [1136]. The source of power for most modern pumps is the mains electricity supply, although some can run off external batteries, e.g. Lifecare 170–C, or be worked manually if the mains power supply fails, e.g. the Cape cuirass pump.

The pumps used for cuirass ventilation have almost invariably been either of the bellows, piston or rotary (fan) type. Bellows pumps were used with Bell's cuirass [3372], the early models of Eisenmenger's Biomotor [87], Steuart's cuirass [3050], the London County Council cuirass respirator [2129], Turner's jacket respirator [2108] and Blanchard's respirator [660]. Eisenmenger's later Biomotors used a rotary pump.

In most bellows pumps the stroke volume of the pump is fixed, but the fraction of this that is extracted from inside the cuirass is controlled by a valve. The respiratory rate and inspiratory/expiratory ratio can be adjusted by altering a gearing system that connects the pump motor to the bellows or piston. The inspiratory waveform can be controlled by spring-loading the valve. Bellows pumps have the advantage

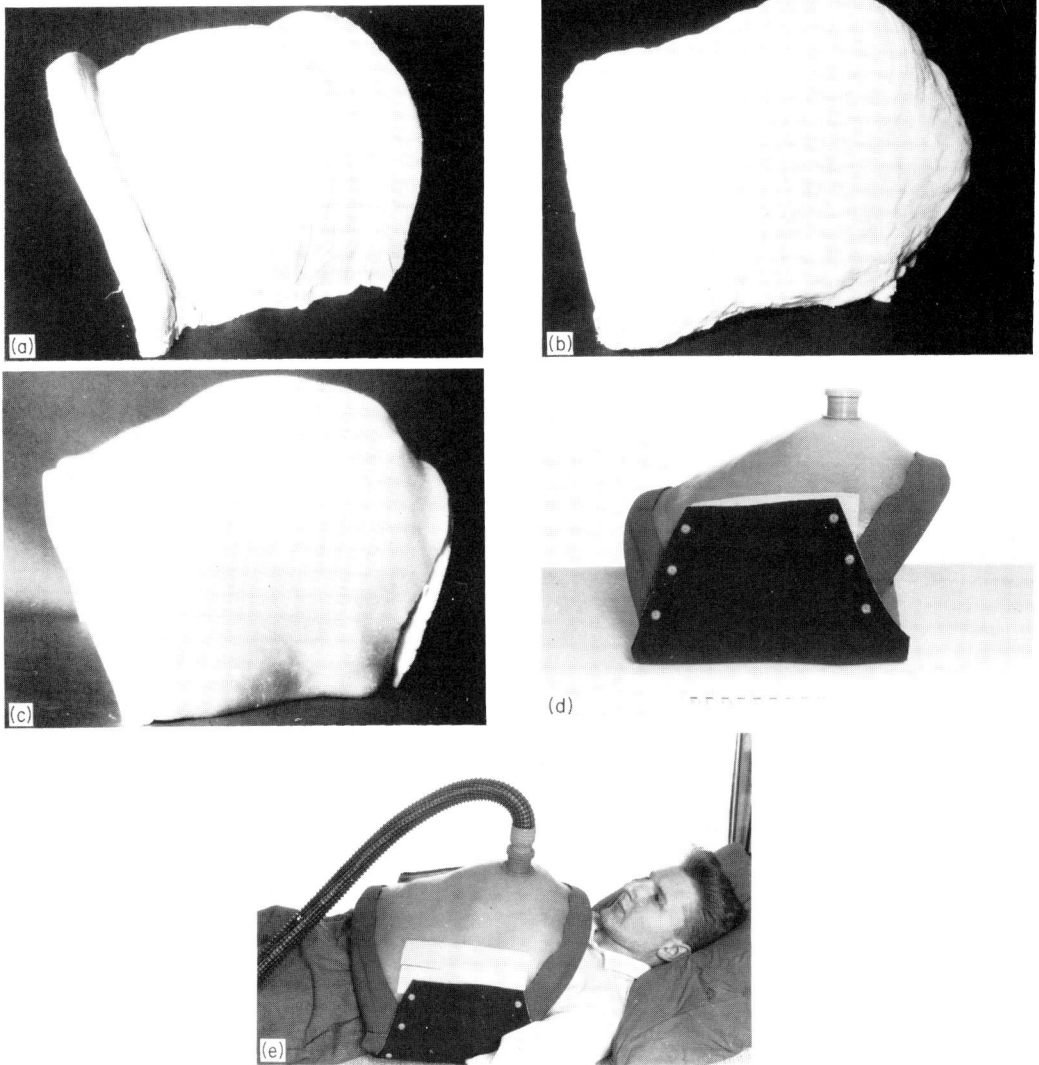

Fig. 17.3. *Stages in construction of individually moulded cuirass: (a) plaster-of-Paris cast of rib cage and abdomen with edges built up, (b) cast after padding to allow for chest wall expansion, (c) vitrathene applied to cast, (d) vitrathene cuirass with edging and back-strap, (e) cuirass applied to patient. Reproduced by courtesy of Mrs L. Brown.*

of being mechanically simple and reliable, but they are large and heavy. They are noisy and mechanically inefficient because the bellows or piston action is the same, irrespective of the volume of air that is extracted from the cuirass.

The rotary pumps work on the principle that as the fan rotates, the pressure behind it falls. By combining many fans in series, a powerful suction pump can be produced. The low-pressure area within the pump is opened intermittently via the connecting tubing to the cuirass by a rotating valve. The pressure waveform can be altered by controlling the movement of this valve.

Both bellows and rotary pumps can be adjusted so that positive as well as negative pressure is applied to the connecting tube. This facility was available on the pumps used for Eisenmenger's Biomotor and the Laffer Lewis, Blanchard and Chestpirator cuirasses. Cuirass positive pressure ventilation is, however, seldom used (p. 241), although this facility may be of value with an abdominal exsufflation belt or even for IPPV.

PROPERTIES OF PUMPS

The pump used for cuirass ventilation should be powerful enough to generate a suffcently negative pressure within the cuirass to assist ventilation. This is usually 30–40 cmH$_2$O peak pressure. It has to overcome the resistance to the air flow by the connecting tubing and any air leaks. The volume of air within the cuirass is usually < 15 l. This is small in comparison with the amount of air that leaks around the edges of the cuirass during inspiration. The volume that the pump has to evacuate from the cuirass therefore reflects the adequacy of the seal between the patient and the cuirass rather than the volume of air within the cuirass itself. At peak negative pressures of less than about 15 cmH$_2$O the air leak increases linearly as the pressure becomes more negative, but above about 15 cmH$_2$O there is little further increase. This is probably because the cuirass moves downward onto the patient or underlying sur-

face, and closes off the air leak. The maximum air leak is around 1300 ml/min with a well-designed cuirass [1685].

The air leak between the patient and the cuirass may vary considerably from moment to moment. Changes in position are frequent during sleep, particularly REM sleep. The Newmarket pump (p. 224) automatically adjusts its output to attain the same negative pressure, to compensate for changes in the air leak. The Cape cuirass pump (p. 224) is unable to adapt in this way but it does have sufficient reserve of stroke volume to be able to compensate for most air leaks. However, it may develop very high intracuirass pressures if the air leak falls [1681].

The negative pressure waveform that is generated by the cuirass pump is in most cases a sine wave, although any waveform can be produced by the Newmarket pump. The large air leak between the patient and the cuirass damps the waveform generated by the pump so that the effects of manipulating the pattern of applied pressure are less than might be anticipated [1675].

CONNECTING TUBING

The diameter of the connecting tubing in some of the early designs of cuirass was 2.5–3.75 cm [449, 1023] but a diameter of at least 5 cm was subsequently recommended [2807]. If air flow is laminar, the resistance to flow varies with the diameter and inversely with the length of the tubing. These relationships do not hold in the presence of turbulent air flow or resonance, which increase the air flow resistance.

The tubing should ideally be short and wide, and should not kink or change in size or shape with pressure changes. It is also desirable that it is light and flexible. Corrugated reinforced plastic 2 m long, with an internal diameter of 4 cm, is usually adequate. With this tubing, the fall in pressure is linearly related to the flow rate [1685]. The flow rate in the tubing at any given pressure is largely determined by the volume of air that leaks between the patient and the cuirass. It therefore varies from subject to subject and with changes in position. With a well-designed cuirass the air leak is usually < 1300 l/min [1685] and the fall in pressure along the tubing is 5–10 cmH$_2$O. It is therefore desirable to measure the pressure inside the cuirass rather than in the pump when assessing the effectiveness of cuirass ventilation.

CURRENTLY AVAILABLE PUMPS

The pumps that are currently most commonly used for cuirass ventilation are:

Newmarket pump (Fig. 17.4)

Available from Si-plan Electronics Research Limited, Avenue Farm Industrial Estate, Birmingham Road, Stratford-upon-Avon, Warwickshire, CV37 OHP. Weight 32.5 kg. Dimensions 47×39.5×35 cm. Cost approx. £2500.

This rotary pump is capable of over 1000 l/min. The negative pressure waveform is normally a sine wave but any waveform can be achieved by changing the control panel program. The movement of the rotary valve is controlled by a negative feedback system so that the pump attains the preset pressure waveform even if the amount of air leaking from the system changes from breath to breath. This automatic adjustment is particularly valuable during sleep, when movement of the patient might otherwise lead to a fall in pressure within the cuirass [1681]. The pump is quieter than bellows pumps since the action of the rotating valve ensures that only the small amount of air required for developing the negative pressures within the cuirass passes through the pump; 50 cmH$_2$O negative and positive pressure can be applied and the pump has a low pressure alarm to indicate failure of the power supply, a pump fault or excessive air leak. The respiratory frequency can be adjusted continuously from 10 to 50 breaths/min and the inspiratory/expiratory ratio can be varied between 2:3 and 3:2.

Cape cuirass pump (Fig. 17.4)

Available from Penlon Limited, Radley Road, Abingdon, Oxford, OX14 3PH. Weight 72 kg. Dimensions 79×61×52 cm. Cost approx. £2500.

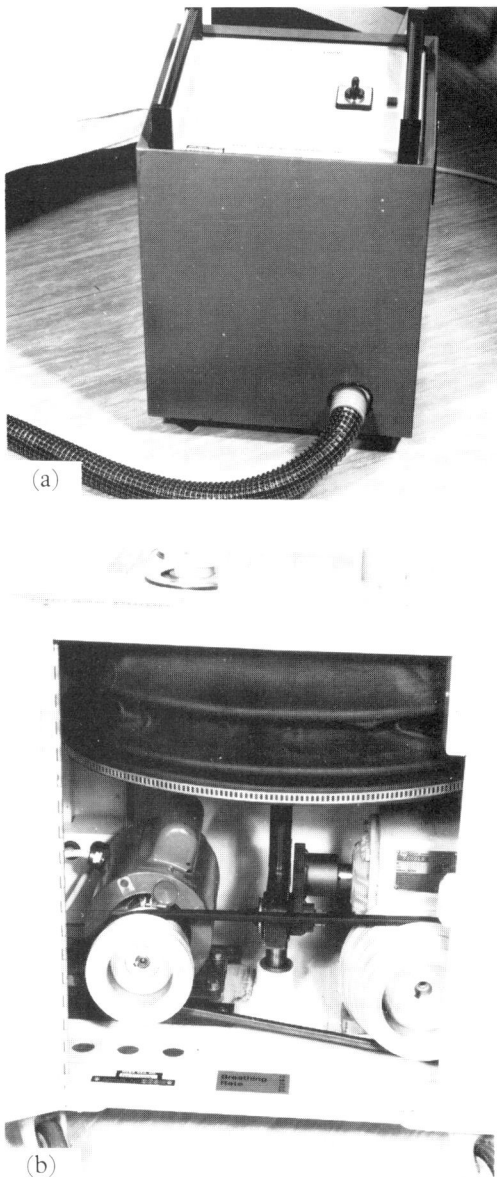

Fig. 17.4. *Cuirass pumps: (a) Newmarket pump and connecting tubing, (b) interior of Cape cuirass pump showing bellows and manually operated gearing system for changing the respiratory frequency.*

This bellows pump was originally designed by Captain Smith Clarke, who was a member of the committee appointed by the Birmingham Regional Hospital Board in 1952 to improve the Both tank ventilator [1081, 2983]. The pump has a stroke volume of 17.6 litres and the pressure waveform is approximately a sine wave. The respiratory frequency can be altered to 13, 16, 19, 22 or 25 breaths/min and the inspiratory/expiratory ratio is fixed at 1:2. This pump is reliable but cumbersome. It can be operated by hand in case of mains power failure.

Emerson chest respirator pump

Available from E & G International Inc., 269 Giralda Avenue, Coral Gables, FL 33134, USA. Weight 10 kg. Dimensions $48 \times 32 \times 28$ cm. Cost approx. £1000.

This rotary pump is able to generate a negative pressure of 60 cmH_2O. The respiratory frequency can be varied from 0 to 40 breaths/min and the inspiratory/expiratory ratio can be adjusted.

Thompson MV Maxivent

Available from Puritan Bennett International Corporation, Heathrow Causeway, 157–176 Great South West Road, Hounslow, Middlesex, TW4 6JS. Weight 16.7 kg. Dimensions $36 \times 27 \times 33$ cm. Cost approx. £4000.

This rotary pump can generate a negative pressure of 70 cmH_2O and a positive pressure of 80 cmH_2O. It has a low-pressure alarm and the respiratory frequency can be adjusted continuously from 8 to 24 breaths/min.

Lifecare 170-C pump

Available from Thomas Respiratory Systems, 3 Cholmeley Crescent, Highgate, London, N6 5EZ. Weight 60 kg. Dimensions $36 \times 41 \times 23$ cm. Cost approx. £4900.

This rotary pump was originally designed and produced by the Monaghan Company. It can generate a negative and positive pressure of 60 cmH_2O. It has a low-pressure alarm and the respiratory frequency can be varied between 10 and 40 breaths/min. It can be used with an external battery as well as mains electricity.

Physiological effects

TIDAL VOLUME

The V_T achieved during cuirass ventilation has been shown in several studies to be almost linearly related to the peak negative intracuirass pressure [431, 611, 1685, 2201, 2497, 2807, 3009] (Fig. 17.5). A levelling off or even a decrease in V_T at high suction pressures has been noted in some studies [611, 2201]. This is probably due to compression of the chest wall by

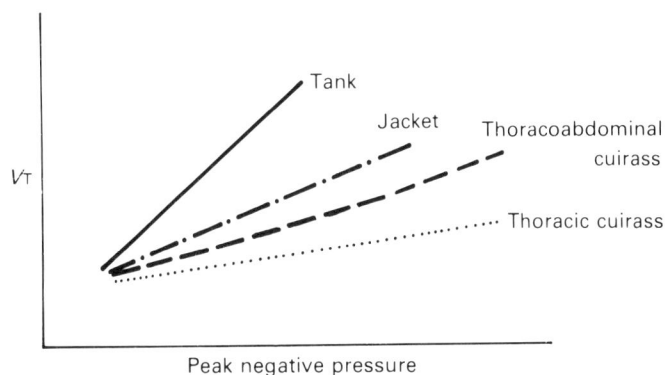

Fig. 17.5. *Relationship between tidal volume (V_T) and peak negative pressure with different methods of negative pressure ventilation. The maximal tidal volume is determined by the slope of this relationship and the maximum pressure that can be tolerated.*

the cuirass but this should be slight in a modern individually-made cuirass [1685].

The V_T attained at any given negative pressure depends not only on the compliance of the lungs and chest wall and the air flow resistance but also on the properties of the cuirass pump and cuirass. The V_T is greatest when as much as possible of the thorax and abdomen is enclosed within the cuirass and exposed to the negative pressure. Long cuirasses that include the abdomen as well as the chest achieve a higher V_T at any given pressure than those that cover the chest alone [611, 2201, 2807, 3322].

The cuirass moves down towards its points of attachment when negative pressure is developed. This may cause pressure sores and prevent expansion, or even cause paradoxical movement of the chest wall at its points of contact. Energy is dissipated in distorting the cuirass and compressing the chest wall rather than in inflating the lungs. The older models of cuirass had back-plates to overcome this defect, e.g. Sahlin-Stille cuirass and Laffer Lewis apparatus, or feet that supported the cuirass on the surface underneath the patient, e.g. Fairchild-Huxley and Technicon-Huxley chest respirators. An alternative is to extend the sides of the cuirass so that they fit directly onto the underlying surface and do not compress the chest wall [416, 2807].

The relative expansion of the rib cage and abdomen during cuirass ventilation is determined by their relative compliances, the area of each of which is exposed to negative pressure, and the regions where the cuirass makes contact with the chest wall. In practice, the expansion of the abdomen increases to a greater extent than that of the rib cage, which may even move paradoxically [1684]. In most of the skeletal disorders causing ventilatory failure, the compliance of the rib cage is lower than that of the abdomen and, in addition, the cuirass probably compresses the ribs and sternum more than the abdomen. It is also possible that reflex inhibition of intercostal muscle activity during assisted ventilation decreases the stability of the rib cage. Cuirass ventilation is able to correct paradoxical

movement of the abdomen due to bilateral diaphragmatic paralysis [416, 1685]. If there is severe abdominal and intercostal muscle weakness, repeated expansion of the chest wall may very rarely lead to a permanent dome-like deformity of the anterior trunk [3218].

RESPIRATORY FREQUENCY

The V_T during cuirass ventilation also varies with the respiratory frequency. The V_T will fall if this is sufficiently fast to prevent the expanding force of the negative pressure and the opposing force of the chest wall and lungs from equilibrating during each breath. The reduction in V_T is usually slight and ventilation increases as the respiratory frequency rises to about 30 breaths/min [1685]. The T_I can be increased by prolonging the inspiratory/expiratory ratio or by adding an end inspiratory pause to the pressure waveform. These manoeuvres may increase V_T slightly [1681] and matching of ventilation and perfusion may improve. The T_E is reduced and, particularly in the presence of air flow obstruction, this may increase the end expiratory volume. Even in the absence of air flow obstruction, cuirass ventilation increases the end expiratory volume slightly [611, 1685], and while this promotes expansion of the bases of the lungs, it may increase the work of respiration and decrease V_T if there is pre-existing hyperinflation.

The increase in ventilation at high respiratory frequencies may be offset by the inability of the patient to coordinate with the rapid changes in pressure. The respiratory frequency that is selected for cuirass ventilation should take into account the patient's comfort and ability to tolerate the respiratory pattern, as well as the effect on V_T and blood gases. An inability to coordinate with the cuirass is an important cause of failure of cuirass ventilation, and reassurance and careful explanation to the patient are essential. Incoordination increases the work of ventilation, since the patient is breathing against the applied pressure and any increase in respiratory muscle activity out of phase with the ventilator decreases the compliance of the chest wall. Triggering of ventilation using changes in the airway pressure [2062] and inspiratory muscle activity [3046] has been attempted, but is technically difficult.

INSPIRATORY MUSCLE ACTIVITY

The negative pressure around the chest wall during inspiration might be expected to inflate the lungs passively, without contraction of the inspiratory muscles. Diaphragmatic EMG studies have demonstrated a reduction in amplitude of the EMG during cuirass ventilation if there is chronic air flow obstruction or a restrictive disorder, but not in normal subjects [1180, 1689, 2680]. It is uncertain why an obstructive or restrictive load is necessary to inhibit inspiratory muscle activity but in a separate study during NREM sleep, EMG activity was eliminated only if the $P\text{CO}_2$ fell below a threshold value [1407]. The oxygen consumption of the respiratory muscles does not change during either cuirass [1689] or jacket ventilation [2062] but the techniques available for its measurement are insensitive.

Inhibition of inspiratory muscle activity would be expected to relieve muscle fatigue and increase the maximal mouth pressures. This has been demonstrated in poliomyelitis [390] and in scoliosis [1685], but there are conflicting results in chronic air flow obstruction [2059, 2503].

BLOOD GASES

Cuirass ventilation is usually able to maintain adequate ventilation in normal subjects and in those whose respiratory muscles have been paralysed by curarization or disease [1179, 2059] such as poliomyelitis [431, 611]. It has even been used to support ventilation continuously in a patient with a zero VC due to severe poliomyelitis [3218]. It may fail to provide adequate ventilation if the compliance is decreased or if air flow resistance is increased, although promising results have been obtained recently [2058, 2059, 2503].

The improvement in blood gases is mainly due to the increase in ventilation [1685] but there may also be changes in ventilation and perfusion matching [285]. These are small but in chronic air flow obstruction the nitrogen washout improves slightly [1023].

EFFECTS DURING SLEEP

Cuirass ventilation is most frequently required at night but there have been surprisingly few studies of its effect on ventilation during sleep. It is usually effective in skeletal and neuromuscular disorders in improving the $P\text{O}_2$ and $P\text{CO}_2$ [453, 1179, 1675, 3158]. The number of apnoeas in NREM sleep falls [1293] and oxygen desaturation during both NREM [1181] and REM [2959] sleep is less severe. It is, however, not invariably effective and failure may be due to:

Incoordination

Coordination with the imposed pattern of ventilation is essential but may not be possible, particularly during REM sleep when the respiratory pattern is irregular [2935]. Triggering of the cuirass from nasal air flow [2062] or inspiratory muscle EMG [3046] has been attempted but is technically difficult.

Abnormal respiratory mechanics

Cuirass ventilation is able to compensate for central apnoeas or consistently low tidal volumes in subjects with normal chest wall and lung mechanics. If there is severe air flow obstruction or a decrease in lung or chest wall compliance, cuirass ventilation may be less successful. Careful attention to the settings of the cuirass pump and the use of equipment such as the Newmarket pump with a sufficient capacity to compensate for air leaks may overcome this problem.

Obstructive sleep apnoeas

Obstructive apnoeas due to inspiratory collapse of the pharyngeal walls are unresponsive to cuirass ventilation. This may even induce obstructive apnoeas, particularly in REM sleep [1181], by causing adduction of the vocal cords. The mechanism is probably similar to the obstructive apnoeas seen with diaphragmatic pacing (p. 275). Cuirass ventilation may inhibit the activity of the laryngeal abductor muscles as part of a generalized inspiratory muscle inhibition, but the loss of the normal synchronization of upper and lower respiratory muscle activation may also be important.

Inadequate cuirass pressure

Cuirass ventilation may fail during sleep because of an inability to generate a sufficiently negative pressure. This may be due to a failure in the power supply to the pump or the pump itself, or to leaks between the connections or in the connecting tubing. The most common cause is an excessive air leak between the patient and the cuirass, which may be intermittent and worsened by movement of the patient during sleep.

CARDIOVASCULAR EFFECTS

The circulatory effects of cuirass ventilation are complex. During inspiration the head and limbs are surrounded by atmospheric pressure whereas the thorax and abdomen are surrounded by subatmospheric pressure. The venous pressure gradient between the periphery and the trunk is therefore maintained, but some blood pools in the abdomen. This decreases the venous return to the heart slightly unless there are compensatory changes in venous tone. The effects on venous return are particularly marked if the T_I/T_{TOT} ratio is increased. Distension of the lungs during ventilation also increases the pulmonary vascular resistance and may lower cardiac output. Conversely, relief of hypoxia and hypercapnia improve myocardial contractility, lessen any pulmonary vasoconstriction and alter the systemic vascular resistance. Studies on dogs during cuirass ventilation have suggested that the cardiac output is increased [1114], and thermographic data have indicated

that this may also be so in humans [3305]. However, direct observation of the cardiac output and pulmonary artery pressure during cuirass ventilation [1675, 1685] and jacket ventilation in patients with emphysema [2062] have shown no significant changes.

Indications

The most important indication for cuirass ventilation is chronic ventilatory failure, but it has been used in a variety of other situations. In the 1950s it was found that ventilation could be adequately supported during bronchoscopy and laryngoscopy under general anaesthesia by a cuirass, except in very obese subjects [206, 1242, 1597, 2964, 3174, 3253]. Cuirasses have also been used post-operatively to increase lung expansion [1484].

Cuirass ventilation has proved disappointing in acute ventilatory failure. It is unsuitable for the unconscious patient because of the risk of aspiration into the trachea and bronchi; if there is air flow obstruction due, for instance, to retained bronchial secretions, it may be impossible to achieve adequate ventilation. Cuirass ventilation is poorly tolerated in acute exacerbations of chronic bronchitis but may be effective during acute bronchitis associated with neuromuscular and skeletal disorders [1891]. Tank ventilation or IPPV are, however, more reliably effective. Cuirass ventilation may be of value in the transitional phase between these more intensive methods of ventilatory support and the establishment of spontaneous respiration. Its use in facilitating weaning from IPPV for acute respiratory failure caused by, for instance, adult respiratory distress syndrome has not been explored fully.

Cuirass ventilation is effective in a variety of neuromuscular and skeletal disorders causing chronic ventilatory failure. It is usually required only during sleep. A tracheostomy is not required unless significant air flow obstruction develops, and does not respond to treatment such as nasal IPPV or the addition of protriptyline or nasal CPAP. Avoiding a tracheostomy is a major advantage over IPPV for long-term treatment. A cuirass is also much simpler for the patient's use in the home than a jacket or tank ventilator.

The benefits of cuirass ventilation in chronic stable air flow obstruction are slight [1023, 1560], although some improvement in respiratory muscle endurance has been demonstrated [687]. It is of most value in disorders of the respiratory drive, in the presence of respiratory muscle weakness, and in skeletal disorders of the thorax. Cuirasses were extensively used during the acute phase of poliomyelitis, until the introduction of IPPV with a cuffed endotracheal tube (see p. 318). The mortality was high with bulbar poliomyelitis because of aspiration into the lungs, but cuirass ventilation is safe and effective in pure acute spinal poliomyelitis [1818, 1819]. It was also of value in the convalescent phase when weaning from more intensive forms of ventilatory support was attempted, and in chronic respiratory failure following poliomyelitis [996, 1061, 1296, 1459, 3218].

The main contraindication to cuirass ventilation in chronic neuromuscular disorders is aspiration of pharyngeal material into the trachea and bronchi. Upper airway obstruction may also prevent adequate ventilation from being attained. Successful long-term treatment has been reported in ventilatory failure due to central alveolar hypoventilation [2357, 3312], bilateral diaphragmatic paralysis from various causes [47, 64, 527, 735, 1459, 1930, 2312, 2786, 3151, 3158], spinal muscular atrophy [735, 1930, 2357], acute idiopathic polyneuropathy [1801], myasthenia gravis [735], Duchenne's muscular dystrophy [8, 58, 147, 696, 1578, 2357], limb-girdle muscular dystrophy [2959], acid maltase deficiency [735, 1556, 1930], nemaline myopathy [2626, 3257], centronuclear myopathy [2357], the sequelae of tuberculosis [1677, 2803] and scoliosis [283, 1293, 1677, 2527, 2569, 3329].

The influence of cuirass ventilation on survival is discussed in Chapter 26. The symptoms of respiratory failure, particularly somnolence, are frequently relieved [1677]. There is no significant change in the VC [1023, 2357] or the lung volumes, except the FRC which increases slightly [1677]. Unless the underlying disorder deteriorates the PI_{max} increases [1677, 1689], but there is no change in PE_{max} since there is no assistance to expiration [1677]. The improvement in PI_{max} probably reflects relief of muscle fatigue, but other factors such as an increase in the compliance of the respiratory system may contribute. The PO_2 and PCO_2 improve [1181, 1677, 1687, 3158], often for a period of 6–9 months [285, 1061, 2357, 2804, 3198] (Fig. 17.6). The fall in PCO_2 does not correlate with the improvement in PI_{max} [1687]. Relief of muscle fatigue is apparent within a few days of start-

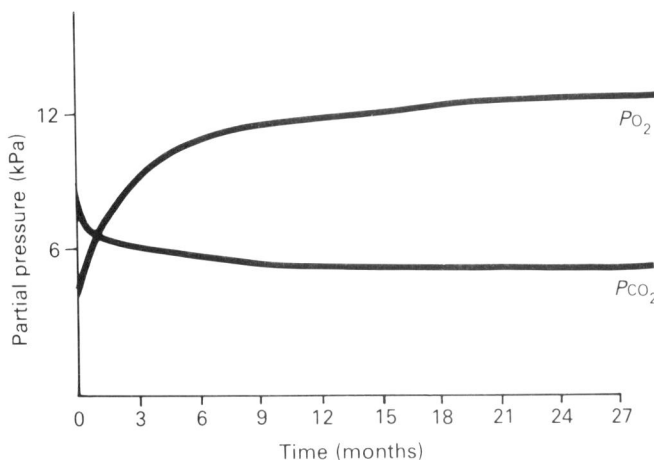

Fig. 17.6. *Pattern of improvement in PaO_2 and $PaCO_2$ in neuromuscular and skeletal disorders during treatment with nocturnal negative pressure ventilatory assistance.*

ing treatment, but the more gradual improvement in the blood gases probably reflects an increase in chest wall compliance due to movement of intervertebral and costovertebral joints that had previously been fixed or had very limited mobility. A further factor contributing to the improvement in blood gases is the change in respiratory drive. The slope of the ventilatory response to hypercapnia improves during cuirass ventilation without any change in the respiratory mechanics, indicating that the central chemoreceptor drive increases [1677, 1680]. The response is proportional to the improvement in the arterial P_{CO_2} and may be mediated by a reduction in the CSF bicarbonate concent-

ration, changes in the cerebral blood flow, improvement in the sleep structure or even a reduction in the central depressant effect of hypercapnia and hypoxia. Relief of hypoxia may be sufficient to relieve polycythaemia and to lower the pulmonary artery pressure [3198].

JACKET VENTILATION

Jacket design

Jacket ventilators were initially used to treat ventilatory failure due to poliomyelitis at a time when the design of cuirasses was unsatisfactory. Jacket ventilators have the advantage that they

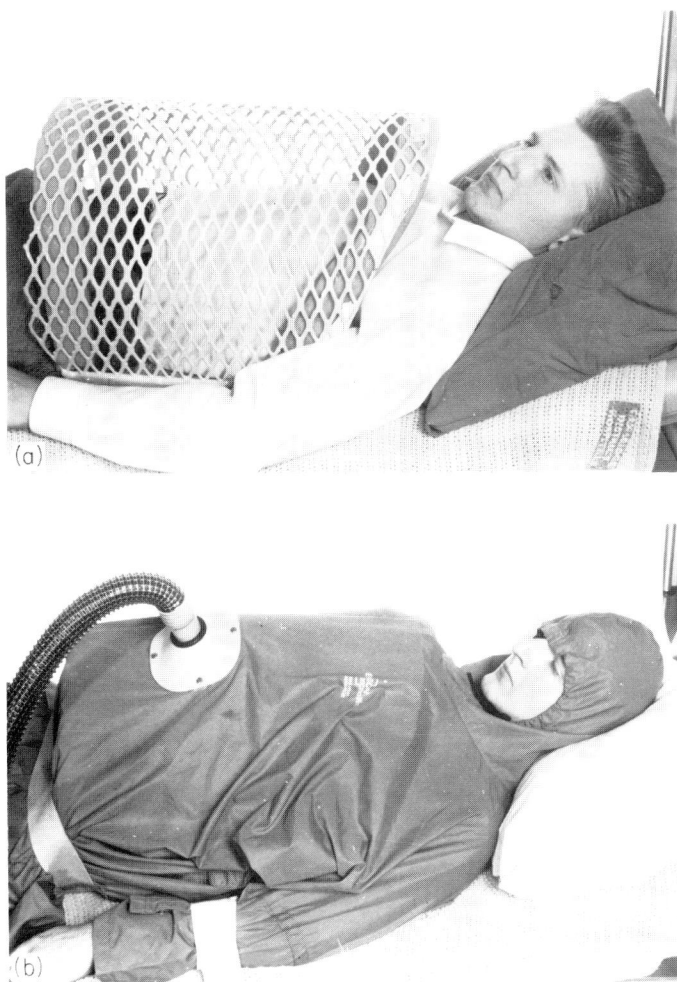

Fig. 17.7. *Jacket ventilator: (a) inner framework in position over rib cage and abdomen, (b) garment applied over framework. Note arm and waist bands and neck tie to minimize air leaks.*

do not have to be individually constructed to fit each patient because the inner framework does not touch the chest wall (Fig. 17.7). The frame should be sufficiently large to enclose the whole of the thorax and abdomen when they expand during inspiration. A back-plate is provided with some models of jacket ventilator for the frame to rest on, but it is often uncomfortable. The jacket itself fits loosely over the inner framework and is made of almost impervious nylon or similar material. The jacket is fastened round the neck, arms and waist to minimize the air leak. This is, nevertheless, considerably greater with all the models of jacket than with a well-designed cuirass. The large air leak often makes the patient feel cold unless the ambient air is very warm.

Since the whole of the rib cage and abdomen is enclosed within the jacket, there is very little restriction of chest wall movement. Both the rib cage and abdomen expand when the negative pressure is applied. Pressure areas are not a problem except occasionally at the site of contact with the back-plate. The disadvantage of enclosing the whole of the chest wall is that jacket ventilators are invariably larger and more cumbersome than a cuirass and may induce claustrophobia. They cannot be used readily with a tracheostomy because of the risk of obstruction of the tracheostome by the neck seal. Jackets are more difficult for the patient to fit and most models require help from another person. They are usually unsuitable for patients who live alone and the need to depend on help may be damaging psychologically.

Equipment

JACKETS

The models of jacket ventilator that are available are remarkably similar. An individually moulded inner framework appears to offer no advantage over the commercially available models [1685]. The most commonly used jacket ventilators are:

Tunnicliffe jacket

Available from Watco Services (Basing Instruments Limited), PO Box 86, Basingstoke, Hants, RG24 ODZ. Cost approx. £350.

The Tunnicliffe jacket was the first effective jacket ventilator to be produced commercially [3009]. The framework consists of a perspex arch that clips onto a plastic back-plate. The jacket itself is largely nylon and the seals are secured by arm bands and an abdominal belt. Two sizes are produced (D and E), but even the large size is too small for many patients with scoliosis.

Emerson chest respirator

Available from E & G International Inc., 269 Giralda Avenue, Coral Gables, FL 33134, USA. Cost approx. £200.

The framework of this jacket is made of metal with a Plastisol coating. The back-plate is plastic, but is not always required. The nylon jacket is sealed by a neck drawstring and elastic straps for the arms and hips. This jacket and grid are produced in three sizes and the back-plate in two sizes.

Lifecare Pulmo-wrap

Available from Thomas Respiratory Systems, 3 Cholmeley Crescent, Highgate, London, N6 5EZ. Cost approx. £500.

The grid and back-plate of this jacket ventilator are enclosed in a synthetic jacket that can be pulled over the head or zipped up. Three sizes are available.

Pneumosuit

Available from Thomas Respiratory Systems, 3 Cholmeley Crescent, Highgate, London, N6 5EZ. Cost approx £500.

This comprises a metal back-plate and an adjustable perforated anterior framework that is coated with nylon. The jacket is also made of nylon and has an anterior zip and belts for the arms and abdomen. Three sizes are available.

JACKET PUMPS

The pumps and connecting tubing that are suitable for cuirass ventilation are also effective with jacket ventilators. The air leak with a jacket is greater than with a cuirass [1685] but all the pumps are able to compensate for this. The change in air leak from breath to breath is probably less in a jacket than in a cuirass because the seals are placed around the neck, upper arms and waist or thigh. The volume of air inside the jacket is greater than that inside a cuirass but the difference is small compared to the air leak around and, to a certain extent, through the jacket.

Physiological effects

The physiological effects of jacket ventilators have been studied less than cuirasses but in general are similar. The differences are mainly due to the lack of restriction of the rib cage and abdominal movement by the jacket. The V_T increases linearly with the peak negative pressure but is slightly greater at any given pressure than in a cuirass [1685, 3009] (Fig. 17.5). The difference is, however, less marked with modern well-designed cuirasses than with older models. The peak negative pressure that can be achieved within a jacket is often lower than in a cuirass so that the maximal tidal volume in a cuirass may even exceed that in a jacket [1685]. The $P_{I_{max}}$ has been shown to increase in bilateral diaphragmatic paralysis [520] and in chronic air flow obstruction [391, 686]. The maximal transdiaphragmatic pressure does not increase [1844], although diaphragmatic EMG activity is reduced [1883].

Indications

The indications for jacket ventilators are similar to those for cuirass ventilators (p. 228). Jackets, like cuirasses, were at one time used during bronchoscopy and laryngoscopy [1402, 1403]. Jacket ventilators may be of value in acute exacerbations of chronic bronchitis and em-

physema [2062], but further study is required.

The main indication for jacket ventilation is chronic ventilatory failure due to neuromuscular and skeletal disorders. In such subjects a cuirass is usually adequate and a jacket, which is larger, more cumbersome and more difficult to fit, is not necessary. However, a jacket should be used if individually-made cuirasses are not available or for occasional patients with severe chest deformities in whom it is impossible to make a satisfactory cuirass. A jacket ventilator may also achieve adequate ventilation in patients with air flow obstruction in whom a cuirass is insufficient.

Jackets have been shown to be of value in central alveolar hypoventilation, both in neonates [2122] and adults [2626], poliomyelitis [1085, 3012, 3198], motor neuron disease [3026], Duchenne's muscular dystrophy [58, 434, 1085, 1578, 1579, 3364], limb-girdle muscular dystrophy [3364], congenital myopathy [2626], the sequelae of tuberculosis [3384] and scoliosis [1085]. Improvements in blood gases [1085, 1181, 2626, 3198, 3384] and pulmonary artery pressure [1085, 2626, 3198] similar to those seen with cuirass ventilation have been reported.

TANK VENTILATION

Historical development

The first tank ventilator was designed by Dalziel in 1838 [712]. He enclosed the patient up to the neck in an airtight box. A manually operated bellows pump was connected to this and was able to evacuate 1/19th of the volume of the box. This equipment was demonstrated to satisfactorily ventilate cadavers [1884] but was never widely used. Woillez proposed a similar apparatus in 1854 [2108] but his first model, termed the Spirophore, was not produced until 1876 [3362]. A metal rod rested on the patient's chest and its movement up and down indicated the amount of chest expansion to the observer. Similar ventilators were designed by Jones in 1864 [1693], Ebersold around 1873 [86], von

Hauke around 1876 [3252, 3372] and Breuillard in 1887 [1136, 1693]. In 1889, Doe described a wooden box designed by Braun for resuscitating neonates and reported success in all fifty patients who were treated [804]. Further tank ventilators were produced early in the 20th century by Davenport in 1905, Hammond in 1905, Severy in 1916 and Schwabe in 1926 [913, 3372, 3373]. Chillingworth and Hopkins designed a body plethysmograph in 1919 that was large enough for a dog and was able to distend its lungs by lowering the internal pressure [556]. A ventilator described by Smith [2987] was constructed of plate-glass but, like these other designs, was never popular.

The principle of tank ventilation was extended by Lord in 1908, who developed a respirator room. This contained several patients whose heads protruded from the room. The air within the room was intermittently evacuated and air was drawn into the lungs from the relatively high pressure outside. In this way, several patients could be ventilated simultaneously [3372]. This principle was copied by Wilson and Drinker at the Children's Hospital, Boston in the 1930s [843, 913], but was never widely used.

The first tank ventilator that was shown to be of value was that developed at the Harvard University Medical School by Drinker, an engineer, in 1928 [843]. His research began in 1926 and was funded by The Consolidated Gas Company of New York City. He produced a sheet-iron welded tank ventilator. This was modified in 1930 so that infants could be treated [2257], and an airtight hood was added for administering oxygen [2886]. Drinker and his colleagues studied the ventilatory response to different negative pressures, the oxygen consumption during ventilation, the chest and abdominal movements, and the clinical results of ventilation in a variety of conditions, particularly poliomyelitis [838, 839, 841, 842, 3330]. Slightly modified versions of Drinker's tank ventilator were subsequently produced and used especially for acute poliomyelitis [2863]. These included the Drinker-Collins ventilator manufactured in the USA, the Drinker respirator manufactured in 1934 by Siebe Gorman in the UK, the sheet-metal Henderson respirator of 1933 [2108] (Fig. 17.8) and the cylindrical Emerson respirator that was produced from 1931 in both adult and infant sizes. A simplified tank ventilator constructed of laminated wood was produced by an Australian engineer, Both, in 1938 [2108] (Fig. 17.9). Drinker also designed a wooden ventilator in 1938 that could be constructed quickly for treating patients with

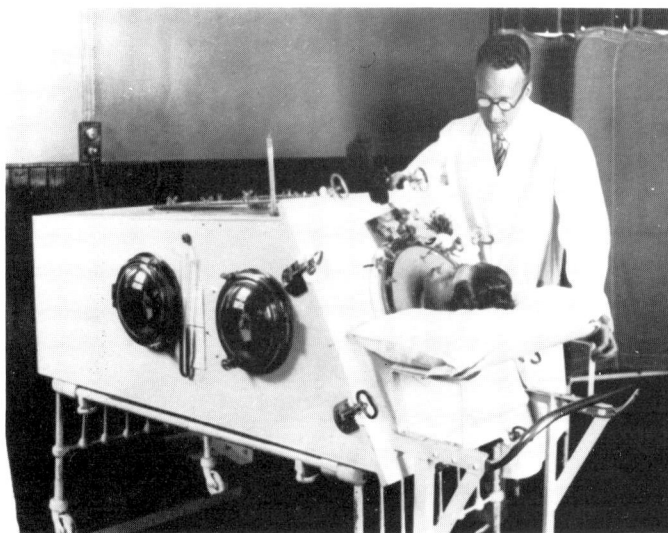

Fig. 17.8. *Henderson respirator. Doctor Henderson pictured in 1933, with the first patient in the UK treated in a tank ventilator of the Drinker type. Reproduced by courtesy of Dr R.G. Henderson.*

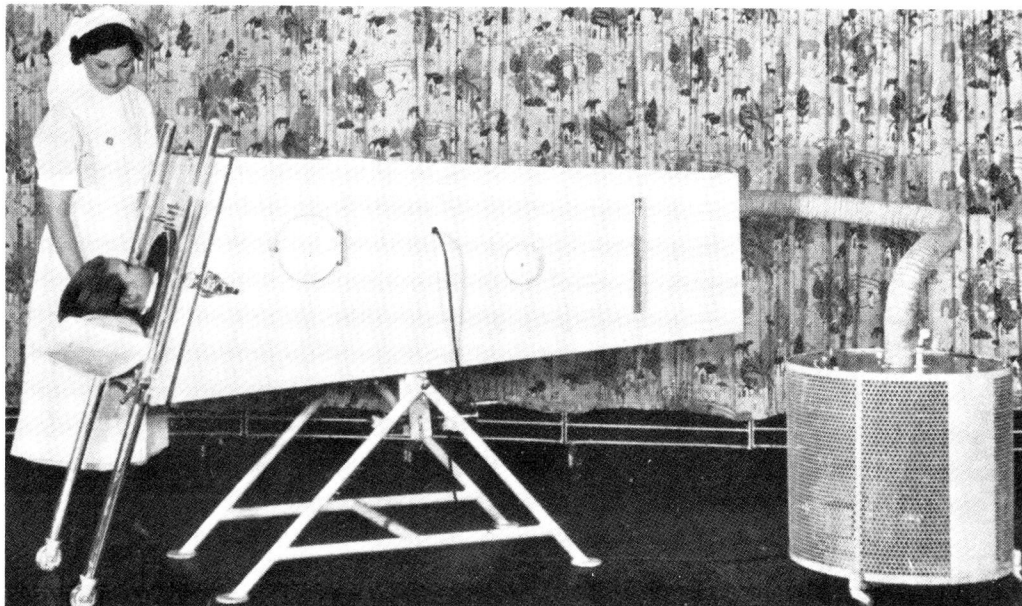

Fig. 17.9. *Both respirator. From the MRC Special Report No. 237, 1939. Reproduced with the permission of the HMSO.*

acute poliomyelitis [840]. A portable half-length cuirass-like metal ventilator was used success-fully by Binet in France around 1948 [284].

In 1938 the Medical Research Council com-missioned a committee to examine the provision of ventilators in the UK [2108], but in that year Lord Nuffield pre-empted its conclusions by offering to donate a Both ventilator to any insti-tution in Great Britain and the British Empire that had a genuine need for one. By March 1939 there were 30 Drinker respirators and 695 Both respirators in the UK, Southern Ireland and the Services [2108]. Many of the latter were hardly, if ever, used.

In 1948 the Ministry of Health set up a Breathing Machines group to advise on the distribution, maintenance and improvement of the existing ventilators [2602]. This led to the drafting of a performance specification for new ventilators in 1951. The Birmingham Regional Hospital Board also drew up a committee, which in 1953 formulated specifications for modifying the many Both ventilators and for new models of tank ventilators [2182].

In that year, Smith reported a modification

of the Both ventilator in which the headpiece was split horizontally [2983]. This principle was carried further by Galpine in 1954 [1081], by splitting the ventilator along its whole length. This 'alligator' ventilator differed from all pre-vious 'telescopic' tank ventilators in which the patient lay on a stretcher that could be pulled in and out of the chamber. The Coventry ven-tilator was designed by Smith-Clarke and was produced in adult and paediatric versions by Cape Engineering Co. Ltd. MacCrae devised the Bristol respirator in 1954, which was similar and had an airtight perspex dome that fitted over the patient's head and enabled positive pressure to be applied [2027]. With the Stan-more model, like the Coventry, positive pres-sure was applied by a face mask or mouthpiece [2602]. A further improvement was reported by Kelleher in 1961, by which the patient could be rotated through 180° so that postural drainage could be carried out [1639] (Fig. 17.10). This enabled 'wet' cases of poliomyelitis, in whom aspiration had occurred, to be reasonably satis-factorily treated.

Ironically, while these improvements were

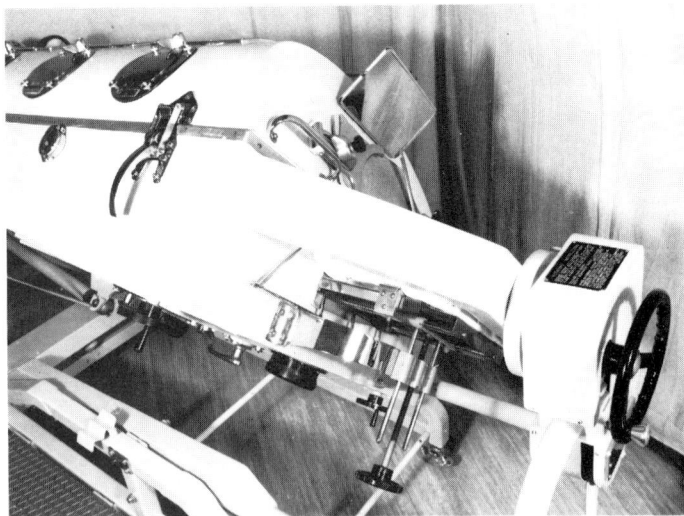

Fig. 17.10. *Kelleher tank ventilator tilted at 45°, showing mechanism for rotating the ventilator.*

being made, experience, particularly of the Copenhagen poliomyelitis epidemic of 1952 [245, 1520, 1817, 1819], had shown that IPPV was more successful than tank ventilation. The use of tanks then declined rapidly. They continued to be employed for a few patients with chronic respiratory failure, particularly due to previous poliomyelitis, but it is only recently with the realization that negative pressure ventilation is effective in many other neuromuscular and skeletal disorders that their use has increased again. Simplified versions of tank ventilators have been developed specifically for use in the home. The models currently available are described on p. 236.

Tank ventilator design and performance

Tank ventilators, unlike cuirasses, do not need to be tailored individually to the patient. In most adult models there is about 178 cm within the tank to enable patients of up to about 191 cm tall to be treated satisfactorily. The size, weight and lack of manoeuvrability of the tank ventilators is the major drawback for their use at home and also in hospital. The newer 'alligator' ventilators require less space than the 'telescopic' models and make it easier and quicker to move the patient in and out of the ventilator. The patient requires help to be placed inside

the conventional models of tank ventilator but this is not always necessary with the newer designs, such as the Cape Warwick portable tank respirator and the Portalung. An alarm system is usually required for tank ventilation in the home.

Tank ventilators are often colloquially referred to as 'iron lungs', possibly because Drinker's original model was made of sheet-iron. Subsequent designs have used steel (e.g. the Drinker-Collins respirator), aluminium (e.g. the Cape alligator ventilator), wood (e.g. the Both and Drinker paediatric respirators) and fibreglass (e.g. the Portalung). It is essential that the body of the tank is sufficiently rigid not to be deformed when negative pressure is developed within it, and it should not only be impervious to air but have efficient seals at each of its joints. The seals are usually made of foam rubber or a similar material, but some air leak is inevitable. The largest leak is usually around the neck of the patient. This is normally covered with padding, which should be neither too tight nor too loose, but newer methods of sealing the neck using either a pneumatic seal or the principle of dilatancy [2105] may prove superior.

The patient is enclosed within the tank up to the neck and is largely inaccessible during treatment. This is less of a problem for home ventilation than it is in hospital where frequent

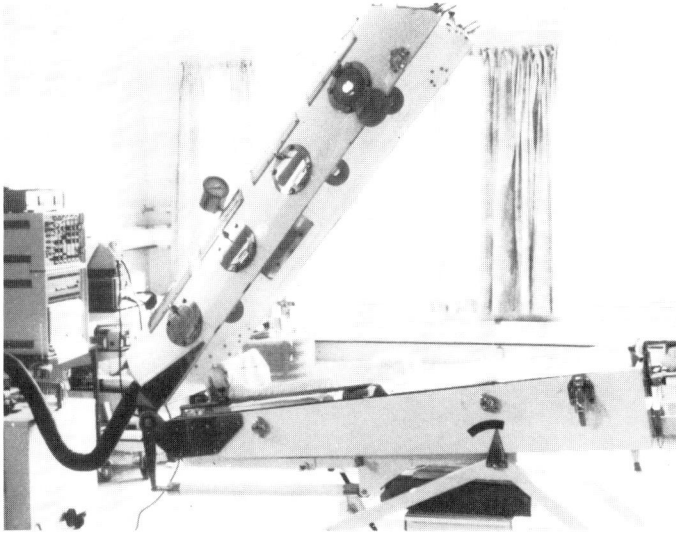

Fig. 17.11. *Cape alligator tank respirator.*

nursing and physiotherapy procedures may be essential. Clinical assessment of the patient is difficult and ventilation may have to be interrupted for medical, nursing or physiotherapy purposes. Some access to the patient is possible through the portholes at the sides of the ventilator. These may also be used for intravenous infusions, urinary catheters and other cannulae. Some of the earlier designs of tank ventilators, such as that of Woillez [3362] and that described by Smith [2987], had a glass front so that the patient could be observed. The more modern designs have windows, which serve the same purpose.

Currently available tank ventilators

Many of the older models of tank ventilator are still in use, although they are not currently in production. A large number are also kept in storage but have not been employed for many years. In the UK, most of these ventilators are Both or Cape ventilators, and in the USA they are mainly Emerson tank ventilators. Since the advent of effective immunization against poliomyelitis there has been a trend towards simpler types of tank ventilator, particularly models that are suitable for home use. The realization that critically ill patients with re-

spiratory failure are better treated by IPPV and more selective use of tank ventilation is largely responsible for this.

The most important models of tank ventilators currently available are:

Cape alligator ventilator (Fig. 17.11)

Available from Penlon Limited, Abingdon, Oxford, OX14 3PH. Cost approx. £15 000.

This tank ventilator has been available since the mid-1950s and is designed on traditional lines. It is constructed of aluminium but has windows to allow inspection of the patient. There are several portholes, which give access to the patient for physiotherapy and through which catheters and cannulae can pass. This ventilator is large, heavy and not portable. Its internal volume is 0.795 m^3. There is a low-pressure alarm.

Cape portable tank respirator (Fig. 17.12)

Available from Penlon Limited, Abingdon, Oxford, OX14 3PH. Cost approx. £11 000.

This simplified model of an alligator tank ventilator was introduced in 1986. It is lighter (weight 220 kg), smaller (dimensions 221×86.4×155 cm) and has an internal volume of $0.61m^3$. It can be dismantled into three sections so that it passes through a doorway. Its internal length is slightly less than the Cape alligator ventilator. There are two models, in one of which the patient can be positioned up to 18° head-down and in the other up to 18° head-up. It is possible for some patients to get in and out of the ventilator unaided. The negative pressure gauge is visible to the patient but there are no low- or high-pressure alarms. Unlike the Cape alligator ventilator, the pump is included in the structure of the ventilator. It is a bellows pump with a slightly greater stroke volume than the Cape Senior pump (p. 238) and can generate about 45 cmH_2O negative pressure in the ventilator. The respiratory frequency can be set at 13, 16, 19, 22 and 25 breaths/min.

Emerson tank ventilator

Available from E & G International Inc., 269 Giralda Avenue, Coral Gables, FL 33134, USA. Cost approx £9000.

These ventilators are no longer in production but reconditioned models are available.

Lifecare Portalung

Available from Thomas Respiratory Systems, 3 Cholmeley Crescent, Highgate, London, N6 5EZ. Cost approx. £4000.

This small, light (weight 46 kg) fibreglass tank ventilator is suitable for home use. Negative pressures of up to 40 cmH_2O can be achieved.

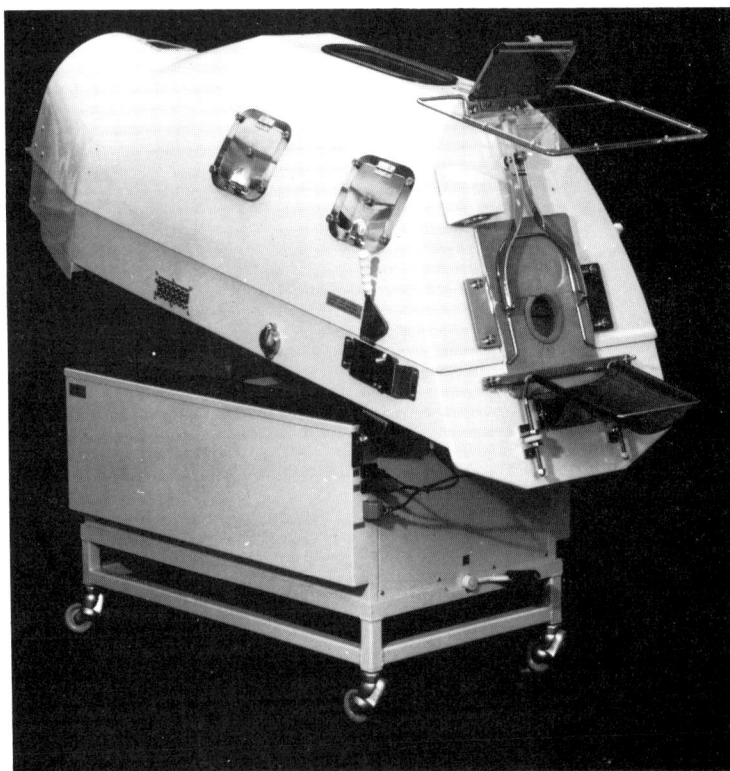

Fig. 17.12. *Cape portable tank respirator, shown in head-down position. Reproduced by courtesy of Penlon Ltd.*

Tank pumps

Some early models of tank ventilator used hand pumps, e.g. Woillez [3362], von Hauke [3372] and Jones [1136]. Schwabe's design was hand-operated by the patient and proved impractical [3373]. Breuillard used a steam ejector pump similar to that for his cuirass [913], but most of the subsequent tank ventilator pumps have been powered by the mains electricity supply. Some, such as the Cape Senior pump, can also be manually operated if the power supply fails.

Bellows pumps were used for most of the early tank ventilators, such as that of Dalziel [712], Drinker's original tank ventilator [842] and the Bristol respirator [2027]. Drinker's paediatric wooden respirator was powered by a rotary pump [840]. The Cape portable and the Emerson tank ventilators have pumps enclosed within the structure of the ventilator. The modern, smaller tank ventilators such as the Portalung can be evacuated by pumps that are suitable for cuirass ventilation, such as the Newmarket pump, MV Maxivent and Lifecare 170-C (p. 224). The Cape alligator tank ventilator, however, requires a higher-capacity pump. The Cape Senior pump, available from Penlon Ltd., Abingdon, Oxford, OX14 3PH, is specifically produced for tank ventilation. It has a stroke volume of 33.8 l and is larger and heavier but otherwise similar to the Cape cuirass pump.

The choice of respiratory frequency, inspiratory/expiratory ratio, pressure waveform and the length and diameter of the connecting tubing are determined by the considerations that have been discussed under cuirass ventilation. The larger capacity of the pump is required to evacuate the volume of air within the tank and to cope with the air leaks. The volume of the newer, simpler tank ventilators is less than that of the older models but the air leaks are often considerable. The majority of the air leak is around the patient's neck rather than at the joints of the ventilator. Most patients can be satisfactorily ventilated with a peak negative pressure of 30 cmH$_2$O, but the capacity to generate a negative pressure of 40–45 cmH$_2$O is useful in some subjects.

Physiological effects

The physiological effects of tank ventilation are, in general, similar to those already described under cuirass ventilation. The most important differences are that tank ventilators are more effective than cuirasses and that they do not limit the expansion of the rib cage or abdomen.

TIDAL VOLUME

The tidal volume achieved in a tank ventilator is, like cuirass and jacket ventilators, linearly related to the peak negative pressure both in restrictive and obstructive disorders [1248, 1364, 2807, 3322]. The V_T is considerably greater than that developed in either cuirass or jacket ventilators [431, 2807], but less than with IPPV [356] (Fig. 17.5). Cuirass and jacket ventilators usually generate between one-third and two-thirds of the V_T of a tank ventilator at any given peak negative pressure [1640, 2201, 2497, 3322]. The V_T within a tank ventilator does not level off at high negative pressures since there is no restriction of the rib cage or abdominal expansion.

INSPIRATORY MUSCLE ACTIVITY

Reduction in diaphragmatic EMG activity during inspiration can be demonstrated, particularly if the peak negative pressure within the tank is greater than about 25 cmH$_2$O [2678, 2680, 2684]. This suggests that tank ventilation may be valuable in relieving inspiratory muscle fatigue. Tank ventilation may also improve the compliance of the chest wall by increasing the range of movement of the intervertebral and costovertebral joints. This lessens the work of the inspiratory muscles.

BLOOD GASES

Tank ventilation is almost always sufficient to maintain adequate ventilation if the lung and chest wall mechanics are normal or if inspiratory muscle weakness is the only abnormality [431,

2502]. Even if there is no spontaneous respiratory effort, the patient can be hyperventilated readily [352]. Hyperventilation may persist for some hours after a period of tank ventilation, both in normal subjects [411] and in those with neuromuscular disorders such as poliomyelitis [26, 679, 1269]. This may be due to resetting of the chemoreceptors and is probably responsible for the breathlessness that occasionally occurs after tank and other forms of negative pressure ventilation.

EFFECTS DURING SLEEP

There is little information on the effect of tank ventilation on sleep apnoeas, although it appears to be similar to cuirass ventilation but more effective [912]. Air flow obstruction at the level of the larynx may develop, as in other forms of negative pressure ventilation [912, 971, 2432, 2809], and this may be severe enough to necessitate either a tracheostomy or an alternative form of treatment.

CARDIOVASCULAR EFFECTS

During tank ventilation the whole body, except the head and neck, is surrounded by subatmospheric pressure during inspiration. The normal venous pressure gradient between the chest and the peripheral veins is lost so that the venous return and the cardiac output are both reduced. 'Tank shock' was recognized during treatment for acute poliomyelitis and was attributed to pooling of blood in the abdominal veins [649]. Tank shock is extremely rare in other conditions and may have been partially due to vasomotor disturbances caused by the poliomyelitis or abnormal blood gases. Venous return can be increased by the addition of positive external pressure during expiration [2049], but this may lead to basal airway closure and mismatching of ventilation and perfusion.

Indications

Tank ventilation was little used until about 1930, but for the next twenty-five years it was widely employed, particularly in poliomyelitis, diphtheria and acute idiopathic polyneuropathy [2108]. It found various other applications, such as treatment of respiratory depression due to drugs [3330], although it has the disadvantage that the airway is not protected. Tank ventilators were used to assist respiration postoperatively [26, 1213, 2307, 2473, 2851]. It has the advantage of avoiding intubation and the need for sedation, and weaning is easier than with IPPV. Tank ventilation was also recommended after a laparotomy, to aid expansion of the lungs and expectoration of retained secretions [1997, 1998, 2262].

The most important uses of tank ventilation are:

ACUTE RESPIRATORY FAILURE

The value of tank ventilation in acute respiratory failure is not yet settled. Tank ventilators have been modified to generate continuous negative pressure to treat, in particular, neonatal respiratory distress syndrome [167, 552, 3149] and pneumocystis pneumonia in childhood [1365, 2784, 2785] and adults [2782]. Neonatal RDS [3047] and viral [797] and bacterial [2159] pneumonias in adults have also been treated successfully with conventional tank ventilation.

The value of tank ventilation in acute exacerbations of chronic bronchitis and emphysema is underestimated. Early studies showed that ventilation often could be adequately supported [354, 464, 1560, 1946, 2922, 3059(b), 3303] and that the need for intubation and IPPV could be avoided. It may enable oxygen to be given without CO_2 retention developing [1978, 3059(b)]. It is much less effective in chronic stable air flow obstruction [1249, 1978], although respiratory muscle endurance may improve [687].

Acute respiratory failure in neuromuscular and skeletal disorders often can be effectively treated by tank ventilation [963, 1619, 1891]. Supplementary oxygen and a respiratory stimulant such as doxapram may be necessary in conjunction with tank ventilation, and it is essential to treat the underlying cause of the acute re-spiratory failure. Tank ventilation is much more effective in this situation than a cuirass or jacket. Intermittent positive pressure ventilation is rarely required unless there is a risk of aspiration into the tracheobronchial tree or tank ventilation is not immediately available.

Acute ventilatory failure is a feature of some neuromuscular conditions, such as poliomyelitis and acute idiopathic polyneuropathy, without any other respiratory condition such as an acute chest infection. In these disorders, tank ventila-tion is satisfactory as long as swallowing and cough is preserved. It is, therefore, of value in spinal poliomyelitis [383, 2973, 3295] and acute idiopathic polyneuropathy if there is no bulbar involvement [1090], and in aiding weaning from IPPV if this is protracted [2938].

Chest infections can also be treated in a tank ventilator, despite the inaccessibility of the pa-tient. Some physiotherapy can be carried out through the portholes and most models of tank ventilator can tilt head-down to 20–25° to enable postural drainage. The Kelleher tank ventilator also rotates to facilitate expectoration of secre-tions [1639]. Unless continuous ventilation is required it is, however, usually best to interrupt ventilation for short periods of physiotherapy with the tank open. A method of assisting coughing by suddenly opening the portholes at the end of inspiration in order to cause a rapid expiration has been described but is not widely used [184, 185, 279, 547, 2307].

CHRONIC VENTILATORY FAILURE

Tank ventilators have an important advantage over IPPV for long-term use in that a tracheos-tomy is not required. This simplifies the nursing care. Humidification is not required since air is drawn in through the upper respiratory tract. There are, nevertheless, several important dis-advantages to tank ventilation. The airway is not protected and the patient is inaccessible within the tank so that it is unsuitable if he is totally ventilator-dependent. Help is required

to get in and out of the ventilator, except with some of the newer, simpler models. Many pa-tients find it uncomfortable to lie on their backs for long periods and claustrophobia may also be a problem. Careful explanation and reassurance is essential, but anxiety or fear may impair the ability to coordinate spontaneous respiration with the ventilator. This not only increases the oxygen consumption of the respiratory muscles but diminishes alveolar ventilation. The simpler types of negative pressure ventilator (cuirasses and jackets) should be tried before long-term tank ventilation is recommended. These are usually effective but if there is air flow obstruc-tion in addition to a neuromuscular or skeletal disorder, tank ventilation may be needed. In many cases this is only required during sleep, but continuous treatment may be necessary if there is severe respiratory muscle weakness. A simpler form of respiratory support, such as IPPB, an exsufflation belt or even diaphragmatic pacing, can be used during the day.

Tank ventilation has been attempted in re-spiratory failure due to obstructive sleep ap-noeas [1031] and obesity [2847] but is of little value, presumably because of upper airway obstruction. It has, however, been shown to be of value in providing long-term ventilatory sup-port in central alveolar hypoventilation both in adults [1085] and neonates [2867], neonatal ap-noeas [2051, 3377], poliomyelitis [1085, 2984, 2985], spinal muscular atrophy [3026], Duchenne's muscular dystrophy [8, 147, 696, 1537, 3026], the sequelae of tuberculosis [1249, 2803] and scoliosis [1085, 3012, 3198].

The influence of long-term tank ventilation on survival is discussed in Chapter 26. The qual-ity of life is impaired, especially if continuous or nearly continuous ventilation is required, be-cause of the limited movement that is possible within the tank. The length of hospital admis-sions may, nevertheless, be decreased [1085] and physiological improvement, such as im-provement in the blood gases [696, 1085, 1537, 1560] and pulmonary artery pressure [3198], may be seen.

Chapter 18
External Positive Pressure Ventilation and Related Treatments

This chapter describes the methods that have been used for applying positive pressure to the chest wall, primarily to assist expiration. Most of these techniques have fallen out of favour because they are less effective than other methods of assisting ventilation and because they decrease the end expiratory volume below the FRC. Basal airway closure with ventilation/perfusion mismatching and hypoxaemia result. Expiration normally occurs largely by elastic recoil with relatively little respiratory muscle contraction so that this type of mechanical assistance is of little benefit in relieving respiratory muscle fatigue. Despite these drawbacks, several of the older techniques do have a limited role in the management of ventilatory failure in skeletal and neuromuscular disorders. The place of newer methods, such as high-frequency chest wall compression, is still uncertain.

THORACIC AND ABDOMINAL POSITIVE PRESSURE VENTILATION

The principle of this method is similar to that of abdominal positive pressure ventilation (p. 242) in that compression of the rib cage and abdomen passively decreases the volume of the chest during expiration. The end expiratory volume falls below the FRC and inspiration occurs passively by elastic recoil, particularly of the chest wall. The difference between these two methods is that the diaphragm is displaced into the chest during abdominal positive pressure ventilation, whereas in this method the compression is applied equally to the rib cage and abdomen. The diaphragm is only displaced if there is a difference of compliance of the two compartments. Positive pressure ventilation applied to both the chest and abdomen does not require the patient to be upright since inspiration occurs through elastic recoil and not by gravitational descent of the abdominal contents.

Equipment

Positive pressure ventilation can be achieved with a cuirass, jacket, or tank ventilator (Chapter 17). Some of the early models of cuirass and pump, such as Eisenmenger's Biomotor [87], the Laffer Lewis apparatus [2108] and the Blanchard [660] and Chestpirator [661] models, were designed to allow positive as well as negative pressure ventilation to be applied. This facility has been retained in some of the pumps currently available for negative pressure ventilation, such as the Newmarket pump, the Thompson MV Maxivent and the Lifecare 170-C (p. 224).

Positive pressure ventilation can be achieved more readily in a tank ventilator than with a cuirass or jacket. The positive pressure tends to blow the cuirass and jacket away from the rib cage and abdomen and this increases the air leak. It is unusual to achieve a positive pressure of more than 5–10 cmH$_2$O with a cuirass, and higher pressures are uncomfortable [1685].

Physiological effects

Expiratory positive pressure is much less effective in increasing the V_T than inspiratory negative pressure [352, 356, 431, 611, 1685, 1686, 3322]. It decreases the end expiratory volume below the FRC [352, 611, 1685, 1686] and this may lead to airway closure and diminish the ventilation to the bases of the lungs. It has been proposed that positive pressure ventilation increases the compliance of the chest wall at low lung volumes [352], but there is no direct evidence for this. Any increase in cardiac output by a similar mechanism to the effect of negative end expiratory pressure (NEEP) used with IPPV [2047, 2048] appears to be slight [1686].

Indications

Positive pressure applied to the thorax and abdomen is rarely used because it is poorly tolerated, has only a small effect on tidal volume and because it can cause airway closure. This occurs even in emphysema if it is used without negative pressure ventilation [1364]. It may nevertheless, be considered:
(a) if the improvement in tidal volume with negative pressure ventilation is just insufficient to maintain adequate ventilation;
(b) if the cardiac output is significantly diminished by negative pressure ventilation;
(c) in subjects with chronic air flow obstruction who develop hyperinflation during negative pressure ventilation.

ABDOMINAL POSITIVE PRESSURE VENTILATION

Compression of the abdomen during expiration has been used for many years in an attempt to increase ventilation. In 1894 Pressey developed an adhesive pad which when compressed was said to elevate the diaphragm, and in 1908 Hofbaur devised an inflatable rubber band which intermittently compressed the abdomen and was driven by a bellows pump [1136]. Other devices, including the Rossbach breathing chair and the Boghean breathing machine, were also developed to intermittently compress the abdomen [53]. However, the first widely used abdominal and rib cage compressor was the Bragg-Paul pulsator (Fig. 18.1). This was originally designed for a friend of Sir William Bragg who had progressive muscular atrophy and who survived for over three years with this equipment [381, 1656, 1657]. Three sizes of Bragg-Paul pulsator were produced and the frequency could be varied between 13 and 27 breaths/min [2108]. Pressures of up to 70 mmHg could be applied and the diaphragm was shown, radiographically, to be elevated by the abdominal com-

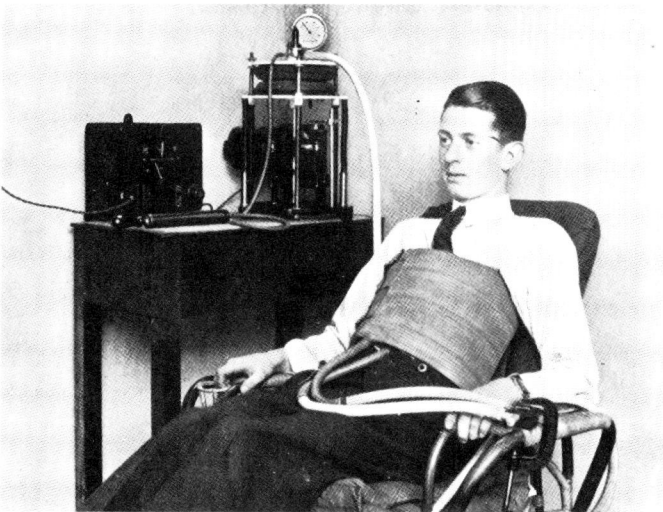

Fig. 18.1. *Bragg-Paul pulsator connected to bellows pump and manometer. Reproduced, with permission, from Paul R.W.* Proc. R. Soc. Med. *1934; 28: 436–8.*

pression [2423]. This apparatus was used successfully for patients with poliomyelitis and diphtheria [1657, 2029, 2030, 2108] but it was less effective than tank ventilation [2108] and was often poorly tolerated [314]. Equipment working on similar principles, particularly Hederer's pulmo-ventilator and Cot's apparatus, were also developed to aid resuscitation [2108].

These abdominal ventilators should be distinguished from abdominal binders (p. 245) in which pressure is applied to the abdomen irrespective of the phase of respiration. The aim of abdominal ventilators is to assist expiration and to elevate the diaphragm so that the end expiratory volume is less than the FRC. Inspiration then occurs passively due to elastic recoil.

Equipment

Abdominal positive pressure ventilation is achieved by inflating a rubber bladder that surrounds the anterior abdominal wall and usually the lower rib cage as well. The bladder is enclosed in an inextensible cloth or canvas binder, which is held securely in place. The bladder is inflated by a positive pressure pump such as the Newmarket pump, Thompson MV Maxivent or the Lifecare 170-C (p. 224).

The two most widely used abdominal ventilators or exsufflation belts are:

Thompson pneumobelt

Available from Puritan Bennett International Corporation, Heathrow Causeway, 152–176 Great South West Road, Hounslow, Middlesex, TW4 6JS. Cost approx. £200.

Three sizes of pneumobelt are produced and a portable battery-powered pump is also available. This has an inspiration/expiration ratio of 2 : 3.

Lifecare exsufflation belt

Available from Thomas Respiratory Systems, 3 Cholmeley Crescent, Highgate, London, N6 5EZ. Cost approx. £270.

This belt is also supplied in three different sizes, but is inefficient and complicated to fit.

Physiological effects

Exsufflation belts are more efficient in the upright position, when gravity causes the abdominal contents to descend during inspiration. Inflation of the belt during expiration raises the intra-abdominal pressure and elevates the diaphragm (Fig. 18.2). Inflation of the bladder tends to move the belt away from the abdomen during expiration rather than to compress it. The efficiency of this equipment is further decreased because part of the energy applied to

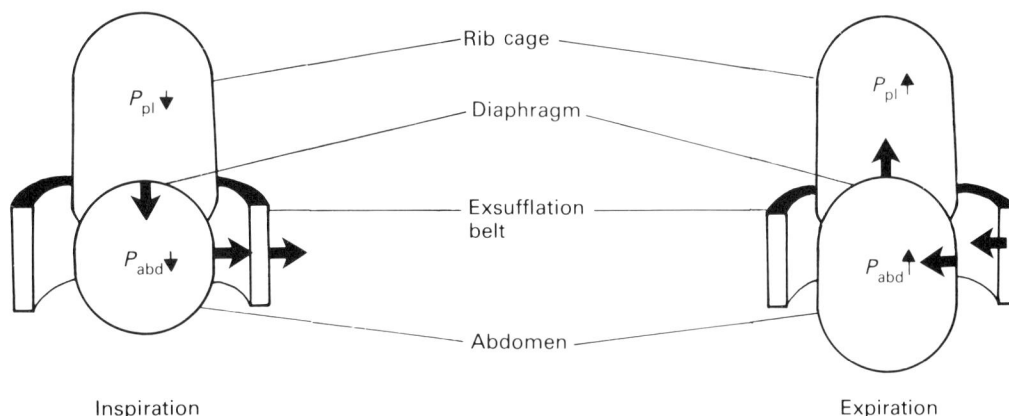

Fig. 18.2. *Diagrammatic representation of the changes in pleural and abdominal pressures, and movements of rib cage, diaphragm and abdomen during treatment with an exsufflation belt.*

the abdominal wall is used to compress the gas within the abdomen rather than to elevate the diaphragm. Peak pressures of around 50 cm-H$_2$O are often required and this may be uncomfortable. The pressure varies with the posture of the patient and an adequate tidal volume can be achieved at lower pressure in the upright position. The tidal volume increases as the inclination of the thorax and abdomen changes from 30° to 75° [16]. The tidal volume is proportional to the peak pressure within the abdominal belt for any individual in a given position, but there is considerable variation between subjects [16]. This is largely related to the degree of relaxation and coordination and to abnormalities of air flow resistance and compliance of the lungs and chest wall.

The exsufflation belts normally enclose not only the abdomen but also the lower rib cage. This approximates to the zone of apposition, which is the region of the rib cage that is exposed to abdominal rather than to intrathoracic pressure (p. 27). Compression of this zone prevents paradoxical expansion of the lower rib cage during expiration [16]. Reduction in the end expiratory volume below the FRC may cause airway closure and ventilation/perfusion mismatching. The effect on the blood gases is variable but improvements during treatment have been documented [493, 1237].

Indications

Abdominal positive pressure ventilators are simple but mechanically inefficient and are only of use in the upright or semi-upright position. They are of no value during sleep if the subject is supine and this has greatly limited their use. The current models of exsufflation belt are not readily portable but the development of smaller pumps may make this possible. Exsufflation belts are of no value in acute respiratory failure, when more reliably effective methods of ventilatory assistance should be employed.

Exsufflation belts have been used as the sole form of respiratory support in limb-girdle muscular dystrophy [2038] but their most common indication is for daytime ventilatory support in patients with severe neuromuscular disorders who require more intensive treatment during sleep. This may be cuirass [166], jacket [2038] or tank [3026] ventilation, diaphragmatic pacing [1147], or IPPV. Exsufflation belts allow the patient to be independent of a ventilator and to use a wheelchair. Beneficial results have been reported in bilateral diaphragmatic paralysis [791, 2200], syringomyelia [204], poliomyelitis [1147], spinal muscular atrophy [3026], motor neuron disease [2957, 3026] and muscular dystrophies [8, 147, 166, 696, 2038, 3026].

An abdominal compressor, the Pinkerton cuirass, was developed to assist ventilation during rigid bronchoscopy, but this is now obsolete [2481]. Exsufflation belts have been used in combination with IPPB to counteract the hyperinflation that this may induce [1237, 2158] and in emphysema to achieve deflation of the lungs [16]. It is probably of little value in this situation and no objective benefit has been demonstrated in anthracosilicosis [1028].

HIGH-FREQUENCY CHEST WALL COMPRESSION

Ventilatory assistance by intermittently compressing the chest wall is conventionally carried out at a frequency similar to that of spontaneous respiration. Promising results have, however, been reported recently with high-frequency chest wall compression. The lower thorax is surrounded by an air-filled cuff and pressures of around 100 cmH$_2$O are generated sonically at frequencies of 3–30 Hz [465, 466, 1110]. The optimal frequency has not been settled but it may depend on the pressure developed and the mechanical properties of the lungs and chest wall, particularly their time constant and resonant frequency.

It is unknown how ventilation is assisted at such high frequencies, but the mechanism may be similar to that of high-frequency ventilation (p. 256). It is thought that the alveolar pressure changes are less than with conventional low-frequency ventilation but it is uncertain how much of the pressure oscillation that is applied to the chest wall is transmitted to the alveoli and airways. The high-frequency compression is an elastic load on the respiratory system and the FRC may decrease slightly [465]. In dogs and cats, high-frequency compression of up to 350 Hz may inhibit inspiratory muscles, particularly the diaphragm, by a supraspinal reflex [2594], but it is not known whether this is of importance in man.

High-frequency chest wall compression is only able to assist ventilation and is insufficient for an apnoeic patient. The high-frequency tidal breaths are superimposed on the normal breathing pattern and they enable a lower spontaneous tidal volume and minute ventilation to maintain adequate blood gases [465, 3397]. High-frequency chest wall compression appears to be as effective as high-frequency oscillation in anaesthetized rats [1357] but data in humans is scanty and the role of this form of treatment in skeletal and neuromuscular disorders is uncertain. It may be of use during the day to assist ventilation in a similar manner to abdominal positive pressure ventilation, but it is unlikely to be reliably effective during sleep, particularly if there are prolonged central sleep apnoeas.

ABDOMINAL SUPPORTS AND ARTIFICIAL PNEUMOPERITONEUM

Abdominal supports have been used for many years in an attempt to elevate the diaphragm into its optimal position for contraction and to diminish air trapping in the lungs [183, 2873]. The same effects can be achieved by inducing an artificial pneumoperitoneum (Fig. 18.3).

Abdominal supports, binders or corsets have been used in a variety of pulmonary conditions [1194], particularly emphysema. An improvement in breathlessness [569, 1194] and an increase in the VC [53, 2532] have been reported, but their use has been limited at least partly by poor compliance with the treatment [2873].

Abdominal supports have been widely used in quadriplegia and severe poliomyelitis [706,

2307], in which the abdominal muscles are paralysed. The support is applied over the abdomen and the lower ribs [1172]. In the upright position the support decreases the compliance of the abdominal wall so that diaphragmatic contraction increases the intra-abdominal pressure and is not dissipated purely by abdominal expansion. In normal subjects abdominal muscle tone performs this function, but this is absent if the abdominal muscles are paralysed. The descent of the diaphragm is limited, therefore, and its force of contraction is not reduced by its fibres shortening excessively. The expansion of the rib cage is increased by abdominal supports and paradoxical movement of the lower rib cage is prevented by enclosing the zone of apposition within the support [1983, 3212]. Abdominal supports are of little value in the supine position since the weight of the abdominal contents is applied to the under surface of the diaphragm and prevents it from descending excessively during inspiration. The VC [68, 931, 1171, 1172, 1494, 2046], transdiaphragmatic pressure [1171, 1172] and cough [1692] improve in the sitting position, but not when supine.

Artificial pneumoperitoneum was most commonly carried out for pulmonary tuberculosis (p. 191) and was shown to decrease the FRC, RV and, to a lesser extent, TLC and VC [1918, 2419, 2912, 3375]. The addition of an abdominal support further decreased the lung volumes [3375]. These principles were applied to subjects with emphysema in order to elevate the diaphragm and lessen air trapping. Elevation of the diaphragm and an improvement in VC, MVV and arterial oxygen saturation during exercise have been demonstrated [464, 505, 1062] but improvement was not invariable [602]. Pneumoperitoneum has not been used in patients with chest wall disorders and is unlikely to be of value.

ROCKING BED

Historical development

The concept of maintaining ventilation for long periods by repeatedly altering the position of the patient arose from Eve's rocking method for artificial respiration [939]. Eve compared the thorax and diaphragm to a cylinder and piston. He emphasized that as the head was lowered, the abdominal contents elevated the diaphragm and air was expired. Inspiration followed as the head was elevated and the abdominal contents descended. This was shown to maintain adequate oxygen saturation and to generate larger tidal volumes than several methods of artificial resuscitation in use at that time, such as the Silvester and Schafer methods [122, 619, 921, 1192, 1668, 1999], but was less effective than the Nielsen method [1191, 1193]. It was used extensively by the British Navy in World War II [619] but it suffered from the need, except in neonates [942], for either two attendants to support and rock the patient [941] or for a stretcher or similar apparatus to tie the patient to [939, 940, 1668]. Specially designed stretchers, such as Riley's rocking resuscitator and the Tor-tilter, were developed [2108].

Eve developed a mechanically-powered rocking bed for longer-term ventilatory assistance, which came into use in 1939 [2108]. This provided up to 35° head-up and head-down tilt. Several other models of rocking bed were manufactured in the USA from the 1940s, such as the Respir-Aid [3376], McKesson [664] and, subsequently, the Emerson rocking beds. In the UK, the Lawson Tait, Sidhill and Coventry models were produced [2602]. The latter, developed by the Cape Engineering Co. Ltd, was manufactured until 1974.

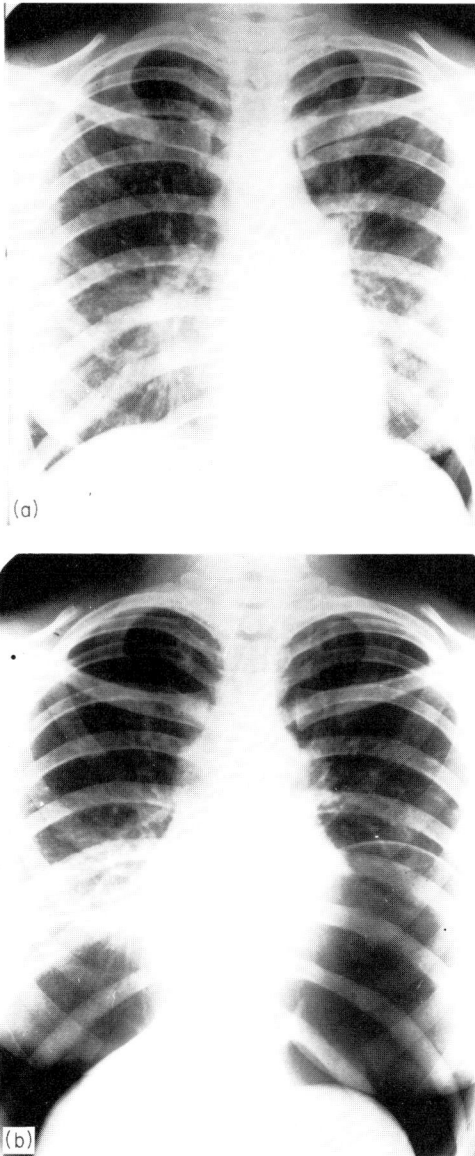

Fig. 18.3. *Chest radiographs at total lung capacity showing position of the diaphragm before (a) and after (b) induction of an artificial pneumoperitoneum.*

Equipment

Rocking beds consist of a surface on which the patient lies and which is pivoted near its centre (Fig. 18.4). The surface is jointed so that back and leg rests can be adjusted for the comfort and stability of the patient. The motor, powered by the mains electricity supply, is situated below the surface on which the patient lies. The number of oscillations per minute (the respiratory frequency) and the angle through which the bed swings can be adjusted readily.

The models of rocking beds currently available for adults are:

Breatheeesy rocking bed

Available from Peter Evans Associates, Golf Course Road, North Road, Bath, BA2 6JG. Cost

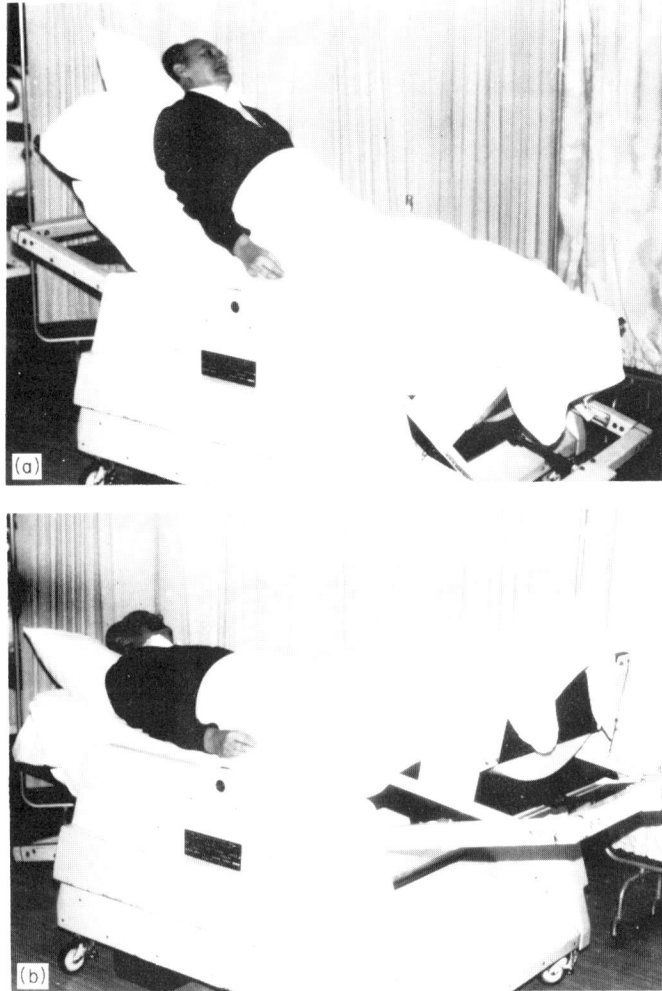

Fig. 18.4. *Rocking bed (a) in head-up position and (b) in head-down position.*

approx. £4400 for standard model and £5300 for deluxe model.

This lightweight rocking bed has a start and stop button that can be operated by either the hands or the feet. It gives a smooth acceleration and deceleration. The angle of swing is adjustable up to $22\frac{1}{2}°$ head-up or head-down. The respiratory frequency can be altered between 13 and 22 breaths/min. The independently adjustable back and knee rests are available on the deluxe model only. The bed uses a power of 400 W.

Emerson rocking bed

Available from E & G International Inc., 269 Giralda Avenue, Coral Gables, FL 33134, USA. Cost approx. £3000 for hospital model and £2000 for home model.

The hospital model tips 30° head-up and 30° head-down, but the home model tips only 15° head-down. The hospital model has adjustable foot boards. A control switch is available for the patient and an alarm rings if rocking ceases.

A rocking bed suitable for neonates is available from SEFAM, Parc d'Activites de Brabois, rue du Bois de la Sivrite, F-54500 Vandoeuvre-les-Nancy, France. The cost is approximately £100 and the unit weighs 2 kg. It fits inside an incubator and the bed rocks about 4° head-up and head-down at a frequency of 15 breaths/min. A bellows placed under one end of the bed is alternately inflated and deflated by movement of a valve that connects it to a reservoir of compressed air or to the atmosphere. The bed tilts when the bellows inflate and a spring reverses this movement when the bellows deflate. The rocking movements provide vestibular stimulation and appear to enhance growth [1738] and reduce the frequency and severity of apnoeas in premature infants [102, 1586, 1733, 1734, 3193]. The small amplitude of the rocking movement does not assist ventilation directly. The rest of this chapter deals only with large-amplitude rocking beds.

Physiological effects

The factors that determine the effectiveness of the rocking bed in assisting ventilation have never been analysed theoretically or investigated adequately. It affects respiration both by altering the posture of the patient and by the rapid changes in posture. It has been recognized for many years that the FRC increases when moving from the supine to the sitting position, but there is relatively little change on moving from the supine to the head-down position [617]. The VC, TLC and RV are also less in the supine than in the sitting position [2014]. These postural changes are largely due to the weight of the abdominal contents, which determine the position of the diaphragm. They may, however, not be realized fully on a rocking bed if there is insufficient inspiratory or expiratory time to achieve a steady state.

The rapid changes in posture lead to gravitational changes in the position and shape of the abdominal contents, lungs and rib cage, which vary with their masses and the velocity of movement. The forces are transmitted across the diaphragm, whose area determines the intra-pleural and abdominal pressures generated by the abdominal and thoracic contents. A source of mechanical inefficiency is that the kinetic energy developed by movement in one direction is dissipated by the subsequent movement in the opposite direction during the next phase of respiration. These theoretical considerations are probably modified considerably by the adaptations of diaphragmatic, intercostal and abdominal muscle activity to the changes in position and with movement. In one early study the oxygen consumption was unchanged during rocking, suggesting that the respiratory muscles remained active [1668]; this has been confirmed by EMG recordings [1180].

The practical application of these principles has never been studied in any depth. There is some evidence that the amplitude of the angle of swing of the bed is important in determining the V_T. This is proportional to the amplitude of the swing in anaesthetized normal subjects [431, 921] and in poliomyelitis [1405, 2000, 2501]. The V_T increases as the amplitude of swing increases to about 90° [3265], unless this is poorly tolerated. It is possible that ventilation could be improved by most of the angle of rock being either from the head-down to the supine position, or more probably from the head-up to the supine position, but direct evidence is lacking.

A respiratory frequency of 10–12 breaths/min was frequently used during short-term resuscitation [939, 1667, 2000]. The V_T falls but ventilation increases even up to respiratory frequencies of 20–22 breaths/min [1668]. As the respiratory frequency increases the T_I and T_E shorten and the rate of movement during each oscillation increases. The inspiration/expiration ratio is fixed at 1:2 on most models of rocking bed, and there is conflicting evidence regarding the importance of varying this ratio [122, 1405]. Fast movement during each phase of respiration increases the importance of the dynamic forces acting on the abdomen and lungs, and influences the ability of the patient to synchronize his breathing with the movement of the bed. Cooperation is essential for assisted ventilation using the rocking bed and careful explanation and attention to the patient's comfort is important. Coordination can be improved if the neck is flexed [1589] and by teaching the patient to inhale as his head rises [2501].

Arterial oxygen saturation can be maintained on a rocking bed in normal subjects who are anaesthetized and intubated [1192], although the V_T is usually < 350 ml [431]. Both the P_{CO_2} and P_{O_2} improve in subjects with neuromuscular disorders [1180].

Ventilation is greater if the patient lies prone rather than supine [431, 2000]. This may be due to a change in the mechanics of the chest wall or to better clearance of secretions from the airways in this position. Both the elastic properties of the chest wall and lungs and the air flow resistance modify the effectiveness of the rocking bed. This has not been studied adequately but clinical experience suggests that rocking beds are ineffective if there is even moderately severe reduction of compliance or increase in air flow resistance.

Circulatory and metabolic benefits have also been claimed for the rocking bed. Oscillatory beds were recommended for promoting the circulation in peripheral vascular disease in the 1940s. Early studies suggested that the venous return improved [940] and that the cardiac output increased [1405, 1668]. These observations need to be confirmed by modern investigative methods.

The loss of muscle mass, nitrogen, calcium and phosphate and the formation of urinary calculi in immobilized subjects is less if they are slowly rocked than if the bed remains horizontal [3306]. These metabolic consequences may be important, particularly in severely disabled patients with chronic neuromuscular disorders,

but they have not been investigated with the more rapidly rocking bed used for ventilatory assistance.

Indications

The rocking bed is a method of assisting ventilation that leaves the patient unencumbered and accessible for nursing procedures. A mouthpiece is not required, although some rocking beds, such as the Coventry model, have attachments whereby IPPB can be administered during or between periods of rocking. Rocking beds are, however, noisy, heavy and cumbersome to move and it may be difficult for the patient to find a comfortable position.

They are only effective if the mechanics of the respiratory system is normal, if the patient is able to coordinate with the rocking movement and if some respiratory muscle activity remains. Early studies suggested that a VC of 200–300 ml [2502] or of $>20\%$ predicted [356] was necessary to maintain adequate ventilation.

Rocking beds have been used in poliomyelitis, particularly in the convalescent phase during weaning from a cuirass [2827] or from a tank ventilator [245, 356, 664, 2501, 2502]. They have also been used to assist quadriplegics in weaning from IPPV [833]. Rocking beds may be of value for long-term treatment, particularly at night, in respiratory failure following poliomyelitis [390, 731], Duchenne's muscular dystrophy [8, 58, 1578] and bilateral diaphragmatic paralysis [791, 939, 1093, 1742, 2406(a), 2957, 3186, 3358]. Their value in central alveolar hypoventilation is controversial. In some reports rocking beds have been effective [1515, 1756, 2852], in others ineffective [432, 2391(b)] but they are often of some benefit, particularly in lowering the P_{CO_2} [193, 2230].

Chapter 19
Intermittent Positive Pressure Ventilation (IPPV)

Tracheostomy has been performed for many centuries but it was only in the nineteenth century that it became widely used, particularly to bypass the upper airway obstruction of diphtheria and inhaled foreign bodies [3266]. The fear of infecting the trachea in the era before antibiotics and the supposed danger of positive pressure on the alveoli delayed the introduction of positive pressure ventilation [351].

A method of positive and negative pressure ventilation that was suitable for neuromuscular disorders and avoided the need for a tracheostomy was devised by Thunberg around 1920 [3159] (Fig. 19.1). The patient was enclosed in a chamber (barospirator) in which the pressure was rhythmically changed from $+55$ to $+70$ mmHg to -55 to -70 mmHg, twenty to thirty times per minute [3321]. These large pressure swings altered the density of the air so that sufficient molecular displacement occurred to ventilate the patient with little or no chest wall movement or inspiratory muscle activity. This method of ventilation proved effective in a variety of neuromuscular conditions, such as head injury, encephalitis lethargica, sedative drug overdose, poliomyelitis, myasthenia gravis and botulism [2451, 2746, 3159]. It was also used in pulmonary tuberculosis in order to 'rest' the lungs [176] but it was never popular because of the complexity, bulk and expense of the apparatus and the inaccessibility of the patient.

Negative pressure ventilators, particularly tank ventilators, remained popular until the severe Copenhagen poliomyelitis epidemic of 1952, in which it was shown that endotracheal intubation with a cuffed tube gave superior re-

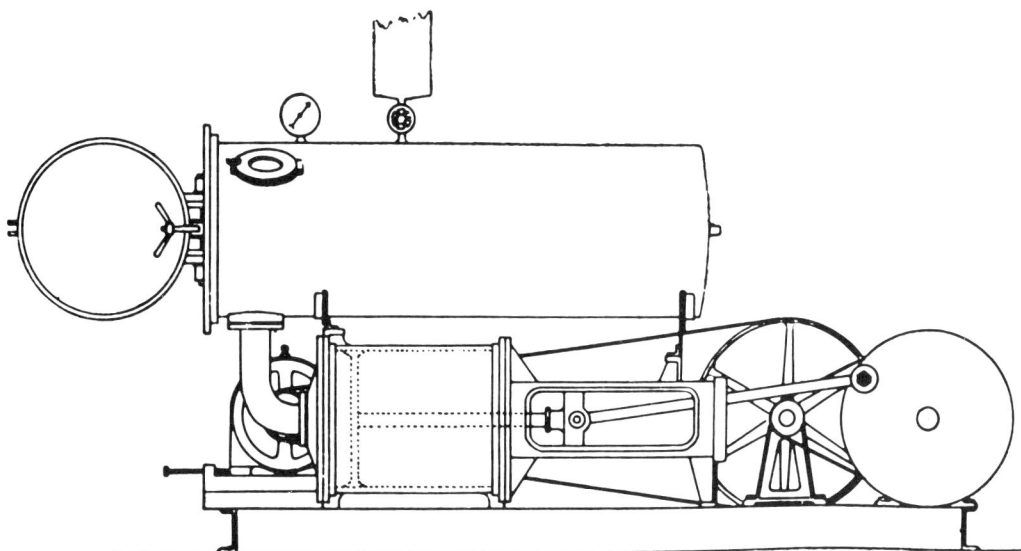

Fig. 19.1. *Thunberg's barospirator. Reproduced, with permission, from Thunberg T. Klin. Wschr. 1925; 4: 536–8.*

sults [245, 1520, 1817, 1819]. Positive pressure ventilation rapidly became accepted and soon superseded negative pressure ventilation.

The construction of a tracheostomy enables any upper airway obstruction to be bypassed and it decreases the anatomical dead space. This may be sufficient to allow some patients to ventilate adequately but IPPV or, occasionally, a negative pressure ventilator is often required to support respiration. The great advantage of a tracheostomy is that the lungs can be protected from aspiration of secretions and other material in the pharynx by the use of a cuffed endotracheal tube. This is especially important in acutely ill and unconscious patients but is also valuable in neuromuscular disorders where swallowing or coughing may be impaired. A tracheostomy also allows direct access to the trachea and bronchi for aspiration of inhaled material or sputum that cannot be expectorated because of a weak cough. A mini-tracheostomy may be sufficient if this is the main indication for a tracheostomy [2090].

Most of the discussion in this chapter concerns the place of tracheostomy and IPPV in providing long-term ventilatory support in neuromuscular and chest wall disorders. IPPV through the mouth and nose is considered separately at the end of this chapter. The management of acute respiratory failure is covered in textbooks of intensive care, anaesthesia and chest medicine and will only briefly be referred to where it is relevant.

EQUIPMENT

Tracheostomy tubes

There are many types of tracheostomy tubes and it is essential to select one of the correct diameter, length and shape for the individual patient. Many of the newer tracheostomy tubes have a fenestration, which permits air to escape from the lungs either through the larynx or through the tracheostome. This is useful to facilitate weaning from mechanical ventilation after an acute illness but the increased air flow resistance may induce inspiratory muscle fatigue [682]. During long-term ventilation it allows speech by directing air through the larynx. Speech can be improved further by deflation of the cuff, a speaking valve or by occlusion of the tracheostome with an inner cannula or a finger.

CUFFED TUBES

The tracheostomy cuff occludes the space between the tracheostomy tube and the trachea and thereby increases the efficiency of IPPV and prevents aspiration of pharyngeal secretions and other material into the lungs. The pressure of

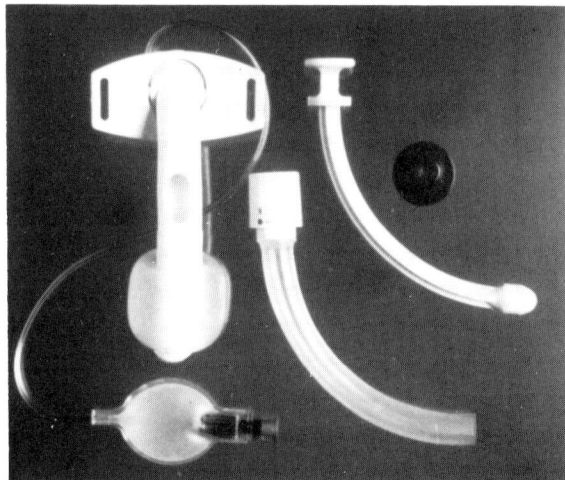

Fig. 19.2. *Shiley cuffed fenestrated tracheostomy set. The outer tracheostomy tube has a large-volume, low-pressure cuff. The inner cannula can be removed easily and cleaned, and the tapered obturator facilitates insertion of the tracheostomy tube. The 'button' occludes the tracheostomy so that respiration can occur solely through the upper respiratory tract. Reproduced by courtesy of Shiley Ltd.*

the cuff on the wall of the trachea can cause considerable damage. Initially, petechiae and granulation tissue appear but sufficient tissue may slough to expose the cartilagenous tracheal rings, which may soften (tracheomalacia). This leads to a floppy segment of the trachea, which moves paradoxically during both inspiration and expiration and causes air flow obstruction. Tracheal stenosis may also develop at a late stage [1104, 2516, 3035]. This is usually mild but may be severe enough to require resection of a length of trachea [1104]. The cuff may even erode through the tracheal wall, either posteriorly to cause a tracheo-oesophageal fistula or laterally into the innominate artery or other major vessel. This may lead to a massive fatal haemorrhage, although it is often preceded by smaller 'warning' bleeds.

Damage to the trachea was particularly common with the older designs of tracheostomy cuff. Until the 1970s, many cuffs were made of stiff rubber, were of low volume and required a high pressure to inflate them. In order to minimize damage to the trachea the cuff had to be deflated regularly, despite the risk of aspiration and the difficulty in ventilating the patient. More recently, thin-walled plastic cuffs have been developed, which contact the trachea over a wide area and are adequately inflated by lower pressures. These low-pressure, high-volume cuffs rarely cause tracheal damage if they are correctly used, unless the patient is debilitated or hypotensive. They do not need to be deflated. They should be filled with sufficient air to permit a slight air leak at the peak inspiratory positive pressure. The pressure within the cuff at this level is usually < 25 cmH$_2$O and some designs, e.g. Shiley and Portex, have a pressure gauge that prevents inflation above a set pressure of around 25 cmH$_2$O. The air leak may be significant if pressures greater than the cuff pressure are required, but aspiration around the cuff is unusual because of the high intratracheal pressure. Suitable cuffs are manufactured by, for instance, Shiley (Fig. 19.2), Portex and Lanz.

The tracheostomy cuff needs to be inflated during IPPV and in order to prevent aspiration of material into the trachea and bronchi. However, during periods when ventilation is not required, the cuff can be deflated if aspiration is not a risk. If this is a problem, the cuff may need to be inflated continuously or for periods of about half an hour after meals and possibly also at night when the risk of aspiration is greatest. The cuff hinders speech but special attachments, such as the Passy-Muir tracheostomy speaking-valve and the 'talk' tube [1707], are of value.

UNCUFFED TUBES

Uncuffed tubes provide no protection against aspiration but, equally, they carry less risk of trauma to the trachea, except from the end of the tracheostomy tube. It is possible to achieve adequate ventilation without a cuff as long as the ventilator is volume-cycled and can deliver about three times the volume of air that would be required with a cuffed tube [136, 141]. This is necessary to compensate for the air leak through the larynx, which can be minimized by using as large a tracheostomy tube as possible [2215]. The high flow rate of air through the upper airways dries the mouth and throat and is often poorly tolerated [2950].

Uncuffed tubes have the advantage that the patient can breathe around the tracheostomy tube if there is a mechanical failure of the ventilator and the patient is unable to disconnect himself from it [136]. This is of value, particularly in the home, since the added resistance of breathing through the ventilator with a cuffed tube may lead to acute ventilatory failure in this situation. The cough can be surprisingly effective with an uncuffed tube. It is possible to control the larynx so that it remains closed during inspiration for a couple of breaths and if it is then opened, secretions can be cleared [1696]. Speech is also possible with an uncuffed tube if there is a speaking-valve attachment (Fig 19.3).

The use of uncuffed tubes for long-term ventilation has been limited by the unpleasantness of large volumes of air escaping through the upper airway and the lack of protection of the airway. Their main place is for patients in whom there is upper airway obstruction, no risk of aspiration and in whom mechanical ventilation is not required. Silver tubes have been popular in the past because they are thin and non-irritant and have an efficient speaking-valve, but the cheaper plastic tubes attach better to ventilator connections.

Positive pressure ventilators for chronic respiratory failure

The requirements of a ventilator for long-term assisted ventilation differ from those for ventilation of the critically ill during an acute illness. Less-complex controls are needed since the ventilatory disability is stable and the lungs are often mechanically almost normal. It is important that the ventilator is not only simple but reliable and in many cases light and portable as well. Both high- and low-pressure alarms are needed to indicate air flow obstruction and disconnection or failure of the ventilator. These alarms must be independent of any external power source, whether this is the mains electricity supply or an external battery. An alarm may need to be specially designed if the patient is severely disabled so that, for instance, it can be operated by the movements of the patient's tongue, chin

or eyes [1089, 3197]. The ventilator, together with an external battery, should be able to fit onto a wheelchair if the patient needs this. Suction equipment and even a source of compressed or liquid oxygen may also have to be supported by the wheelchair.

The most suitable ventilators for long-term assisted ventilation, particularly in the home, are:

THOMPSON M-25B ASSIST MINILUNG PORTABLE VOLUME VENTILATOR

Available from Puritan Bennett International Corporation, Heathrow Causeway, 152–176 Great South West Road, Hounslow, Middlesex, TW4 6JS. Weight 10.9 kg. Dimensions 40.6×20.3×22.9 cm. Cost approx. £4500.

This volume-cycled ventilator has a metal case and is both small and easily portable. It can run off the mains electricity supply or an external battery. It also has an internal battery, which provides ventilation for at least 20 min if the external power source fails. The tidal volume can be varied between 300 and 2500 ml and the respiratory frequency between 5 and 20 breaths/min. Inspiratory time varies from 1.5 to 5.0 sec. The inspiratory pressure waveform is a sine wave. There is a high- and low-pressure alarm.

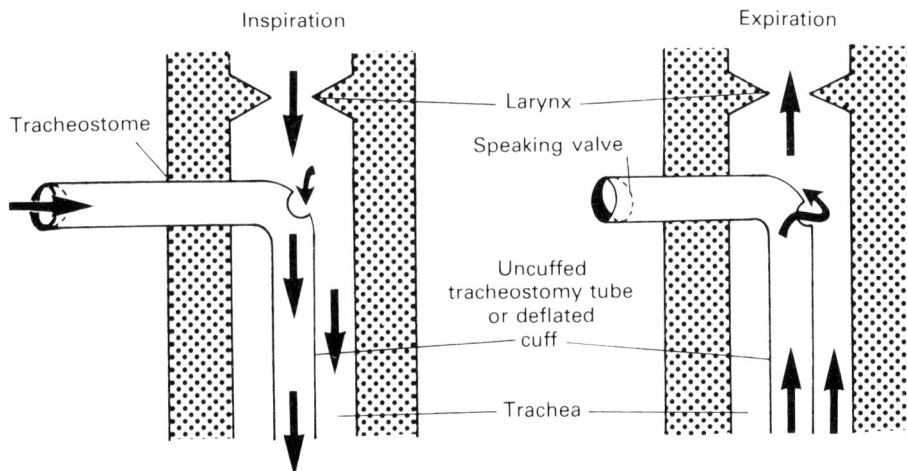

Fig. 19.3. *Mechanism of speech with a fenestrated tracheostomy tube and speaking-valve. The arrows indicate the direction of air flow during inspiration and expiration.*

LIFECARE PLV-100

Available from Thomas Respiratory Systems, 3 Cholmeley Crescent, Highgate, London, N6 5EZ. Weight 12.8 kg. Dimensions 22.9×31.1×31.1 cm. Cost approx. £4900.

This ventilator is light and portable and is powered either by the mains electricity supply or an external battery. It also has an internal battery for use if the external power source fails. The tidal volume can be varied from 50 to 3000 ml and the respiratory frequency from 2 to 30 breaths/min. The inspiratory flow rate and inspiration/expiration ratio can be varied and there is a facility for patient triggering and synchronized intermittent mandatory ventilation. There is a high- and low-pressure alarm.

COMPANION 2800 PORTABLE
VOLUME VENTILATOR (Fig. 19.4)

Available from Puritan Bennett International Corporation, Heathrow Causeway, 152–176 Great South West Road, Hounslow, Middlesex, TW4 6JS. Weight 14.1 kg. Dimensions 29.0×30.5×25.5 cm. Cost approx. £6900.

This ventilator is more complex than the preceding models but can also be powered either by the mains electricity supply, an external bat-

tery or by an internal battery. The range of tidal volumes is 50 to 2800 ml and respiratory frequency can be varied from 1 to 69 breaths/min. The inspiration/expiration ratio can be altered and there is a facility for introducing sighs, for patient-triggering and for synchronized intermittent mandatory ventilation. There is a high- and low-pressure alarm.

THOMPSON MV MAXIVENT (see p. 225)

LIFECARE 170-C (see p. 225)

EAST RADCLIFFE RP4, M2 AND
B2 VENTILATORS

Available from H. G. East and Company Limited, Littlemore, Oxford, OX4 5JT. Cost approx. £3200 for RP4 and £1200 for M2 or B2.

The RP4 [2731] requires either a mains electricity supply or an external battery. It is not readily portable but it can be used in the home. There is a choice of six respiratory frequencies.

The M2 and B2 ventilators are powered by the mains electricity supply or an external battery, respectively. They are light, portable, volume-cycled bellows ventilators but have only a single fixed respiratory frequency. The tidal volume can be increased to 1250 ml as long as the

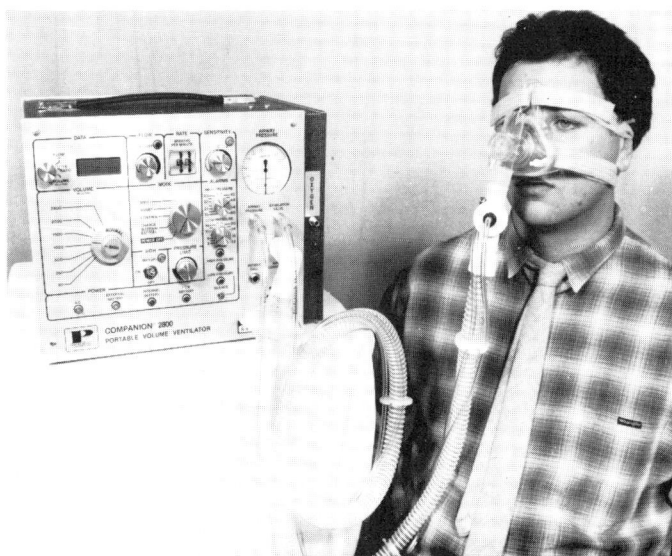

Fig. 19.4. *Nasal IPPV system illustrating the tight-fitting nasal mask and portable ventilator suitable for home use.*

peak pressure required is < 40 cmH$_2$O. The inspiration/expiration ratio can be varied between 1:1 and 1:8 by altering the tidal volume. These ventilators are suitable for short-term ventilation but, because of the fixed respiratory frequency and small range of tidal volumes, they are too inflexible for long-term ventilation unless used in combination with the RP4 ventilator.

TRACHEOSTOMY CARE

The importance of prevention of the early complications [1396, 3036] of a tracheostomy is well recognized. The late complications can be minimized by attention to the following aspects of tracheostomy care.

Tube changes

Modern plastic tracheostomy tubes have an inner cannula, which should be changed and cleaned twice daily. The outer cannula need only be changed about once a month. The technique of changing the tube should be understood by the patient and his relatives, but until the tracheostomy track is fully developed the outer cannula should only be removed by experienced medical or nursing staff. Occasional mild bleeding from the stoma is common. The outer cannula should be secured correctly so that the tip of the tracheostomy tube does not rub against the wall of the trachea.

Tracheal suction

The tracheostomy cuff interrupts the flow of mucus towards the larynx, and secretions tend to collect in the large airways. The cough is, however, surprisingly effective with a tracheostomy, particularly if an uncuffed tube is used or the cuff is deflated. Some patients do not require tracheal suction.

The suction catheter should be cleaned between each aspiration and the patient should be taught the correct technique of suctioning. Disposable catheters may be used but these are more expensive. The quantity of secretions that cannot be expectorated determines how often suctioning is required.

Suctioning may cause trauma to the trachea and main bronchi, and occasionally haemoptysis. Severe hypoxia may develop if the patient is completely ventilator-dependent. In this situation, pre-oxygenation may be valuable and suctioning should be limited to around 15–20 sec. Cardiac dysrhythmias may be triggered by contact with the tracheal and bronchial mucosa, particularly in the presence of hypoxia.

Humidification

The normal humidifying surface of the upper airway is bypassed by the tracheostomy. In acutely ill patients humidification of the inspired air is required but with long-term tracheostomies it is not usually needed. If it is required, the most satisfactory type of humidifier is a heat and moisture exchanger (artificial nose), such as the Pall Ultipor BB5OT [274]. This works on the principle that the water vapour in the expired gas condenses and gives up heat to the exchanger so that the heat and humidity can be transferred to the inspired air of the next breath. The humidity of dry air is usually raised to 50–80% relative humidity. The resistance to air flow is very low and these humidifiers largely avoid the problems of other humidifiers, such as condensation in the circuit and bacterial colonization.

Control of infection

Bacterial colonization of the tracheostome and tracheostomy tube is common during long-term ventilation but clinically significant infection is rare. This contrasts with the frequent occurrence of tracheostomy infections in intensive-care units. Regular and careful changing of the inner tracheostomy cannula and, if necessary, suctioning and humidification all reduce the risk of infection.

Filtering of inhaled particles

Inhalation of particles into the lungs can be reduced by avoiding dusty or smoky areas and shielding the tracheostomy with a cover such as a scarf. These measures are not necessary if a heat and moisture exchanger is used, since this is an effective filter.

PHYSIOLOGICAL EFFECTS

During IPPV the intrapleural pressure rises relative to the atmospheric pressure as air enters the lungs. The distribution of the inspired air is partly determined by the compliance and air flow resistance of each lung unit. The product of these two factors, the time constant, determines how quickly equilibration occurs. This is more complete and ventilation is more even throughout the lungs if the inspiratory time is prolonged. Conversely, if the mean inspiratory flow rate is too rapid, the distribution of ventilation is uneven and the physiological dead space increases. If the lungs are normal, an inspiratory time of 1.0 sec is usually adequate. An end inspiratory hold may improve the distribution of ventilation but this is worsened if there is a subatmospheric (negative) end expiratory pressure (NEEP), which causes basal airway closure and mismatch of ventilation and perfusion. The inspiratory pressure waveform has little effect on the distribution of ventilation [157, 158]. The expiratory time should be sufficient to prevent air trapping and an expiratory retard will hold the airways open for longer. The oxygen consumption of the respiratory muscles can be reduced by IPPV if the patient can synchronize with the ventilator.

The increased intrapleural and alveolar pressure has profound effects on the circulation. The distribution of perfusion within the lungs is altered because the pressure gradient between the pulmonary arteries and the alveoli is decreased. At the apices of the lungs (or anteriorly in the supine position) the alveolar pressure exceeds the arterial pressure and the capillaries are compressed. The reduced perfusion to the apices increases the physiological dead space and the pulmonary vascular resistance, and thereby decreases the cardiac output. This is also lessened because the pressure gradient between the veins within the thorax and in the periphery is altered. During a spontaneous inspiration the intrathoracic pressure is subatmospheric and venous return to the chest increases. During the inspiratory phase of IPPV the pressure gradient is reversed and venous return falls. This is partially compensated by an increase in the venous tone as long as the autonomic control of the circulation is intact and the blood volume is adequate.

The fall in cardiac output is most closely related to the mean inflation pressure. The waveform of the pressure during inspiration is unimportant [255] but an increase in inflation pressure or in inspiratory time, which improve the ventilation of the lungs, decreases the cardiac output. Negative end expiratory pressure improves cardiac output but causes airway closure [2047, 2048]. The cardiac output may also fall if the P_{CO_2} is decreased, if the pulmonary vascular resistance is increased by hyperinflation and also by less-well-identified humoral mechanisms that impair myocardial contractility [2669].

In practice, a compromise between the ventilator settings that are best for ventilation and for the circulation has to be reached. The inspiration/expiration ratio is usually close to 1:2, and the peak inspiratory pressure is adjusted so that a tidal volume is achieved that is adequate to maintain the arterial blood gases. High inflation pressures are avoided by increasing the respiratory frequency if the compliance of the lungs or chest wall is decreased.

The technique of high-frequency ventilation has been introduced because it develops a lower mean intrathoracic pressure and, therefore, has fewer circulatory complications. The respiratory frequency may be as rapid as 50 Hz but is usually < 10 Hz. The tidal volume is less than the usually accepted physiological dead space, although recent studies have shown that it falls progressively as the frequency is increased so that above 80 breaths/min the dead space is only 1.1 ml/kg [525] (Fig. 19.5). Nevertheless, the mechanisms by which inspired air reaches the

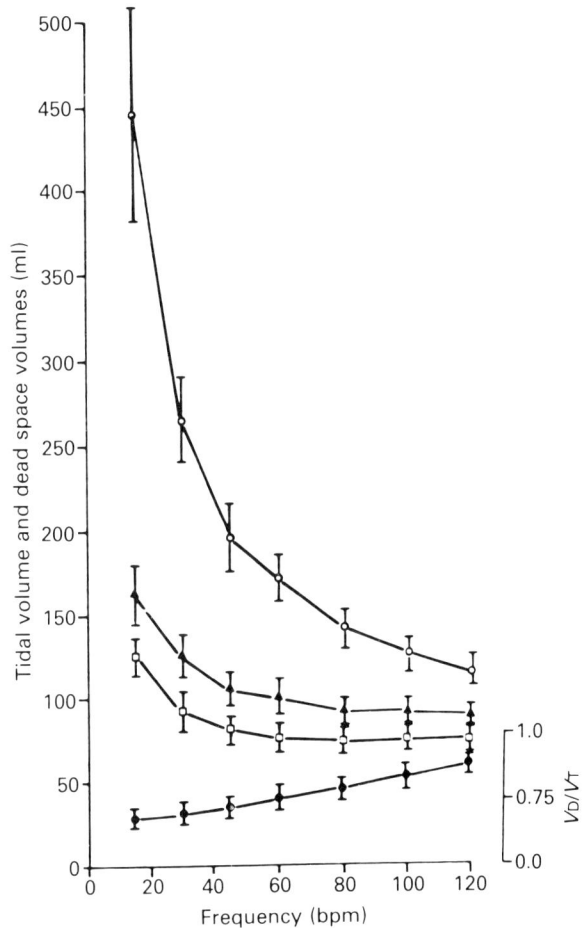

Fig. 19.5. *Changes in dead space and tidal volume (○) during high-frequency ventilation, with* Pa_{CO_2} *maintained within the normal range. (▲) Physiological dead space, (□) anatomical dead space, (●) measured* V_D/V_T *ratio. Reproduced, with permission, from Chakrabarti M.K. Br. J. Anaesth., 1986;* **58:** *14.*

alveoli during high-frequency ventilation are still uncertain [1050, 1108, 1720, 3128]. Convective gas flow, which is normally responsible for movement of gas in the large airways, appears to be unimportant but other mechanisms, including streaming of gas in the centre of the bronchi, augmented diffusion, expiratory mixing of gases and resonance of the air columns, may all play a part.

INDICATIONS

The main indications for IPPV are:

Acute respiratory failure

Respiratory failure may appear to be acute in patients with neuromuscular and skeletal disorders but it is frequently superimposed on mild chronic respiratory failure. The ventilatory management of both acute and acute on chronic respiratory failure is similar. Intermittent positive pressure ventilation is the most effective form of mechanical ventilation and has advantages over other methods in that it protects the airways if aspiration is a problem and gives direct access to the tracheobronchial secretions. Confusion and occasionally coma due to the blood gas abnormalities or to the acute illness itself predispose to aspiration and may prevent coordination with other forms of ventilatory support.

Initially, a nasotracheal or orotracheal tube should be used. A tracheostomy should be avoided if possible since even a slight degree of tracheomalacia or tracheal stenosis may impede spontaneous or assisted ventilation after the acute episode. If a tracheostomy is required it should be sited as high as possible if long-term treatment with a cuirass is considered. A temporary mini-tracheostomy may avoid the need for a traditional tracheostomy, particularly if sputum retention is the predominant problem [2090].

Weaning from IPPV may be difficult in the presence of neuromuscular and skeletal disorders; a transitional phase of assisted ventilation with a negative pressure ventilator, such as a tank ventilator or cuirass, may be required. The need for long-term ventilatory support should be assessed carefully after any episode of acute respiratory failure.

Upper airway obstruction

A permanent tracheostomy may be required to bypass an obstruction to the upper airway and after laryngectomy. Intermittent positive pressure ventilation is not normally required. Tracheostomy was the first effective form of treatment for severe obstructive sleep apnoeas but its indications have declined with the development of newer, simpler treatments. It is, nevertheless, probably the most effective method of improving daytime somnolence [592, 594, 1301, 2738, 3216] and the personality changes of chronic hypoxia [1301, 2738]. The sleep pattern returns to normal [1525], oxygen desaturation during sleep is lessened [1279, 2233], the frequency and mean duration of obstructive apnoeas falls [592, 1279, 1525, 2233] and the ventilatory response to hypercapnia increases [126]. Central sleep apnoeas appear when the tracheostomy is constructed [594, 3163] but become less frequent over the months following the tracheostomy [1279]. Their cause is uncertain. If the tracheostomy is closed, obstructive sleep apnoeas recur [592, 594, 1301].

The P_{O_2} and P_{CO_2}, while awake, improve following tracheostomy for obstructive sleep apnoeas [1525, 3216]. The pulmonary artery pressure falls [592, 594, 1301, 2233] and right heart failure diminishes [3216]. Systemic blood pressure may also fall [1301, 2233] if hypoxia is relieved. Cardiac dysrhythmias may be helped by a tracheostomy [592, 3163] but recur when this is blocked [3163].

These benefits of tracheostomy have to be weighed against the psychological and physical problems that it causes [872]. Depression, divorce and loss of employment often follow tracheostomy for obstructive apnoeas, despite an improvement in somnolence and personality [635]. Stomal problems may develop, particularly in the obese [633, 635, 1301]. Tracheostomies should, therefore, be limited to patients with severe obstructive sleep apnoeas in whom other forms of treatment have proved ineffective, or occasionally where there are life-threatening complications such as intractable cardiac dysrhythmias and other treatments are not immediately available.

Chronic respiratory failure

The two main advantages of IPPV, i.e. effective ventilation and airway protection, have to be balanced against the disadvantages of a tracheostomy and ventilator. The social disadvantages of a tracheostomy and the loss of normal speech are considerable. The need to care for the tracheostomy at home places a severe strain on both the patient and his family. Their ability to cope with the skilled nursing requirements of a tracheostomy needs to be assessed carefully before this form of treatment is initiated. In neuromuscular disorders, in particular, there may be other physical disabilities that prevent the patient from looking after his tracheostomy, and trained attendants may be necessary (p. 323).

Ventilatory support with a long-term tracheostomy is almost always given in the form of IPPV. Occasionally, however, negative pressure ventilation or diaphragmatic pacing are preferable. Jacket and tank ventilation is often impossible with a tracheostomy because the neck seal blocks the tracheostome. Cuirass ventilation can be achieved without difficulty but it is preferable for the tracheostomy to be sited as high as possible [2447]. Both diaphragmatic pacing and cuirass ventilation can maintain adequate ventilation if the respiratory mechanics are normal once a tracheostomy has been constructed but, conversely, both forms of treatment occasionally require a tracheostomy to be constructed because they can induce upper airway obstruction.

In many cases ventilatory support is only required during sleep, but occasionally it may be needed continuously for short periods, particularly during intercurrent illnesses such as a chest infection. In more severely disabled subjects, IPPV may be needed almost continuously and some subjects, particularly those with quadriplegia, extensive poliomyelitis and end-stage muscular dystrophies, may be completely ventilator-dependent. In this last group, IPPV has the advantage over negative pressure ventilators in that ventilation need not be interrupted for ordinary nursing procedures, whereas the negative pressure ventilators render the patient, to some extent, inaccessible during treatment.

The impairment of the physical, social and psychological quality of life with a permanent tracheostomy limits its use for long-term ventilatory support. It should be reserved for those patients in whom other simpler methods of ventilatory assistance are not suitable. Adequate ventilation can be achieved usually by negative pressure ventilators, unless the air flow resistance or compliance of the lungs or chest wall are very abnormal. In some cases, a severe chest deformity such as scoliosis may make it impossible to construct a cuirass that is effective, but in practice the main indication for a permanent tracheostomy and IPPV is aspiration of pharyngeal secretions into the lungs or an inability to expectorate sputum. These various indications for IPPV often coexist in the same patient, particularly in neuromuscular disorders. A permanent mini-tracheostomy should be considered, since this reduces the anatomical dead space, gives good access to retained secretions

and enables supplementary oxygen to be given [168]. It does not protect the airway against aspiration.

An alternative to conventional or low-frequency IPPV is high-frequency ventilation (p. 256). The high-frequency oscillations can be generated either by a jet source of gas or sonically, for instance, by a loudspeaker. The high frequency can be applied to the tracheostome or to the mouth. It has not yet been used to assist ventilation in neuromuscular and skeletal disorders but may prove to be of value for short periods during the day, particularly during exercise, and for nocturnal ventilation. It is less effective than conventional IPPV but it reduces the degree of spontaneous ventilation that is needed to maintain normal blood gases [1111]. In chronic air flow obstruction it has been shown to increase the exercise tolerance and diminish breathlessness [1109].

Conventional IPPV has been used for long-term ventilatory support in chronic air flow obstruction and parenchymal lung disease [271, 273, 341, 855, 961, 990, 1112, 1527, 2405, 2643, 2644, 2648, 2951, 3191], as well as in skeletal and neuromuscular disorders. It has been used successfully in neonates [1021] and in older children [446, 1036], as well as in adults. It has proved effective in, for example, central alveolar hypoventilation and central sleep apnoeas [446, 872, 1294, 2867, 2950, 3024], syringomyelia with vocal cord palsy [3342], quadriplegia [1216, 1696, 3024, 3033], motor neuron disease [42, 1427, 1696, 1853, 2312, 2327, 2949–2952, 2957], poliomyelitis [136, 141, 566, 990, 1342, 1441, 1696, 1819, 2038, 2373, 2646], multiple sclerosis [446, 2949, 2950], spinal muscular atrophy [3024], diaphragm paralysis [2955], myasthenia gravis [136, 3024], Duchenne's muscular dystrophy [58, 147], dystrophia myotonica [458, 3024], limb-girdle muscular dystrophy [166, 2038], acid maltase deficiency [427, 781, 3186], nemaline myopathy [1973], congenital myopathy [446], the sequelae of tuberculosis particularly thoracoplasty [271, 990, 1722, 2038, 2405, 2643, 2646, 2648, 2949–2951], and scoliosis [136, 271, 426, 990, 1112,

1441, 1526, 1722, 2038, 2643, 2646, 2648, 2649, 2949–2951].

Adequate ventilation usually can be achieved in these groups of subjects and improvement in blood gases has been recorded in scoliosis [1441, 2649], poliomyelitis [566] and in a mixed group of restrictive disorders [271, 273]. Marked hyperventilation with P_{CO_2} values as low as 1.6 kPa may occur and may be tolerated for many years [566, 1342, 2373]. The blood gases may continue to improve for up to a year after IPPV has been started [272, 2649], possibly because of a gradual improvement in chest wall compliance. As a consequence of the better oxygenation, the haemoglobin concentration may decrease [1441], right heart failure may improve [1112, 1441, 2646] and the need for diuretics may lessen [2951]. Exercise tolerance frequently increases [1112, 1441, 2951] and there are fewer episodes of acute respiratory failure and less time spent in hospital [271, 1526, 2646]. The effect on survival is discussed in Chapter 26.

NASAL INTERMITTENT POSITIVE PRESSURE VENTILATION

The development of comfortable and airtight nasal masks has enabled IPPV to be delivered through the nose (Fig. 19.4). The same masks are used as with nasal CPAP (p. 267), but intermittent rather than continuous positive pressure is applied. Most of the ventilators that are used for IPPV through a tracheostomy are suitable for nasal IPPV. Either patient-triggered ventilation or controlled ventilation may be satisfactory.

No humidification is required and the need for a tracheostomy is avoided. Nasal IPPV also has the advantage over negative pressure ventilation and diaphragmatic pacing of not inducing upper airway obstruction. The nasal masks may, however, be uncomfortable and cause pressure sores. The peak pressure is usually around 20 cmH$_2$O and this may induce earache and other upper respiratory symptoms. The risk of aspira-

tion pneumonia remains, since the airway is not protected. The ventilator has to deliver a large volume of air through the nose because of leakage through the mouth. If this is excessive an elastic tape around the forehead, cheeks and chin may hold the mouth closed or, alternatively, adhesive tape may be applied across the upper and lower lips. Air leaks around the edges of the nasal mask can usually be controlled by careful positioning and selection of the correct size of the mask.

Initial experience with nasal IPPV during sleep has been promising. Improvements in ventilatory failure have been recorded in chronic air flow obstruction [503], central alveolar hypoventilation [1654], spinal muscular atrophy [912], motor neuron disease [1654], poliomyelitis [912, 2831], myopathies [1850], muscular dystrophies [912, 1654, 2831], the sequelae of tuberculosis [1850] and scoliosis [1850]. Oxygen saturation during sleep improves [503, 912, 2831] and sleep is less fragmented [2831]. Symptoms such as somnolence and early-morning headache may disappear [1654] and the arterial blood gases during wakefulness [503, 1654, 1850], pulmonary artery pressure [1850] and maximal inspiratory pressure, and FVC [1653] may improve. A reduction in hospital admissions after treatment has also been documented [1850].

MOUTH INTERMITTENT POSITIVE PRESSURE VENTILATION

IPPV delivered through the mouth continuously for several hours should be distinguished from IPPB (Chapter 20) in which ventilatory support is only provided for short periods. The delivery of IPPV through the mouth has been limited by difficulties in achieving an adequate mouth seal. This is particularly a problem during sleep, if there is weakness of the orbicularis oris muscle, or if lung disease increases the peak inspiratory pressure. Lip seals, e.g. Bennett, have proved reasonably satisfactory [146(b)]. The nose is not covered but elevation of the soft palate during the inspiratory phase closes off the nasopharynx and limits the air leak through the nose. The ventilators that are used for nasal IPPV are also suitable for IPPV delivered through the mouth.

Mouth IPPV is usually used only to support ventilation during sleep, but it can also be effective during wakefulness. If air leaks develop during sleep or if there is a significant risk of displacement of the lip seal, nasal IPPV can be substituted and mouth IPPV used during the day. Mouth IPPV may fail if the soft palate does not prevent air from leaking through the nose. This is usually due to weakness of the soft palate as part of the neuromuscular disorder

that requires ventilatory assistance. If the cricopharyngeal sphincter is incompetent, air may enter the oesophagus and abdominal distension may develop [146(b)]. Long-term use of the lip seal may also lead to abnormalities of bite and, since the airway is not protected, the risk of aspiration pneumonia persists.

Despite these problems, ventilatory assistance using mouth IPPV can be of value. Improvements in ventilatory failure due to syringomyelia [204], poliomyelitis [146(b)] and other neuromuscular disorders [912], as well as the sequelae of tuberculosis [3384], have been recorded.

Chapter 20
Intermittent Positive Pressure Breathing (IPPB)

Intermittent positive pressure breathing (IPPB) was introduced in 1936 to treat pulmonary oedema [2522]. It was thought to have several advantageous actions, such as decreasing the work of the breathing and air flow resistance, improving the distribution of inspired gas, increasing alveolar ventilation and enabling bronchodilators to be administered efficiently [2891]. It became increasingly widely used until around 1975 [161, 2514]. The early encouraging results were, however, not confirmed by later studies [182] and the use of IPPB has steadily declined. Experience with this form of treatment has been gained mainly in patients with air flow obstruction, but it has been used also in neuromuscular and skeletal disorders and still has a small place in their management.

EQUIPMENT

Intermittent positive pressure breathing is usually delivered to the patient by a mouthpiece but a tight-fitting face mask can be used. It may be impossible to maintain a tight seal around the mouthpiece if the patient is confused or drowsy, if there is weakness of the orbicularis oris muscle (as in many of the neuromuscular disorders) or if a high positive pressure is delivered. The inspired gas traverses the upper respiratory tract so that humidification is not required. Compressed air is usually given but this may be enriched with oxygen if necessary and nebulized drugs, especially bronchodilators, may be administered.

Many models of IPPB apparatus have been used in the past. A modified Dustette vacuum cleaner [2028] was used as long ago as 1936 [2522] and in several subsequent studies [1336,

1803, 2028]. The IPPB ventilators that are currently most commonly used are:

BENNET AP-5B

Available from Puritan Bennett International Corporation, Heathrow Causeway, 152–176 Great South West Road, Hounslow, Middlesex, TW4 6JS. Cost approx. £600.

This is a pressure-cycled ventilator that has a flow-sensitive valve. It can be triggered by the patient and positive end expiratory pressure may be added. The maximal inspiratory pressure is 35 cmH$_2$O and the maximal inspiratory flow rate is 90 l/min.

BIRD MARK 7 RESPIRATOR

Available from Medical & Industrial Equipment Ltd, Falcon Road, Sowton Industrial Estate, Exeter, Devon, EX2 7NA. Cost approx. £1500.

This is a pressure-cycled ventilator, which can be patient-triggered or have a fixed respiratory rate. The sensitivity of the trigger, inspiratory flow rate, expiratory time and maximum inspiratory pressure can all be varied [1091].

CAPE TC 50 PORTABLE VENTILATOR

Available from Penlon Limited, Abingdon, Oxford, OX14 3PH.

This is a volume-preset, time-cycled ventilator. The tidal volume can be varied in the range 0–1200 ml, the respiratory frequency at 10–50 breaths/min and the inflation pressure at 10–70 cmH$_2$O.

PHYSIOLOGICAL EFFECTS

It might be anticipated that IPPB would inflate the lungs without the action of the respiratory muscles. Since expiration is largely passive, it would be expected that the oxygen consumption of respiration and any respiratory muscle fatigue would be reduced. In practice, these benefits are often not obtained because of an inability to coordinate respiration with the IPPB. This is particularly a problem with acutely ill patients. A failure to synchronize with the equipment may itself lead to agitation and increase the oxygen consumption. Extra inspiratory and expiratory effort is also required to combat the applied positive pressure [146(a)]. It has been demonstrated that the diaphragm is active during inspiration and the abdominal muscles are active during expiration, when positive pressure is applied [32, 298, 299, 423].

Coordination with IPPB is only possible if the pressure applied is comfortable for the patient. It is particularly difficult if there is a high peak inspiratory pressure or if the inspiratory flow rate is too low. A peak inspiratory pressure of $10-15$ cmH$_2$O is usually optimal but in some studies considerably higher pressures have been used [747, 1803]. The best-tolerated inspiratory waveform is the reversed ramp (in which the pressure falls throughout inspiration after an initial peak) without a negative expiratory phase [1587]. Incoordination can be overcome partially by patient-triggering of the ventilator, instead of using a fixed respiratory frequency [1587, 3092].

The positive inspiratory pressure may cause hyperinflation of the lungs. This is most marked if high inspiratory pressures are used [1587] or if there is air flow obstruction [550]. Hyperinflation is detrimental since it both shortens the inspiratory muscles and decreases the compliance of the chest wall and lungs. It is, however, uncommon in pure chest wall disease as long as the expiratory time is not greatly shortened [642, 747]. Intermittent positive pressure breathing increases the physiological dead space [1587, 3092], although the nitrogen washout time is unchanged [3180]. The ventilation to the bases appears to be reduced during IPPB [456] and the high alveolar pressure compresses the capillaries and alters the regional blood flow within the lungs. The cardiac output falls, particularly if the mean intrathoracic pressure is high [2891]. This disadvantage can be overcome partially by the addition of a negative expiratory phase, although this can lead to basal airway closure and is rarely used [1587, 1615]. The arterial oxygen saturation and PCO$_2$ may improve [260, 916] or deteriorate [293, 1198, 1615, 3092], but these changes reflect the degree of coordination with IPPB more than any changes in the distribution of ventilation and perfusion.

Measurement of the changes in compliance following IPPB have given conflicting results. The dynamic compliance of the lungs has been found to increase after IPPB in scoliosis [2947], and in a separate study the increase was greatest in those with the lowest initial compliance and the lowest TLC [642]. The dynamic compliance reflects air flow resistance as well as the elastic properties of the lungs and it is likely that the improvements that have been recorded are due to opening of basal airways by the deep breaths induced by the IPPB. In other studies, particularly in neuromuscular disorders such as the muscular dystrophies, a standardized number of deep breaths were taken before any measurements were made, and no effect of IPPB on compliance was detected [747, 1982] (Fig. 20.1). Any benefit of IPPB, therefore, appears to be due to the increase in tidal volume. An improvement in compliance would only be expected if spontaneous deep breaths and sighs are impossible for neurological reasons, because of severe respiratory muscle weakness or because of a markedly decreased compliance of the lungs or chest wall.

Opening of the basal airways not only improves ventilation and perfusion matching, but decreases the work of the respiratory muscles by improving the lung compliance. It is uncertain how long these benefits are maintained but in one study the improvements were still present two and a half hours after treatment [2947]. The

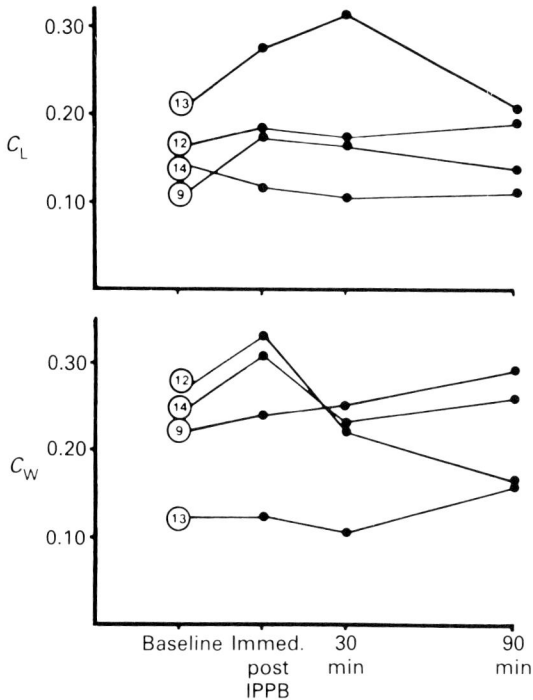

Fig. 20.1. *Effect of IPPB on lung (C_L) and chest wall (C_W) compliance. Any small initial improvements are not maintained. Reproduced, with permission, from McCool F.D. et al. Chest 1986;* **90**: *546–52.*

improvement in compliance is related to the increase of tidal volume during IPPB [2947]; volume rather than pressure-cycled ventilators are therefore more reliably effective [2075, 2936].

INDICATIONS

The most common situations in which IPPB is considered are:

Acute respiratory failure

Intermittent positive pressure breathing is of little value in acute respiratory failure because of the difficulties of coordination experienced by patients who are seriously ill, particularly if they are confused. In this situation, IPPB is tiring [1615] and often confers no physiological benefit. It can only be used intermittently and rarely avoids the need for more effective ventilation such as IPPV or tank ventilation.

Chronic respiratory failure

The value of IPPB in chronic respiratory failure is limited because, in contrast with the various forms of IPPV, it can only be used for short periods of time and while the patient is awake. It is usually administered for about 15 min four times a day, but can be used for longer periods.

Intermittent positive pressure breathing has been used widely in chronic respiratory failure due to neuromuscular and skeletal disorders, but its value has not been demonstrated convincingly. Its main benefit appears to be to increase the lung compliance by opening basal airways in a similar way to frog breathing (p. 286) and incentive spirometry (p. 283). This may be of value if the respiratory muscles are weak or if there is an inability to sigh. Intermittent positive pressure breathing probably has little effect on hypoxia and hypercapnia during sleep, and nocturnal ventilatory support is frequently needed in addition to IPPB during the day [857, 989, 996, 2803]. Intermittent positive pressure breathing can be of value in quadriplegics when IPPV or diaphragmatic pacing is discontinued for short periods in the daytime. It can be used in conjunction with an abdominal exsufflation belt if the action of these two forms of equipment is synchronized [1237]. Intermittent positive pressure breathing has been used to provide respiratory support so that oxygen can be given without the danger of the P_{CO_2} rising [1027], but other more reliable methods of ventilatory assistance are preferable.

In quadriplegics IPPB can increase the $P_{I_{max}}$ and $P_{E_{max}}$, TLC, VC, MVV and the expiratory reserve volume [1054, 1494] and is of use particularly during chest infections since it increases the strength of the cough [259, 1054]. Early studies in poliomyelitis showed that the symptoms of respiratory failure [1336], VC [2028], and FRC and blood gases [1803] all improved. Intermittent positive pressure breathing has been used extensively in Duchenne's muscular dystrophy [8, 58, 147, 434, 1578, 1984] but there is very little evidence regarding its effectiveness. It is of no benefit in dystrophia myotonica [595, 596]. It has been reported to be of value in selected patients with the sequelae of tuberculosis [1722, 3198] and scoliosis [260, 1722], although recent work has not confirmed these findings [1441, 2400].

Intermittent positive pressure breathing has been used widely in chronic air flow obstruction but it has been shown to be of no benefit in the long term when it is used without nebulized drugs [699, 1932, 2400, 3157]. It is less certain whether it has any long-term benefit in skeletal and neuromuscular disorders. There are several reports, particularly from France, indicating that the blood gases can improve, time spent in hospital lessened, and survival prolonged by IPPB [271, 273, 1627, 1722, 1880, 2199]. However, all these studies are uncontrolled and include patients with a variety of restrictive disorders, often with chronic air flow obstruction as well.

Bronchodilator administration

Intermittent positive pressure breathing has been used for many years as an effective way of administering nebulized drugs, particularly bronchodilators [2231, 2891]. However, its value has recently been doubted [2326, 2892] and careful trials have shown that it has no benefit over air compressors [550, 1532].

Post-operatively

Intermittent positive pressure breathing is still used widely, particularly in the USA [2349] to prevent post-operative pulmonary complications. There is very little evidence for its value [2514]. The VC may increase with IPPB [538] but this is rarely any greater than that which can be achieved by verbal encouragement to breathe deeply and by conventional physiotherapy exercises [1980].

Chapter 21
Nasal Continuous Positive Airway Pressure (CPAP)

Continuous positive airway pressure (CPAP) can be delivered orally or nasally. Oral CPAP has been used widely but is limited by difficulties with the mouth seal and because the airway is not protected [676, 1702]. Nasal CPAP has been feasible for several years [1624, 1625] but it was not until 1981 that it was shown to be effective in eliminating obstructive sleep apnoeas [3099]. Closure of the upper airway is prevented as long as an adequate positive pressure is maintained within the airway during the respiratory cycle.

EQUIPMENT

The delivery of air to the nasal airway under pressure is achieved by fitting either a flexible mask or a moulded nosepiece closely to the face (Fig. 21.1). Nasal catheters [3063] are not as satisfactory and nasal foam cannulae, although comfortable, do not sustain CPAP reliably be-

cause of the considerable air leakage [3336]. Thin nasopharyngeal cannulae that are inserted beyond the soft palate have, however, been used successfully [1705]. A nasal mask or nosepiece must be fixed securely over the nose so that it is not dislodged during sleep.

The nasal attachment is connected by tubing to a pump that compresses the inspired air. This should be capable of flow rates of about 100 l/min. These high flow rates are required so that even when the inspiratory flow rate is greatest the ventilation of the subject remains a small proportion of the output of the pump and makes little difference to the applied pressure. The pump should be able to maintain as nearly a constant pressure as possible despite any change in flow rates, but it should not be able to generate high pressures if air flow is obstructed.

The inspiratory resistance of the system should be low in order to prevent upper airway collapse induced by strong inspiratory efforts to overcome the resistance. A high inspiratory resistance is analogous to a raised upper airway resistance in the way that it predisposes to downstream collapse of the upper airway (p. 66). The resistance of the system can be gauged by measuring the pressure swings in the nose during breathing. These should be around 1 cmH_2O [3098].

The pressure within the system is controlled by altering the resistance to expiration. A positive end expiratory pressure valve or, more simply, a clip on the expiratory tubing that can be altered manually, are satisfactory. It is not usually necessary to warm or humidify the inspired gas, despite the high flow rates.

The most satisfactory nasal CPAP systems currently available are:

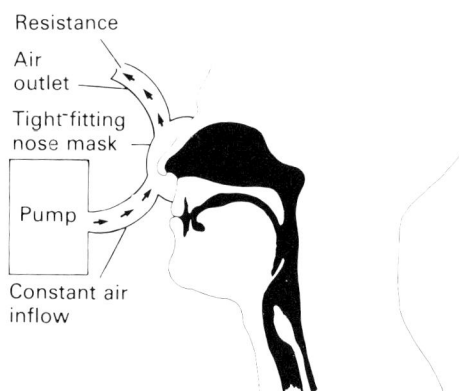

Fig. 21.1. *Diagrammatic representation of nasal CPAP system.*

Resistance
Air outlet
Tight fitting nose mask
Pump
Constant air inflow

Respironics Sleepeasy Nasal CPAP System

Available from Medic-Aid Limited, Hook Lane, Pagham, Sussex, PO21 3PP. Cost approx. £800.

The nasal mask is comfortable and efficient. It is supplied in three sizes and is easily secured to the head. The rotary pump is capable of flow rates of over 150 l/min and has a satisfactory pressure–flow relationship. It is fitted with an air filter and the maximum pressure is 20 cmH$_2$O. The expiratory resistance is controlled by valves that provide 5, 7.5, 10.0, 12.5 or 15 cmH$_2$O pressure. The original PVC mask has been superseded by a silicone mask. A 'Sanders circuit' is available. This reduces the volume of air delivered to the patient but maintains the present pressure.

Pression +

Available from SEFAM, Parc d'Activites de Brabois, rue du Bois de la Sivrite, F-54500 Vandoeuvre-les-Nancy, France. Cost approx. £1400.

The nasal mask adapts to the contours of the patient's face and is held in place by straps that are fixed behind the ears. The masks are light and are supplied in three sizes. The rotary pump is quiet and capable of 72 l/min. The circuit has a low resistance and pressure is continuously adjustable in the range 3–16 cmH$_2$O.

CPAP circuit

Available from Thomas Respiratory Systems, 3 Cholmeley Crescent, Highgate, London, N6 5EZ. Cost approx. £550.

The SEFAM nasal mask is used with a rotary pump, which is large and has an air filter. The expiratory resistance valve is spring-loaded.

PHYSIOLOGICAL EFFECTS

Nasal CPAP increases the pressure in the upper airway and prevents its collapse during inspiration. Its most important action is to act as a 'pneumatic splint', opposing the forces that favour occlusion of the airway (Chapter 6). The pressure required is determined for each patient and is usually 5–15 cmH$_2$O, measured at end expiration. A safety margin of 1–2 cmH$_2$O should be allowed above the pressure required to abolish apnoeas. An adequate airway pressure has to be maintained throughout inspiration and in all phases of sleep. A higher pressure is required during REM than during NREM sleep because the tone of the upper airway muscles is reduced.

Nasal CPAP may fail if large volumes of air leak out of the mouth, since this dissipates the pressure within the upper airway. The soft palate and tongue are pushed away from the posterior pharyngeal wall when the pressure is applied, so that they meet to provide a seal. This may not be complete in normal subjects but in those with frequent obstructive sleep apnoeas an adequate seal is almost always achieved. If high pressure develops in the upper airway for any reason, breathing can continue through the mouth since the pressure is applied only to the nose. In rare cases, however, hypoxaemia worsens [1766], probably because the epiglottis is blown downwards so that it obstructs the airway [79].

The primary action of nasal CPAP is, therefore, to hold the upper airway open. Positive airway pressure applied purely during expiration has been reported to be equally effective [2034], although this would not be expected to influence directly the size of the upper airway during inspiration. This observation has not been confirmed. Nevertheless, positive airway pressure may initiate or alter upper airway reflexes that influence respiratory drive or muscle tone (p. 10). These reflexes could change the balance of activation between the dilators and the constrictors of the upper airway and between the upper airway and chest wall muscles, particularly the diaphragm, or it could alter the coordinated activity of these muscles (p. 33). Various aspects of respiratory drive, including V_T/T_I and V_T/T_E, are modified by positive pressure breathing [300], and changes in the EMG activity of the genioglossus [2561] but not of the alae nasi [3083] have been noted.

Continuous positive airway pressure also increases the end expiratory volume. This effect is less than might be expected from the expiratory pressure because of changes in respiratory muscle tone [300] and abdominal muscle reflex activity [298, 299]. The changes in lung volume may alter the matching of ventilation and perfusion.

The high intrathoracic pressure during CPAP diminishes venous return and cardiac output [2465, 3228], but this complication appears to be of little importance. High pressure in the upper airway can cause mucosal changes in the nose and barotrauma to the ears, but these are infrequent [2598]. The cricopharyngeal sphincter can normally withstand at least 20 cmH_2O positive pressure and prevents gastric distension. There is, however, a risk of gastric distension if this sphincter is weak or in the presence of oesophageal disease, especially when high pressures are applied.

INDICATIONS

Nasal CPAP suffers from the disadvantage that some patients find the nasal attachments uncomfortable and are unable to tolerate the treatment for long. The high flow rates of air dry the upper respiratory tract and the positive pressure itself may be poorly tolerated [2769, 3251]. Air leaks around the mask may cause corneal ulceration and the pressure of the mask may ulcerate the skin of the nose. Nevertheless, the majority of patients are able to continue with treatment in the long term [1049, 1541, 1763, 2768, 2769, 3097].

The main indication for nasal CPAP is for patients with complications of obstructive sleep apnoeas, such as somnolence, respiratory failure and right heart failure. It usually leads to an immediate and dramatic improvement. It is effective in the obese [268, 3096] but may not be of value after UPPP because an adequate seal between any remaining soft palate and the tongue may not be obtainable. Daytime somnolence can be relieved [2554, 2773, 3095, 3096, 3100], often after only one or two night's treatment.

Snoring is usually completely abolished [268] with a pressure as low as 2–6 cmH_2O [1544, 1546]. The sleep pattern improves with a return of REM sleep and stages 3 and 4 NREM sleep [1763, 2554, 2562, 2773]. Computerized tomography scans have shown that the pharynx is wider during nasal CPAP than without treatment [2561] and obstructive and mixed sleep apnoeas become less frequent and shorter [1541, 1990, 2554, 2561, 2768, 2771, 3095, 3099]. The degree of oxygen desaturation during these apnoeas is diminished [2554, 2768] but central apnoeas may persist [1541, 2768, 2771, 3099, 3251] unless high pressures are applied (see below). The haemoglobin concentration falls if hypoxia is abolished [1049] and the ventilatory response to hypercapnia may improve within a few days if hypercapnia is present during wakefulness [270] (Fig. 21.2).

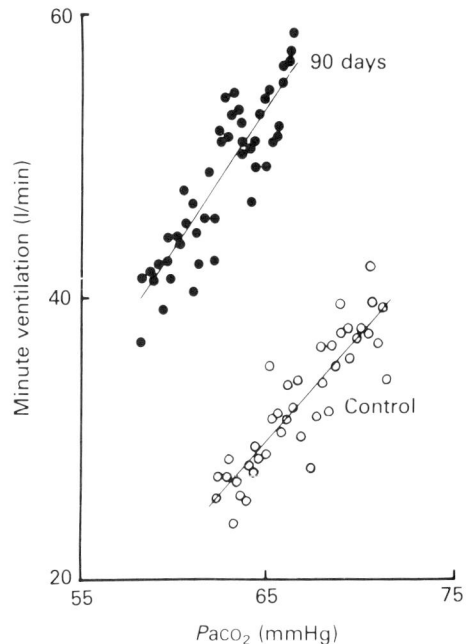

Fig. 21.2. *Breath-by-breath ventilatory responses to rebreathing CO_2 in one patient before and after 90 days treatment with nasal CPAP. Reproduced, with permission, from Berthon-Jones M. & Sullivan C.E. Am. Rev. Respir. Dis. 1987; 135: 144–7.*

The rapid improvement in symptoms is often an incentive to continue with treatment, but some patients prefer not to use nasal CPAP once they feel better. In some reports a course of 2–5 weeks' treatment has been sufficient to initiate a remission, which is maintained for a considerable period [3095, 3096]. However, obstructive sleep apnoeas may reappear immediately after the cessation of treatment [2770] unless the cause of the apnoea, such as obesity, is treated, and nasal CPAP is usually required indefinitely [3100].

Nasal CPAP has also been recommended for central sleep apnoeas [1447, 1764, 3098]. It may not be reliably effective at pressures of < 15 cmH$_2$O, which are usually sufficient to abolish obstructive sleep apnoeas [2554]; pressures as high as 20 cmH$_2$O may be required [1546]. The increase in upper airway pressure may prevent central apnoeas by reflexly increasing upper airway tone or changing the respiratory drive through stimulation of mechanoreceptors.

Chapter 22
Diaphragmatic Pacing (Electrophrenic Respiration)

HISTORICAL DEVELOPMENT

Electric currents have been employed thera-peutically in a wide variety of respiratory and other conditions [2811, 2848]. Phrenic nerve stimulation was used by Ure in 1818 in order to contract the diaphragm and produce abdom-inal movement in a cadaver. Prior to this, it had been employed in dogs in 1756 by Caldani in an attempt to achieve artificial respiration, and had been proposed for neonatal asphyxia by Hufeland in 1783 [2811]. Interest in phrenic nerve stimulation revived in the middle of the nineteenth century and it was applied success-fully to humans by Duchenne in 1871 [848]. He stimulated the phrenic nerve in the neck by an external electrode and interrupted the cur-rent to allow expiration. This technique was utilized by Israel from 1927 [1538, 1539] and subsequently by Cross [689], to maintain venti-lation in neonates.

In 1937 Waud showed that phrenic nerve stimulation could maintain ventilation in rabbits [3267] but it was the work of Sarnoff and his colleagues that laid the foundations for dia-phragmatic pacing in man. In a series of studies commencing in 1948, they described many of the physiological effects of phrenic nerve stimu-lation [2789–2791, 2794, 3323]. They also dem-onstrated the 'motor point' of the phrenic nerve on the anterior surface of the anterior scalene muscle under the sternomastoid muscle [2793]. They used a 'thimble' electrode placed on the index finger for locating the phrenic nerve and stimulating it percutaneously [2788]. They even implanted an electrode in one patient [3323]. This demonstrated that long-term phrenic nerve stimulation was a possibility, but it was not until

1966 that this was first achieved by Glenn and his colleagues [1596]. Since that date, phrenic nerve stimulation has been introduced as a diag-nostic technique (p. 101–102), as well as for ventilatory support.

The equipment and methods of stimulation have been refined but stimulation of the phrenic nerve has remained superior to other techniques that have been proposed for diaphragmatic pac-ing. Direct stimulation of the diaphragm has been shown to be possible [1581, 2244, 2321] but has not been widely used. After injury to the phrenic nerve, anastomosis to the vagus and subsequent electrical stimulation of the vagus has been proposed [3344], but this has not been tried in humans. A similar technique for anas-tomosing the phrenic to the brachial nerve has been successful in cats [1749]. Electrical stimu-lation of the spinal cord is not feasible in man, although it is effective in animals such as dogs [2388, 2389].

SURGICAL TECHNIQUE

Phrenic nerve stimulation is best achieved by surgical implantation of an electrode around the phrenic nerve. Transvenous pacing, although effective, has never proved popular [926, 2485, 3044, 3219] and, in any case, it is only possible to stimulate the right phrenic nerve through the lateral aspect of the superior vena cava. Pacing of the left hemidiaphragm can be achieved by placing an electrode in the pulmonary artery, but carries the risk of ventricular fibrillation if it is displaced [1063].

The technique of electrode implantation is well established [1139, 1145, 1150]. The phrenic nerve is most easily explored in the neck and the electrode is carefully secured around it. However, it is common for accessory phrenic nerves to join the main trunk below the clavicle (p. 27) and escape stimulation. Electrical stimulation may also spread to the brachial plexus, causing troublesome contractions of the muscles of the arm or hand. For these reasons a thoracic approach is preferable, especially if there is any doubt about the normal functioning of the phrenic nerve or diaphragm [1145].

The best approach to the phrenic nerve is by an incision through the 2nd intercostal space anteriorly. A median sternotomy gives good access to both phrenic nerves, but the morbidity is greater with this incision. A lateral thoracotomy gives a poor view of the phrenic nerve but a low anterior incision is satisfactory. There is a small risk of ventricular fibrillation, however, if the electrode is implanted over the pericardium. Bilateral electrodes can be implanted simultaneously, although this carries a small risk of infection of both phrenic nerves [2016]. Prophylactic antibiotics should be given

pre-operatively and for 24 h after surgery. It is essential to minimize any trauma to the nerve at the time of electrode implantation and not to damage the fine blood vessels that surround it.

The electrode is connected to a receiver, which is placed subcutaneously (Fig. 22.1). The best site for implantation of the receiver is over the rib cage laterally, where it is accessible, where there is little hair and where it can be more securely fixed than over the abdomen. The radio frequency output from the transmitter may interfere with demand cardiac pacemakers and the receiver should be implanted at a distance of at least 5 cm and preferably >10 cm from the pacemaker [3326]. The risk of interference is less with bipolar than with monopolar electrodes.

The receiver is controlled by an external transmitter, which determines the electric current that is generated around the phrenic nerves by the implanted electrodes. None of the available diaphragm pacing systems include an implantable transmitter because the energy required for phrenic nerve stimulation is so great

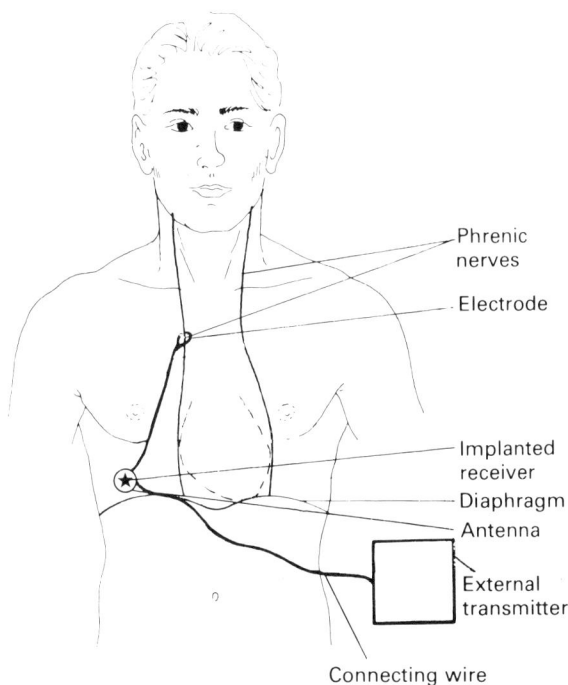

Fig. 22.1. *Diaphragmatic pacing system. The electrode is shown applied to the right phrenic nerve and is connected to an implanted subcutaneous receiver. The antenna is placed on the skin and linked to the external transmitter.*

Phrenic nerves

Electrode

Implanted receiver

Diaphragm

Antenna

External transmitter

Connecting wire

that frequent battery changes would be necessary. Implantable radioactive sources of energy, such as plutonium-238 with a half-life of 89 years, have been used in experimental animals [1063] but would not be suitable for humans. The development of miniaturized but powerful and long-lasting batteries may soon enable the whole pacing system to be implanted. The system could then be controlled by changes in arterial blood gas levels while retaining the facility to program it externally.

EQUIPMENT

Electrodes

The electrical properties of the phrenic nerve are described quite accurately by conventional cable theory, so that it can be regarded as having a conducting core and a high-resistance sheath. Depolarization of the axons within the phrenic nerve takes place only at the nodes of Ranvier [1968]. The resting potential within the axon is negative and depolarization occurs at the cathode electrode. This requires a voltage that generates sufficient flow of current across the cell membrane to change the potential by about 15 mV. Depolarization takes place most readily if the current passes parallel to the axis of the nerve [2729].

The electrodes that are used for phrenic nerve stimulation contain platinum, to minimize corrosion and polarization [3044], and are nontoxic. Damage to the phrenic nerves may be caused by electrochemical reactions due to the flow of current. Electrodes that encircle the phrenic nerve probably restrict its growth and should be avoided in children. Growth may also lead to tension developing in the implanted components unless a loop of the connecting wire is loosely coiled, for instance, inside a Teflon bag situated subcutaneously. A biphasic current enables depolarization to be achieved with no net flow of current and probably decreases the risk of tissue damage [1140, 1617]. The risk of electrical damage to the phrenic nerve is small but is thought to be reduced by minimizing the amount of current delivered to each axon within the nerve. If a monopolar electrode is used, most or all of the axons are stimulated with each pulse of current, but if a bipolar or even quadripolar electrode is implanted, the frequency of stimulation of each axon is reduced. Each of the two or four implanted electrodes is activated in rotation and is thought to stimulate half of a quadrant of the nerve. The interval between each stimulation, therefore, is longer. This lessens the risk of diaphragmatic fatigue (see below) as well as phrenic nerve damage.

Receiver

The stimulating electrode is connected to a receiver that is implanted subcutaneously. The receiver is enclosed in an epoxyresin case, which is inert and hermetically seals it. There are no batteries within the receiver and it does not need to be replaced unless there is a mechanical or electrical fault.

The receiver converts the radio frequency electromagnetic waves from the transmitter to an electric current. Capacitors within the receiver store the electrical energy and produce a pulse of current after the radio frequency stimulation has ceased.

Transmitter

The activity of the implanted electrode and receiver is controlled by an external transmitter. This may be powered by the mains electricity supply or by a battery which enables the patient to be mobile. The transmitter signal is coupled to the implanted receiver by an antenna, which is placed on the skin overlying it.

The transmitter emits radio frequency waves as an interrupted pulse train. The duration of each pulse determines the amount of current that is applied to the phrenic nerve and the interval between each pulse determines the frequency of electrical stimulation. The pulse amplitude is a poor method of coupling the antenna to the receiver, since it decreases as the distance between them increases. Both the pulse duration and pulse interval can be varied within a single inspiration, to achieve a physiological pattern of air flow (see below). The respiratory frequency, T_I and, less directly, the tidal volume can be controlled by altering the transmitter settings. Expiration occurs passively but can be retarded by maintaining some stimulation of the phrenic nerve early in expiration. Deep breaths ('sighs') can be introduced. If bilateral electrodes are implanted each hemidiaphragm may be stimulated for a period or on alternate breaths, or the whole diaphragm may be made to function with each respiration.

Diaphragmatic pacing systems are available from:

1 Avery Laboratories AG, Fraumunsterstrasse 13, CH-8001, Zurich. Cost approx. £15 000. Monopolar and bipolar electrodes and a portable transmitter powered by a 9-V battery are available. Receiver failure is common between 18 months and 5 years after implantation.

2 Atrotech OY, SF-38300, Kiikka, Finland. Cost approx. £15 000. This system is battery powered. The quadripolar electrode is arranged so that the four stimulating points surround the phrenic nerve and excite most of the axons with a lower current than is possible with a monopolar or bipolar electrode. This not only leads to an almost simultaneous contraction of the whole diaphragm but lessens the risk of phrenic nerve damage. The frequency of stimulation of each axon is slower so that diaphragmatic fatigue can be avoided, even with continuous stimulation.

3 MedImplant, Biotechnisches Labor, Laudongasse 10, A-1080 Vienna VIII, Austria. Cost approx. £15 000. This system can be powered either by mains electricity or battery. The quadripolar electrodes provide a sequential stimulation of the phrenic nerve axons.

PHYSIOLOGICAL EFFECTS

Force of diaphragmatic contraction

The force of diaphragmatic contraction during phrenic nerve stimulation is determined by the type of electrode and its closeness to the nerve, the frequency of stimulation, the current applied by the electrode, the contractile properties of the diaphragm and its length and configuration. As the frequency of stimulation increases, the individual diaphragmatic twitches fuse into a smooth tetanic contraction. The frequency–force curve of the diaphragm is similar to that of other skeletal muscles (Chapter 2). The force increases with the frequency up to about 30 Hz, but above this there is little further change. As the flow of current is increased, more motor neurons are stimulated and the force of contraction increases. This is analogous to the physiological recruitment of motor neurons during spontaneous breathing when the strength of diaphragmatic contraction increases. The difference is that with electrical stimulation the larger axons supplying type 2 muscle fibres are stimulated at lower currents than the smaller axons to the type 1 fibres. This results in a reversal of the normal sequence of activation so that the more easily fatiguable fibres are stimulated most readily.

The pattern of the diaphragmatic contraction is dependent on the rate of change of the radio frequency stimulation [785, 2181]. A smooth increase in the force of contraction is most effective and best tolerated, and is achieved by gradually increasing the current and the stimulation frequency applied to the phrenic nerve.

Diaphragmatic fatigue

Electrical stimulation of the phrenic nerve is capable of causing diaphragmatic fatigue (Fig. 22.2). The susceptibility of the diaphragm to fatigue may decrease once pacing is established. Experimental studies have shown that muscle fibres can change their properties according to their frequency of stimulation. Ultrastructural, histochemical and physiological changes appear and type 2 fibres can convert to type 1 fibres with prolonged low-frequency stimulation [2760, 2761]. The resistance to fatigue increases [575] and microcirculatory and other changes seen with endurance training also develop (p.

Waveform: Bidirectional (Lilly)
Electrode: Monopolar
Current level: Maximal Stim.
Respiratory rate: 20/min.

Stimulating frequency;

●——● 13 – 11 Hz (5 studies)

〈——〈 26 – 24 Hz (5 studies)

×——× 36 – 29 Hz (5 studies
          except as noted
          ■ 4 studies, ■■ 3 studies)

Waveform: Bidirectional (Lilly)
Electrode: Monopolar
Current level: Maximal Stim.
Stimulating frequency:
≈ 25 Hz (P.I. = 40 msec)

Respiratory rate:

●——● 10/min (3 studies)

○——○ 20/min (3 studies)

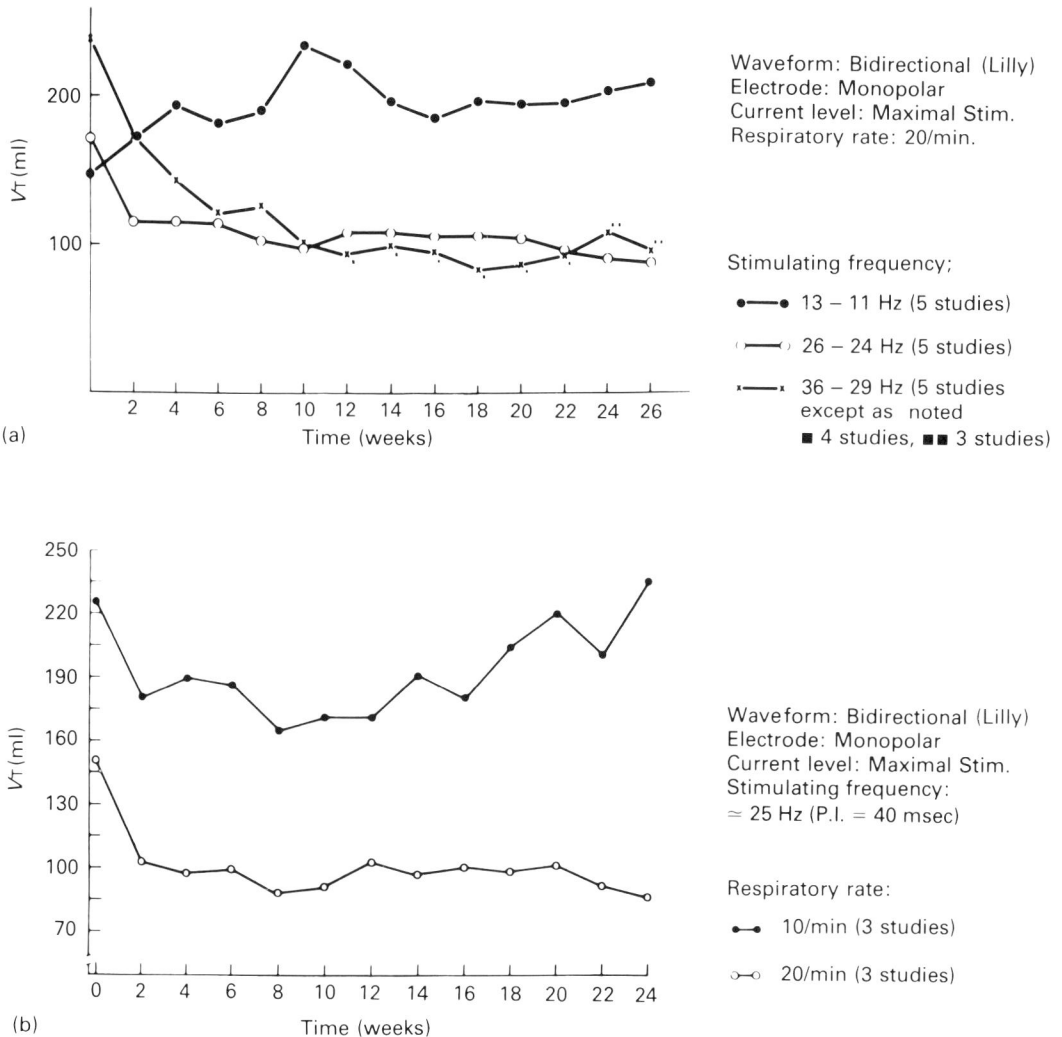

Fig. 22.2. *Development of diaphragmatic fatigue, indicated by a fall in tidal volume, during phrenic nerve stimulation. (a) Effect of electrical stimulation frequency, (b) effect of respiratory frequency. Reproduced, with permission, from Oda T. J.Surg.Res. 1981;* **30:,** *147.*

287). Muscle fibre adaptation is an important aspect of prolonged low-frequency phrenic nerve stimulation and can alter the frequency–transdiaphragmatic pressure curve and the stimulation frequency at which a tetanic contraction is seen [2323]. Endurance increases but the maximal force that can be exerted by the diaphragm is reduced.

Diaphragmatic fatigue used to be common if pacing was continued for more than 12 h

continuously but with better realization of the factors responsible, continuous pacing is now possible without fatigue appearing. Fatigue is especially a problem with high stimulation frequencies, if the T_I/T_{TOT} ratio increases, or if the current applied is close to that which gives the maximal tidal volume [2348]. The T_I/T_{TOT} usually increases with respiratory frequency because T_E shortens more than T_I. With a monopolar electrode a stimulation frequency of

< 20 Hz, with a respiratory frequency of about 10–12 breaths/min or even slower and a maximal or near maximal tidal volume, is satisfactory [1140, 1144]. With quadripolar electrodes, fatigue appears to be less of a problem [1617]. A higher respiratory frequency of around 14 breaths/min is tolerated and T_1 can be prolonged to about 1.6 sec without fatigue developing.

Inhibition of respiratory muscle activity

The early observations of phrenic nerve stimulation suggested that inspiratory muscle activity ceased in all the other respiratory muscles including the contralateral hemidiaphragm [2790, 2793, 3323]. This acts as if it were paralysed and moves paradoxically during inspiration [1501, 2016, 2789]. The rib cage may also move paradoxically [373], particularly in children in whom it is more compliant than in adults.

This inhibition of respiratory muscle activity is independent of the respiratory frequency, P_{O_2} or P_{CO_2} [2794] but probably has a similar mechanism to the relief of inspiratory muscle activity that is seen during tank and cuirass ventilation (p. 227). This may also explain the frequent failure of contraction of the abductor muscles of the vocal cords during phrenic nerve stimulation [1521]. The pressure within the trachea is less than atmospheric pressure during the inspiratory phase and the vocal cords adduct. This obstructs the upper airway and can prevent adequate ventilation from being achieved [1139, 1141, 1143, 1501, 1514]. Because the air flow obstruction occurs at the level of the larynx, treatments such as nasal CPAP, which are effective in obstructive apnoeas due to pharyngeal obstruction, may not always be effective. A tracheostomy may be required.

Alveolar ventilation

Unilateral diaphragm pacing is usually sufficient to maintain adequate ventilation [402, 3323] but if the phrenic nerve or diaphragm are partially damaged, bilateral pacing is required [2612]. This is also needed if there is air flow obstruction or a low compliance of the lungs or chest wall or paradoxical movement of the chest wall.

During unilateral pacing, the pleural pressure falls bilaterally but to a greater extent on the stimulated side [713, 2180]. The ventilation of the contralateral lung is, nevertheless, almost as great as that on the side of the pacing [1596, 2789, 2793] and the mediastinal shift that is seen in children [1139] is uncommon in adults [1751, 2789]. Ventilation/perfusion matching is maintained in both lungs, even during unilateral pacing [923, 1016, 2179]. The fall in pulmonary artery pressure is not purely due to relief of hypoxic pulmonary arterial vasoconstriction since it cannot be reproduced by breathing oxygen [1147, 1809]. It seems probable that better expansion of the bases of the lungs is associated with increased perfusion because of recruitment of previously closed blood vessels, and that this lowers the pulmonary vascular resistance.

INDICATIONS

Phrenic nerve stimulation is an alternative to other methods of ventilatory support, particularly negative pressure ventilation and IPPV. The relative merits of each of these methods of treatment should be considered carefully before phrenic nerve stimulation is attempted. Ventilatory failure should not only be sufficiently severe to require treatment but should also be required in the long term. Phrenic nerve stimulation has been employed temporarily to assist the rehabilitation of patients with severe muscle weakness, particularly with quadriplegia [402], but other forms of treatment that do not require a surgical approach are usually preferable. Nevertheless, many of the patients who require phrenic nerve stimulation are otherwise completely dependent on mechanical ventilation, and the relative freedom that this allows can increase the quality of their lives as well as the potential for rehabilitation. A tracheostomy is often required because of adduction of the vocal cords during diaphragmatic pacing, but frequently this has already been constructed to enable IPPV to be carried out before phrenic nerve stimulation is considered.

Phrenic nerve stimulation may be indicated if there is:

Normal phrenic nerve function

The axons in the phrenic nerve degenerate if either the phrenic nerve nucleus in C3–C5 segments of the spinal cord or the nerve itself are damaged. With lesions higher in the cervical cord, in the medulla or in other regions of the brain, the viability of the phrenic nerve axons is retained. Phrenic nerve stimulation is, therefore, not effective following trauma or other damage to the spinal cord at the C3–C5 level or to the phrenic nerve itself. The methods of testing nerve function, such as the phrenic nerve conduction time, are described in Chapter 9. Diaphragmatic pacing is usually possible if the conduction time is normal or slightly prolonged, as long as it is < 14 msec [2887]. Serial measurements of the phrenic nerve conduction time are useful in assessing phrenic nerve damage both before [1897] and after implantation of the pacing electrode.

Normal diaphragmatic function

Weakness of the diaphragm may be due to failure of phrenic nerve activation, to an intrinsic disorder of the diaphragm itself, or to the diaphragm working at a mechanical disadvantage because of changes in its length or configuration. Phrenic nerve stimulation is only effective in the first of these situations. It is of no value in the primary disorders of muscles, such as the myopathies. The methods of assessing diaphragmatic function have been described in Chapter 9, but some of these tests may be impossible to carry out in patients who are being considered for phrenic nerve stimulation. The amplitude of the diaphragmatic EMG during phrenic nerve stimulation is of limited value because only part of the nerve may be stimulated [2887]. Descent of the diaphragm by 5 cm or more on fluoro-scopic examination usually indicates that phrenic nerve pacing will be successful [1145].

Normal respiratory mechanics

Diaphragmatic pacing is much less effective if there is air flow obstruction or a decreased lung or chest wall compliance than if the lung and chest wall mechanics are normal. The position of the diaphragm appears to be particularly important in determining the force generated during stimulation [1362]. Patients with ventilatory failure due to chronic air flow obstruction obtain little benefit from phrenic nerve stimulation, but further experience is required in skeletal disorders of the thorax.

These criteria for pacing are most commonly fulfilled by patients with central alveolar hypoventilation or frequent central sleep apnoeas and those with high cervical cord lesions. These form the vast majority of the 600 subjects who have been treated by phrenic nerve stimulation [1151]. It has, however, also been employed in chronic air flow obstruction to enable oxygen to be administered without the risk of hypercapnia developing [1139, 1142, 1146], in chronic diaphragmatic myoclonus [3323] and in intractable hiccough [1012].

Phrenic nerve stimulation has been successful in both neonatal [1501, 1521, 1922, 2113, 2122, 2546] and adult onset central alveolar hypoventilation [955, 1141], whether this is idiopathic or due to encephalitis [1139], cerebral ischaemia [1013, 1143], brain stem cysts and tumours [3389], multiple system atrophy [2016], following trauma to the posterior fossa [1139] or with foramen magnum abnormalities [1013, 1139, 1938]. Improvements in the P_{O_2} and P_{CO_2}, ventilatory response to hypercapnia, pulmonary artery pressure, right heart failure and polycythaemia have been demonstrated [955, 1146, 1147, 1515, 1596, 1809].

The majority of subjects with high cervical spinal cord lesions who benefit from phrenic nerve stimulation have suffered cervical cord trauma [462, 1011, 1139, 1145, 1148, 1149,

1948, 2341, 3033] but it is equally effective in other situations, such as following cordotomy [554, 1139, 2507] or in syringomyelia [1139, 1145, 1149]. Diaphragmatic pacing is occasionally of value in poliomyelitis [146(b), 1139, 1147, 2787, 2792] but only if the ventilatory failure is predominantly due to failure of the medullary respiratory centres rather than inspiratory muscle weakness or scoliosis.

It is usual to treat ventilatory failure in cervical cord injuries with IPPV until it is clear how much respiratory muscle function will recover. Phrenic nerve stimulation is occasionally employed to facilitate rehabilitation in the early phase after the injury [402], but IPPV is usually continued for 3–6 months until respiratory function is stable. Effective pacing is achieved in only about one-third of quadriplegic subjects [1149], possibly because of damage to the phrenic nerve nucleus at the time of injury. An abdominal binder is required in the upright position (p. 245). In quadriplegics the chest wall is flaccid due to intercostal muscle paralysis, and paradoxical movement will be exacerbated by phrenic nerve stimulation [2100]. If pacing is attempted unilaterally, the contralateral hemidiaphragm will also move paradoxically. Bilateral pacing, therefore, is usually required and a fail-safe alarm triggered, for instance, by movements of the head or tongue is required [65, 1140].

PACING SCHEDULES

The success or failure of diaphragmatic pacing requires close attention to the details of the pacing schedule. Damage to the phrenic nerve, diaphragmatic fatigue and inadequate ventilation are usually avoidable. The most important aspects of the pacing regimen are:

Duration of pacing

At the time of implantation of the electrode around the phrenic nerve, there is always an inflammatory reaction and it is usual to delay pacing for 10–14 days from the time of operation.

In subjects with brain stem disorders in whom there has been spontaneous diaphragmatic contraction before implantation of the electrode, the duration of phrenic nerve stimulation can be increased rapidly as long as fatigue does not develop. This can be detected by EMG and other techniques (Chapter 9) or more simply by estimating the V_T or minute ventilation before and after a period of pacing. Three hours of pacing can usually be tolerated initially and, if fatigue does not develop, overnight pacing can be attempted.

In high cervical cord lesions the diaphragm is usually atrophied because of prolonged disuse. Phrenic nerve stimulation needs to be introduced slowly to prevent muscle fatigue [1149]. It is usual to pace for about 10 min/h initially and to gradually increase the duration if fatigue does not develop. It may be several months before continuous pacing can be achieved. During this time, the repeated low-frequency stimulation induces fatigue resistance in the diaphragm. There is, however, some experimental evidence which indicates that intermittent electrical stimulation damages skeletal muscle, and it may prove preferable to pace the diaphragm continuously at very low frequencies initially and to gradually increase the frequency of stimulation.

Unilateral or bilateral pacing

The decision whether to stimulate one or both phrenic nerves depends on the age of the patient, whether pacing is required during wakefulness as well as during sleep, on the function of the phrenic nerves and diaphragm, and on the mechanics of the respiratory system (Table 22.1). Unilateral stimulation is sufficient for adult patients with central sleep apnoeas and central alveolar hypoventilation which is severe only at night. If treatment is required during the day as well, there is a risk of diaphragmatic fatigue with conventional pacing schedules. This can be avoided by alternating the stimulation of the two phrenic nerves at 12-hourly intervals. Alternatively, a single phrenic nerve can be stimulated during the day and mechanical

Table 22.1. *Indications for unilateral and bilateral diaphragmatic pacing*

Disorder	Unilateral	Bilateral
Central alveolar hypoventilation Central sleep apnoeas	1 Nocturnal pacing in adults 2 Continuous pacing in adults with newer pacing schedules 3 Daytime pacing in adults with conventional pacing schedules combined with nocturnal mechanical ventilation	1 All children 2 Continuous pacing in adults with conventional pacing schedules
High cervical cord lesions	Only in adults with no damage to C3–C5 segments and insignificant paradox induced by pacing	Most
Air flow obstruction or diminished lung or chest wall compliance	None	All

ventilation employed at night. If a tracheostomy is required, IPPV is usually used but negative pressure ventilation is preferable if a tracheostomy has not been constructed. With modern pacing schedules, it is possible to stimulate a single phrenic nerve continuously without causing phrenic nerve damage or diaphragm fatigue, thus avoiding bilateral implants and mechanical ventilation.

Some quadriplegics can also be ventilated continuously with alternating unilateral phrenic nerve stimulation, but paradoxical movement of the rib cage and of the contralateral diaphragm often necessitates bilateral simultaneous pacing. Bilateral stimulation is needed if damage to C3–C5 segments of the spinal cord impairs phrenic nerve function. With conventional pacing schedules an additional form of ventilatory assistance will be required for 12 h each day, but with modern electrodes and pacing schedules it may be possible to stimulate both phrenic nerves continuously without risking diaphragmatic fatigue.

In children, the compliant chest wall and contralateral diaphragm move paradoxically if unilateral pacing is attempted and bilateral implants are always required [462]. Bilateral stimulation is also required in adults if the air flow resistance is increased or if the lung or chest wall compliance is decreased, but even this may not maintain adequate ventilation.

Transmitter settings

The output from the transmitter can be altered so that the respiratory pattern is, to a large extent, controllable. These should be adjusted so that ventilation is adequate to maintain normal blood gases, usually measured continuously and non-invasively (p. 94), and should also minimize the risk of phrenic nerve damage or diaphragmatic fatigue. It is essential to reassess the transmitter settings at regular intervals after phrenic nerve stimulation has been initiated.

PACING FAILURE

Failure of the diaphragm pacing system may be manifested by a recurrence of the presenting symptoms or physical signs. It is essential to check that the patient understands the principles of the equipment, the controls of the transmitter and how to use the antenna. Malfunction of the pacing system may be indicated by a rising threshold for stimulation or a fall in V_T or transdiaphragmatic pressure, or a deterioration in the arterial blood gases with a given pattern of stimulation. It is, however, normal for the stimulation threshold to rise slightly during the first six months after implantation and then to fall slowly. The functioning of the pacing system should be reassessed regularly to detect any faults at an early stage.

Mechanical failure of the system is uncommon but may occur at any time after implantation of the electrodes. It is important to check that the battery is properly inserted into the transmitter and is fully charged, and that the connection with the mains electricity supply is functioning. The transmitter can be tested by placing an AM transistor radio close to it. When this is tuned to the frequency of the transmitter, a series of clicks should be heard in time with the radio frequency output of the transmitter. The antennae should be accurately centred over and securely fixed to the skin above the implanted receivers. The material encapsulating the receiver is not completely impervious and ingress of water occasionally causes it to fail. This may present during pacing as a sudden pain, referred to the neck from the phrenic nerve [1013, 1149]. Problems with the electrode and the wires between the receiver and the electrode are very uncommon, although the wire may break occasionally. This is usually detectable on a chest radiograph. Displacement of the electrode occurs particularly during the first two weeks after its insertion.

In the absence of these mechanical or electrical faults, the most common causes of failure of the pacing system soon after implantation are:

Incorrect patient selection

Patients with disorders of the phrenic nerve nuclei, phrenic nerve, diaphragm or with abnormal respiratory mechanics may not benefit from diaphragmatic pacing. An error in assessing the severity of these factors may be responsible for failure of pacing.

Phrenic nerve damage

The phrenic nerve may be damaged during implantation of the electrode because of trauma either to the nerve or to its blood supply during dissection or when securing the electrode. Damage may be permanent but, more frequently, phrenic nerve function returns within twelve to sixteen months [1149]. This represents the time for remyelination to take place. It would be anticipated that this would occur sooner with a thoracic than with a cervical approach, since the length of nerve that has to regrow is less. The phrenic nerve may also be damaged by postoperative infection.

Inappropriate pacing schedule

The pacing schedule has to be adjusted according to the state of the diaphragm. This has usually atrophied in quadriplegics, and pacing should be introduced more gradually than with disorders of the medullary respiratory centres.

Upper airway obstruction

Phrenic nerve stimulation may induce upper airway obstruction, which reduces ventilation. A tracheostomy may be necessary but other measures, such as nasal CPAP, may be effective.

Late failure of phrenic nerve stimulation is most commonly due to:

Diaphragmatic fatigue

This has been discussed on p. 273.

Phrenic nerve damage

The factors leading to phrenic nerve damage have been discussed on p. 272. Demyelination may be extensive and damage to the phrenic nerve may be permanent [1501, 1669, 1922]. Damage to the phrenic nerve not only causes a rising threshold for stimulation but also lengthens the phrenic nerve conduction time [1149, 2887]. Phrenic nerve damage and diaphragm fatigue can normally be avoided by the use of a suitable electrode and pacing schedule.

Displacement of electrode

Late displacement of the electrode is uncommon but has been recorded in a subject with a neurofibroma on the phrenic nerve [2611].

Newly acquired respiratory disorders

Pacing failure may also be due to the development of lung or chest wall disorders after the implantation of the electrodes. It is important to regularly assess the patient's condition as well as the functioning of the pacing system.

Chapter 23
Physiotherapy and Physical Training

The value of physiotherapy in respiratory failure has been belittled in recent years largely because of the lack of evidence for its efficacy. This is partly because several types of physical therapy are often given either simultaneously or sequentially. It has proved difficult to analyse how each component of the treatment works and which aspects are the most valuable. The decline in the popularity of physiotherapy has been paralleled by the development of effective mechanical equipment for assisting ventilation, but the benefits from physiotherapy can be considerable [1135].

The success of physiotherapy and physical training depends on the skill of the therapist in communicating with and encouraging the patient, and on the motivation of the patient. It is essential to practice the techniques and exercises regularly and to continue with them after the formal course of teaching has ceased [2169].

Physiotherapy techniques need to be tailored to the individual type of ventilatory disorder. Patterns of breathing, such as pursed-lips breathing, that are of value in air flow obstruction, especially emphysema, are not indicated in neuromuscular and skeletal disorders. Only the methods of treatment applicable to these conditions are considered in this chapter.

EXPECTORATION OF SECRETIONS

Sputum retention and inhalation of material from the pharynx are common features of several neuromuscular disorders in which the cough is weak or swallowing is inefficient. Assistance with the expectoration of secretions is one of the most important functions of the physiotherapist [1695, 2260]. Huffing, vibration, percussion, postural drainage and assistance with coughing may all be of value [1092]. In the forced expiration (huffing) technique, repeated forced expirations from around the FRC with an open glottis cause dynamic compression of airways deeper in the lungs than with the conventional method of coughing [2104]. This enables the smaller airways to be cleared of secretions [1695, 2539, 3119].

IMPROVING EFFICIENCY OF MOVEMENT

The oxygen required to carry out a given task varies considerably from person to person. It depends partly on the weight of the subject [724] but also on the efficiency of their movements. In scoliosis [1909], paraplegia [994], hemiplegia [190, 994] and multiple sclerosis [2358], the oxygen consumption during walking is greater than normal. In scoliosis this can be improved by spinal fusion, which both lessens the work of breathing and the amount of energy required to maintain a satisfactory posture while walking [1909]. Other activities such as bicycling are also performed inefficiently in neuromuscular disorders [501].

It is an important role of the physiotherapist to recognize inefficient patterns of movement and to teach the patient how to correct them. Muscular coordination can be improved by exercise training so that tasks can be carried out without necessarily any increase in the strength of the muscles [707, 1439, 2315]. Coordination of respiratory movements with those of the arms and legs is often beneficial. Exercise using the arms disrupts the coordination of the respiratory muscles to a greater extent than leg exercise since the accessory muscles of respiration are needed simultaneously both for the exercise and for respiration [674]. Synchronization of respiratory movements with leg movements may also increase the exercise ability. The best pattern of breathing is often to inspire while taking one or two steps and to breathe out for two or three steps.

The physiotherapist has an important role in improving the confidence of the patient and achieving relaxation. This reduces the oxygen consumption of the skeletal muscles and the compliance of the chest wall increases as the respiratory muscles relax. The effect of relaxation exercises may, however, be short-lived [482].

Patients are often unaware of how to carry out everyday activities in the home with the least energy expenditure. It is important not to move too fast and it may be helpful to rest between activities. The provision of suitable aids to minimize energy consumption may be invaluable and simple measures such as sitting down rather than standing up while cooking may be of help. Advice about posture is often valuable. It is usually preferable to sit leaning forward or to stand bending forward and rest the arms on a support [947].

'DIAPHRAGMATIC' BREATHING

In patients with extensive muscular weakness, exercises to improve the strength of the accessory muscles of the neck may be valuable and training of the abdominal muscles can improve the cough [22, 2169]. Physiotherapy to increase chest expansion and spinal flexibility is of value in ankylosing spondylitis [1593] and possibly in scoliosis. Specific respiratory muscle training is, however, most frequently directed at the diaphragm [947]. The patient is asked to put his dominant hand on the epigastrium and his other hand over his sternum [178, 2169, 2735]. During inspiration he should feel the dominant hand moving but his other hand remaining stationary. Diaphragmatic breathing exercises are usually

carried out while sitting, but the supine or even head-down position may be preferable. The addition of weights on the abdomen [22, 2735] or even a special spring-loaded abdominal belt [177] has been recommended to aid learning.

The term 'diaphragmatic' breathing implies that the diaphragm can be contracted selectively and the assumption is made that this is physiologically beneficial. The ability to selectively control the activity of the diaphragm has been disputed but is probably extremely rare [3248]. A few subjects can acquire the ability not to contract their diaphragm during inspiration [751, 3055] and it is even possible to learn to move only one side of the chest wall [2715]. Diaphragmatic breathing exercises are, in reality, exercises in which abdominal rather than rib cage expansion is encouraged. Abdominal expansion is determined not only by diaphragmatic contraction but also by abdominal muscle and, indirectly, intercostal and accessory muscle activity.

The second assumption that diaphragmatic breathing is more efficient than any other form of breathing has not been substantiated. The oxygen consumption of the respiratory muscles depends partly on whether the diaphragm is in the optimal position at the end of expiration. It has been suggested that in emphysema the trained diaphragm can be elevated to a greater extent at the end of expiration [183], but there is no direct evidence for this. In chronic air flow obstruction an increase in abdominal expansion may induce asynchronous or even paradoxical movement of the rib cage and abdomen [2737, 3339].

It has been proposed that diaphragmatic breathing improves the matching of ventilation and perfusion by increasing the ventilation to the bases of the lungs where the perfusion is greatest. Regional ventilation depends on the time constant (the product of compliance and air flow resistance) of the lung and on the regional transpulmonary pressure. Diaphragmatic breathing would not be expected to alter either compliance or air flow resistance. The regional transpulmonary pressure increases towards the bases of the lungs because of their weight. In dogs, the basal intrapleural pressure can be decreased by electrical stimulation of the phrenic nerves [2179, 2180], but the stiffer chest wall in man is not so easily distorted by diaphragmatic contraction and little change in the distribution of ventilation would be expected [1231]. Nitrogen washout and xenon studies have confirmed that there is no change in the distribution of ventilation during 'diaphragmatic' breathing [1231, 1257, 2739, 2889].

'Diaphragmatic' breathing exercises have been used widely but have been subjected to little critical study. In emphysema, the symptoms may improve [178] and some early reports showed encouraging physiological changes [2168]. Subsequent studies have not confirmed these changes [1864, 2875]. Any benefit from 'diaphragmatic' breathing may be psychological or related to reassurance, relaxation or the ability to control the respiratory rate rather than to control the diaphragm.

DEEP BREATHING EXERCISES

It has been shown that even a few deep breaths can increase the lung compliance [897, 2101, 2261]. This is thought to be due to opening of previously closed small airways, particularly at the bases of the lungs. These basal airways are exposed to the highest pleural pressure and readily close, particularly if there is air flow obstruction or a decreased elastic recoil of the lungs. The closing volume may be above the FRC, particularly in the supine position, but the airways reopen with inflation of the lungs above this volume.

The compliance of the lungs has been demonstrated to increase after a few deep breaths in patients with poliomyelitis [970] and obesity [2747]. The increased lung compliance lessens the work of the respiratory muscles and opening of the basal airways improves ventilation/perfusion matching and arterial oxygenation. The recommendation to increase the tidal volume by breathing deeply is usually accompanied by a fall in the respiratory frequency in order that

the alveolar ventilation remains constant. This breathing pattern reduces the dead space and, since T_E is prolonged more than T_I, the inspiratory muscle duty cycle decreases. This relieves inspiratory muscle fatigue. At low inspiratory flow rates, the regional ventilation is altered so that the bases of the lungs are preferentially ventilated [1254].

Sighing has similar effects on lung compliance as taking deep breaths [243]. Since sighs are only intermittent they have little effect on dead space or on the inspiratory muscle duty cycle, but they reduce the risk of chest infections by keeping the basal airways open and enabling the cough to be more effective because of the higher end inspiratory volume [2002]. Sighs occur regularly in normal subjects at rest, but are absent or reduced in frequency in disorders of the carotid body [199], vagus nerve [1152] and in quadriplegia [2002].

The benefits of deep breathing exercises or encouraging the patient to sigh are, therefore, similar to those of frog breathing (p. 286) and IPPB (p. 263). A variety of other mechanical aids to deep breathing have been developed. Incentive spirometry is the most popular, especially in the USA [2349] (Fig. 23.1). A sustained deep inspiration is required to reach a target and the patient can see whether or not this has been achieved [553]. There is little difference in the efficacy of the various models of incentive spirometer [1840]. They are used particularly peri-operatively, but have not been demonstrated convincingly to be of any benefit [2514]. They have not been evaluated adequately in patients with chronic neuromuscular and skeletal disorders but, like IPPB, may be of benefit in selected patients.

Blow bottles have also been recommended to aid inspiration, but they primarily provide a resistance to expiration. They increase the airway and pleural pressure in a similar manner to a Valsalva manoeuvre and may cause muscle fatigue, a decreased cardiac output and an increased FRC [610, 2514]. Their only benefit is that a deep inspiration is usually taken prior to exhaling against the expiratory resistance. Their

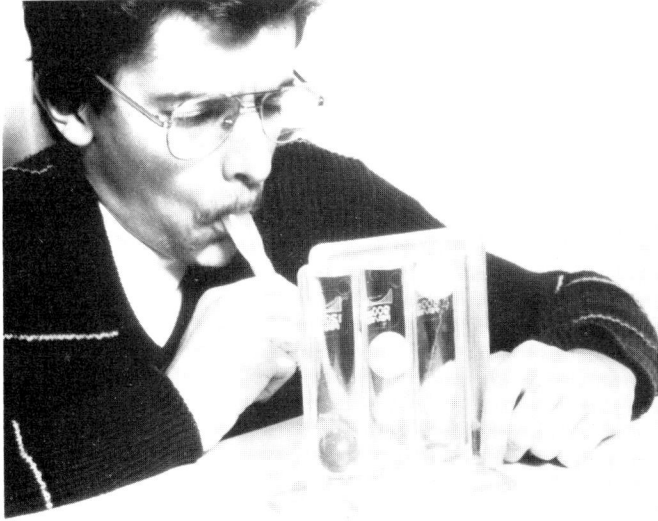

Fig. 23.1. *Incentive spirometer. The inspiratory effort of the subject has lifted two balls but is insufficient to lift the third.*

disadvantages outweigh the possible benefits [1529, 2514].

FROG BREATHING (GLOSSOPHARYNGEAL RESPIRATION)

Frog breathing is a technique whereby the muscles of the mouth and pharynx pump air into the trachea and inflate the lungs. Its value was first realized by Dail [705], who noticed that some of his patients with poliomyelitis had developed this technique to increase their tidal volume. Its use increased steadily during the 1950s, particularly for patients with poliomyelitis [24, 708, 2256] and subsequently in quadriplegics [2132, 2203]. However, interest in frog breathing waned when acute poliomyelitis became less common in developed countries, and it is now relatively little used.

Technique (Fig. 23.2)

Frog breathing is also known as glossopharyngeal respiration or amphibian breathing, because its essence is that mouthfuls of air are gulped into the trachea through the open larynx. The larynx is then closed, acting as a valve to prevent the escape of air. This process is repeated rapidly so that the lungs are inflated often well above the TLC that can be achieved by the normal inspiratory muscles. Frog breathing is different from oesophageal speech practised after laryngectomy, in which air is swallowed into the oesophagus when the cricopharyngeal shincter relaxes and is subsequently regurgitated.

Frog breathing is easily learned as long as the patient is cooperative and motivated [708, 2256], although the speed at which it is mastered varies considerably. Some patients frog-breathe naturally without being taught [708]. It is completely independent of the chest wall muscles and can be performed even by patients whose VC is zero [705]. An ability to contract and coordinate the muscles of the mouth, tongue and larynx is, however, essential. If the patient is learning to frog-breathe while he is ventilated through a tracheostomy, the tracheostomy tube must be fenestrated and the tracheostome plugged while practising. The patient must be able to tolerate about 30 sec without mechanical ventilation while he is frog breathing. These

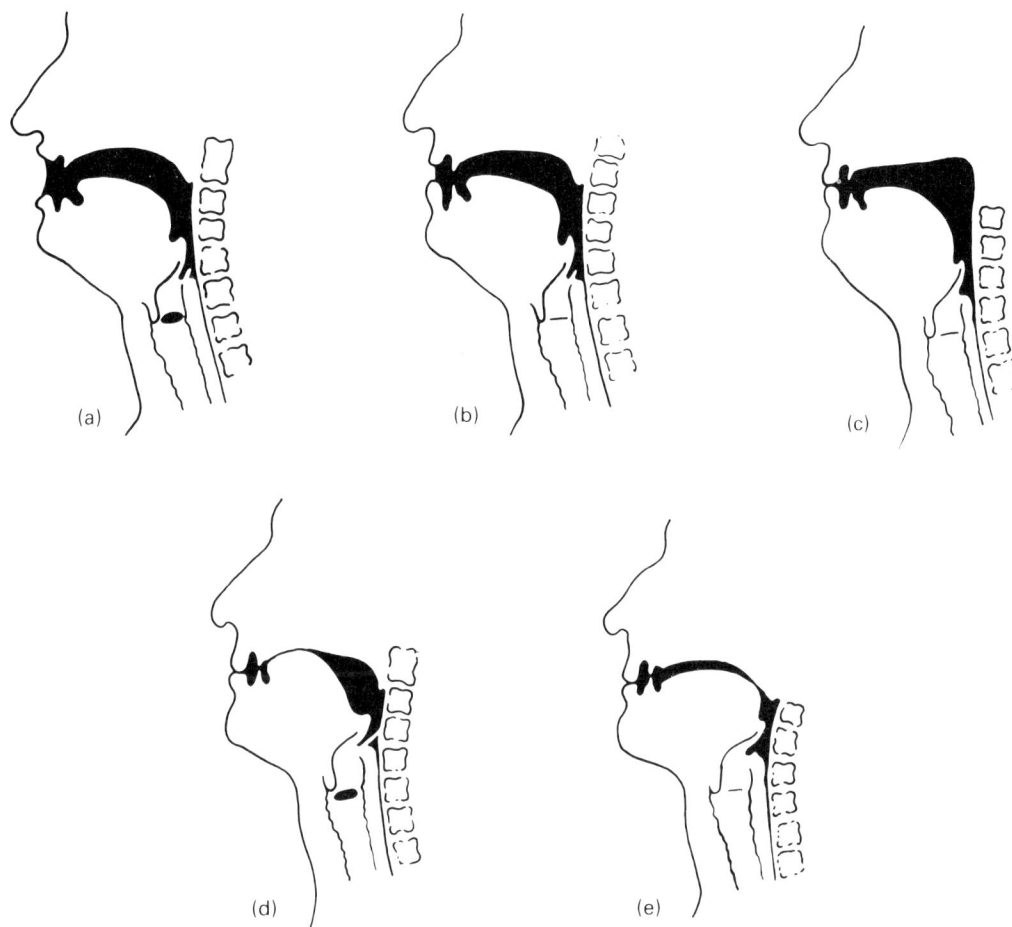

Fig. 23.2. *Stages in frog breathing: (a) normal inspiration, (b) mouth filled with air, (c) air pushed backwards towards closed larynx, (d) air enters trachea as larynx opens, (e) larynx closes.*

difficulties usually prolong the time required to become proficient in the technique [587].

The first actions in frog breathing are to take a deep breath in to TLC and then to fill the mouth with air and depress the tongue, jaw and larynx. The lips are then closed and the soft palate raised to block these two possible exits of air from the mouth. The floor of the mouth, jaw and the larynx is raised and the tongue rolled backwards so that air is pushed through the open larynx into the trachea. The larynx is then closed and the process repeated. It may be difficult initially to learn to raise the soft palate,

and pinching the nose with the fingers is a useful alternative.

Physiological effects

The stroke volume of each gulp varies from patient to patient and is determined by the size of the mouth, the strength of the mouth muscles, the intratracheal pressure and the skill in frog breathing that has been acquired. Stroke volumes of 50–80 ml are usual [27, 708, 959, 1559] but analysis of flow volume loops has shown that the volume of each gulp may de-

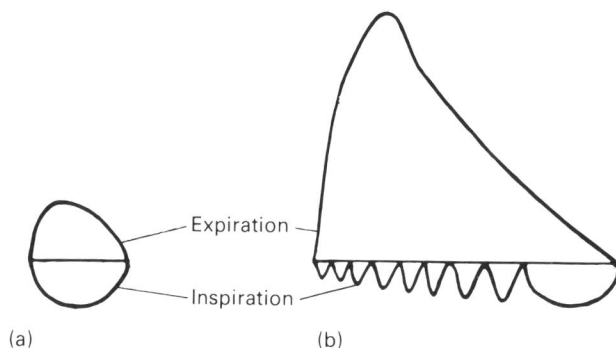

Fig. 23.3. *Flow volume loops in respiratory muscle weakness: (a) using normal respiratory muscles; (b) during frog breathing. After a deep inspiration, several smaller gulps enable the vital capacity to be increased and improve expiratory flow rates.*

crease as the lung volume increases (Fig. 23.3). The intratracheal pressure rises at high lung volumes to as much as $30\,cmH_2O$ [1925] because of the elastic recoil of the lungs and chest wall. This pressure opposes the positive pressure in the mouth and the volume of each gulp, although initially constant [1559], may fall as the lung volume rises [2097]; 10–20 gulps are usually taken between each expiration [27, 708, 1832, 2097] but up to 40 may be needed. Each gulp usually takes 0.3–1.0 sec [708] so that a respiratory frequency of about 6 breaths/min is commonly adopted [705, 1832].

Frog breathing is a form of positive pressure breathing with a greatly prolonged inspiratory phase. The duration of inspiration depends both on the time taken for each gulp and on the number of gulps. It has been postulated that this positive pressure diminishes the venous return and the cardiac output [612, 708]. There is very little direct evidence for this but light-headedness may occur towards the end of a prolonged inspiration [1641] and this side-effect can be avoided by limiting the number of gulps per inspiration.

Frog breathing may greatly increase the VC in conditions such as quadriplegia [587, 2132, 2203] and poliomyelitis [26, 959], particularly in those subjects with the smallest VC breathing normally [708, 1579, 3218]. Improvements of about a litre are common.

This ability to take a deep breath almost certainly increases the compliance of the lungs by opening small airways and preventing subsegmental collapse. It may also prevent a deterioration in the compliance of the chest wall [708, 2204], which is probably common with respiratory muscle weakness. Direct evidence is lacking except in poliomyelitis where the increase in compliance of the respiratory system is related to the VC attained during frog breathing [2256].

The ability to take a deep breath also improves the strength of the cough [68, 2002]. The $P_{E_{max}}$ increases [1559], probably because the TLC is increased, and the peak expiratory flow rate may be more than doubled [612, 1832, 2203], particularly if the compliance of the lung is normal [959].

Indications

Frog breathing is a form of positive pressure breathing, which has the advantage that no equipment is needed. It can be carried out at almost any time but it is not possible to frog-breathe during sleep. It may be dangerous during meals because of the risk of aspiration of food and fluid into the lungs [1641]. Frog breathing has been used particularly in patients with poliomyelitis [24, 401, 708, 1885, 2256], quadriplegia [814, 1559, 2002, 2132, 2203] and Duchenne's muscular dystrophy [58, 147, 1579], but it is probably of value in a much wider range of neuromuscular and chest wall disorders.

Its main indications are to:

Frog breathing may enable spontaneous respiration to maintain adequate blood gases for several hours without ventilatory support in patients who otherwise would require ventilatory assistance [27]. Frog breathing may increase the exercise tolerance so that basic activities, such as moving from a bed to a chair, or dressing, are possible [1579]. The psychological benefits may be considerable [1363, 1925] and the patient's quality of life greatly enhanced. Frog breathing also enables patients who are completely ventilator-dependent to call loudly for help if the ventilator fails [2203], as well as being able to breathe spontaneously for some time. This is particularly valuable if the patient is receiving assisted ventilation at home.

RELIEVE MUSCLE FATIGUE

The usual inspiratory muscles are rested during frog breathing since the work of respiration is carried out by the muscles of the mouth, tongue and larynx. The probable improvement in chest wall and lung compliance also decreases the work of breathing and reduces the risk of respiratory muscle fatigue. Regular frog breathing may, therefore, be useful in neuromuscular and chest wall disorders either as an adjunct to nocturnal ventilatory support or to delay the necessity for this.

AID COUGH AND SPEECH

The beneficial effects of frog breathing on coughing and in preventing basal airway closure have been described above. It decreases the frequency of chest infections in quadriplegics [2002, 2203] and enables speech to be louder and longer sentences to be enunciated.

PHYSICAL TRAINING

Training of the respiratory muscles so that the ability to ventilate the lungs is improved has recently become popular. The respiratory muscles require coordination, strength and endurance to function normally. Strength is needed for sudden respiratory movements such as coughing and sneezing, and brief spells of extreme exertion, whereas endurance is necessary for more prolonged exercise or to overcome an increase in air flow resistance or a decrease in compliance.

Physical training can improve either of these attributes independently [1859]. An increase in strength is accompanied by muscle hypertrophy; the maximal tension increases but the tension per unit cross-sectional area of muscle remains constant. Endurance training does not increase the size or number of the muscle fibres or lead to muscle hypertrophy, but there are structural, biochemical and functional changes in the muscle fibres. The size and number of mitochondria, the amount of myoglobin, and the ability to oxidize carbohydrates, fats and ketones all increase [1324, 1456, 1457, 2761]. The ability to extract oxygen from the blood also increases, partly because of the increase in cardiac output and changes in the autonomic control of the microcirculation, and also because of an increase in the density of capillaries and the ability of the muscle cells to utilize oxygen [1324, 1457, 2761].

The changes in the muscle fibres are due to alterations in the stimulation frequency of the α motor neurons. Constant low-frequency stimulation induces similar changes [2761], and adaptation of muscle fibre functioning is also seen with phrenic nerve stimulation (p. 273). Physical training causes less-marked functional changes since the low-frequency stimulation is only intermittent and the frequency is more variable. The changes in the muscle fibres render them less susceptible to fatigue.

Training methods

For a respiratory muscle training programme to be successful, the load on the muscles must be greater than that which they are normally presented with. The most effective training schedules provide frequent but short periods of exercise, which alternate with longer periods of rest [48]. The duration should be increased more than the intensity of the exercise, in order to improve endurance. The optimal frequency and duration of each session is unknown, but is likely to vary considerably between individuals according to their respiratory muscle and pulmonary function. The intensity of training can be increased by inhaling oxygen during the exercise in order to prevent hypoxia [179, 1135, 1935, 2476, 3371] (p. 308).

The training programme must be continued in order to prevent the muscles returning to their previous state. Physical training is often arduous for the patient and motivation is essential if it is to be successful [2131, 2306]. The criteria that should be used to assess the response to training depend on the patient's presenting problem and whether strength or endurance is required. Improvement may be seen purely from the effect of practice or because of close medical or technical supervision, independently of any increase in the strength or endurance of the respiratory muscles or improvement in the cardiovascular capacity. The most commonly employed methods of physical training are:

ADDITION OF AN INSPIRATORY RESISTANCE

An added inspiratory resistance, such as the P-flex inspiratory trainer [581, 1564, 2308, 2842, 3052] has been widely used but the extra inspiratory resistance may induce dangerous respiratory muscle fatigue [1564] with a rise in the P_{CO_2} [2361]. It provides a form of strength rather than endurance training. The benefit is partly determined by the respiratory pattern adopted in response to the respiratory resistance. Better results are seen if T_I is prolonged and the mean inspiratory flow rate is slow [235].

ISOCAPNIC HYPERVENTILATION [232, 1858]

In this method the patient attempts to maintain a target ventilation for a period of, for instance, 10–15 min while the P_{CO_2} is kept constant. Spe-

cial training devices are available [1858]. Isocapnic hyperventilation is more similar to exercise than inspiratory resistance training in that a volume rather than a pressure load is placed on the respiratory system. This leads to an increase in respiratory frequency, shortening of T_I and an increase in the mean inspiratory flow rate.

ADDITION OF AN ELASTIC LOAD

An elastic load may be applied by binding the chest or abdomen, or by breathing from an airtight container. This method has been little used.

WHOLE-BODY EXERCISE

Exercises employing especially the upper arm muscles [3052] or the leg muscles [1849, 2620, 3245] have been recommended to improve respiratory function. They can be as effective in increasing respiratory muscle endurance as the more specific respiratory muscle training exercises [1636], but have been superseded largely by the methods described above. Nevertheless, bicycle exercise in patients with chronic air flow obstruction can improve the EMG signs of diaphragmatic fatigue [1230]. Whole-body exercise also increases the cardiovascular fitness and, by training the leg muscles, may improve mobility as much or more than specific training of the respiratory muscles [2131]. Physical unfitness is common in both neuromuscular [1969] and skeletal disorders but this type of training has only been studied adequately in scoliosis (p. 212).

Indications

The indications for respiratory muscle training are not settled. It may be of value if exercise is limited by respiratory muscle strength or if there is a risk of respiratory muscle fatigue, particularly if this would lead to hypoventilation during sleep. Cough may be more effective if muscle strength can be improved. Metabolic disorders influencing muscle contractility, such as malnutrition, should be corrected before or during training. The best results of physical training are seen if the muscles are unfit but otherwise normal. The scope for improvement is limited in primary disorders of the muscles, such as muscular dystrophies, and clinically significant benefits are unlikely if factors such as air flow obstruction rather than respiratory muscle contractility limit respiratory function.

Most experience with respiratory muscle training has been gained in the following conditions.

CHRONIC AIR FLOW OBSTRUCTION

Training of the respiratory muscle strength is dangerous in the presence of air flow obstruction because it may precipitate respiratory failure by causing respiratory muscle fatigue [1564, 3000]. Endurance training benefits about 40% of subjects [2681] but the response is very variable [233]. The EMG signs of muscle fatigue may lessen [80, 2402], the maximal sustainable ventilation may increase [234, 1877] and the heart rate during exercise [2131], maximum voluntary ventilation [950], exercise tolerance [950, 1876, 2306, 2620, 3001] and maximal oxygen uptake [2402, 2403, 3245] may all improve.

CYSTIC FIBROSIS

Training programmes designed to increase the ventilatory endurance in cystic fibrosis have shown slight improvements in the $P_{I_{max}}$, the maximal inspiratory resistance that can be tolerated without fatigue, and other criteria of ventilatory endurance [110, 1636]. Exercise ability is, however, hardly influenced because it is limited by factors other than muscle fatigue, such as air flow obstruction and widespread intrapulmonary disease.

QUADRIPLEGIA

Muscle fatigue can be demonstrated in quadriplegia (p. 132), although the degree of exercise that is possible is greatly limited. Training

schedules against an inspiratory resistance over a period of 4–8 weeks have been studied. The VC and $P_{I_{max}}$ increase [1263, 1264, 1494] and low-frequency fatigue becomes less prominent [1262].

POLIOMYELITIS

Exercises against resistance have been recommended in poliomyelitis [962] but there are no adequate studies of respiratory muscle training. In one report, patients breathed through a narrow airway as part of a comprehensive rehabilitation programme for the respiratory muscles. The VC improved but no control group was studied [3052].

MUSCLE DISORDERS

Respiratory muscle training has been attempted, particularly in the muscular dystrophies, but most of the training schedules would be considered inadequate by modern standards. Some improvement in muscle strength has been seen particularly in limb-girdle and facioscapulohumeral muscular dystrophy rather than in Duchenne's muscular dystrophy [3232]. Several trials of respiratory muscle training using exercises such as blowing musical instruments, breath-holding contests and games involving blowing, have shown that in Duchenne's muscular dystrophy muscle coordination can be improved but with no increase in muscle strength [1439]. This has been confirmed in subsequent studies of respiratory muscle training exercises [934, 2069]. The VC has remained unchanged in some studies [1473, 2069, 2889] but has increased in others [15, 934, 1439, 2916]. Any alteration in the VC could be due to factors such as a change in diaphragmatic position secondary to an increase in abdominal muscle activity rather than to a direct effect on the function of the diaphragm or intercostal muscles themselves.

In contrast, respiratory muscle endurance can be improved [934, 2069]. The benefit is greatest in those whose VC is largest, suggesting that

their muscle strength is better preserved [794].
In acid maltase deficiency, inspiratory resistance
training has been shown to reduce breathlessness, muscle fatigue and nocturnal desaturation
and to increase $P_{I_{max}}$ and $P_{E_{max}}$ [2077].

WEANING FROM MECHANICAL VENTILATION

The respiratory muscles are often wasted when
weaning is attempted from mechanical ventilation, because of a combination of the catabolic
influence of acute illness and because of prolonged rest during ventilation. Encouraging
initial results have been reported in aiding weaning with respiratory muscle training [48, 232].

Chapter 24
Ventilatory Stimulants and Inotropic Drugs

VENTILATORY STIMULANTS

The idea of increasing the ventilatory drive with stimulant drugs is attractive. It may be beneficial not only if the respiratory drive is impaired but also if the respiratory muscles are weak, or if the mechanics of the chest wall or lungs are abnormal. The older drugs used for this purpose frequently caused side-effects because of generalized stimulation of the central nervous system, but with the newer compounds the complications are fewer. None of these, however, is able to increase the voluntary respiratory drive except non-specifically by raising the level of consciousness. The hypoxic and hypercapnic drives can be improved but, in practice, the benefits are slight. The value of ventilatory stimulants has been the subject of considerable debate over the years [67, 280, 2741, 3370] but none has yet been studied adequately in neuromuscular and chest wall disorders.

Physiological effects

The ventilatory stimulants all act by influencing the automatic control of respiration or altering the level of consciousness (Fig. 24.1). The degree of selectivity of this stimulant effect varies considerably. Analeptic drugs in particular cause generalized central nervous system stimulation, one manifestation of which is stimulation of respiration. They increase the activity of skeletal muscle so that oxygen uptake and CO_2 production rise. This may offset any benefits from the increase in ventilation. The work of respiration also rises as the ventilation is increased but this is a relatively minor factor unless air flow resistance is increased or the lung and chest wall compliance reduced. The hypoxic and hypercapnic drives increase in parallel with the metabolic rate (pp. 8 and 177), in addition to any direct pharmacological action of the stimulant drug. The more selective ventilatory neurostimulants that have been developed do not have these actions, but they all have other side-effects. These are discussed in the sections on the individual drugs.

The ventilatory stimulants increase the automatic drive to respiration in a variety of ways. Doxapram and almitrine act specifically on the carotid body chemoreceptors but, conversely, the hypercapnic drive is increased, particularly by aminophylline and the carbonic anhydrase inhibitors. Some of the compounds have several different modes of action but for some it is uncertain how ventilation is increased. Both the mean inspiratory flow rate and the timing of inspiration and expiration may be altered. Almitrine, for instance, increases the intensity of the drive but respiratory timing is also altered by doxapram and progesterones.

In neuromuscular and skeletal disorders the need for ventilatory stimulation is greatest during sleep. The actions of most of the drugs are preserved in sleep except for the progesterones. Protriptyline is unusual in that its main action is to alter the structure of sleep so that less time is spent in REM sleep. The number of apnoeas and episodes of oxygen desaturation are correspondingly reduced. The little-used analeptic drugs cause arousal and would also be expected to lessen sleep apnoeas and episodes of desaturation, but at the cost of sleep deprivation.

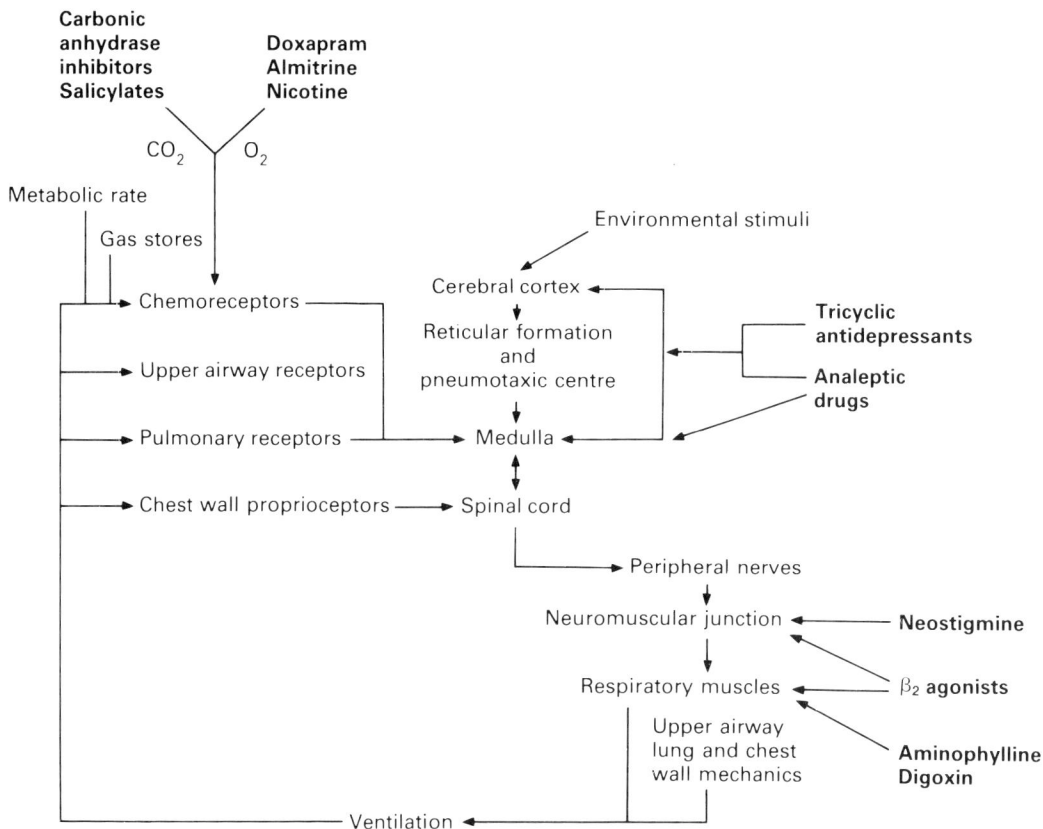

Fig. 24.1. *Sites of action of ventilatory stimulants and inotropic drugs.*

Individual ventilatory stimulants

The most important compounds that have been used to stimulate ventilation are:

ANALEPTIC DRUGS

The early analeptic drugs such as camphor and strychnine are ineffective and are no longer used, and the others have been almost completely superseded by safer ventilatory stimulants. All the analeptic drugs cause generalized central nervous system stimulation, possibly through an action on the brain stem reticular formation. The low toxic/therapeutic ratio limits their usefulness because the appearance of side-effects often prevents the dose from being increased to effective levels. Fits are the most serious complication but other problems include an increase in muscle tone, muscle twitching, itching, coughing, sneezing, hiccoughs, laryngospasm, asthma, hypertension and tachycardia [3355]. The raised level of consciousness and coughing are often beneficial since they help to expectorate retained secretions and improve ventilation.

Ventilation is stimulated by a direct action on the medullary respiratory centres. The ventilatory response to hypercapnia increases because of a lowering of the threshold of the ventilatory response [2683]. The V_T increases rather than the respiratory frequency [551, 2170, 2748, 2899, 3355] but the generalized increase in muscle activity raises the oxygen consumption considerably [551, 2688] and largely offsets the benefits of respiratory stimulation.

The most widely used analeptic drugs were

nikethamide, ethamivan, prethcamide and be- megride. Nikethamide and ethamivan were the most satisfactory and were considerably more effective than the others [888, 3355]. Nikethamide is a derivative of nicotinic acid and, like nicotinic acid, it may have an effect on the carotid bodies as well as on the respiratory centres. The same may also be true for ethami- van, which is a benzoic acid derivative. Both these drugs were only effective when given parenterally [2688, 2899].

Analeptic drugs have been used to treat over- doses of sedative drugs with some success since both the level of consciousness and the blood gases improve [551, 2170, 2688]. The tidal vol- ume and blood gases may improve in hypoven- tilation due to obesity [551, 2748] and there is a report of a response in scoliosis with air flow obstruction [2170]. Ventilatory failure as- sociated with chronic air flow obstruction also improved temporarily in most studies [551, 2688, 2748, 2899] but not in all [2245]. None of these drugs has found a place in the long-term management of ventilatory failure.

AMPHETAMINES

Amphetamines, such as methylphenidate, have been demonstrated to stimulate ventilation [998] and to be of value in central alveolar hypoven- tilation [2543], but their addictive properties and the development of other effective ventilat- ory stimulants has led to their abandonment.

SALICYLATES

Salicylates have been known for many years to stimulate ventilation sufficiently to cause a re- spiratory alkalosis. This is thought to be due partly to a pharmacological effect on the medul- lary respiratory centres and partly to the metabolic acidosis that they induce. Their action is independent of both carotid body function [3147] and of the increase in oxygen consump- tion that they generate [2172]. Salicylates in- crease the ventilatory response to hypercapnia and act rapidly so that the P_{CO_2} may fall within

an hour of intravenous administration [2766, 3274].

Salicylates can be effective in acute ventilatory failure but are not often used because the large doses that are required frequently cause side- effects. Tolerance develops with prolonged ad- ministration and they have been little used in chronic respiratory failure.

CAROTID BODY STIMULANTS

Doxapram

Doxapram increases respiration in low doses by stimulating the carotid bodies and in high doses by acting on the medullary respiratory centres. In cats, its ability to increase ventilation is abolished by carotid body denervation [2190]. Its stimulant effects are increased by hypoxia but not affected by hyperoxia [2190]. The rapid- ity of the response following intravenous ad- ministration also suggests that it acts on the carotid bodies [2838].

The frequency of afferent impulses in the carotid sinus nerve at any given P_{O_2} increases with the dose of doxapram but about 90% of the maximal response is seen at a dose of 2 mg/kg body weight [2190]. The usual dose by continuous infusion is 0.5–4.0 mg/min. In high doses the ventilatory response to hypercapnia also increases, even under hyperoxic conditions [443, 469], raising the possibility that it is acting directly on the brain stem.

Doxapram increases the tidal volume to a greater extent than the respiratory frequency [443, 1500]. The T_I/T_E ratio and $P_{0.1}$ rise as the tidal volume increases. Both the intensity of the respiratory drive and the timing of inspiration and expiration are, therefore, altered.

Doxapram has a much higher toxic/therapeu- tic ratio than the analeptic drugs; respiratory stimulation is achieved much more selectively. The side-effects of analeptic drugs may, how- ever, appear at high doses. Irritability, agitation, an inability to sleep, muscular twitching, cough- ing, sweating, tachycardia, hypertension and oc- casionally fits may be seen [3355]. Pulmonary hypertension may also develop [629] and the level of consciousness increases, particularly at high doses.

Doxapram is more effective than the intravenous analeptic drugs [3355]. It is used to counteract post-operative respiratory depression and has the advantage over naloxone in that the analgesia of opiate drugs is not lost [1307]. It may also be of value following overdoses of sedative drugs [856] and in acute on chronic air flow obstruction where it increases ventilation and may prevent or reduce hypercapnia during oxygen administration [489, 490, 2226, 2635]. It is also effective in acute infections superimposed on chronic neuromuscular and skeletal disorders, but is of very limited use in chronic respiratory failure because it has to be administered intravenously. A temporary improvement in hypoventilation secondary to obesity or central alveolar hypoventilation [1474, 1959] has been recorded, but in neonates with the latter condition prolonged administration is limited by side-effects [1500]. Obstructive sleep apnoeas are terminated at a higher P_{O_2} with doxapram so that the duration and degree of oxygen desaturation, but not the frequency of the apnoeas, are reduced [3114].

Almitrine

Almitrine is a piperazine derivative that can be given orally or intravenously and has a long half-life. Like doxapram, it acts on the carotid body to increase ventilation, particularly during hypoxia rather than hypercapnia. Its effects are abolished by bilateral carotid body resection [150] or denervation [1820] and it hardly alters ventilation in normal subjects who are not hypoxic [1820, 3031]. It raises the ventilatory response to hypoxia [2092, 3032] and, to a lesser extent, to hypercapnia [2092, 3032, 3065], in keeping with stimulation of the carotid body chemoreceptors. It does not appear to have any direct effect on the medullary respiratory centres.

Almitrine increases ventilation by raising the mean inspiratory flow rate [2092] and, to a lesser

extent, by altering the T_I/T_E ratio [2092, 3070]. The ventilatory responses do not correlate closely with the blood level of almitrine [624, 3031, 3065] and, interestingly, its effect on ventilation can be detected after its blood level has fallen considerably. This may be due to an active metabolite that is not detected by the almitrine assay or to persistence of the drug in the tissues.

The improvement in arterial P_{O_2} is often out of proportion to the improvement in the P_{CO_2}. This suggests that almitrine improves the ventilation/perfusion matching as well as increasing ventilation. It has been suggested that this is partly the result of changes in the timing and rate of inspiration [3070] but, in addition, almitrine is a pulmonary vasoconstrictor and alters the distribution of perfusion within the lungs. It has no effect on the distribution of ventilation [2124, 2622]. The A–a gradient is reduced [2124, 2939, 2940, 3070] and blood flow to the bases of the lungs is diminished and redirected to the apices [2622].

Right heart catheterization has confirmed that the pulmonary artery pressure and pulmonary vascular resistance rise during both oral [2018, 2124] and intravenous administration [854]. The right ventricular ejection fraction [2018] and cardiac output fall and the right ventricular stroke work increases [854]. Pulmonary vasoconstriction may be caused by the potentiation of hypoxic pulmonary vasoconstriction [1789] but is probably due to a reflex initiated by carotid body stimulation since it is abolished by carotid body removal [150].

Almitrine may be of use both in acute and chronic respiratory failure but its benefits have to be balanced against the side-effects, particularly a peripheral neuropathy. This appears to be related to the plasma almitrine concentration. It is likely to be of most value if hypoxia is more severe than hypercapnia, since its ability to increase ventilation is limited. The improvement in ventilation/perfusion matching may disproportionately increase the P_{O_2} as long as the right ventricular function is sufficient to cope with an increased pulmonary arterial pressure. It can improve the blood gases both during the day and at night in long-term use in chronic bronchitis and emphysema [624, 3070], but little benefit is seen in the 'sleep apnoea syndrome' [1761, 1762], congenital central alveolar hypoventilation [2376] or central sleep apnoeas, whether given orally [823] or intravenously [2266].

Nicotine

Nicotine probably stimulates both the carotid body chemoreceptors and receptors on the ventrolateral surface of the medulla that are closely linked with the CO_2 receptors [2191]. Injection of nicotine into the lateral ventricles increases the electrical activity in the hypoglossal nerve [1386, 1387]. In cats, intravenous nicotine increases the EMG activity in the genioglossus muscle to a greater extent than in the diaphragm [1387]. These observations led to the suggestion that it might be useful in maintaining a patent upper airway in subjects with obstructive sleep apnoeas. Nicotine decreases the upper airway resistance in dogs [3080], and in humans the number of obstructive sleep apnoeas falls during the first 2 h of sleep after chewing nicotine gum [1199]. This effect may, however, have been due to the stimulant action of nicotine reducing the amount of stages 3 and 4 NREM and REM sleep rather than to any primary effect on the upper airway muscles. Smokers take longer to fall asleep and remain awake for longer periods during the night than non-smokers [2998]. A disadvantage of nicotine in the treatment of obstructive sleep apnoeas is that its action is only transient and there are no preparations that are effective throughout the night.

METHYLXANTHINES

Both aminophylline and caffeine have been used as respiratory stimulants. Caffeine increases ventilation and the slope of the ventilatory response to hypercapnia [3355] but it does not reverse the respiratory depression of opiate drugs [230]. It probably acts on the cerebral cortex at low doses, the medulla at high doses and the spinal cord at even higher doses [3355].

The site of action of aminophylline is uncertain. It may act directly on the respiratory centres in the medulla [908] but it also increases ventilation by reducing the cerebral blood flow because of an increase in the cerebrovascular resistance [1077, 2241, 3271]. Aminophylline increases the ventilatory response to hypoxia [1795, 2767] (Fig. 24.2), but its main effect is to lower the threshold of the ventilatory response to hypercapnia without altering the slope of this response [830, 1795, 2613, 2767] (Fig. 24.3). The resulting increase in ventilation is dose-dependent [2767] and is largely achieved by an increase in tidal volume [2613]. These effects have been most clearly demonstrated with intravenous aminophylline but are also seen with oral preparations [2767].

Aminophylline increases the heart rate more than other ventilatory stimulants [3355] and at high doses causes gastro-oesophageal reflux, nausea, headaches and an inability to sleep. It

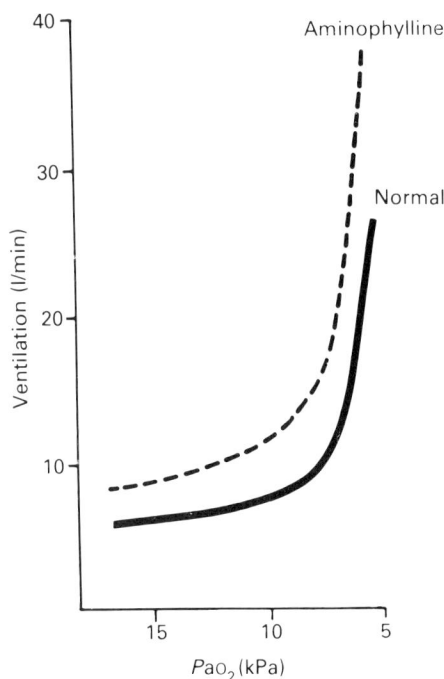

Fig. 24.2. *Effect of aminophylline on the ventilatory response to hypoxia.*

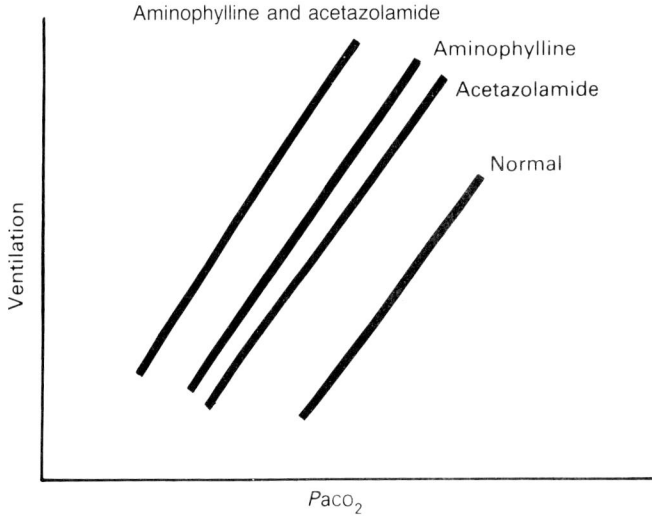

Fig. 24.3. *Effect of aminophylline and acetazolamide on the ventilatory response to* CO_2. *The combination of the two drugs is more effective than either drug alone.*

does, however, have other actions that are often beneficial, including bronchodilatation, an increase in cardiac contractility [795] and a beneficial effect on respiratory muscle contractility (p. 301). It is also a pulmonary vasodilator if pulmonary vasoconstriction is already present. This lowers the pulmonary artery pressure but may increase the shunting of blood through the lungs and lead to hypoxaemia, despite an increase in cardiac output [1574].

Aminophylline rapidly abolishes Cheyne-Stokes respiration [830], possibly because of its effect on cerebral blood flow or, more probably, because the lower threshold for the ventilatory response to hypercapnia enables the respiratory centre to respond more promptly when the $P\text{CO}_2$ rises. Central sleep apnoeas are reduced in severity [554, 2547]. Aminophylline is widely used as a ventilatory stimulant in apnoea associated with prematurity [214], but its value in other situations has not been studied adequately. In emphysema it leads to little increase in ventilation [830] and, although oral theophylline may decrease the number of apnoeas and hypoxic episodes [2093], it would appear to be of little value in obstructive sleep apnoeas [1287].

CARBONIC ANHYDRASE INHIBITORS

Acetazolamide and dichlorphenamide are both carbonic anhydrase inhibitors but their exact mechanism of action in stimulating ventilation is uncertain. They increase renal bicarbonate loss and thereby induce a metabolic acidosis. This would be expected to decrease the CSF bicarbonate and so to increase the central CO_2 receptor sensitivity to hypercapnia. Bicarbonate loss can be demonstrated within 4 h of administering acetazolamide [1076]. Acetazolamide also leads to chloride retention but dichlorphenamide retains its respiratory stimulant activity without this action and despite inducing less metabolic acidosis [2271]. Both drugs decrease the CSF flow and pressure [1077] and may have a direct action on the respiratory centres.

They increase the ventilatory response to hypercapnia [1077, 2271, 3315] (Fig. 24.3) and the mean inspiratory flow rate [2960]. The increase in ventilation is seen more rapidly with intravenous than with oral administration in normal subjects [463].

Acetazolamide is usually prescribed as 250 mg tds or qds orally and dichlorphenamide as

100 mg bd orally. Acetazolamide may cause paraesthesiae and headaches; nausea, anorexia and epigastric discomfort can be problems with dichlorphenamide [2019]. Both drugs have a weak diuretic action, which may be of benefit if there is cardiac failure.

Acetazolamide abolishes Cheyne-Stokes respiration [1322, 3117] and also decreases the frequency and severity of central sleep apnoeas [3315], possibly by inducing a metabolic acidosis (p. 126). The central apnoeas may be replaced by obstructive apnoeas, which can cause even more severe episodes of oxygen desaturation [2877]. These are not invariable [3314, 3315] but may be caused by the increase in respiratory drive to the diaphragm and intercostal muscles exceeding that to the upper airway muscles, so that the stability of the upper airway is lost [2876, 2909]. Acetazolamide is also useful in acute mountain sickness [1815], probably because of both its diuretic action and the stimulation of ventilation that relieves the hypoxaemia. Both acetazolamide and particularly dichlorphenamide are able to lower the P_{CO_2} in at least some patients with emphysema [1076, 2019, 2271], but are ineffective in scoliosis [2271]. There are no studies of their long-term use in neuromuscular or skeletal disorders.

PROGESTERONES

It has been recognized for many years that hyperventilation is characteristic of pregnancy and the luteal phase of the menstrual cycle. This has been attributed to the increased progesterone level [2535]. The site of action of progesterones within the central nervous system is uncertain, but the respiratory alkalosis that they induce lowers the CSF bicarbonate and increases the response to hypercapnia. The threshold of this response is reduced but the sensitivity (slope) is not altered [691]. The arterial P_{CO_2} consequently falls in normal subjects while they are awake [1187, 1672, 2962]. Studies in subjects with chronic air flow obstruction have shown that the mean inspiratory flow rate,

$P_{0.1}$ and V_T increase, and T_I falls [2960, 2962]. This indicates that changes in both the timing and intensity of the medullary respiratory drive can be achieved. There are no changes in the amount of sleep or in the structure of sleep [2960], or changes in cerebral blood flow that might account for these observations.

Progesterone 50–100 mg daily was initially used as a ventilatory stimulant but this has been replaced largely by medroxyprogesterone acetate 20 mg tds orally. Some response to medroxyprogesterone acetate is detectable within 24 h, but its maximal effect is seen within about one week [2963, 3082]. The side-effects of the progesterones are inseparable from their endocrine functions and include nitrogen loss, as part of their catabolic action, and a decrease in libido. They are weak diuretics because of their anti-aldosterone action.

Progesterones have less effect on ventilation during sleep than during wakefulness. The response in hypoventilation associated with obesity is variable and probably reflects the individual differences in the mechanical properties of the lungs and chest wall and abnormalities of the ventilatory drive [3116]. The P_{O_2} and P_{CO_2} while awake may improve considerably, although the blood gases revert to their original state after stopping treatment [1971]. The improvement in ventilation during sleep is much less marked. In one study no change was detected in the frequency or duration of apnoeas, or the severity of hypoxaemia during sleep [2379]. In a minority of patients the number of apnoeas may fall, with an improvement in daytime somnolence [3082] and sufficient relief of hypoxia to decrease the pulmonary artery pressure [3116]. In non-obese subjects with frequent obstructive sleep apnoeas the P_{CO_2} may fall during wakefulness but there is little change in the frequency or duration of apnoeas, or oxygen saturation, during sleep [328, 2551, 2552, 3078].

Medroxyprogesterone acetate decreases the P_{CO_2} during wakefulness in some subjects with chronic air flow obstruction [808, 2961, 2962, 3206]. The benefit is greatest if the P_{CO_2} can be lowered by voluntary hyperventilation and if mechanical factors are less important than the defect in the ventilatory drive. The response may depend on the ability to raise the V_T sufficiently to overcome the increased physiological dead space [2960, 2962]. In a few subjects the oxygen saturation during sleep improves [2962], but this has not been confirmed in an unselected group of patients [808].

TRICYCLIC ANTIDEPRESSANTS

Imipramine [648] and monochlorimipramine [1760, 1778] have been tried as ventilatory stimulants but protriptyline has been most widely used because it is non-sedating and may even increase arousal [2817]. Like other tricyclic antidepressants it acts on the brain stem reticular formation to decrease the duration of REM sleep. It thereby diminishes the number and severity of apnoeas and oxygen desaturations occurring in REM sleep. Its beneficial effects may also be explained partly by weight loss and by its cardiovascular actions, which include an increase in cardiac output. It has also been postulated that it increases the upper airway muscle tone and so stabilizes the airway. There is no evidence for this in humans but stimulation of the upper airway muscles exceeds that of the diaphragm when protriptyline is given to vagotomized decerebrate cats [343].

Protriptyline has a long half-life and it may take up to three weeks before a steady state is reached. It is usually given as 5 mg nocte initially, increasing gradually to a dose of up to 20 mg nocte. Its side-effects are similar to those of other tricyclic antidepressants and include tachycardia, a dry mouth, urinary hesitancy and retention, constipation and impotence. These complications are related to the dose and the rate at which this is increased.

Somnolence improves partly because of the arousal effect of protriptyline and partly because of improvement in respiration during sleep. Protriptyline has been recommended in narcolepsy and cataplexy [2817]. Obstructive sleep apnoeas become less numerous in some subjects [585, 636] but this and any lessening of noctur-

nal hypoxia are proportional to the reduction in REM sleep time [420, 421, 2981]. In chest wall disorders the small improvement in blood gases during wakefulness also correlates with the decrease in REM sleep time [2937].

Improvement in sleep apnoeas is more marked if there is no anatomical cause for upper airway obstruction and if the apnoeas are only mild or moderately severe. Any benefits from protriptyline are maintained for at least six months without tolerance developing [420, 421] but troublesome side-effects may prevent successful long-term treatment [632].

OPIATE ANTAGONISTS

The opiate drugs decrease the ventilatory response to hypercapnia and it has been postulated that endogenous opiates (endorphins), which are present in large quantities in the medulla, may be responsible for depression of respiration in certain circumstances. This led to the examination of a competitive opiate antagonist, naloxone, as a respiratory stimulant.

Naloxone is able to relieve respiratory depression caused by morphine and other opiates, although it has no agonist action of its own [1307]. In a single patient with acute on chronic respiratory failure it initially increased ventilation, although after a few weeks no response was detectable [145]. This suggests that in the acute but not in the chronic phase, either excessive endorphin production or sensitivity to endorphins was partly responsible for respiratory failure. In Leigh's syndrome the amount of endorphin in the brain and CSF is raised and naloxone both increases the level of consciousness and diminishes the number of apnoeas [385].

Naloxone also has a minor effect on respiration in other situations. It decreases the fluctuations in tidal volume in Cheyne-Stokes respiration [523]. In subjects with chronic air flow obstruction, breathing against an inspiratory resistance, the $P_{0.1}$, increases following naloxone dosing [2781]. However, in normal subjects there is no change in ventilation, $P_{0.1}$,

VT/TI or $TI/TTOT$ during hypoxia and hypercapnia [1003]. Obstructive sleep apnoeas are not improved [789, 1287] except through a reduction in the duration of REM sleep [125].

Indications

Ventilatory stimulants have the advantage that they require little equipment other than, in some cases, an intravenous infusion. They are, therefore, more widely available than many of the other methods of treatment but they suffer from the disadvantage that they are not very effective. Their use requires considerable judgement since it may be more appropriate to rest the respiratory muscles by assisting ventilation than to increase their activity, particularly if muscle fatigue is present. Ventilatory stimulants are said to be of limited value in the presence of a mechanical cause for ventilatory failure [2064], whether this is airway obstruction in the upper respiratory tract or within the lungs, or a decreased chest wall or lung compliance. Increasing the respiratory drive may even increase upper airway obstruction (Chapter 6). It has also been proposed that these drugs are less effective in neuromuscular disorders where the respiratory muscle strength is limited [3370], but unless muscle fatigue is present ventilation often improves when the ventilatory drive is augmented.

ACUTE VENTILATORY FAILURE

Ventilatory stimulants used in acute and acute on chronic respiratory failure are not curative but are only supportive, like mechanical ventilation. It is essential to treat the underlying cause of the deterioration in respiratory function as early and energetically as possible. The most common indications for ventilatory stimulants are post-operative respiratory depression, overdose with sedative drugs, and acute exacerbations of chronic respiratory failure. None of these drugs protect the airway and this limits their usefulness in unconscious patients. They

may, however, enable oxygen to be given without hypercapnia developing and, in this way, avoid the need for mechanical ventilation [489, 490, 2226, 2635]. They may also be used in conjunction with some forms of mechanical ventilation, particularly negative pressure ventilation, with or without oxygen.

Intravenous drugs are preferable to oral drugs and the most satisfactory is doxapram. This can be continued as an intravenous infusion for several days or even weeks if necessary [1474]. Aminophylline may be required for other reasons, such as bronchoconstriction, and although its ventilatory stimulant action is useful, it is rarely prescribed for this reason alone.

CHRONIC VENTILATORY FAILURE

Most experience with ventilatory stimulants has been gained with chronic air flow obstruction and there are little data on the use of these drugs in neuromuscular and skeletal disorders. None of the intravenous stimulants is suitable for long-term administration unless a tunnelled central intravenous line is inserted. Intravenous stimulants are more commonly used to treat acute exacerbations of chronic ventilatory failure (see above).

Acetazolamide and dichlorphenamide decrease the frequency of central apnoeas but they may be replaced by obstructive apnoeas. None of the ventilatory stimulants has been shown to be of value in central alveolar hypoventilation [432, 571, 603, 648, 773, 1004, 1302, 1325, 1515, 2689, 2852, 2978, 3312]. Protriptyline decreases the duration of REM sleep and of apnoeas in this phase of sleep. It appears to be of most value when obstructive apnoeas are mild or of moderate severity, and in combination with negative pressure ventilation (p. 228). Cheyne-Stokes respiration can be abolished by aminophylline, acetazolamide and dichlorphenamide, and modified by naloxone, but treatment is rarely required. It is possible that almitrine or the carbonic anhydrase inhibitors may be of value in muscular and skeletal disorders, but further studies are required. Protriptyline may be beneficial in these conditions if oxygen desaturation occurs, particularly during REM sleep, but progesterone is unlikely to be of value in nocturnal hypoventilation, whatever its cause.

INOTROPIC DRUGS

Weakness of the respiratory muscles may be improved by drug treatment directed at its cause, such as thyrotoxicosis or Cushing's syndrome. Correction of malnutrition and metabolic factors, such as hypokalaemia and hypomagnesaemia, and relief of hypoxia may also improve respiratory muscle function. Bronchodilator and other drug treatments may relieve hyperinflation and improve the mechanical efficiency of the inspiratory muscles. Several drugs have also been used in an attempt to increase the contractility of the respiratory muscles. They should be distinguished from the ventilatory stimulant drugs that increase the respiratory drive but do not alter the properties of the respiratory muscles themselves (Fig. 24.1).

Individual inotropic drugs

There is no totally satisfactory drug for increasing contractility of the respiratory muscles. The most important drugs that have been used are:

NEOSTIGMINE

This has been shown to increase the contractility of the fatigued diaphragm in dogs [1479].

β_2-AGONISTS

Adrenaline and isoprenaline have been shown to enhance the transmission at the neuromuscular junction and to increase the maximal twitch tension [362]. There are β_2-receptors in the diaphragm [363] and isoprenaline increases the contractility of the dog's diaphragm during low-frequency stimulation [1480]. Terbutaline also increases the contractility of the fatigued dog diaphragm and this effect is abolished by β-

blockade [133, 134]. Propranolol diminishes inspiratory muscle endurance in humans [2242]. Terbutaline increases the isometric strength of the quadriceps muscle but does not improve the endurance or alter the recovery from fatigue [1810].

β_2-Agonists have not been widely used in clinical practice but salbutamol has been shown to increase the VC significantly in a patient with SLE, presumably by increasing inspiratory muscle contractility [3152].

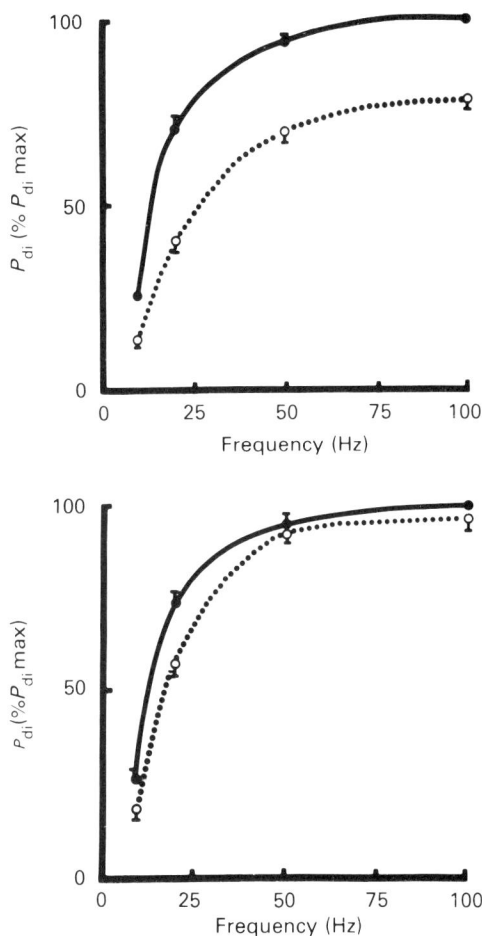

Fig. 24.4. *Stimulation frequency: transdiaphragmatic pressure curves before fatigue (●) and five minutes after fatigue (○). Top figure shows curve before aminophylline and lower figure shows improvement during intravenous aminophylline infusion. Reprinted, by permission of* N. Engl. J. Med. 1981; *305: 251.*

METHYLXANTHINES

Aminophylline improves myocardial contractility, as indicated by an increase in the peak left ventricular pressure and the rate of rise of pressure [795]. A similar effect on skeletal muscle has been observed in several studies. The rate of rise of twitch tension and the peak twitch tension increase, but the duration of the twitch and its rate of relaxation are not affected [795, 1478, 1480, 1582, 2923]. Its actions on cardiac muscle are thought to be due to changes in the movement of calcium into the muscle fibres [795] but there is less certainty about its mechanism of action on skeletal muscle [131, 795, 3109].

Some studies have shown an increase in diaphragmatic contractility and reduction or prevention of low-frequency fatigue, and that these benefits are dose-dependent [132, 795, 1480, 3108, 3234] (Fig. 24.4). Caffeine has similar but more marked effects on contractility *in vitro* [3110] and on transdiaphragmatic pressure *in vivo* [131, 3108].

Recent work has, however, thrown doubt on the clinical value of the methylxanthines, particularly aminophylline. There are no changes in the contractile properties of the adductor pollicis muscle [2237, 3332] and there is no increase in the transdiaphragmatic pressure after supramaximal phrenic nerve stimulation [2237] or improvements in the ventilatory response to exercise [639]. There are no changes in the diaphragmatic EMG activity after isocapnic hyperpnoea sufficient to cause muscle fatigue [2096], and it does not prevent low-frequency fatigue of the sternomastoid muscle [1887].

These conflicting results may be due partly to species and technical differences, such as the methods of producing muscle fatigue. The significance of any clinical benefits from the methylxanthines in increasing respiratory muscle contractility is still uncertain.

DIGOXIN

Digoxin has a positive inotropic action on the heart through its effect on calcium transport across the cell membrane. The diaphragm has several biochemical similarities to heart muscle, and digoxin appears to increase its contractility. In dogs, the maximal transdiaphragmatic pressure generated by electrical stimulation is increased by > 20% [135]. A similar result has been obtained in patients with chronic air flow obstruction during episodes of acute respiratory failure [130].

Chapter 25
Oxygen Therapy

The investigations of Lavoisier and Priestley in the 1770s led to the recognition of oxygen and that it was necessary to support animal life. Oxygen was subsequently used therapeutically, particularly by Beddoes [2734], but few of its indications were soundly based. Oxygen treatment fell into disrepute, although it continued to be used for respiratory conditions and was recommended for respiratory failure due to scoliosis as early as 1884 [3230]. The ability to estimate the arterial oxygen saturation and to measure the oxygen and carbon dioxide content of alveolar air in the early twentieth century enabled oxygen to be used more precisely and the importance of hypoxia as a ventilatory stimulant to be appreciated [1331].

It was soon realized that oxygen therapy was not a simple antidote to hypoxaemia but that it could have serious consequences. Hypercapnia during oxygen administration was demonstrated [188] and the risk of carbon dioxide narcosis in chronic respiratory disease gradually became appreciated [175]. This was thought to be due to stimulation of the metabolism by oxygen and for this reason it was often given only intermittently [1476]. The risk of carbon dioxide retention still limits the use of oxygen in chronic respiratory failure and in many cases ventilatory support is safer.

SOURCES OF OXYGEN

The main sources of oxygen for long-term treatment are:

Compressed oxygen cylinders

These have been available for many years and are supplied in the UK by the British Oxygen Corporation Limited, Chertsey Road, Windlesham, Surrey, GU20 6HJ.

Oxygen cylinders for home use are prescribable by the patient's general practitioner and contain 1360 litres when full (F size cylinder). Each cylinder will last for about 11 h if used at 2 l/min, although the flow rate falls when the cylinder is nearly empty. Smaller cylinders containing about 110 or 230 litres of oxygen are also available and can be refilled from the standard F size cylinders. They supply no more than 2 h of oxygen at 2 l/min.

Oxygen cylinders are expensive and bulky and there is a risk of explosion because of the quantity of oxygen stored in the cylinder.

Oxygen concentrators

Oxygen concentrators filter nitrogen from the ambient air through a crystal lattice composed of metallic aluminosilicates (zeolites) (Fig. 25.1). Zeolites are unable to separate argon (which comprises almost 1% of the atmosphere) from oxygen. They can deliver over 90% oxygen at flow rates of 3–4 l/min but the concentration falls as the flow rate increases because the air is in contact with the zeolite for a shorter time (Fig. 25.2). Oxygen concentrators working on the principle of a semipermeable membrane that selectively allows the passage of oxygen and water have been developed but are less satisfactory than the concentrators that contain zeolites [1211].

Modern oxygen concentrators are reliable, small, light and portable. They can be linked to the patient by long connecting tubing, which enables oxygen to be supplied throughout the home. They require a mains electricity supply and use about 400 W. An oxygen cylinder

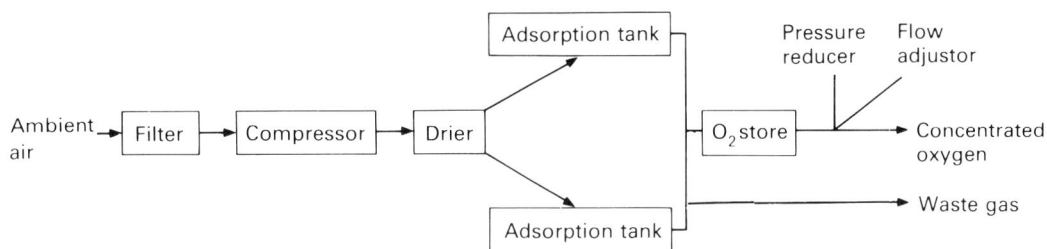

Fig. 25.1. *Schematic representation of the components of an oxygen concentrator.*

should be kept in reserve in the home in case the power supply fails. Oxygen concentrators could theoretically concentrate potentially harmful atmospheric contaminants, such as carbon monoxide and hydrocarbons, in certain circumstances. They are cheaper than oxygen cylinders if more than about 3–4 h of oxygen is required per day.

Liquid oxygen

This is not generally available in the UK but a Union Carbide oxygen walker is used in the USA and is cheaper than oxygen cylinders. Liquid oxygen sources are heavy but portable equipment has been devised.

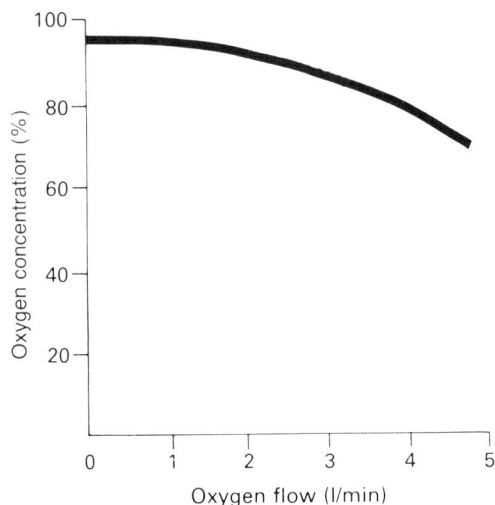

Fig. 25.2. *Typical oxygen concentrations delivered at different flow rates by an oxygen concentrator.*

Chemical reactors

Oxygen may be produced by chemical reactors such as the Oxyquick apparatus [1576]. This contains sodium carbonate peroxyhydrate, which reacts with manganic oxide to provide up to 30 min of oxygen per sachet.

DELIVERY OF OXYGEN

The delivery of oxygen from one of these sources to the patient can be achieved in several ways. A tube-and-funnel method was originally used [2734] and, later, oxygen chambers and oxygen tents were popular [477]. Oxygen is now usually delivered to the patient by:

Face mask

The inspired oxygen concentration cannot be controlled accurately with some face masks but this has been partially overcome by the use of the Venturi principle [475]. A hole in the mask entrains air into the stream of oxygen as it enters the mask. The air dilutes the oxygen to an extent that is determined by the oxygen flow rate and the size of the hole. This enables concentrations of oxygen to be delivered fairly precisely so that the risk of carbon dioxide narcosis can be minimized. A dead space that leads to re-breathing of the expired CO_2 is unavoidable with face masks, but is small in most modern designs. Oxygen concentrations of between 24% and about 60% can be delivered by mask.

Face masks are often poorly tolerated and

cannot be worn during meals. They are inconvenient during conversation and may give a feeling of claustrophobia.

Nasal cannulae

The original form of nasal cannula was the metal Tudor Edwards spectacle, but there are now several varieties of soft plastic nasal cannulae that are much more comfortable. They can be worn both during sleep and in the daytime, and are more convenient than a face mask. There is no dead space but the inspired concentration cannot be controlled accurately since it varies with the volume of air inspired and, to a lesser extent, whether it is inspired through the mouth or nose. Flow rates of 2–4 l/min of oxygen are usually adequate and provide an inspiratory concentration of oxygen of approximately 30%.

The conventional type of nasal cannula supplies oxygen both during inspiration and expiration. This is wasteful and several types of inspiratory-phased cannulae have been developed [506, 1209, 1210, 2211, 2634, 3161, 3360] (Fig. 25.3). They either store oxygen in a reservoir during expiration and deliver it as a bolus early in inspiration when the flow rate is greatest, or have a sensor that detects the onset of inspiration and times the release of the oxygen. They are as effective as the conventional cannulae but use about half the volume of oxygen. This is of no advantage with an oxygen concentrator but it prolongs the life of oxygen cylinders, thus decreasing the cost of oxygen treatment.

Transtracheal catheter

This method of oxygen delivery has become practicable with the development of fine Teflon

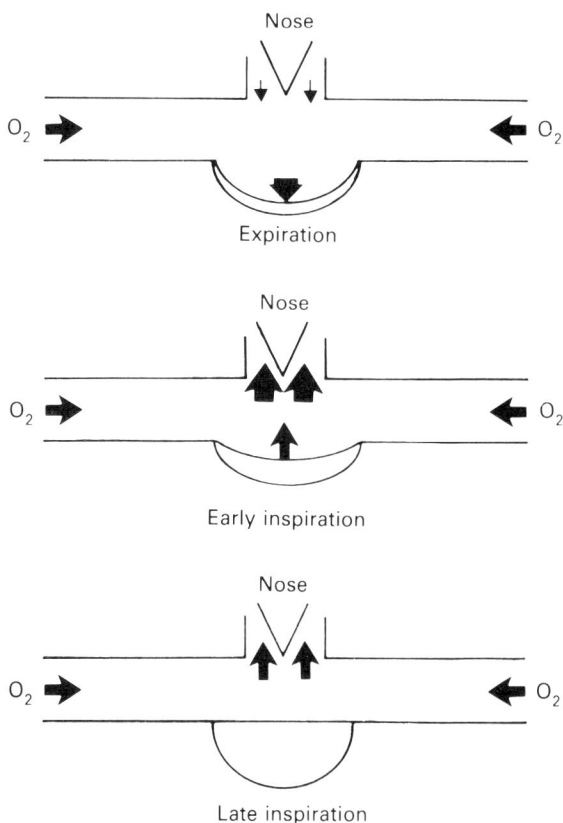

Fig. 25.3. *Inspiratory-phased oxygen cannulae. During expiration the reservoir fills with oxygen, which is utilized in the early part of inspiration. Later in inspiration, sufficient oxygen is delivered despite the collapse of the reservoir.*

catheters. They can be inserted between the 2nd and 3rd tracheal cartilages and are an effective method of administering oxygen [168]. The volume of oxygen required is about half that used by conventional nasal cannulae [169, 570, 1445]. The dead space is reduced by delivering the oxygen directly into the trachea and there is no wastage of oxygen, as is inevitable with conventional nasal cannulae. The transtracheal catheters are surprisingly well tolerated because they interfere less with activities such as eating and washing than other methods of oxygen administration. Subcutaneous emphysema and cough may be troublesome at the time of insertion. The most important late complications are displacement, fracture or blockage by secretions of the catheter, and staphylococcal infections at the catheter site.

PHYSIOLOGICAL EFFECTS

The primary objective of supplemental oxygen is to relieve hypoxaemia. The extent to which this is achieved depends on:

Inspired oxygen concentration and flow rate, and efficiency of administration

The oxygen consumption at rest is around 0.25 l/min whereas 2–4 l/min of oxygen are usually supplied either by a face mask or nasal cannulae. This allows for the wastage of oxygen that is delivered close to the mouth and nose but not inspired, and the oxygen that enters the dead space but does not reach the alveoli. Transtracheal administration of oxygen is more efficient.

Alveolar ventilation

The alveolar ventilation determines how much inspired oxygen is accessible to the alveolar capillary membrane. The simplified alveolar air equation states that

$$P_{A_{O_2}} = P_{I_{O_2}} - \frac{P_{A_{CO_2}}}{R}$$

where R is the respiratory exchange ratio, which is normally about 0.8. From this equation, it is apparent that if the P_{CO_2} remains constant, the alveolar P_{O_2} increases by about 1.5 kPa for each kPa of increase in inspired P_{O_2}. In other words, a small increase in the inspired oxygen concentration leads to a relatively large rise in the alveolar and, therefore, the arterial P_{O_2} [476, 1330].

Oxygen uptake

The oxygen uptake in the lungs is limited by the adequacy of ventilation/perfusion matching. This may be impaired if there is disease of the lungs or if there is basal airway closure due to a restrictive defect or a fall in the FRC, for instance, during sleep. Alterations in the oxyhaemoglobin dissociation curve and the metabolic rate also determine the oxygen uptake in the lungs.

Relief of hypoxaemia lessens the severity of its complications, such as pulmonary hypertension, polycythaemia, systemic hypertension and cardiac dysrhythmias. The function of organs such as the brain, liver and kidney, which are particularly sensitive to hypoxia, improves. A different P_{O_2} is probably required to relieve each of these complications. A P_{O_2} of > 8.0 kPa while awake and at rest is usually recommended, but this is only a crude estimate of what is needed.

Chronic hypoxia early in life may reduce the hypoxic ventilatory drive. There are no studies on the effect of oxygen administration in childhood on the ventilatory drive but it has no effect on this in adults with chronic air flow obstruction [1002]. Administration of oxygen to subjects with a chronically raised P_{CO_2} may, however, raise the P_{CO_2} still further. The increase in CSF bicarbonate concentration reduces the hypercapnic ventilatory drive. When hypoxia is relieved there is no chemical stimulus to breathe, and extremely high P_{CO_2} levels may develop. From the alveolar air equation it would be predicted that a P_{CO_2} above about 12.0 kPa would be very unusual while breathing air, but levels as high as around 20.0 kPa can be achieved while breathing oxygen. This is a risk particularly during sleep or if respiratory sedatives are prescribed. Carbon dioxide retention during oxygen administration is best avoided by careful observation of the patient's clinical condition, monitoring of the blood gases, provision of low inspired oxygen concentrations and supportive treatment such as ventilatory stimulants [489, 490, 2226, 2635] or mechanical ventilation if required.

INDICATIONS

The main indications for oxygen treatment are:

Acute respiratory failure

Acute respiratory failure in the absence of any previous lung or chest wall disease may be treated safely with a high concentration (60%) of oxygen by face mask, without any risk of carbon dioxide retention. If the arterial P_{O_2} does not rise above about 8.0 kPa, mechanical ventilation and supplemental oxygen may be necessary. Pulmonary oxygen toxicity is seen particularly with acutely and severely ill patients who require an inspiratory oxygen concentration of > 60% for more than 24 h [1551].

Acute on chronic respiratory failure

Severe hypoxaemia may result from acute exacerbations of chronic respiratory failure. The concentration of inspired oxygen has to be adjusted carefully to maintain an adequate P_{O_2} without hypercapnia developing [1509]. The observations and treatment required have been outlined above. In chronic neuromuscular and skeletal disorders, IPPV may be avoided by combining oxygen and a ventilatory stimulant, such as doxapram, with tank ventilation.

Chronic respiratory failure

Long-term oxygen therapy can decrease the mortality of patients with chronic air flow obstruction [90, 641, 1873, 2324, 2603]. Nasal or tracheal cannulae with flow rates of about

2 l/min are usually used. At least 15 h per day appears to be necessary and the improvement in survival increases as the duration of treatment approaches 24 h per day. The basic 15 h should include the period of sleep [1006] and is usually taken between around 6 p.m. and 9 a.m. In this way it is still possible to carry out a full-time occupation, but many patients find that this treatment is incompatible with a reasonable quality of life. Compliance with long-term oxygen treatment is poor unless the patient is highly motivated.

The pulmonary artery pressure falls during long-term oxygen treatment for chronic air flow obstruction [9, 1008, 1873, 3165, 3287], although this has not been demonstrated clearly in some studies [641, 2324, 2603]. The extent of the immediate fall in pulmonary artery pressure with oxygen may be able to predict which patients will survive longer with oxygen than if they were left untreated [114]. The cardiac output and pulmonary capillary wedge pressure do not alter, but the pulmonary vascular resistance falls [9, 3287]. These changes are probably due to the relief of hypoxic pulmonary vasoconstriction and regression of the muscular hyperplasia of the small pulmonary arteries. The haematocrit and red cell mass also diminish during long-term oxygen treatment [1851].

None of the trials of long-term oxygen treatment have included a placebo group receiving, for instance, compressed air and none have taken into account the changes in smoking habits of patients treated by oxygen. It is, therefore, difficult to assess the value of the oxygen treatment itself and, while mortality may be diminished, the duration of hospitalization and the ability to continue in work are not improved. Carbon dioxide retention is uncommon in patients with chronic air flow obstruction treated with long-term oxygen, but it often develops in patients with neuromuscular and chest wall diseases. It may be necessary to supply as little as 0.5 l/min by nasal cannulae, in order to minimize the risk of hypercapnia and yet improve the arterial oxygen saturation (Fig. 25.4).

The indications for oxygen therapy in chronic

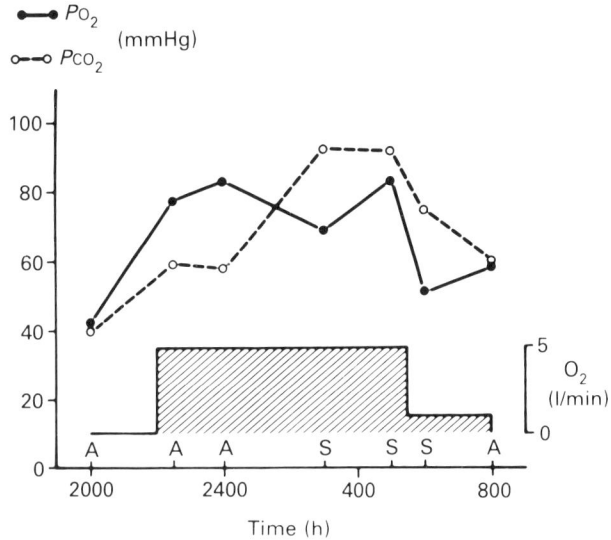

Fig. 25.4. *Changes in P_{CO_2} and P_{O_2} during oxygen therapy in central alveolar hypoventilation. (A = awake. S = asleep.) Reproduced, with permission, from* Am. Rev. Resp. Dis. *1978;* **118**: *950.*

air flow obstruction are not yet clear, but a P_{O_2} below 7.3–8.0 kPa at rest, while awake, should be demonstrated in the stable state and there should be evidence of hypoxic complications such as polycythaemia or right heart failure [89, 325]. Some patients with neuromuscular and skeletal disorders who fulfil these criteria are satisfactorily treated by oxygen but hypercapnia often worsens and most are more safely treated with mechanical ventilatory support.

Sleep apnoeas

Treatment with nocturnal oxygen for obstructive sleep apnoeas usually improves the baseline oxygen saturation and lessens desaturation during apnoeas in NREM sleep. There is no benefit during REM sleep [1159, 2982]. The frequency and duration of sleep apnoeas lessens [1159, 2076] but the changes are often small and may reflect an improvement in the central and mixed apnoeas rather than in the obstructive apnoeas [2982]. Severe bradycardias seen during prolonged obstructive apnoeas can be prevented by oxygen administration [3407], although this improvement is not invariable [59].

The danger of oxygen administration for obstructive sleep apnoeas is that the abolition of the hypoxic stimulus to arousal may prolong the apnoeas and lead to carbon dioxide retention and acidosis [432, 1084, 1182, 2232]. This is particularly likely when the oxygen concentration is high and the patients have severe obstructive sleep apnoeas together with lung disease, such as chronic air flow obstruction [59, 1633].

There are little data on the value and safety of oxygen administration for central sleep apnoeas. In one study the baseline oxygen saturation and the falls in saturation improved during the apnoeas, but the central apnoeas were replaced by obstructive apnoeas [1158]. In a single subject with reduced hypercapnic and hypoxic ventilatory responses, central apnoeas were not prolonged with oxygen treatment and the quality of sleep and daytime somnolence improved [2020]. These benefits may have been due to relief of hypoxic depression of the brain stem but it is not clear from either of these studies whether the central apnoeas were pathological or represented Cheyne-Stokes respiration for which oxygen is known to be effective [1561, 3103]. Nocturnal oxygen administration in central alveolar hypoventilation may raise the P_{CO_2} considerably [193].

Exercise

Hypoxia can develop rapidly during exercise because the body's stores of oxygen are small. Oxygen should be given during exercise rather than before or after. In one study, predosing with oxygen increased the exercise ability [3369], but this has not been substantiated.

Unfortunately, none of the sources of oxygen are easily portable. Small cylinders and the liquid oxygen walker can be used during exercise. Exercise ability is only improved if they are not carried by the patient [1852], since the additional oxygen consumption of carrying the equipment outweighs the advantages of receiving additional oxygen. Nasal cannulae are usually used during exercise [1935] and the newer inspiratory-phased cannulae and transtracheal catheters require less oxygen and prolong the life of portable oxygen cylinders [506, 570, 3161].

Evaluation of portable oxygen is complicated by the large placebo element in this treatment. This may be as important as the effect of the oxygen itself [3264]. The improvement in exercise ability is very variable but oxygen is of benefit in some patients with chronic air flow obstruction [656, 1852]. The relief of hypoxia during exertion reduces the ventilation at any given oxygen uptake [1852], which is valuable if exercise is limited by ventilatory factors. The patients with chronic air flow obstruction who benefit most are those with severe disease who have the worst prognosis [655], but this may not be applicable to those with neuromuscular and skeletal disorders.

Exercise training

The improvements in respiratory function during exercise training are discussed in Chapter 23. Oxygen administration should be considered if severe hypoxia prevents a course of exercise training from being safely undertaken [179, 1135, 3371]. Hypoxia during exercise may be eliminated [1935], ventilation during exercise reduced, and the exercise ability improved by the course of training [2476].

Symptomatic treatment

Most of the oxygen used in the home in the UK is prescribed to treat breathlessness. It is usually taken intermittently and makes little impression on the overall severity of hypoxaemia. This type of treatment is the least-well-documented indication for oxygen treatment and any benefit may be due largely to a placebo effect. There is, nevertheless, some evidence that administration of oxygen to hypoxic patients, particularly during exercise, may relieve breathlessness independently of any decrease in exercise ventilation or any increase in the distance they are able to walk [14, 3264]. The mechanism of this is obscure, but it may involve reflexes mediated by the carotid body.

Chapter 26
Long-term Assisted Ventilation

INDICATIONS

The wide variation in the use of long-term ventilatory assistance for neuromuscular and skeletal disorders reflects both the patchy provision of facilities and uncertainty about the exact indications for initiating treatment. It is often difficult to decide when this is required, but there are a series of questions that should be asked before treatment is begun. Some of these may have to be bypassed if the patient presents with acute respiratory failure and requires assisted ventilation urgently. It may not be possible to wean him completely from this and chronic ventilatory support may have to be instituted.

Does the neurological or skeletal disorder have respiratory complications?

The patient should be observed closely once a diagnosis of a disorder that has respiratory complications, especially ventilatory failure, has been made. It is essential to be aware of the problems that are likely to be encountered in each particular disease so that they can be recognized early on. The clinical features of the most important of these disorders have been described in Chapters 10–16.

Is ventilatory failure present?

The most important information in deciding whether ventilatory support is needed is the knowledge of the arterial blood gases. Samples taken during the day may be of value, but in many disorders ventilatory failure is only present during sleep. A continuous recording of the oxygen saturation (or Po_2) and the Pco_2 is invaluable (Chapter 9).

What is the cause of ventilatory failure?

The cause of ventilatory failure has to be assessed accurately but is often multifactorial. For instance, in poliomyelitis the respiratory drive may be defective, the respiratory muscles weak, scoliosis severe, aspiration pneumonia a constant risk and the upper airway obstructed, particularly during sleep. In obesity the upper airway obstruction, the elastic load of the adipose tissue on the respiratory system, and functional impairment of the diaphragm all contribute to ventilatory failure and, once this is established, secondary abnormalities in respiratory drive appear. Lung disease often coexists with chest wall disease and should be distinguished carefully from this.

Is ventilatory failure severe enough to require treatment?

Treatment is usually indicated if the respiratory failure is sufficiently severe to cause troublesome symptoms, potentially serious complications such as polycythaemia or pulmonary hypertension, or is likely to lead to these problems or even to premature death. Several symptoms are due to the abnormalities of the blood gases, and indicate severe respiratory failure (Chapter 4). Similarly, complications such as polycythaemia or pulmonary hypertension reflect the severity and duration of hypoxia.

The prognosis without treatment may be difficult to assess. Treatment is obviously required to support life if respiratory failure is so severe that the patient is virtually completely dependent on a ventilator. Conversely, the prognosis may be good without treatment if respiratory failure is mild and the underlying disease is not progressive. Many cases, however, fall between these two extremes. There have been no adequate studies of the natural history of chronic ventilatory failure in neuromuscular and skeletal disorders. There is some information on the prognosis after an isolated episode of acute respiratory failure and for chronic ventilatory failure once treatment has been started (p. 311). In chronic lung disease the prognosis depends on age and the degree of physical activity that is possible after the initial episode of respiratory failure [119, 1572].

How effective will treatment be?

Ventilatory support is only effective in certain groups of patients with respiratory failure and the likelihood of success must be assessed carefully before it is started. Assisted ventilation is rarely of benefit if respiratory failure is due predominantly to lung disease. Alveolar ventilation may be increased marginally but hypoxaemia will persist if there is a large A–a oxygen gradient. In contrast, ventilatory support may be highly effective if respiratory failure is due

Table 26.1. *Beneficial effects of treatment on respiratory drive and mechanics*

Type of treatment	Improved automatic ventilatory drive	Reduced upper airway resistance	Increased chest wall and lung compliance	Improved respiratory function
Ventilatory stimulants	+ +			
Remove sedatives	+ +			
Negative pressure ventilation	+		+ +	+ +
External positive pressure ventilation				+
Abdominal supports				+
IPPV	+	+	+ +	+ +
IPPB			+	
Nasal CPAP		+		
Diaphragmatic pacing				+
Physiotherapy techniques			+	+
Respiratory muscle training				+
Nutritional support				+
Inotropic drugs				+
Oxygen				+
Relief of hyperinflation			+	+
Surgery—spinal fusion			+ +	+
—for obstructive apnoeas		+		
—tracheostomy		+ +		
—diaphragm plication			+	+ +

+ + = The most important effect; + = additional effect.

purely to inadequate alveolar ventilation because of a defective respiratory drive, weak respiratory muscles or an abnormality of the chest wall. Upper airway obstruction may also respond dramatically to appropriate treatment.

A trial period of treatment may be needed after the initial assessment in order to decide whether it will be effective in the long term. The response to treatment can be gauged from the improvement in symptoms such as somnolence, physical signs such as those of muscle weakness, respiratory failure or right heart failure, or the results of investigations such as the blood gases during sleep, maximal mouth pressures and the 6-min walking distance (Chapter 9).

Will the prognosis be improved?

The probability of improving the prognosis is difficult to assess because the prognosis without treatment is uncertain. Most subjects who present with ventilatory failure and are left untreated die of this, often during a chest infection or other acute illness, or with right heart failure. If assisted ventilation is effective, it should prevent death from chronic respiratory failure and at least prevent the progression of right heart failure. The patient remains vulnerable to acute illnesses unless prompt and intensive treatment is provided.

The prognosis once long-term assisted ventilation has been started has been the subject of several studies. They all have defects that make them difficult to interpret. Respiratory and right heart failure are often not defined clearly, the age of the patients is not taken into account, control groups are absent, patients with different diagnoses and types of treatment are included in the same study, there is no stratification according to the severity of the respiratory failure and there are probably differences in medical treatment between patients in each of the studies. Most of these reports originate from France and the USA [271, 273, 341, 764, 815, 1112, 1214, 1596, 1722, 1879, 2246, 2405, 2513, 2643, 2644, 2646–2649].

Early experience with poliomyelitis showed that long-term survival with negative pressure ventilation was possible. One patient remained in the same tank ventilator from 1931 to 1949, before dying with a pyonephrosis secondary to renal calculi [2984, 2985]. Experience with poliomyelitis in larger series revealed good survival figures with IPPV over a period of more than 20 years [566, 1342, 1819]. Similar results have been obtained in other reports, which include a variety of neuromuscular and skeletal disorders [3025]. A one-year survival of 88% has been achieved using cuirass ventilation at night in adults [1677] and an 84% one-year survival in children who required either negative or positive pressure ventilation [1036]. Other studies have shown promising results with negative pressure ventilation, although inadequate data are presented to make any conclusions [1085, 2803, 2804]. In the more progressive disorders, such as Duchenne's muscular dystrophy, survival for a few years with negative pressure ventilation or similar equipment can be achieved [58, 696].

The French studies have concentrated on treatment with IPPV and IPPB. There appears to be little difference in their survival figures from those using negative pressure ventilators. Both IPPV and negative pressure ventilation are probably equally effective as long as the blood gases are improved to the same extent for a sufficient period during each day and night [2647].

There appears to be a high early mortality after starting assisted ventilation, but this initial phase is succeeded by a period with a better outlook [764, 1036, 1819, 2405]. In general, the prognosis is better in younger subjects, except for those with congenital central alveolar hypoventilation and spinal cord injuries [3024]. The prognosis of patients with chronic air flow obstruction and other pulmonary disorders has been shown to be worse than in chest wall and neurological conditions in most studies [341, 702, 990, 1112, 2643, 2644, 2647, 2648] but not all [271, 1596, 1916, 2513] (Fig. 26.1).

Patients with scoliosis and non-progressive

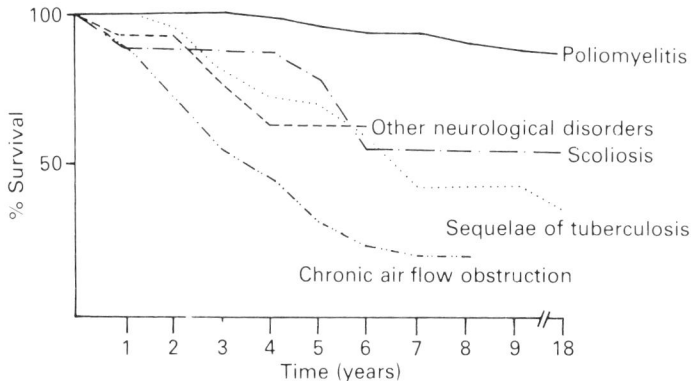

Fig. 26.1. *Actuarial survival during treatment with ventilatory assistance for ventilatory failure.* (———) *Poliomyelitis,* (— — —) *other neurological conditions,* (— · —) *scoliosis,* (......) *sequelae of tuberculosis,* (·· — ·· —) *chronic air flow obstruction. Reproduced, with permission, from Robert D. et al. Rev. Fr. Mal. Resp. 1983;* **11**: 923–36.

neuromuscular disorders have a better prognosis than those with previous tuberculosis or progressive neuromuscular disorders [1214]. It is impossible to give accurate survival figures for these diagnostic groups because of the differences between the various studies. The 1-, 3-, 5- and 10-year survival figures for patients with chronic air flow obstruction are approximately 75, 60, 50 and 30%, and for the restrictive disorders approximately 90, 80, 70 and 60%, respectively. The prognosis in some of these conditions is not determined by the respiratory failure but by factors such as pulmonary hypertension, which may be only partially reversible even if hypoxia is satisfactorily treated. Survival may also be limited by non-respiratory factors, such as renal failure secondary to immobilization in quadriplegics and those with severe poliomyelitis (p. 141), muscular dystrophy, or a cardiomyopathy associated with the underlying disorder, as in Friedreich's ataxia.

Will the quality of life be improved?

The quality of life improves if the symptoms due to respiratory failure can be relieved. In many cases, the exercise ability is increased [990, 2951] and the duration of time spent in hospital is reduced [990, 1526, 2645, 2646]. These benefits must be balanced against the disadvantages of the treatment itself. All forms of treatment interfere to some extent with the activities of normal life. This may be very slight

if, for instance, a ventilatory stimulant drug or physiotherapy is needed, although all the ventilatory stimulants do have side-effects. Assisted ventilation may cause psychological problems and retardation of mental development in children, but the severity of their disease may leave no alternative but to initiate treatment. Some forms of ventilatory support, such as IPPB, are only required intermittently during the day, but most are required either regularly at night or continuously. Nocturnal respiratory support intrudes much less on the patient's life than continuous treatment and is preferable if it is sufficiently effective.

The duration of treatment is, however, not the only factor that influences the patient's lifestyle. Intermittent positive pressure ventilation requiring a tracheostomy is a serious social and psychological handicap. It requires considerable nursing care and interferes with the patient's speech. Some ventilators can be fitted to wheelchairs so that the patient is mobile and can leave his home even if IPPV is required during the day. The wheelchair can be motorized but this makes it heavier and it may be preferable for the attendant to push it. Supplemental oxygen and suction equipment are often necessary and can be fitted to the wheelchair [2037, 2038].

Negative pressure ventilation is preferable to IPPV if it is effective, since a tracheostomy is not usually required. A cuirass can usually be fitted by the patient himself but a jacket normally requires help from another person. Traditional tank ventilators also require assistance and are large and inconvenient. The smaller, modern tank ventilators have been designed specifically for home use and can usually be operated by the patient if his limbs are of normal strength. Nasal or mouth IPPV are alternatives to negative pressure ventilators.

The decision to initiate assisted ventilation can cause ethical difficulties in subjects whose condition is likely to deteriorate progressively. This is particularly a problem in certain neuromuscular conditions, such as Duchenne's muscular dystrophy and motor neuron disease, in which the prognosis ultimately depends on the rate of progress of the disease. Ventilatory assistance is only supportive and eventually the patient's general muscular weakness may be profound. It is advisable to plan the sequence of treatment before assisted ventilation is initiated and to decide in advance whether invasive treatment such as a tracheostomy and IPPV will be considered under any circumstances, such as an acute deterioration following a chest infection. It may be helpful to discuss these problems with the patient or the patient's relatives. The patient may not wish to receive invasive treatment when his disease has progressed and his view must be respected. In motor neuron disease in particular, aspiration pneumonia is normally a terminal complication. Intermittent positive pressure ventilation with a cuffed endotracheal tube may prevent this, whereas negative pressure ventilation may accelerate this natural phase of the disease.

PRINCIPLES FOR CHOOSING THE METHOD OF VENTILATORY ASSISTANCE

In many cases, several methods of ventilatory assistance are likely to be effective. The choice of treatment will, to some extent, depend on the experience of the doctor and the facilities available, but there are certain principles that should guide the selection of the method of treatment. The treatment should be:

Simple and well tolerated

The method of treatment should be adjusted to the physical and psychological capacities of the patient so that compliance with the treatment is maintained. It is important to preserve the patient's independence and, ideally, treatment should not require help or supervision from another member of the family or an attendant. Treatment with drugs, such as ventilatory stimulants, is simpler than using mechanical appliances, even if these are straightforward. Nasal CPAP and IPPV are easy to administer but are poorly tolerated by some patients. Negative pressure ventilators necessitate greater alteration in the patient's lifestyle but, in this respect, a cuirass is preferable to a jacket ventilator. Rocking beds are tolerated quite well by some patients but are not suitable for the patient's partner. Diaphragmatic pacing is simple for the patient to use once the electrodes have been inserted, but it often requires a tracheostomy. This is also the main disadvantage of conventional IPPV, which should be reserved for situations where other simpler treatments are not effective or when aspiration is a problem and the airway needs to be protected.

Reliable

It is essential that any mechanical method of ventilatory assistance is reliable. This is particularly important if the patient is completely dependent on a ventilator. Disconnection of any component of the ventilator may be fatal. A high- and low-pressure alarm should be provided and a patient-activated alarm may be of value. The ventilator should have a battery that is independent of the mains electricity supply in case of an unavoidable mains power failure.

Effective

Simple treatments such as IPPB may be useful for patients with relatively mild respiratory failure. More severely affected subjects frequently require more complex equip-

ment, such as a negative pressure ventilator or
IPPV. It may even be necessary for more than
one type of ventilatory assistance to be given.

Safe

The complications of each type of treatment
have been discussed in detail in Chapters 17–25.
They have to be balanced against the potential
benefits of the treatment and the risks and benefits of alternative forms of treatment.

Portable

Most patients need to leave their home during
the day and in many cases travel considerable
distances, for instance, on holiday. It is an advantage if the equipment required for ventilatory assistance at night is small and light enough
to fit into a car. Rocking beds and tank ventilators are not portable but cuirass and jacket
ventilators powered by small pumps such as the
Newmarket pump are readily portable. Diaphragmatic pacing equipment presents no problems with travelling but a mains electricity
supply may be necessary. Ventilators used for
IPPV in the home should be light and portable
and, if necessary, fit onto a wheelchair.

Cheap

The capital cost of ventilatory support together
with the cost of disposable accessories, its
maintenance and the nursing requirements are
discussed on p. 324.

PHYSIOLOGICAL EFFECTS
OF TREATMENT

The details of the physiological effects of the
individual methods of assisting ventilation have
been discussed in Chapters 17–25. These are
shown in Table 26.1 and briefly summarized
below.

Lung volumes

Most of the neuromuscular and skeletal disor-

ders cause a restrictive defect. This may be improved by either strengthening the inspiratory
and expiratory muscles (see below) or by increasing the compliance of the chest wall or
lungs (see below). Some forms of treatment,
such as IPPV and IPPB, may cause hyperinflation, particularly in the presence of air flow
obstruction, and this will decrease the efficiency
of the respiratory muscles.

Chest wall and lung compliance

The chest wall compliance may be reduced
because of skeletal abnormalities, obesity or stif-
fening of the soft tissues of the chest wall secondary to a restricted range of tidal respiratory
movements. Surgery may be useful, particularly
spinal fusion for scoliosis and stabilization of
the rib cage in the presence of a flail segment.
It is likely that most forms of ventilatory assistance improve the compliance of the chest wall
if the duration of the treatment is long enough,
but there is little direct evidence for this.

The lung compliance may be decreased because of pulmonary disease but is also reduced
if the lung volume is small, secondary to the
chest wall disorder. Any treatment that opens
the basal airways will increase lung compliance.
This includes IPPB, frog breathing, deep-brea-
thing exercises, sighing or even negative pressure ventilation or IPPV.

Respiratory muscles

The cause of respiratory muscle weakness
should be treated, and nutritional and metabolic
disorders should be corrected. Muscle strength
may be improved by inotropic drugs, exercise
training, and the adaptation that follows
prolonged low-frequency stimulation, as in diaphragmatic pacing. The coordination of the
respiratory muscles may be improved by
physiotherapy techniques. The length of the
muscle and its rate of shortening determine the
force that is developed. Diaphragmatic length
can be optimized by a variety of treatment, such
as abdominal positive pressure ventilation,

thoracic and abdominal positive pressure ventilation, abdominal supports, 'diaphragmatic' breathing, diaphragmatic plication and probably spinal fusion in selected cases. Hyperinflation due to air flow obstruction should be treated, and the load on the respiratory muscles should be decreased by other methods, such as weight loss, where appropriate.

If these measures fail to improve respiratory muscle function or if muscle fatigue persists, it may be necessary to rest the muscles. Intermittent positive pressure ventilation and negative pressure ventilation appear to be the most effective measures. The EMG activity is reduced and these methods of ventilation usually abolish paradoxical movement of the rib cage and abdomen.

Upper airway obstruction

This may be induced by negative pressure ventilation and diaphragmatic pacing, unless these can be synchronized with spontaneous respiratory efforts. A tracheostomy may be needed. In other cases, upper airway obstruction causing, in particular, obstructive sleep apnoeas may be overcome by weight loss, lying on the side rather than supine [510], withdrawal of sedative drugs and alcohol, or the addition of protriptyline. A mandibular positioning device [85], a tongue retainer or a nasopharyngeal tube [79, 1705] may be useful and stimulation of upper airway dilator muscles, electrically [2154] or by strychnine [2596], has been recommended. Nasal CPAP is, however, the most valuable form of treatment if simple measures are insufficient. Supplementary oxygen may lead to hypercapnia and surgical treatments should not be carried out before the anatomy of the upper respiratory tract has been assessed carefully. In most cases, nasal CPAP is preferable but surgery such as UPPP is occasionally indicated. The construction of a tracheostomy to bypass the upper respiratory obstruction is rarely needed [369] and is often technically difficult in the obese [3079].

Oxygen consumption

The oxygen consumption of the respiratory muscles is increased in most skeletal disorders of the chest wall and by many of the ventilatory stimulant drugs. Inotropic drugs also probably increase the oxygen requirements, and refeeding of malnourished subjects has a similar effect. The oxygen consumption of the respiratory muscles can be reduced by improving the mechanical efficiency of their contraction and by optimizing their length (see above). Respiratory support, particularly by negative pressure ventilation or IPPV, rests the respiratory muscles and reduces their oxygen requirements. Reduction of the chest wall or lung compliance and of air flow resistance has a similar effect.

Voluntary respiratory control

This may be improved by reversing any depression of the level of consciousness and treating the underlying disorder.

Automatic respiratory control

The automatic ventilatory drive is reduced in many disorders of the brain stem. It is also depressed by severe hypoxia and chronic hypercapnia, which increases the CSF bicarbonate concentration and reduces the hypercapnic drive. Disruption of the sleep structure due to hypoxic or hypercapnic arousal also reduces respiratory drive. These abnormalities may be corrected by successfully treating the respiratory failure and by withdrawing any sedative drugs. Ventilatory stimulants may be of value, particularly in acute respiratory failure, but mechanical assistance to ventilation is often needed.

Ventilation/perfusion matching

Ventilation/perfusion mismatching may be due to basal airway closure as a result of the restrictive defect. Disease within the lung and, to a lesser extent, pulmonary hypertension have a similar effect. Correction of pulmonary hypertension may be of benefit and careful attention to position if the diaphragm or abdominal muscles are paralysed may improve the matching of ventilation and perfusion. Techniques by which some of the respiratory muscles are selectively contracted, such as diaphragmatic pacing or 'diaphragmatic' breathing exercises, have remarkably little effect on the distribution of ventilation or perfusion.

Blood gases

The arterial blood gas levels reflect the balance of the metabolic rate and transfer of gases across the alveolar capillary membrane. Hypercapnia may be relieved by increasing the ventilatory drive, respiratory muscle strength or the chest wall compliance. Ventilation increases and, if the tidal volume enlarges, the physiological dead space will be reduced and alveolar ventilation improved. These changes may be seen both with negative pressure ventilation and IPPV if treatment is continued for a sufficient duration. Improvement in chest wall compliance probably continues for several weeks or months.

Hypoxia usually improves as the level of CO_2 falls, but it may be necessary to increase the inspired oxygen concentration. If the cardiac output is low, the oxygen extraction in the tissues will be increased and the mixed venous oxygen saturation reduced. This worsens the arterial hypoxaemia but is correctable if the cardiac output can be increased. The oxygen consumption and carbon dioxide production vary with the metabolic rate, and the activity of the respiratory muscles can, particularly in exercise, form a considerable proportion of this (see above).

Polycythaemia

Polycythaemia develops in response to hypoxia. It can be corrected by venesection or plasmapheresis but it is more important to treat the underlying cause so that the hypoxia is relieved.

Pulmonary hypertension

This develops in response to hypoxia or if the pulmonary vascular bed is damaged. The pulmonary vascular resistance also increases if the lung volume rises. Pulmonary hypertension is best corrected by relieving hypoxia but if ventilatory support, particularly IPPV, increases the mean intrathoracic pressure, the cardiac output will fall.

SELECTION OF METHOD OF VENTILATORY ASSISTANCE

The selection of the method of ventilatory assistance should be guided by the principles described earlier in this chapter. However, the final choice is also governed by whether ventilatory failure is acute or chronic, its severity, the nature of the cause of the ventilatory failure and the presence of other complications, such as difficulty in swallowing or an inadequate cough. Some of the factors guiding the choice of ventilatory assistance will be considered here.

Acute ventilatory failure

It is essential to recognize and to treat the cause of the ventilatory failure, as well as to provide mechanical support. A chest infection or asthma is often responsible, and prompt treatment should be given. Reduction of the patient's temperature will lower the metabolic rate and reduce the oxygen consumption and carbon dioxide production. The latter can also be decreased by a low carbohydrate diet [675, 2764].

Supplementary oxygen usually increases the $P\text{CO}_2$ in the presence of neuromuscular and skeletal disorders and should only be given if the patient is observed regularly and the blood gases are estimated either directly or non-invasively. A flow rate of oxygen of as little as 0.5 l/min by nasal cannulae may sufficiently improve the oxygen saturation or $P\text{O}_2$. A continuous doxapram infusion may be required, even with this low flow rate, to prevent carbon dioxide retention.

Considerable skill is required in judging when ventilatory assistance is needed. Careful clinical assessment is essential and should be combined with regular blood gas monitoring and VC measurement. In poliomyelitis [972, 1885, 3254] and acute idiopathic polyneuropathy [1416, 2209, 2305], a fall in the VC to 25–35% predicted or around 1 litre usually indicates that ventilatory support will be needed. It may be possible for acute ventilatory failure to be managed successfully without mechanical support [1891, 2977], but this should always be available.

Intermittent positive pressure ventilation is more frequently the best method of support than it is for chronic ventilatory failure. The disadvantages of sedating the patient and the need for a tracheostomy if ventilation is prolonged, are often outweighed by the advantages of protection of the airway, access to the tracheobronchial secretions and achieving adequate ventilation.

It is usually possible to wean patients with neuromuscular and skeletal disorders from IPPV. This contrasts with those with chronic bronchitis and emphysema, in whom muscle fatigue has been shown to be prominent [1126, 2155, 2523, 3124, 3171].

Weaning may require a phase of negative pressure ventilation before spontaneous breathing is resumed. Tank ventilation is effective in this transitional period but, in less severe cases, cuirass or jacket ventilation may be sufficient. Wherever possible, weaning to a negative pressure ventilator or nasal IPPV should be attempted before a tracheostomy is performed since this often leads to tracheomalacia or tracheal stenosis, which, even if slight, may be critical in determining whether or not ventilatory support is required in the long term.

Tank ventilation may be sufficient in acute ventilatory failure without IPPV. Cuirass and jacket ventilators, external positive pressure, IPPB and the rocking bed are usually inadequate. Acute exacerbations of ventilatory failure are now the most important indication for tank ventilation, since other simpler methods of support are usually effective for long-term assisted ventilation. Tank ventilators also appear to be effective for acute exacerbations of chronic bronchitis and emphysema (p. 239) and do not present the difficulties in weaning that are experienced with IPPV.

The prognosis in neuromuscular and skeletal disorders after an episode of acute respiratory failure depends largely on the nature of the underlying disorder. In general, the prognosis is considerably better [819, 1613, 1891] than in patients requiring mechanical ventilation for acute respiratory failure due to pulmonary diseases [120, 2135, 2448] or other reasons [690, 2228, 2339]. These series, however, included a large percentage of patients who were ventilated for acute conditions, such as myasthenia gravis and acute idiopathic polyneuropathy. Further episodes of acute ventilatory failure or progression to chronic ventilatory failure are likely if there is an underlying disorder, such as a muscular dystrophy, that is likely to deteriorate. In conditions that are at least outwardly static, such as scoliosis, the prognosis probably lies between these two extremes, although there are very little data. In one group of scoliotics, the survival without ventilatory support after a median follow-up period of six years was 50–67%, but during this period a mean of 2.4 further episodes of acute ventilatory failure occurred [1891]. The need for long-term ventilatory assistance should always be considered after acute ventilatory failure, particularly if the deterioration was caused by only a mild acute illness.

Chronic ventilatory failure

Ventilatory assistance is often the mainstay of treatment for chronic ventilatory failure, but it is complimentary to other more general aspects of treatment. The cause of the ventilatory failure should, of course, be treated if possible and complications such as cardiac failure and polycythaemia should be assessed carefully. Coexisting lung disease, such as asthma, may contribute to ventilatory failure by impairing the function of the respiratory muscles, and should be treated energetically.

The value of the newer forms of ventilatory assistance, such as high-frequency ventilation and nasal IPPV, are not settled but the benefits of most of the longer-established treatments are well documented. The development of these techniques is illustrated by the changes in treatment for poliomyelitis between 1930 and the late 1950s. The poliomyelitis epidemics were the main stimulus to the development of mechanical ventilation in the first half of the twentieth century. Thunberg's barospirator was tried without success but Drinker's tank ventilator proved effective in purely spinal cases [382, 383, 2973, 2984, 3295, 3348]. Cuirass ventilation was also of value [256] but the mortality in bulbar poliomyelitis remained extremely high [382, 922, 1800, 2310, 3348]. The use of a tracheostomy, particularly in the late 1940s, enabled secretions to be aspirated from the chest [356, 1078–1080], but a cuffed endotracheal tube was first employed in the Copenhagen epidemic of 1952 [245, 922, 1520, 1817, 1819]. It reduced the mortality of bulbar poliomyelitis considerably. Intermittent positive pressure ventilation quickly superseded negative pressure ventilation, although this remained effective for patients without bulbar involvement. Weaning from IPPV in the convalescent phase was usually possible and cuirass ventilation and rocking beds proved of most value. Improvement continued for up to two years after the acute illness but a small number of patients required long-term ventilation (p. 143).

The value of IPPV with a cuffed endotracheal tube in acute poliomyelitis with bulbar involvement overshadowed the effectiveness and relative simplicity of negative pressure ventilators if bulbar function was normal. Little attention was paid to negative pressure ventilation and the other older techniques of ventilatory support for about twenty-five years after the disappearance of the poliomyelitis epidemics from the developed countries. Recently, however, their value in a variety of other neurological and skeletal disorders has been appreciated and they are again becoming more widely used.

The selection of the method of ventilation depends on the severity of the ventilatory failure. This may alter gradually or quite suddenly after ventilation has started so that the type of treatment required needs to be continually reassessed. For instance, a deterioration in respiratory drive, muscle strength or lung and chest wall compliance may necessitate IPPV through a tracheostomy after years of satisfactory control with a negative pressure ventilator. Conversely, obstructive sleep apnoeas may improve when weight is lost and treatment with nasal CPAP may no longer be required.

The choice of treatment also varies according to the anatomical site of the damage to the respiratory pump or its control.

DISORDERS OF VOLUNTARY RESPIRATORY CONTROL

Most of the disorders of voluntary respiratory control do not require long-term ventilatory support.

DISORDERS OF AUTOMATIC RESPIRATORY CONTROL

The respiratory dysrhythmias that do not cause chronic ventilatory failure do not need mechanical assistance. However, medullary and cervical cord disorders that lead to central sleep apnoeas or central alveolar hypoventilation frequently require treatment. Hypoventilation is worse during sleep and nocturnal mechanical support is often sufficient. Rocking beds are not reliably effective and negative pressure ventilation, nasal IPPV or diaphragmatic pacing are usually most suitable. A cuirass or jacket is preferable to a tank ventilator for long-term treatment. Infants with frequent central sleep apnoeas or central alveolar hypoventilation may need almost continuous assisted ventilation because they sleep for long periods. Intermittent positive pressure ventilation through a tracheostomy is most suitable, but diaphragmatic pacing or negative pressure ventilation in a small tank ventilator are alternatives.

DISORDERS OF SPINAL CORD

Cervical cord disorders may involve either the automatic or voluntary respiratory pathways, or both. Their treatment has been described above. In other cases, the predominant feature is weakness of the respiratory muscles. Negative pressure ventilation or nasal IPPV may be adequate but IPPV through a tracheostomy is preferable if the patient is completely ventilator-dependent. Diaphragmatic pacing should be considered if the lesion is above the level of the phrenic nerve nuclei.

RESPIRATORY MUSCLE WEAKNESS

This may be due to disorders of the peripheral nerves, neuromuscular junction or the respiratory muscles themselves. Ventilatory support is not required if only the expiratory muscles are affected. Assisted ventilation may, however, be valuable if the inspiratory muscles, particularly the diaphragm, are weak. Nasal IPPV or negative pressure ventilators such as a cuirass or jacket are usually sufficient. They may be required only at night but continuous support may be needed in more severe cases. Diaphragmatic pacing is ineffective and IPPV should be reserved for those patients who require continuous ventilatory assistance, protection of their airway, or who have upper airway obstruction as well. The rocking bed may be of value if the respiratory mechanics are normal. Combinations of treatment, such as nocturnal negative pressure ventilation and IPPB during the day, or nocturnal IPPV with abdominal positive pressure ventilation during the day, may be needed.

SKELETAL DISORDERS

Ventilatory failure is rare in many of the skeletal disorders of the thorax but it does occur, particularly in scoliosis and following a thoracoplasty. The principles of treatment are similar to those of respiratory muscle weakness. Ventilatory failure occurs particularly during sleep and, although IPPB during the daytime may aid lung expansion, nocturnal ventilatory support is usually required. Diaphragmatic pacing, rocking beds and abdominal positive pressure ventilators are of little value. Nasal IPPV or negative pressure ventilators such as a cuirass or jacket are suitable for most patients, but long-term treatment in a tank ventilator or even by IPPV through a tracheostomy is occasionally needed.

UPPER AIRWAY OBSTRUCTION

Nasal CPAP is effective in treating obstructive sleep apnoeas due to occlusion of the airway above the larynx. Tracheostomy is now rarely required.

Chapter 27
Organization of Assisted Ventilation Service

HISTORICAL DEVELOPMENT

The provision of services for patients requiring long-term assisted ventilation has been neglected for many years in the UK as well as in many other countries. A report from the Royal College of Physicians on disabling chest disease as recently as 1981 mentioned that IPPB may be of benefit but provided no other details of the requirements of this group of patients [2725]. A further report in 1986 on physical disabilities omitted any provision for respiratory care units [2]. Before the Second World War when poliomyelitis and diphtheria were common, the need for assisted ventilation was more widely recognized. The MRC working party set up in 1938 recommended that regional centres should be established for treating patients with ventilatory failure [2108]. However, Lord Nuffield offered to donate a Both tank ventilator to any hospital in Great Britain and the British Empire that had a genuine need for one, with the result that care became fragmented.

The need for long-term mechanical assistance to ventilation declined when poliomyelitis and diphtheria immunizations became effective in the 1950s. Many of the patients with poliomyelitis who required treatment continued to be cared for by the Phipps Unit at the South Western Hospital, London, which provided a centralized service [1164]. Only recently have the principles of treatment used successfully for both poliomyelitis and diphtheria been applied to other neuromuscular and skeletal disorders. Special units at the National Hospital for Nervous Diseases (London), Brompton Hospital (London) and Newmarket General Hospital (Newmarket) have been established. These, together with the Phipps Unit, supervise the treatment of the large majority of patients requiring negative pressure ventilation and related types of treatment. A few other centres provide a nasal CPAP service. Specialized units have also been established for the care of certain conditions, such as spinal injuries and muscular dystrophies, but these have remained largely separate from the mainstream of respiratory medicine.

The March of Dimes campaign was initiated in 1938 by President Roosevelt, who had himself contracted poliomyelitis in 1921. The National Foundation for Infantile Paralysis led to the setting up of specialized units in the USA for the care and rehabilitation of patients with poliomyelitis. These units continued until the 1950s when some were disbanded and others were converted to care particularly for the increasing number of patients with spinal cord injuries. Some of these old poliomyelitis centres, such as the Goldwater Memorial Hospital (New York), Rancho los Amigos Hospital (California) and the Texas Institute for Rehabilitation and Research (TIRR, Houston), together with new units at, for instance, Boston University and Bethesda Lutheran Hospital (Minnesota), now provide long-term assisted ventilation to a wider range of patients. A specialized programme for children is in existence in Illinois [1163, 2604]. These centres also care for patients with chronic lung disease who cannot be weaned from IPPV after an acute exacerbation [2454]. This is more frequently a problem in the USA than elsewhere.

Only France has a centrally organized programme for assisted ventilation. This had its origins in local organizations, particularly in Montpellier, Paris (ADEP) and Lyons (ALLP) [1161]. These centres initially cared especially for patients with respiratory muscle weakness and those requiring a tracheostomy. Intermittent positive pressure breathing later became increasingly frequently used but has recently waned in popularity. Negative pressure ventilators are hardly employed in France at present. A national organization, Association Nationale de Traitement a Domicile des Insuffisants Respiratoires (ANTADIR), has been established to coordinate and help the regional groups. It has medical, technical and social sub-committees and encourages research and the formation of Patient Associations [1162].

The organization of assisted ventilation services is relatively poorly developed in other countries. There are a few exceptions, such as the Montreal Respiratory Home Care Service, which covers a population of around 2 000 000 people [211]. The main interest in most other countries has been to provide long-term oxygen therapy, particularly for patients with severe chronic lung rather than chest wall disease.

SIZE OF THE NEED FOR ASSISTED VENTILATION

It is very difficult, for several reasons, to assess the number of patients who require assisted ventilation. Firstly, many patients who require treatment are not recognized because of lack of awareness of the symptoms and signs of ventilatory failure and that effective treatment is available. At present there are only about 500 patients in the UK who are treated with negative or positive pressure ventilators, diaphragmatic pacing or a rocking bed. Larger numbers receive domiciliary oxygen. In the USA, over 3000 had mechanical ventilatory assistance in their home in 1983 [2953] compared with only 1271 in 1959 [1822] and an estimated 6500 (2.8/100 000 population) in 1986 [2036]. In 1985, 495 of these were known to be under the care of muscular dystrophy clinics [604]. About 300 tank ventilators were estimated to be in use in the USA

in 1985 [843]. About 600 patients have had diaphragmatic pacing electrodes implanted [1151] and almost all of these have been provided in the USA. It was estimated that in France, in 1979, about 1000 patients had tracheostomies, 7000 required long-term oxygen treatment and 3000 needed other forms of mechanical assistance for breathing [2742].

These geographical differences largely reflect variations in medical care rather than the needs of the population. There are, however, true geographical differences in the prevalence of certain conditions. An example is respiratory failure due to obstructive sleep apnoeas. This is much more frequently recognized in the USA than in the UK, probably reflecting the greater prevalence of obesity in the USA as well as a greater awareness of the condition.

The number of patients requiring ventilatory assistance fluctuates from decade to decade for many disorders. More patients with muscular dystrophies are developing respiratory failure amenable to long-term treatment because they are now surviving long enough to develop this complication. Improvements in antenatal genetic screening may reduce the number of subjects born with muscular dystrophies but will not eliminate this problem since, for instance, about one-third of patients with Duchenne's muscular dystrophy are mutations and give no family history that would indicate a need for antenatal screening. The number of cervical cord injuries that require assisted ventilation has increased and is likely to increase further in the future. A large number of patients who underwent thoracoplasty for tuberculosis before 1960 are now developing ventilatory failure, but this is a temporary phenomenon since thoracoplasty is now hardly ever carried out.

In contrast, the need for assisted ventilation is now less in some conditions than formerly. Mechanical ventilation was frequently needed during poliomyelitis epidemics but nowadays it is the relatively small number of patients who had poliomyelitis many years ago who require long-term assisted ventilation. In 1951 it was estimated that about 500 patients in the USA required mechanical aids to breathing, most of whom would have had poliomyelitis [29]. The number of patients who had poliomyelitis and who required respirators at home in 1979 in the USA was between 800 and 1000 [487], but this number is likely to fall steadily. Ventilatory failure in scoliosis will probably also become less frequent if spinal fusion is carried out in the high-risk patients.

These examples highlight some of the problems of predicting the requirements for an assisted ventilation service. They do, however, provide a basis from which such an estimate could, and should, be derived so that adequate facilities can be provided.

ROLE OF SPECIALIZED CENTRES

The number of patients requiring long-term assisted ventilation is too few for every hospital to obtain enough experience to be able to provide the care that is required. There is, therefore, a need for specialized centres where the patients can be assessed accurately, appropriate treatment can be supplied and long-term follow-up can be carried out. At present, three of the four main centres in the UK are situated in London, and the fourth at Newmarket. This unsatisfactory arrangement should be replaced by a national network of specialized units.

It is difficult to assess how many such units are required. If there are too many each will gain insufficient experience and be expensive to run. Conversely, if there are too few centres, both the patients and their relatives have to travel long distances, the care of acute exacerbations has to be largely delegated to the local non-specialized hospitals and there is a risk that the centre will provide an impersonal service. Communications become more difficult and the provision of community services is less satisfactory if the centre is too far from the patient's home and local hospital.

Treatment of acute respiratory failure outside the specialized centres is less of a drawback than might be anticipated, because IPPV is a satisfactory method of treating most exacerbations if

tank ventilators and other facilities are not available. The patient can be transferred if necessary to the specialized unit while still intubated, so that weaning using a tank ventilator can be attempted before a tracheostomy is considered. One specialized centre per one or two health regions in the UK may be the optimal number, but this largely depends on the size of the populations within each region.

The specialized centres will remain dependent on and require close collaboration with the less-specialized respiratory units, irrespective of how many centres are created. The local hospitals will always have to deal with some of the acute exacerbations of respiratory failure as well as the initial assessment of patients before assisted ventilation is considered. It is essential that there is an interchange of ideas between the specialized and less-specialized centres. It may also be possible to share the supervision of individual patients, although this is not always satisfactory.

The initial assessment of patients who may need ventilatory assistance may be carried out in the less-specialized hospitals. The most important screening tests for respiratory failure are the estimation of the blood gases while awake and monitoring of the $P\text{CO}_2$ and $P\text{O}_2$ (or oxygen saturation) while asleep. This facility should be available at all major hospitals and should not be restricted to the specialized units. Referral to the latter should be considered after the initial assessment because of the complexity of the interrelated factors that lead to ventilatory failure and the specialized nature of their treatment.

FACILITIES OF SPECIALIZED CENTRES

The specialized centres should have the ability to provide all or at least most of the types of mechanical ventilatory support that have been discussed in this book. A comprehensive rehabilitation programme may be necessary, according to the type of patients that are referred to the unit. Some types of treatment, such as tank ventilators, are available in very few hospitals in the UK and even fewer in the rest of Europe. Diaphragmatic pacing is a specialized technique that should perhaps be available in one or only a small number of centres in the UK, which would provide a supraregional service.

The doctor in charge of the unit should have a wide knowledge both of respiratory medicine and of the disorders that may cause ventilatory failure. Experience in anaesthetics is valuable but the recommendation that only anaesthetists should be in charge of such a unit [1928] fails to recognize the wider aspects of patient care. Mechanical ventilation is only one aspect of the treatment of these patients. The doctor should have a sympathetic, caring attitude to the physical, psychological and social problems that these chronic disorders impose on his patients. It is desirable that a single doctor should be responsible for the patient and should see him during each admission so that any minor changes in his condition can be recognized. Continuity of care may be difficult to preserve in the larger specialized centres.

Support from well-trained nurses is essential. The nursing of patients with tracheostomies, for instance, who may require IPPV or tank ventilation is a specialized and highly skilled task. Physiotherapy techniques are also invaluable and the construction of a cuirass is best carried out by physiotherapists who are used to working with plaster-of-Paris and similar materials. A social worker should be available for advice and help, including claiming for allowances such as the Attendance Allowance, Invalid Care Allowance, Mobility Allowance and Severe Disablement Allowance, which may be payable to the patient and his relatives [774]. The unit should have a physiological measurement laboratory with suitably trained technical staff. There should be a programme of equipment maintenance and the facility to visit the patient in his home if the equipment fails.

HOME OR HOSPITAL CARE?

Many subjects who require IPPV are initially nursed on intensive-care units but this is an expensive use of resources for long-term ventilation. As a result, intermediate-care units or progressive respiratory care units have evolved [1165, 1527, 1528]. These offer more comprehensive rehabilitation programmes than most intensive-care units. The length of time required in such units depends on the severity of the patient's respiratory failure, his other medical conditions and the type of equipment that he requires for ventilatory support.

There are several advantages in transferring the patient from hospital to home once his medical condition is stable [1683]. The patient's quality of life is better at home, morale is higher, medical care is cheaper and the patient is usually as safe as in hospital. This is almost certainly true for the less-invasive forms of ventilatory assistance, such as negative pressure ventilation, nasal CPAP and rocking beds. The main problem is with patients who have a tracheostomy and require IPPV. Deaths do occasionally occur at home, particularly during the first few days, but these are remarkably few and usually could not have been prevented even if the patient was in hospital [990, 1161, 1492, 3024].

The success of treatment in the home depends on the patient and his family or other attendants being physically able to manage the equipment and to understand how to cope with any problems that may arise. Many patients who require domiciliary assisted ventilation are disabled in other ways and have, for instance, weakness or deformities of their limbs, which prevent them from managing their equipment unaided. Careful planning and assessment of the physical needs of each patient is essential before discharge from hospital.

The psychological state of the patient and the support from his family are particularly important. The patient's personality and his previous ability to cope with stress are factors that determine the likelihood of success of long-term mechanical ventilatory assistance. This is particularly true with the more invasive forms of treatment, such as tracheostomy and IPPV or tank ventilation. Simpler methods, such as cuirass ventilation and nasal CPAP or IPPV, may fail not because of an inability of the patient or family to manage the treatment, but because of a lack of motivation. Encouragement from the staff of the assisted ventilation unit and explanation of why the treatment is needed is essential.

The transfer of care to the home helps to maintain the independence of the patient and his family. This is an important facet of treatment. The patient and his relatives should be encouraged as far as possible to be responsible for the patient's care, even if this requires special skills, such as looking after a tracheostomy. If necessary, provision for attendants to be present in the home, either part-time or continuously, should be made. This is rarely necessary with cuirass ventilation but is often required with other forms of negative pressure ventilation and IPPV, particularly if the patient has no relatives.

These aspects of domiciliary care should be assessed fully before discharge of the patient from hospital [989, 1133, 1683, 2040–2042, 2351, 2777]. This requires cooperation between the doctors, nurses, physiotherapists and social workers of the central unit and the staff based in the community [2039]. The central unit should ideally run its own community unit comprising skilled staff, such as nurses, who can visit the patients in their homes. The review of the patient's condition after discharge from hospital is best carried out partly in his home and partly at the central unit. The community-based staff can provide information about the patient's needs and progress, which cannot be obtained in hospital.

It is possible for some degree of physiological assessment to be carried out in the patient's home with modern portable transcutaneous monitors [2479], oximetry, spirometry and other techniques. This may be of value but is not a substitute for regular clinical assessment. The frequency with which the patient should return to the central unit varies according to the severity of the respiratory failure, the response to treatment, the progression of the underlying cause of the respiratory failure and the psychological and social needs. It is important that the patient should know who to contact if his equipment fails or if there is any deterioration in his condition. Prompt access to the central unit should be available in these situations.

COST OF ASSISTED VENTILATION

The provision of ventilatory assistance for patients with severe respiratory failure is expensive but this has to be balanced against the cost of other forms of treatment and prolonged periods in hospital if this specialized treatment is withheld.

It has been shown in the USA, France and in the UK that it is much cheaper to provide care at home than in hospital, particularly if IPPV is required. Even the cost of an intermediate-care unit can save up to 30% of the cost of care on a normal intensive-care unit [1165]. Several series have shown that long-term IPPV in the home costs between 2% and 50% of the same care provided in hospital [166, 446, 680, 961, 1164–1166, 1528, 2038, 2604, 2645, 3024, 3183, 3191]. The main saving is on the salaries of hospital staff required to look after the patient, although if an attendant is required in the home, some of this saving is lost [860, 2650].

The reduction in the duration of time spent in hospital is responsible for most of the saving with negative pressure ventilation [1677, 3025]. Domiciliary treatment with cuirass ventilation in subjects with both skeletal and neuromuscular disorders costs about 10% of that of continuous hospital care [1676]. The number of home visits from the general practitioner and the need for drugs, such as diuretics, are reduced [1676, 2951].

The capital cost of the equipment is an important but, in the long term, a relatively minor expense. Equipment for IPPB costs around £600, for a cuirass ventilator and pump around £2500, for an IPPV ventilator £4000–5000, for a nasal CPAP pump about £700, for a rocking bed about £2500 and for diaphragm pacing equipment about £15 000. A suction pump and disposable items, such as suction catheters, may also be needed and equipment such as a modified wheelchair and oxygen cylinders and concentrators need to be taken into account [2650]. The patient's home may also need to be altered to accommodate the equipment.

The funding for both the capital and the revenue costs of providing an assisted ventilation service should be planned in accordance with the needs of the community served by the specialized centre. The method of funding varies from country to country, depending on the administration of the local health services [828, 1220]. In the UK there is no standard method of financing this type of treatment. This is unsatisfactory but is not surprising, considering the neglect from which this form of treatment has suffered from the medical profession since the end of the poliomyelitis epidemics in the 1950s. A comprehensive service is unlikely to be organized or financed until it is more widely recognized that ventilatory failure is an important facet of many neurological and skeletal disorders and that its treatment is effective.

References

1 A National Cooperative Study. J Am Med Assoc 1982; 247: 997–1003.
2 A report of the Royal College of Physicians. J Coll Physicians 1986; 20: 160–94.
3 Aaro S, Dahlborn M. Spine 1981; 6: 460–7.
4 Aaro S, Dahlborn M, Svensson L. Acta Radiol (Diagn) 1978; 19: 990–2.
5 Aaro S, Ohlund C. Spine 1984; 9: 220–2.
6 Abbey Smith R. Thorax 1982; 37: 161–8.
7 Abbott OA, Hopkins WA, Guilfoil PH. J Thorac Surg 1950; 20: 571–83.
8 Aberion G, Alba A, Lee MHM, Solomon M. NY State J Med 1973; 73: 1206–7.
9 Abraham AS, Cole RB, Bishop JM. Circ Res 1968; 23: 147–57.
10 Abrahamson ML. Lancet 1959; 1: 449–50.
11 Ackerman LV, Kasuga K. Am Rev Tuberc 1941; 43: 11–30.
12 Ackroyd RS, Finnegan JA, Green SH. Arch Dis Childh 1984; 59: 217–21.
13 Adams FH, Gyepes MT. J Pediatr 1971; 78: 119–21.
14 Adams L, Chronos N, Guz A. Clin Sci 1982; 63: 17P.
15 Adams MA, Chandler LS. Phys Ther 1974; 54: 494–6.
16 Adamson JP, Lewis LL, Stern JD. J Am Med Assoc 1959; 169: 1613–7.
17 Addington WW, Pfeffer SH, Gaensler EA. Respiration 1969; 26: 214–25.
18 Adelman S, Dinner DS, Goren H, Little J, Nickerson P. Arch Neurol 1984; 41: 509–10.
19 Adey WR, Bors E, Porter RW. Arch Neurol 1968; 19: 377–83.
20 Adhikari PK, Bianchi FA, Boushy SF, Sakamoto A, Lewis BM. Am Rev Respir Dis 1962; 86: 823–31.
21 Adickes ED, Buehler BA, Sanger WG. Hum Gen 1986; 73: 39–43.
22 Adkins HV. Phys Ther 1968; 48: 577–81.
23 Adorno AR, White RD. Am Heart J 1945; 29: 440–8.
24 Affeldt J. J Am Med Assoc 1954; 156: 12–15.
25 Affeldt JE, Bower AG, Dail CW, Arata NN. Arch Phys Med Rehabil 1957; 38: 290–5.
26 Affeldt JE, Collier CR, Crane MG, Farr AF. Curr Res Anesth Analg 1955; 34: 41–53.
27 Affeldt JE, Dail CW, Collier CR, Farr AF. J Appl Physiol 1955; 8: 111–3.
28 Affeldt JE, West HF, Landauer KS, Wendland LV, Arata NN. Clin Orthop 1958; 12: 16–21.
29 Affeldt JE, Whittenberger JL, Mead J, Ferris BG. N Engl J Med 1952; 247: 43–7.
30 Agnew HW Jnr, Webb WB, Williams RL. Psychophysiol 1966; 2: 263–6.
31 Agostoni E. J Appl Physiol 1961; 16: 1055–9.
32 Agostoni E. J Appl Physiol 1962; 17: 215–20.
33 Agostoni E. J Appl Physiol 1963; 18: 30–6.
34 Agostoni E, Sant'Ambrogio G, Carrasco H del P. J Appl Physiol 1960; 15: 1093–7.
35 Agostoni E, Torri G. J Appl Physiol 1962; 17: 427–8.
36 Ahmad M, Cressman M, Tomashefski JF. Arch Intern Med 1980; 140: 29–30.
37 Aicardi J, Conti D, Goutieres G. J Neurolog Sci 1974; 22: 149–64.
38 Ainger LE. Br Heart J 1968; 30; 356–62.
39 Alajouanine T, Bouchet M, Pialoux P, Lhermitte F. Rev Neurol 1953; 89: 157–8.
40 Alajouanine T, Thurel R, Blatrix C. Rev Neurol 1950; 82: 280–1.
41 Alba A. In: Olson DA, Henig E, eds. Proceedings of an international symposium. Whatever happened to the polio patient? Chicago, 1979: 101–5.
42 Alba A, Pilkington A, Kaplin E, et al. Respir Ther 1976; 6: 49–56; 102–5.
43 Alcala H, Dodson WE. Neurology 1975; 25: 875–8.
44 Alcock AJW, Hildes JA, Kaufert PA, Kaufert JM, Bickford J. Univ Manitoba Med J 1980; 50: 83–93.
45 Alcock AJW, Hildes JA, Kaufert PA, Kaufert JM, Bickford J. Can Med Assoc J 1984; 130: 1305–10.
46 Al-din ASN, Jamil AS, Shakir R. Br Med J 1985; 291: 535–6.
47 Aldrich TK, Herman JH, Rochester DF. J Pediatr 1980; 97: 988–91.
48 Aldrich TK, Karpel JP. Am Rev Respir Dis 1985; 131: 461–2.
49 Aldridge LM. Br J Anaesth 1985; 57: 1119–30.
50 Alesen LA. J Am Med Assoc 1925; 84: 730–1.
51 Alex CG, Onal E, Lopata M. Am Rev Respir Dis 1986; 133: 42–5.
52 Alexander C. Clin Radiol 1966; 17: 79–83.
53 Alexander HL, Kountz WB. Am J Med Sci 1934; 187: 687–92.
54 Alexander J. Ann Intern Med 1930; 4: 348–60.
55 Alexander J. The collapse therapy of pulmonary tuberculosis. London: Bailliere Tindall and Cox, 1937.

56 Alexander JK. Am J Cardiol 1964; 14: 860–5.

57 Alexander JK, Amad KH, Cole VW. Am J Med 1962; 32: 512–24.

58 Alexander MA, Johnson EW, Petty J, Stauch D. Arch Phys Med Rehabil 1979; 60: 289–92.

59 Alford NJ, Fletcher EC, Nickeson D. Chest 1986; 89: 30–8.

60 Alix JA, Alba M, Aleman G, Nunez E. Rev Clin Esp 1960; 76: 279–89.

61 Allard P, Danserau J, Thiry PS, Geoffroy G, Raso JV, Duhaime M. Can J Neurol Sci 1982; 9: 105–11.

62 Allen SM, Hunt B, Green M. Br J Dis Chest 1985; 79: 267–71.

63 Alpert M, Feldman F. Radiology 1964; 82: 872–5.

64 Al-Shaikh B, Kinnear W, Higenbottam TW, Smith HS, Shneerson JM, Wilkinson I. Br Med J 1986; 292: 1325–6.

65 Alstad B, Fodstad H. Scand J Rehabil Med 1984; 16: 137–8.

66 Altman M, Robin ED. N Engl J Med 1969; 281: 1347–8.

67 Altose MD, Hudgel DW. Clin Chest Med 1986; 7: 481–94.

68 Alvarez SE, Peterson M, Lunsford BR. Phys Ther 1981; 61: 1737–45.

69 Amad KH, Brennan JC, Alexander JK. Circulation 1965; 32: 740–5.

70 Ambler R, Gruenewald S, John E. Arch Dis Childh 1985; 60: 170–2.

71 American Thoracic Society Respiratory Therapy Committee. Am Rev Respir Dis 1977; 115: 893–5.

72 Aminoff MJ, Sears TA. J Physiol 1971; 215: 557–75.

73 Amis TC, Ciofetta G, Hughes JMB, Loh L. Clin Sci 1980; 59: 485–92.

74 Anagnostakis D, Economu-Mavrou C, Moschos A, Vlachos P, Liakakos D. Arch Dis Childh 1973; 48: 977–9.

75 Anch AM, Remmers JE. Am Rev Respir Dis 1980; 121: Suppl 310.

76 Anch AM, Remmers JE. Am Rev Respir Dis 1981; 123: Suppl 185.

77 Anch AM, Remmers JE, Bunce H III. J Appl Physiol 1982; 53: 1158–63.

78 Ancoli-Israel S, Kripke DF, Mason W, Messin S. Sleep 1981; 4: 349–58.

79 Andersen APD, Alving J, Lildholdt T, Wulff CH. Chest 1987; 91: 621–3.

80 Andersen JB, Dragsted L, Kann T, et al. Scand J Respir Dis 1979; 60: 151–6.

81 Andersen JB, Kann T, Rasmussen JP, Howardy P, Mitchell J. Am Rev Respir Dis 1978; 117: Suppl 89.

82 Anderson JP, Keal EE. Br J Dis Chest 1969; 63: 222–6.

83 Anderson PR, Puno MR, Lovell SL, Swayze CR. Acta Anaesth Scand 1985; 29; 186–92.

84 Andrew BL. J Physiol 1955; 130: 474–87.

85 Andrews JM, Guilleminault C, Holdaway RA. Bull Eur Physiopath Respir 1983; 19: 611.

86 Anonymous. Lancet 1876; 2: 436–7.

87 Anonymous. Lancet 1904; 1: 515.

88 Anonymous. Lancet 1985; 1: 84–5.

89 Anonymous. Lancet 1985; 2: 365–7.

90 Anthonisen NR. Clin Chest Med 1986; 7: 673–8.

91 Anthonisen NR, Kryger MH. Am Rev Respir Dis 1982; 126: 1–2.

92 Apps MCP. Br J Hosp Med 1983; 31: 339–47.

93 Apps MCP, Empey DW, Kennard C. Am Rev Respir Dis 1983; 127: Suppl 262.

94 Apps MCP, Empey DW, Kennard C. Clin Sci 1983; 64: 31–2P.

95 Apps MCP, Kopelman PG, Cope T, Empey DW. Am Rev Respir Dis 1983; 127: Suppl 233.

96 Apps MCP, Sheaff PC, Ingram DA, Kennard C, Empey DW. J Neurol Neurosurg Psychiatr 1985; 48: 1240–5.

97 Arborelius M, Lilja B, Senyk J. Respiration 1975; 32: 253–64.

98 Arborelius M, Lilja B, Senyk J. Bull Physiopath Respir 1975; 11: 147–9P.

99 Arce-Gomez E, Palma-Garcia S, Yanez JL et al. Angiology 1964; 15: 407–10.

100 Argov Z, Mastaglia FL. N Engl J Med 1979; 301: 409–13.

101 Arkinstall WW, Nirmel K, Klissouras V, Milic-Emili J. J Appl Physiol 1974; 36: 6–11.

102 Arnould JP, Didelon J, Duvivier C, Monin P. Innov Tech Biol Med 1982; 3: 490–5.

103 Aronow WS, Stemmer EA. Chest 1972; 61: 187–8.

104 Arora NS, Gal TJ. J Appl Physiol 1981; 51: 494–8.

105 Arora NS, Rochester DF. Chest 1979; 76: 344.

106 Arora NS, Rochester DF. Clin Res 1979; 27: 394A.

107 Arora NS, Rochester DF. Am Rev Respir Dis 1982; 126: 5–8.

108 Arora NS, Rochester DF. J Appl Physiol 1982; 52: 64–70.

109 Aserinsky E. Science 1965; 150: 763–6.

110 Asher MI, Pardy RL, Coates AL, Thomas E, Macklem PT. Am Rev Respir Dis 1982; 126: 855–9.

111 Ashok PP, Ahuja GK, Manchanda SC, Jalal S. Acta Neurol Scand 1983; 68: 113–20.

112 Ashour M, Campbell IA, Umachandran V, Butchart EG. Thorax 1985; 40: 394–5.

113 Ashutosh K, Gilbert R, Auchincloss JH Jnr, Peppi D. Chest 1975; 67: 553–7.

114 Ashutosh K, Mead G, Dunsky M. Am Rev Respir Dis 1983; 127: 399–404.

115 Ashworth B, Hunter AR. Proc R Soc Med 1971; 64: 489–90.

116 Askanazi J, Nordenstrom J, Rosenbaum SH, et al. Anesthesiology 1981; 54: 373–7.

117 Askanazi J, Weissman C, LaSala PA, Milic-Emili J, Kinney JM. Anesthesiology 1984; 60: 106–10.

118 Askanazi J, Weissman C, Rosenbaum SH, Hyman AI, Milic–Emili J, Kinney JM. Crit Care Med 1982; 10: 163–72.

119 Asmundsson D, Kilburn KH. Ann Intern Med 1974; 80: 54–7.

120 Asmundsson T, Kilburn KH. Ann Intern Med 1969; 70: 471–85.

121 Asmussen E. Acta Physiol Scand 1977; 99: 85–90.

122 Asmussen E, Nielsen M. J Appl Physiol 1950; 3: 95–102.

123 Asplund K, Fugl–Meyer AR, Engde M, Eriksson S, Strand T. Scand J Rehabil Med 1983; Suppl 9: 103–7.

124 Atarashi H, Saito H, Aoki H, Hayakawa H. Jpn Circ J 1981; 45: 763–8.

125 Atkinson RL, Suratt PM, Wilhoit SC, Recant L. Int J Obesity 1985; 9: 233–9.

126 Aubert–Tulkens G, Willems B, Veriter C, Coche E, Stanescu DC. Bull Eur Physiopath Respir 1980; 16: 587–93.

127 Aubier M, Farkas G, de Troyer A, Mozes R, Roussos C. J Appl Physiol 1981; 50: 538–44.

128 Aubier M, Murciano D, Lecocguic Y, et al. N Engl J Med 1985; 313: 420–4.

129 Aubier M, Murciano D, Lecocguic Y, Viires N, Pariente R. J Appl Physiol 1985; 58: 58–64.

130 Aubier M, Murciano D, Viires N, Lebargy F, Curran Y, Seta J–P, Pariente R. Am Rev Respir Dis 1987; 135: 544–8.

131 Aubier M, Murciano D, Viires N, Lecocguic Y, Pariente R. J Appl Physiol 1983; 54: 460–4.

132 Aubier M, Troyer A de, Sampson M, Macklem PT, Roussos C. N Engl J Med 1981; 305: 249–52.

133 Aubier M, Viires N, Medrano G, Murciano D, Lecocguic Y, Pariente R. Am Rev Respir Dis 1983; 127: Suppl 231.

134 Aubier M, Viires, N, Murciano D, Medrano G, Lecocguic Y, Pariente R. J Appl Physiol 1984; 56: 922–9.

135 Aubier M, Viires N, Murciano D, Seta J–P, Pariente R. J Appl Physiol 1986; 61: 1767–74.

136 Auchincloss JH, Gilbert R. Am Rev Respir Dis 1973; 108: 373–5.

137 Auchincloss JH Jnr, Cook E, Renzetti AD. J Clin Invest 1955; 34: 1537–45.

138 Auerbach O. J Thorac Surg 1941; 11: 21–42.

139 Auerbach O. Am Rev Tuberc 1949; 60: 604–20.

140 Austen FK, Carmichael MW, Adams RD. N Engl J Med 1957; 257: 579–90.

141 Avery EE, Morch ET, Benson DW. J Thorac Surg 1956; 32: 291–311.

142 Axen K. J Appl Physiol 1984; 56: 1099–103.

143 Axen K, Bergofsky EH. J Appl Physiol 1977; 43: 339–46.

144 Axen K, Pineda H, Shunfenthal I, Haas F. Arch Phys Med Rehabil 1985; 66: 219–22.

145 Ayres J, Rees J, Lee T, Cochrane GM. Br Med J 1982; 284: 927–8.

146 (a) Ayres SM, Kozam RL, Lukas DS. Am Rev Respir Dis 1963; 87: 370–9.
(b) Bach JR, Alba AS, Bohatiuk G, Saporito L, Lee M. Chest 1987; 91: 859–64.

147 Bach J, Alba A, Pilkington LA, Lee M. Arch Phys Med Rehabil 1981; 62: 328–31.

148 Bachmann M. Bibl Med Abteilung D 1899; 1: 4.

149 Backer OG, Brunner S, Larsen V. Acta Radiol 1961; 55: 249–56.

150 Backer W de, Bogaert E, Maele R van, Vermeire P. Eur J Respir Dis 1983; 64: Suppl 126: 239–42.

151 Bader ME, Bader RA. Am J Med 1960; 28: 333–6.

152 Bagg LR, Hughes DTD. Thorax 1979; 34: 224–8.

153 Bain SH, Helms P, Warner JO. Thorax 1983; 38: 710.

154 Bainton CR, Kirkwood PA, Sears TA. J Physiol 1978; 280: 249–72.

155 Bake B, Bjure J, Kasalicky J, Nachemson A. Thorax 1972; 27: 703–12.

156 Bake B, Fugl–Meyer AR, Grimby G. Clin Sci 1972; 42: 117–28.

157 Baker AB, Babington PCB, Colliss JE, Cowie RW. Br J Anaesthesia 1977; 49: 1207–20.

158 Baker AB, Colliss JE, Cowie RW. Br J Anaesthesia 1977; 49: 1221–34.

159 Baker AB, Matzke HA, Brown JR. Arch Neurol Psychiatr 1950; 63: 257–81.

160 Baker AS, Dove J. J Bone Joint Surg 1983; 65B: 472–3.

161 Baker JP. Am Rev Respir Dis 1974; 110: Suppl 170–7.

162 Baker NH, Messert B. Neurology 1967; 17: 559–66.

163 Baker SR, Ross J. Arch Otolaryngol 1980; 106: 486–91.

164 Balcerzak SP, Bromberg PA. Semin Hematol 1975; 12: 353–82.

165 Balk RA, Hiller C, Lucas EA, Scrima L, Wilson FJ, Wooten V. Am Rev Respir Dis 1985; 132: 929–30.

166 Banaszak EF, Travers H, Frazier M, Vinz T. Respir Care 1981; 26: 1262–8.

167 Bancalari E, Garcia OL, Jesse MJ. Pediatrics 1973; 51: 485–93.

168 Banner NR, Govan JR. Thorax 1985; 40: 709.

169 Banner NR, Govan JR. Br Med J 1986; 293: 111–4.

170 Bannister R, Gibson W, Michaels L, Oppenheimer DR. Brain 1981; 104: 351–68.

171 Bannister R, Oppenheimer DR. Brain 1972; 95: 457–74.

172 Banta JV, Park SM. Spine 1983; 8: 765–70.

173 Banzett RB, Inbar GF, Brown R, Goldman M, Rossier A, Mead J. J Appl Physiol 1981; 51: 654–9.

174 Banzett RB, Inbar GI, Brown R, Goldman MD, Rossier A, Mead J. Fed Proc 1979; 38: 1300.

175 Barach AL. Ann Intern Med 1938; 12: 454–81.
176 Barach AL. Am Rev Tuberc 1940; 42: 586–613.
177 Barach AL. Arch Phys Med Rehabil 1955; 36: 379–90.
178 Barach AL. J Chronic Dis 1955; 1: 211–5.
179 Barach AL. Dis Chest 1959; 35: 229–41.
180 Barach AL. Bull NY Acad Med 1973; 49: 666–73.
181 Barach AL. Chest 1974; 66: 112–3.
182 Barach AL. J Am Med Assoc 1975; 231: 1141–2.
183 Barach AL, Beck GJ. Am J Med 1954; 16: 55–60.
184 Barach AL, Beck GJ, Bickerman HA, Seanor HE. J Am Med Assoc 1952; 150: 1380–5.
185 Barach AL, Beck GJ, Bickerman HA, Seanor AG, Smith W. J Appl Physiol 1952; 5: 85–91.
186 Barach AL, Bickerman HA, Petty TL. Respir Care 1975; 20: 627–42.
187 Barach AL, Woodwell MN. Arch Intern Med 1921; 28: 421–5.
188 Barach AL, Woodwell MN. Arch Intern Med 1921; 28: 394–420.
189 Barbeau M. Can J Neurol Sci 1976; 3: 389–97.
190 Bard G. Arch Phys Med Rehabil 1963; 44: 368–70.
191 Bardenwerper HW. J Am Med Assoc 1962; 179: 763–6.
192 Barkve T, Stavem P. Acta Med Scand 1966; 180: 295–300.
193 Barlow PB, Bartlett D Jnr, Hauri P, et al. Am Rev Respir Dis 1980; 121: 141–5.
194 Barnes ND, Hull D, Milner AD, Waterston DJ. Arch Dis Childh 1971; 46: 833–7.
195 Barnhart BJ, Reynolds JW, Lees MH. Clin Res 1980; 28: 120A.
196 Barr R. Can Med Assoc J 1966; 95: 912–7.
197 Barrera F, Hillyer B, Ascanio G, Bechtel J. Am Rev Respir Dis 1973; 108: 819–30.
198 Barth PG, Wijngaarden GK van, Bethlem J. Neurology 1975; 25: 531–6.
199 Bartlett D Jnr. Respir Physiol 1971; 12: 230–8.
200 Bartlett D Jnr, Remmers JE, Gautier H. Respir Physiol 1973; 18: 194–204.
201 Barwick DD, Walton JN. Am J Med 1963; 25: 646–60.
202 Bashour F, Winchell P, Reddington J. N Engl J Med 1955; 252: 768–70.
203 Bateman DN, Cooper RG, Gibson GJ, Peel ET, Wandless I. Br Med J 1981; 283: 190–1.
204 Baum J, Alba A, Schultheiss M, Pilkington LA, Lee M, Ruggeieri A. Respir Ther 1975; 5: 43–50.
205 Baxter DW, Olszewski J. J Neurophysiol 1955; 18: 276–87.
206 Bayuk AJ. Anesthesiology 1957; 18: 135.
207 Beals RK, Kenney KH, Lees MH. Clin Orth Rel Res 1972; 89: 112–6.
208 Beamish D, Wildsmith JAW. Br Med J 1978; 2: 1607–8.
209 Bear SE, Priest JH. J Oral Surg 1980; 38: 543–9.
210 Beaupere-Duval G, Grossiord A. Press Med 1967; 75: 2375–80.
211 Beaupre A. Bull Eur Physiopath Respir 1986; 22: Suppl 93–4S.
212 Beckerman R, Meltzer J, Sola A, Dunn D, Wegmann M. Arch Neurol 1986; 43: 698–701.
213 Bedell GN, Rosenberg RS. J Appl Physiol 1961; 16: 928–33.
214 Bednarek FJ, Roloff DW. Pediatrics 1976; 58: 335–9.
215 Beer SI, Avidan G, Viure E. J Am Med Assoc 1980; 244: 2728.
216 Beevor CE. Br Med J 1898; 2: 976–7.
217 Begin R, Bureau MA, Lupien L, Bernier J–P, Lemieux B. Am Rev Respir Dis 1982; 125: 312–8.
218 Begin R, Bureau MA, Lupien L, Lemieux B. Am Rev Respir Dis 1980; 121: 281–9.
219 Begin R, Bureau M–A, Lupien L, Lemieux B. Am J Med 1980; 69: 227–34.
220 Begin R, Lupien L, Bureau MA, Labbe J, Lemieux B. Can J Neurol Sci 1979; 6: 159–65.
221 Beiser GD, Epstein SE, Stampfer M, Goldstein RE, Noland SP, Levitsky S. N Engl J Med 1972; 287: 267–72.
222 Belcher JR. Br J Dis Chest 1961; 55: 77–85.
223 Bell EJ, Riding MH, Grist NR. Br Med J 1986; 293: 193–4.
224 Bellamy D, Davis JMN, Hickey BP, Benatar SR, Clark TJH. Am Rev Respir Dis 1975; 112: 867–73.
225 Bellamy R, Pitts FW, Stauffer ES. J Neurosurg 1973; 39: 596–600.
226 Bellemare F, Bigland–Ritchie B. Respir Physiol 1984; 58: 263–77.
227 Bellemare F, Grassino A. J Appl Physiol 1982; 53: 1190–5.
228 Bellemare F, Grassino A. J Appl Physiol 1982; 53: 1196–206.
229 Bellemare F, Grassino A. J Appl Physiol 1983; 55: 8–15.
230 Bellville JW, Wang KC, Wallenstein SL, Howland WS. Anesthesiology 1958; 19: 95–6.
231 Bellville JW, Whipp BJ, Kaufman RD, Swanson GD, Aqleh KA, Wiberg DM. J Appl Physiol 1979; 46: 843–53.
232 Belman MJ. Eur J Respir Dis 1981; 62: 391–5.
233 Belman MJ. Clin Chest Med 1986; 7: 585–97.
234 Belman MJ, Mittman C, Weir R. Am Rev Respir Dis 1980; 121: 273–80.
235 Belman MJ, Thomas SG, Lewis MI. Chest 1986; 90: 662–9.
236 Belmusto L, Brown E, Owens G. J Neurosurg 1963; 20: 225–32.
237 Belmusto L, Woldring S, Owens G. J Neurosurg 1965; 22: 277–83.
238 Benady SG. Dev Med Child Neurol 1978; 20: 746–57.
239 Benaim S, Worster–Drought C. Med Illust 1954; 8: 221–6.
240 Bendall MJ. Br Med J 1976; 2: 981–2.
241 Bender AN, Bender MB. Neurology 1977; 27: 206–12.

242 Bender S. Br Med J 1965; 2: 1166.

243 Bendixen HH, Smith GM, Mead J. J Appl Physiol 1964; 19: 195–8.

244 Beneux J, Rigault P, Pouliquen JC, Duval–Beaupere G, Pasteyer J, Durand Y. Rev Chir Orthoped 1976; 62: 781–92.

245 Bengtsson E, Werneman H. Acta Med Scand 1956; Suppl 316: 55–62.

246 Benton JG, Kriete BC. J Chronic Dis 1956; 4: 516–26.

247 Berend N, Marlin GE. Pathology, 1979; 11: 485–91.

248 Berendes J, Miehlke A. Arch Otolaryngol 1973; 98: 63–5.

249 Berg RA, Kaplan AM, Jarrett PB, Molthan ME. Am J Dis Child 1980; 134: 390–3.

250 Berge JE. J Obstet Gynaecol Br Commonwealth 1962; 69: 81–98.

251 Berger AJ, Mitchell RA, Severinghaus JW. N Engl J Med 1977; 297: 194–201.

252 Berger AJ, Mitchell RA, Severinghaus JW. N Engl J Med 1977; 297: 138–43.

253 Berger AJ, Mitchell RA, Severinghaus JW. N Engl J Med 1977; 297: 92–7.

254 Bergfeldt L, Edhag O, Vallin H. Acta Med Scand 1982; 212: 217–23.

255 Bergman NA. J Appl Physiol 1963; 18: 1049–52.

256 Bergman R. Acta Paediatr 1948; 36: 470.

257 Bergofsky EH. J Appl Physiol 1964; 19: 698–706.

258 Bergofsky EH. Arch Phys Med Rehabil 1964; 45: 575–80.

259 Bergofsky EH. Ann Intern Med 1964; 61: 435–47.

260 Bergofsky EH, Turino GM, Fishman AP. Medicine 1959; 38: 263–317.

261 Bergofsky EH. Am Rev Respir Dis 1979; 119: 643–69.

262 Berman JS, Woodford DM. In: Brody JS, Snider GL, eds. Current Topics in the Management of Respiratory Diseases, Vol 2. New York: Churchill Livingstone, 1985: 1–30.

263 Bernstein C, Loeser WD, Manning LE. Radiology 1958; 70: 368–72.

264 Bernstein L, Kazantzis G. Thorax 1954; 9: 326–39.

265 Berra A, Reggiani A. Minerva Med 1960; 51: 1253–8.

266 Berrettini WH. Am J Psychiatr 1980; 137: 493–4.

267 Berry DTR, Webb WB, Block AJ. Chest 1984; 86: 529–31.

268 Berry RB, Block AJ. Chest 1984; 85: 15–20.

269 Berthon–Jones M, Sullivan CE. Am Rev Respir Dis 1982; 125: 632–9.

270 Berthon–Jones M, Sullivan CE. Am Rev Respir Dis 1987; 135: 144–7.

271 Bertrand A, Michel FB, Diet J, et al. Rev Fr Mal Resp 1978; 6: 365–72.

272 Bertrand A, Milane J. Munch Med Wschr 1977; 119: 1647–51.

273 Bertrand A, Milane J. Rev Fr Mal Resp 1979; 7: 341–52.

274 Bethune DW. Anaesthesia 1985; 40: 210–1.

275 Beutler L, Karacan I, Thornby JI, Ware JC, Chambliss S. Sleep Res 1978; 7: 181.

276 Bevegard S. Acta Med Scand 1962; 171: 695–713.

277 Bhatia ML, Misra SC, Prakash J. J Laryngol Otol 1966; 80: 412–7.

278 Bianchi AL, Denavit–Saubie M, ed. Neurogenesis of central respiratory rhythm. Lancaster: MTP Press Ltd, 1985.

279 Bickerman HA, Beck GJ, Gordon C, Barach AL, Itkin S. J Appl Physiol 1952; 5: 92–8.

280 Bickerman HA, Chusid EL. Chest 1970; 58: 53–6.

281 Bicknell PG. J Laryngol Otol 1973; 87: 123–7.

282 Bienenstock H, Lanyi VF. Arch Otolaryngol 1977; 103: 738–9.

283 Binet L, Bochet M. Presse Med 1961; 69: 2040–1.

284 Binet L, Bochet M, Bour H. Biol Med 1948; 37: 1–38.

285 Binet L, Bour H, Bochet M, Schaison G, Melhen R. Presse Med 1961; 69: 1737–40.

286 Biot MC. Lyon Med 1876; 23: 517–28, 561–7.

287 Birath G, Bergh N–P, Swenson EW. Am Rev Tuberc Pulm Dis 1957; 75: 710–23.

288 Birath G, Caro J, Malmberg R, Simonsson BG. Scand J Respir Dis 1956; 47: 27–36.

289 Birath G, Malmberg R, Simonsson BG. Clin Sci 1965; 29: 59–72.

290 Birath G, Soderholm B. Am Rev Tuberc Pulm Dis 1957; 75: 724–9.

291 Birath G, Swenson EW, Ander L, Bergh NP. Am Rev Tuberc Pulm Dis 1957; 76: 983–7.

292 Bird CE. J Am Med Assoc 1927; 89: 101–2.

293 Birnbaum ML, Cree EM, Rasmussen H, Lewis P, Curtis JK. Am J Med 1966; 41: 552–61.

294 Birns JW. Ann Otol Rhinol Laryngol 1984; 93: 447–51.

295 Biscoe TJ, Sampson SR, Purves MJ. Nature 1967; 215: 654–5.

296 Biscoe TJ, Willshaw P. In: Hornbein TF, ed. Regulation of Breathing. Part 1. New York: Marcel Dekker, 1981: 321–45.

297 Bisgard JD. Arch Surg 1934; 29: 417–45.

298 Bishop B. J Appl Physiol 1963; 18: 37–42.

299 Bishop B. J Appl Physiol 1964; 19: 224–32.

300 Bishop B, Hirsch J, Thursby M. J Appl Physiol 1978; 45: 495–501.

301 Bishop HC, Koop CE. Pediatrics 1958; 22: 1088–96.

302 Bixler EO, Kales A, Soldatos CR, Vela–Bueno A, Jacoby JA, Scarone S. Res Commun Chem Pathol Pharmacol 1982; 36: 141–52.

303 Bjork L. Acta Radiol 1973; 14: 412–6.

304 Bjork VO, Carlens E. J Thorac Cardiovasc Surg 1959; 38: 209–14.

305 Bjorkman S, Carlens E. Acta Med Scand 1951; Suppl 259: 63–8.

306 Bjure J, Grimby G, Kasalicky J, Lindh M, Nachemson A. Thorax 1970; 25: 451–6.

307 Bjure J, Grimby G, Nachemson A. Scand J Clin Lab Invest 1968; 21: 190–2.

308 Bjure J, Grimby G, Nachemson A. Acta Orthop Scand 1969; 40: 325–33.

309 Bjure J, Grimby G, Nachemson A, Lindh M. Acta Orthop Scand 1969; 40: 325–33.

310 Bjure J, Nachemson A. Clin Orthop Rel Res 1973; 93: 44–52.

311 Black LF, Hyatt RE. Am Rev Respir Dis 1969; 99: 696–702.

312 Black LF, Hyatt RE. Am Rev Respir Dis 1971; 103: 641–50.

313 Black WC, Ravin A. Arch Pathol 1947; 44: 176–91.

314 Blackwell U. Lancet 1949; 2: 99–101.

315 Blades B, Beattie EJ Jnr, Elias WS. J Thorac Surg 1950; 20: 584–97.

316 Blair E, Hickam JB. J Clin Invest 1955; 34: 383–9.

317 Bland JW Jnr, Edwards FK, Brinsfield D. Am J Cardiol 1969; 23: 830–7.

318 Blanloeil Y, Rochedreux A, Arnould JF, Souron R, Dixneuf B. Ann Fr Anesth Reanimation 1984; 3: 303–5.

319 Blau I, Casson I, Lieberman A, Weiss E. Arch Neurol 1980; 37: 384–5.

320 Bledsoe SW, Hornbein TF. In: Hornbein TF, ed. Regulation of Breathing. Part 1. New York: Marcel Dekker, 1981: 341–427.

321 Blesa MI, Lahiri S, Rashkind WJ, Fishman AP. N Engl J Med 1977; 296: 237–41.

322 Block AJ. Heart Lung 1980; 9: 1011–24.

323 Block AJ. Heart Lung 1981; 10: 90–6.

324 Block AJ, Boysen PG, Wynne JW, Hunt LA. N Engl J Med 1979; 300: 513–7.

325 Block AJ (Chairman), Burrows B, Kanner RE, Lilker ES, Mithoefer JC, Petty TL. Am Rev Respir Dis 1977; 115: 897–9.

326 Block AJ, Faulkner JA, Hughes RL, Remmers JE, Thach B. Chest 1984; 86: 114–22.

327 Block AJ, Wexler J, McDonnell EJ. J Am Med Assoc 1970; 212: 1520–2.

328 Block AJ, Wynne JW, Boysen PG, Lindsey S, Martin C, Cantor B. Am J Med 1981; 70: 506–10.

329 Blom–Bulow B, Jonson B, Bauer K. Semin Arthritis Rheum 1963; 13: 174–81.

330 Blossom RA, Affeldt JE. Am J Med 1956; 20: 77–87.

331 Bluestone CD, Delerme AN, Samuelson GH. Ann Otol 1972; 81: 778–83.

332 Blumbergs PC, Byrne E, Kakulas BA. J Neurol Sci 1984; 65: 221–9.

333 Blythe JA, Griffin JP, Gonyea EF. Arch Intern Med 1977; 137: 1455–7.

334 Bofenkamp B. Arch Otolaryngol 1958; 68: 165–72.

335 Boffa P, Stovin P, Shneerson J. Thorax 1984; 39: 681–2.

336 Bohan A, Peter JB, Bowman RL, Pearson CM. Medicine 1977; 56: 255–86.

337 Bohlman ME, Haponik EF, Smith PL, Allen RP, Bleecker ER, Goldman SM. Am J Roentgenol 1983; 140: 543–8.

338 Bohmer D. Zeitschrift fur Orthopadie 1973; 111: 822–7.

339 Bokinsky GE, Hudson LD, Weil JV. N Engl J Med 1973; 288: 947–8.

340 Bollinger MS, Menkes HA, Benjamin JJ, Ball WC Jnr. Am Rev Respir Dis 1974; 110: 803–6.

341 Bollot JF, Robert D, Chemorin B, et al. Munch Med Wschr 1977; 119: 1641–6.

342 Bonnett C, Brown JC, Perry J, et al. J Bone Joint Surg 1975; 57A: 206–15.

343 Bonora M, St John WM, Bledsoe TA. Am Rev Respir Dis 1985; 131: 41–5.

344 Bonvallet M, Bobo EG. Electroencephalogr Clin Neurophysiol 1972; 32: 1–16.

345 Boor JW, Johnson RJ, Canales L, Dunn DP. Arch Neurol 1977; 34: 686–9.

346 Borowiecki B, Pollak CP, Weitzman ED, Rakoff S, Imperato J. Laryngoscope 1978; 88: 1310–3.

347 Bosch MW, Hirdes JJ, Olthof GKA, Beumer HM. Dis Chest 1962; 41: 49–60.

348 Bosma JF. Pediatrics 1957; 19: 1053–79.

349 Bossen EH, Shelburne JD, Durham NC, Verkauf BS, Bragg F. Arch Pathol 1974; 97: 250–2.

350 Botha GSM. Thorax 1957; 12: 50–6.

351 Boulton TB, Mulvein JT. Proc R Soc Med 1970; 63: 825–31.

352 Bourdillon RB, Davies–Jones E, Stott SD, Taylor LM. Br Med J 1950; 2: 539–47.

353 Bouree P, Bouvier JB, Passeron J, Galanaud P, Dormont J. Br Med J 1970; 1: 1047–9.

354 Boutourline–Young HJ, Whittenberger JL. J Clin Invest 1951; 30: 838–47.

355 Bowen TE, Zajtchuk R, Albus RA. Ann Thorac Surg 1982; 33: 184–8.

356 Bower AG, Bennett VR, Dillon JB, Axelrod B. Ann West Med Surg 1950; 4: 686–716.

357 Bowers VM Jnr, Danforth DN. Am J Obstet Gynecol 1953; 65: 34–9.

358 Bowes G, Andrey SM, Kozar LF, Phillipson EA. J Appl Physiol 1982; 52: 863–8.

359 Bowes G, Andrey SM, Kozar LF, Phillipson EA. J Appl Physiol 1983; 54: 1195–201.

360 Bowes G, Townsend ER, Kozar LF, Bromley SM, Phillipson EA. J Appl Physiol 1981; 51: 40–5.

361 Bowes G, Woolf GN, Sullivan CE, Phillipson EA. Am Rev Respir Dis 1980; 122: 899–908.

362 Bowman WC, Goldberg AAJ, Raper C. Br J Pharmacol Chemother 1962; 19: 464–84.

363 Bowman WC, Raper C. Br J Pharmacol Chemother 1964; 23: 184–200.

364 Boyd DHA, Rogan MC. Br J Dis Chest 1962; 56: 206–11.

365 Boye E, Bastrup–Madsen P. Acta Haematol 1959; 21: 224–31.

366 Boysen PG, Block AJ, Wynne JW, Hunt LA, Flick MR. Chest 1979; 76: 536–42.

367 Brach BB. Chest 1979; 75: 648–50.

368 Brackett NC Jnr, Cohen JJ, Schwartz WB. N Engl J Med 1965; 272: 6–12.

369 Bradley D, Phillipson EA. Am Rev Respir Dis 1983; 128: 583–6.

370 Bradley TD, Brown IG, Grossman RF, et al. N Engl J Med 1986; 315: 1327–31.

371 Bradley TD, Brown IG, Zamel N, Phillipson EA, Hoffstein V. Am Rev Respir Dis 1987; 135: 387–91.

372 Bradley TD, Chartrand DA, Fitting JW, Killian KJ, Grassino A. Am Rev Respir Dis 1986; 134: 1119–24.

373 Bradley TD, Day A, Hyland RH, et al. Am Rev Respir Dis 1984; 130: 678–80.

374 Bradley TD, McNicholas WT, Rutherford R, et al. Am Rev Respir Dis 1986; 134: 217–21.

375 Bradley TD, Rutherford R, Grossman RF, et al. Am Rev Respir Dis 1985; 131: 835–9.

376 Bradley TD, Rutherford R, Lue F, et al. Am Rev Respir Dis 1986; 134: 920–4.

377 Bradley TD, Rutherford R, Popkin J, McNicholas WT, Phillipson EA. Am Rev Respir Dis 1985; 131: Suppl A103.

378 Bradley WG. Ann Neurol 1983; 13: 466.

379 Brady L, Wilson WJ. J Urol 1948; 61: 381–8.

380 Brage D. Rev Clin Esp 1959; 72 30–8;.

381 Bragg WH. Br Med J 1938; 2: 254.

382 Brahdy MB. NY State J Med 1936; 36: 1147–50.

383 Brahdy MB, Lenarsky M. Am J Dis Child 1933; 46; 705–29.

384 Brancatisano T, Collett PW, Engel LA. J Appl Physiol 1983; 54: 1269–76;.

385 Brandt NJ, Terenius L, Jacobsen BB, et al. N Engl J Med 1980; 303: 914–6.

386 Branthwaite MA. Br J Dis Chest 1986; 80: 360–9.

387 Brashear RE, Martin RR, Glover JL. Am Rev Respir Dis 1971; 104: 245–8.

388 Braun NMT, Arora NS, Rochester DF. J Appl Physiol 1982; 53: 405–12.

389 Braun NMT, Arora NS, Rochester DF. Thorax 1983; 38: 616–23.

390 Braun NMT, Faulkner J, Hughes RL, Roussos C, Sahgal V. Chest 1983; 84: 76–84.

391 Braun NMT, Marino WD. Chest 1984; 85: Suppl 59S.

392 Braun NMT, Rochester DF. Am Rev Respir Dis 1979; 119 Suppl: 123–5.

393 Braun SR, Giovannoni R, Levin AB, Harvey RF. Am J Phys Med 1982; 61: 302–9.

394 Bredin CP. Am Rev Respir Dis 1984; 129: A275.

395 Bridger GP. Arch Otolaryngol 1970; 92: 541–53.

396 Bridger GP, Proctor DF. Ann Otol Rhinol Laryngol 1970; 79: 481–8.

397 Brille D, Hatzfeld C, Lejeune F. J Fr Med Chir Thor 1963; 17: 181–90.

398 Briskin JG, Lehrman KL, Guilleminault C. In: Guilleminault C, Dement WC, eds. Sleep Apnea Syndromes. New York: AR Liss Inc, 1978: 317–22.

399 Broadbent WH. Lancet 1877; 1: 307–9.

400 Brodkin HA. Arch Surg 1958; 77: 261–70.

401 Brody AW, O'Halloran PS, Connolly JJ Jnr, Wander HJ, Schwertley FW. Dis Chest 1964; 46: 263–75.

402 Broggi G, Franzini A, Borroni V. Acta Neurochir 1980; 51: 273–8.

403 Brostoff J. Br Med J 1966; 2: 1571–2.

404 Brouillette RT, Hahn YS, Noah ZL, Ilbawi MN Wessel HU. J Ped Surg 1986; 21: 63–5.

405 Brouillette RT, Hunt CE, Gallemore GE. Am Rev Respir Dis 1986; 134: 609–11.

406 Brouillette RT, Ilbawi MN, Hunt CE. J Pediatr 1983; 102: 32–9.

407 Brouillette RT, Thach BT. J Appl Physiol 1979; 46: 772–9.

408 Brouillette RT, Thach BT. J Appl Physiol 1980; 49: 801–8.

409 Brown AL. J Thorac Surg 1939; 9: 164–84.

410 Brown AL. Dis Chest 1951; 20: 378–91.

411 Brown EB Jnr, Campbell GS, Johnson MN, Hemingway A, Visscher MB. J Appl Physiol 1948; 1: 333–8.

412 Brown HW, Plum F. Am J Med 1961; 30: 849–60.

413 Brown IG, Bradley TD, Phillipson EA, Zamel N, Hoffstein V. Am Rev Respir Dis 1985; 132: 211–5.

414 Brown JC, Swank SM, Matta A, Barras DM. J Pediatr Orthop 1984; 4: 456–61.

415 Brown JR, Baker AB. J Nerv Ment Dis 1949; 109: 54–78.

416 Brown L, Kinnear W, Sergeant K–A, Shneerson J. Physiotherapy 1985; 71: 181–3.

417 Brown MM, Wade JPH, Marshall J. Brain 1985; 108: 81–93.

418 Brown SE, Casciari RJ, Light RW. South Med J 1983; 76: 194–8.

419 Brownell AKW, Gilbert JJ, Shaw DT, Garcia B, Wenkebach GF, Lam AKS. Neurology 1978; 28: 1306–9.

420 Brownell LG, Perez–Padilla R, West P, Kryger MH. Bull Eur Physiopath Respir 1983; 19: 621–4.

421 Brownell LG, West P, Sweatman P, Acres JC, Kryger MH. N Engl J Med 1982; 307: 1037–42.

422 Browning RJ. Proc Staff Meetings Mayo Clin 1961, 36: 537–43.

423 Bruce EN. Am Rev Respir Dis 1979; 119: Suppl 61–3.

424 Bruce T. Acta Tuberc Scand 1945; 19: 142–52.

425 Bruce T. Acta Tuberc Scand 1946; 20: 68–88.

426 Bruderman I, Stein M. Ann Intern Med 1961; 55: 94–102.

427 Brunel D, Fanjoux J, Raphael JC, Goulon M. Presse Med 1984; 13: 2322–3.

428 Bryan AC, Muller NL. Sleep 1980; 3: 401–6.

429 Bryan MH. Am Rev Respir Dis 1979; 119: Suppl 137–8.

430 Bryant S, Edwards RHT, Faulkner JA, Hughes RL, Roussos C. Chest 1986; 89: 116–24.

431 Bryce–Smith R, Davis HS. Anesth Analg 1954; 33: 73–84.

432 Bubis MJ, Anthonisen NR. Am Rev Respir Dis 1978; 118: 947–53.

433 Buchem FS van, Nieveen J. Acta Med Scand 1963; 174: 657–63.

434 Buchsbaum HW, Martin WA, Turino GM, Rowland LP. Neurology 1968; 18: 319–327.

435 Bucy PC, Case TJ. J Nerv Ment Dis 1936; 84: 156–68.

436 Buhlmann A, Gierhake W. Schweiz Med Wschr 1960; 90: 1153–5.

437 Buhlmann AA, Neuenschwander R. Schweiz Med Wschr 1977; 107: 802–7.

438 Bulow K. Acta Physiol Scand 1963; 59: Suppl 209: 1–110.

439 Bunch WH, Smith D, Hakala M. Clin Orthop Rel Res 1977; 128: 107–12.

440 Bureau MA, Berthiaume Y, Begin R, Shapcott D, Lemieux B, Cote M. Can J Neurol Sci 1978; 5: 97–9.

441 Bureau MA, Ngassam P, Lemieux B, Trias A. Can J Neurol Sci 1976; 3: 343–7.

442 Burke SS, Grove NM, Houser CR, Johnson DM. Am J Dis Child 1971; 121: 230–4.

443 Burki NK. Chest 1984; 85: 600–4.

444 Burns BD. Br Med Bull 1963; 19: 7–9.

445 Burnstein SL, Weinstein JN, Miota DJ, Melnicoff IL. J Am Osteop Assoc 1979; 78: 723–6.

446 Burr BH, Guyer B, Todres ID, Abrahams B, Chiodo T. N Engl J Med 1983; 309: 1319–23.

447 Burrows B, Harrison RW, Adams WE, Humphreys EM, Long ET, Reimann AF. Am J Med 1960; 28: 281–97.

448 Burrows DL, Hart RW, Onal E, Clancy M, Lopata M. Am Rev Respir Dis 1984; 129: Suppl A246.

449 Burstall AF. Br Med J 1938; 2: 611–2.

450 Burwell CS, Robin ED, Whaley RD, Bickelmann AG. Am J Med 1956; 21: 811–8.

451 Butler J. Clin Sci 1960; 19: 55–62.

452 Butler WJ, Bohn DJ, Bryan AC, Froese AB. Anesth Analg 1980; 59: 577–84.

453 Bye PTP, Ellis ER, Donnelly PD, Issa FG, Sullivan CE. Am Rev Respir Dis 1985; 131: Suppl A108.

454 Bye PTP, Esau SA, Walley KR, Macklem PT, Pardy RL. J Appl Physiol 1984; 56: 464–71.

455 Byers RK, Banker BQ. Arch Neurol 1961; 5: 140–64.

456 Bynum LJ, Wilson JE III, Pierce AK. J Appl Physiol 1976; 41: 341–7.

457 Byrne–Quinn E, Weil JV, Sodal IE, Filley GF, Grover RF. J Appl Physiol 1971; 30: 91–8.

458 Cadieux RJ, Kales A, McGlynn TJ Jnr, Jackson D, Manders EK, Simmonds MA. Arch Otolaryngol 1984; 110: 611–3.

459 Cadieux RJ, Kales A, Santen RJ, Bixler EO, Gordon R. J Clin Endocrinol Metab 1982; 55: 18–22.

460 Cady RB, Bobechko WP. J Pediatr Orthop 1984; 4: 673–6.

461 Cahill JL, Lees GM, Robertson HT. J Pediatr Surg 1984; 19: 430–3.

462 Cahill JL, Okamoto GA, Higgins T, Davis A. J Pediatr Surg 1983; 18: 851–4.

463 Cain SM. Proc Soc Exp Biol Med 1961; 106: 7–10.

464 Callaway JJ, McCusick VA. N Engl J Med 1951; 245: 9–13.

465 Calverley PMA, Chang HK, Vartian V, Zidulka A. Chest 1986; 89: 218–23.

466 Calverley PMA, Chang HK, White D, Zidulka A. Thorax 1984; 39: 235.

467 Calverley PMA, Ewing DJ, Campbell IW, et al. Clin Sci 1982; 63: 17–22.

468 Calverley PMA, Porta D la, Fleury B, Comptois A, Grassino A. Thorax 1984; 39: 716.

469 Calverley PMA, Robson RH, Wraith PK, Prescott LF, Flenley DC. Clin Sci 1983; 65: 65–9.

470 Cameron GS, Scott JW, Jousse AT, Botterell EH. Ann Surg 1955; 141: 451–6.

471 Campbell D. Anaesthesia 1959; 14: 331–8.

472 Campbell EJM. J Physiol 1952; 117: 222–33.

473 Campbell EJM. J Anat 1955; 89: 378–86.

474 Campbell EJM. J Physiol 1957; 136: 556–62.

475 Campbell EJM. Lancet 1960; 2: 12–14.

476 Campbell EJM. Lancet 1960; 2: 10–11.

477 Campbell EJM. Br J Dis Chest 1964; 58: 149–57.

478 Campbell EJM. Br Med J 1965; 1: 1451–60.

479 Campbell EJM. In: Howell JBL and Campbell EJM, eds. Breathlessness. Oxford: Blackwell Scientific Publications, 1966: 55–64.

480 Campbell EJM, Agostoni E, Newsom Davis J. The Respiratory Muscles. Mechanics and Neural Control. London: Lloyd–Luke, 1970.

481 Campbell EJM, Freedman S, Clark TJH, Robson JG, Norman J. Clin Sci 1967; 32: 425–32.

482 Campbell EJM, Friend J. Lancet 1955; 1: 325–9.

483 Campbell EJM, Godfrey S, Clark TJH, Freedman S, Norman J. Clin Sci 1969; 36: 323–8.

484 Campbell EJM, Green JH. J Physiol 1953; 122: 282–90.

485 Campbell EJM, Guz A. In: Hornbein TF, ed. Regulation of Breathing. Part 2. New York: Marcel Dekker, 1981: 1181–95.

486 Campbell EJM, Westlake EK, Cherniack RM. J Appl Physiol 1957; 11: 303–8.

487 Campbell JC. In: Olson DA, Henig E, eds. Proceedings of an international symposium. Whatever happened to the polio patient? Chicago, 1979: 87–90.

488 Cannon PJ. Am J Med 1962; 32: 765–75.

489 Canter HG. Am Rev Respir Dis 1963; 87: 830–5.

490 Canter HG, Luchsinger PC. Am J Med Sci 1964; 248: 206–11.

491 Cape CA, Fincham RW. Neurology 1965; 15: 191–3.

492 Carbone JE, Barker D, Stauffer JL. Chest 1985; 87: 401–3.

493 Cardus D, Vallbona C, Spencer WA. Dis Chest 1966; 50: 297–306.

494 Carlin L, Biller J. J Neurol Neurosurg Psychiatr 1975; 44: 852–3.

495 Caro CG, DuBois AB. Thorax 1961; 16: 282–90.

496 Caro CG, Gucker T III. Am Rev Tuberc 1958; 78: 326.

497 Caroll JE, Zwillich C, Weil JV, Brooke MH. Neurology 1976; 26: 140–6.

498 Carpenter RJ III, McDonald TJ, Howard FM Jnr. Otolaryngology 1978; 86: 479–84.

499 Carratu L, Marangio E, Pesci A, Censi A, Sofia M. Torace 1978; 21: 93–105.

500 Carroll D. Am J Med 1956; 21: 819–24.

501 Carroll JE, Hagberg JM, Brooke MH, Shumate JB. Arch Neurol 1979; 36: 457–61.

502 Carroll JE, Zwillich CW, Weil JV. Neurology 1977; 27: 1125–8.

503 Carroll N, Branthwaite MA. Thorax 1987; 42: 723.

504 Carskadon MA, Dement WC. J Gerontol 1981; 36: 420–3.

505 Carter MG, Gaensler EA, Kyllonen A. N Engl J Med 1950; 243: 549–58.

506 Carter R, Williams JS, Berry J, Peavler M, Griner D, Tiep B. Chest 1986; 89: 806–10.

507 Carter RE. Paraplegia 1979; 17: 140–6.

508 Carter RE. Adv Neurol 1979; 22: 261–9.

509 Cartwright R, Lilie J. Sleep Res 1985; 14: 149.

510 Cartwright RD. Sleep 1984; 7: 110–4.

511 Cartwright RD, Samelson CF. J Am Med Assoc 1982; 248: 705–9.

512 Castile RG, Staats BA, Westbrook PR. Am Rev Respir Dis 1982; 126: 564–8.

513 Caton R. Br Med J 1889; 1: 358.

514 Catterall JR, Calverley PMA, Shapiro CM, Flenley·DC, Douglas NJ. Am Rev Respir Dis 1985; 132: 86–8.

515 Catterall JR, Douglas NJ, Calverley PMA, et al. Am Rev Respir Dis 1983; 128: 24–9.

516 Caughey JE, Gray WG. Thorax 1954; 9: 67–70.

517 Caughey JE, Pachomov N. J Neurol Neurosurg Psychiatr 1959; 22: 311–3.

518 Cavrot E, Richards J. Brux Med 1957; 37: 1366–73.

519 Celli BR. Clin Chest Med 1986; 7: 567–84.

520 Celli BR, Corral R, Rassulo J, Gilmartin M, Beer DJ. Am Rev Respir Dis 1985; 131: A319.

521 Celli BR, Rassulo J, Berman JS, Make B. Am Rev Respir Dis 1985; 131: 178–80.

522 Ceriana G, Locatelli G. Minerva Med 1969; 60: 2507–32.

523 Chadha TS, Birch S, Sackner MA. Chest 1985; 88: 16–23.

524 Chadha TS, Watson H, Birch S, et al. Am Rev Respir Dis 1982; 125: 644–9.

525 Chakrabarti MK, Gordon G, Whitwam JG. Br J Anaesth 1986; 58: 11–17.

526 Chamberlain DA, Millard FJC. Q J Med 1963; 32: 341–50.

527 Chan CK, Mohsenin V, Loke J, Virgulto J, Sipski ML, Ferranti R. Chest 1987; 91: 567–70.

528 Chandler KW, Rozas CJ, Kory RC, Goldman AL. Am J Med 1984; 77: 243–9.

529 Chang KC, Morrill CG, Chai H. Chest 1978; 73: 667–9.

530 Chanson P, Timsit J, Benoit O, et al. Lancet 1986; 1: 1270–1.

531 Chapman EM, Dill DB, Graybiel A. Medicine 1939; 18: 167–202.

532 Chapman KR, Liu FLW, Watson RM, Rebuck AS. Chest 1986; 89: 540–2.

533 Charles BM, Hosking G, Green A, Pollitt R, Bartlett K, Taitz LS. Lancet 1979; 2: 118–20.

534 Chau W, Lee KH. J Obstet Gynaecol Br Commonwealth 1970; 77: 1098–1102.

535 Chaudhary BA, Elguindi AS, Giacomini K, Speir WA. Am Rev Respir Dis 1982; 125: Suppl 101.

536 Chaudhary BA, Elguindi AS, King DW. South Med J 1982; 75: 65–7.

537 Chausow AM, Kane T, Levinson D, Szidon JP. Am Rev Respir Dis 1984; 130: 142–4.

538 Cheney FW Jnr, Nelson EJ, Horton WG. Am Rev Respir Dis 1974; 110: Suppl 183–7.

539 Chennebault JM, Masson C, Dumont AM, Alquier P. Nouv Presse Med 1980; 9: 2848.

540 Cherniack NS. J Am Med Assoc 1974; 230: 57–8.

541 Cherniack NS. New Engl J Med 1981; 305: 325–30.

542 Cherniack NS. J Clin Invest 1984; 73: 1501–6.

543 Cherniack NS, Altose MD. In: Hornbein TF, ed. Regulation of Breathing. Part 2. New York: Marcel Dekker, 1981: 905–64.

544 Cherniack NS, Euler C von, Homma I, Kao FF. Respir Physiol 1979; 37: 185–200.

545 Cherniack NS, Longobardo GS. Physiol Rev 1970; 50: 196–243.

546 Cherniack NS, Longobardo GS. N Engl J Med 1973; 288: 952–7.

547 Cherniack RM. J Clin Invest 1953; 32: 1192–6.

548 Cherniack RM, Adamson JD, Hildes JA. J Appl Physiol 1955; 7: 375–8.

549 Cherniack RM, Ewart WB, Hildes JA. Ann Intern Med 1957; 46: 720–7.

550 Cherniack RM, Svanhill E. Am Rev Respir Dis 1976; 113: 721–8.

551 Cherniack RM, Young G. Ann Intern Med 1964; 60: 631–40.

552 Chernick V. Pediatrics 1973; 52: 114–5.

553 Cheshire DJE, Flack WJ. Paraplegia 1978; 16: 162–74.

554 Chevrolet J–C, Reverdin A, Suter PM, Tschopp J–M, Junod AF. Chest 1983; 84: 112–5.

555 Chick DW, deHoratius RJ, Skipper BE, Messner RP. J Rheumatol 1976; 3: 262–8.

556 Chillingworth FP, Hopkins R. J Lab Clin Med 1919; 4: 555–63.

557 Chin EF. Br J Surg 1957; 44: 360–76.

558 Chin EF, Lynn RB. J Thorac Surg 1956; 32: 6–14.

559 Chisholm JC Jnr, Gilson A. J Nat Med Assoc 1980; 72: 997–8.

560 Chodoff P, Imbembo AL, Knowles CL, Margand PMS. Surgery 1977; 81: 399–403.

561 Chokroverty S, Sachdeo R, Masdeu J. Arch Neurol 1984; 41: 926–31.

562 Chokroverty S, Sharp JT. J Neurol Neurosurg Psychiatr 1981; 44: 970–82.

563 Chokroverty S, Sharp JT, Barron KD. J Neurol Neurosurg Psychiatry 1978; 41: 980–6.

564 Chong KC, Letts RM, Cumming GR. J Pediatr Orthop 1981; 1; 251–4.

565 Chopra JS, Banerjee AK, Murthy JMK, Pal SR. Brain 1980; 103: 789–802.

566 Christensen MS, Kristensen HS, Hansen EL. Acta Med Scand 1975; 198: 409–13.

567 Christensen P. Thorax 1959; 14: 311–9.

568 Christie AB. Br Med J 1954; 2: 663–5.

569 Christie RV. J Clin Invest 1934; 13: 295–321.

570 Christopher KL, Spofford BT, Brannin PK, Petty TL. Am Rev Respir Dis 1986; 133: A209.

571 Chuan PS. Singapore Med J 1970; 11: 125–9.

572 Chudley AE. Am J Dis Child 1979; 133: 1182–5.

573 Chung HD, DeMello DE, D'Souza N, Estrada J. Neurology 1982; 32: 441–4.

574 Church SC. Arch Intern Med 1967; 119: 176–81.

575 Ciesielski TE, Fukuda Y, Glenn WWL, Gorfien J, Jeffery K, Hogan JF. J Neurosurg 1963; 58: 92–100.

576 Cirignotta F, Lugaresi E. Sleep 1980; 3: 225–6.

577 Cisler I. Arch Int Laryngol 1927; 6: 1054–7.

578 Citrin DL, Boyd G, Bradley GW. Scot Med J 1973; 18: 109–13.

579 CJST. Br Med J 1912; 1: 843–5.

580 Clague HW, Hall DR. Thorax 1979; 34: 523–6.

581 Clanton TL, Dixon G, Drake J, Gadek JE. Chest 1985; 87: 62–6.

582 Clanton TL, Dixon GF, Drake J, Gadek JE. J Appl Physiol 1985; 59: 1834–41.

583 Clark FJ, Euler C von. J Physiol 1972; 222: 267–95.

584 Clark RW, Boudoulas H, Schaal SF, Schmidt HS. Neurology 1980; 30: 113–9.

585 Clark RW, Schmidt HS, Schaal SF, Boudoulas H, Schuller DE. Neurology 1979; 29: 1287–92.

586 Clements PJ, Furst DE, Campion DS, et al. Arthritis Rheum 1978; 21: 62–71.

587 Clough P. Arch Phys Med Rehabil 1983; 64: 384–5.

588 Coates EO Jnr, Brinkman GL, Noe FE. Ann Intern Med 1958; 48: 50–9.

589 Cobb JR. Am Acad Orthop Surg 1948; 5: 261–75.

590 Cobb S, Forbes A. Am J·Physiol 1923; 65: 234–51.

591 Cobham IG, Davis HS. Anesth Analg 1964; 43: 22–9.

592 Coccagna G, Donato G di, Verucchi P, Cirignotta F, Mantovani M, Lugaresi E. Arch Neurol 1976; 33: 769–76.

593 Coccagna G, Mantovani M, Brignani F, Parchi C, Lugaresi E. Bull Physiopath Respir 1972; 8: 1159–72.

594 Coccagna G, Mantovani M, Brignani F, Parchi C, Lugaresi E. Bull Physiopath Respir 1972; 8: 1217–27.

595 Coccagna G, Mantovani M, Parchi C, Mironi F, Lugaresi E. J Neurol Neurosurg Psych 1975; 38: 977–84.

596 Coccagna G, Martinelli P, Lugaresi E. Acta Neurol Belg 1982; 82: 185–94.

597 Cohen CA, Zagelbaum G, Gross D, Roussos C, Macklem PT. Am J Med 1982; 73: 308–16.

598 Cohen FL. J Neurosurg 1973; 39: 589–95.

599 Cohen MI. Am J Physiol 1964; 206: 845–54.

600 Cohen MI. Physiol Rev 1979; 59: 1105–73.

601 Cohen MI, Hugelin A. Arch Ital Biol 1965; 103: 317–34.

602 Cohn JE, Carroll DG, Riley RL. Am J Med 1954; 17: 447–63.

603 Cohn JE, Kuida H. Ann Intern Med 1962; 56: 633–44.

604 Colbert AP, Schock NC. Arch Phys Med Rehabil 1985; 66; 760–2.

605 Cole P, Fastag O, Forsyth R. J Otolaryngol 1980; 9: 309–15.

606 Cole P, Haight JSJ. Am Rev Respir Dis 1984; 129: 351–4.

607 Cole P, Haight JSJ, Love L, Oprysk D. Am Rev Respir Dis 1985; 132: 1229–32.

608 Cole S, Lindenberg LB, Galioto FM Jnr, et al. Pediatrics 1979; 63: 13–17.

609 Coleman RF, Thompson LR, Niehuis AW, Munsat TL, Pearson CM. Arch Pathol 1968; 86: 365–76.

610 Colgan FJ, Mahoney PD, Fanning GL. Anesthesiology 1970; 32: 543–50.

611 Collier CR, Affeldt JE. J Appl Physiol 1954; 6: 531–8.

612 Collier CR, Dail CW, Affeldt JE. J Appl Physiol 1956; 8: 580–4.

613 Collins D, Scoggin CH, Zwillich CW, Weil JV. Clin Res 1977; 25: 132A.

614 Collins VP. Arch Neurol Psychiatr 1942; 48: 774–88.

615 Collis DK, Ponseti IV. J Bone Joint Surg 1969; 51A: 425–45.

616 Colp C, Kriplani L, Nussbaum M. Chest 1980; 77: 218–20.

617 Colville P, Shugg C, Ferris BG Jnr. J Appl Physiol 1956; 9: 19–24.

618 Comroe JH, Botelho S. Am J Med Sci 1947; 214: 1–6.

619 Comroe JH, Dripps RD. J Am Med Assoc 1946; 130: 381–3.

620 Comroe JH Jnr. Am Rev Respir Dis 1975; 111: 689–92.

621 Comroe JH, Wood FC, Kay CF, Spoont EM. Am J Med 1951; 10: 786–9.

622 Conn HO. Am J Med 1960; 29: 647–61.

623 Conn HO, Dunn JP, Newman HA, Belkin GA.
     Am J Med 1957; 22: 524–33.

624 Connaughton JJ, Douglas NJ, Morgan AD, et al.
     Am Rev Respir Dis 1985; 132: 206–10.

625 Conner LA. Am J Med Sci 1911; 141: 350–60.

626 Conner LA, Stillman RG. Arch Intern Med
     1912; 9: 203–19.

627 Conomy JP, Levinsohn M, Fanaroff A. J Pediatr
     1975; 87: 428–30.

628 Contamin F, Lissac J, Nick J. Presse Med 1966;
     74: 1939–42.

629 Conti F, Bertoli L, Bertoli M, Mantero O.
     Pharmacol Res Commun 1976; 8: 243–51.

630 Conway W, Fujita S, Zorick F, et al. Chest 1985;
     88: 385–7.

631 Conway W, Fujita S, Zorick F, Roth T, Hartse
     K, Piccione P. Am Rev Respir Dis 1980; 121:
     Suppl 121.

632 Conway W, Roth T, Zorick F. Am Rev Respir
     Dis 1982; 125: Suppl 102.

633 Conway W, Victor L, Fujita S, Zorick F, Roth
     T. Am Rev Respir Dis 1980; 121: Suppl 122.

634 Conway WA, Bower GC, Barnes ME. J Am Med
     Assoc 1977; 237: 2740–2.

635 Conway WA, Victor LD, Magilligan DJ Jnr, et
     al. J Am Med Assoc 1981; 246: 347–50.

636 Conway WA, Zorick F, Piccione P, Roth T.
     Thorax 1982; 37: 49–53.

637 Cook CD, Barrie H, DeForest SA, Helliesen PJ.
     Pediatrics 1960; 25: 766–74.

638 Coombs CF. Br J Surg 1930; 18: 326–8.

639 Cooper CB, Davidson AC, Cameron IR. Bull
     Eur Physiopath Respir 1987; 23: 15–22.

640 Cooper CB, Trend PStJ, Wiles CM. Thorax
     1985; 40: 633–4.

641 Cooper CB, Waterhouse J, Howard P. Thorax
     1987; 42: 105–10.

642 Cooper DM, Rojas JV, Mellins RB, Keim HA,
     Mansell AL. Am Rev Respir Dis 1984; 130:
     16–22.

643 Cooper KR, Phillips BA. J Appl Physiol 1982;
     53: 855–8.

644 Corda M, Euler C von, Lennerstrand G. J
     Physiol 1965; 178: 161–77.

645 Corda M, Euler C von, Lennerstrand G. J
     Physiol 1966; 184: 898–923.

646 Cormack RS, Cunningham DJC, Gee JBL. Q J
     Exp Physiol 1957; 42: 306–19.

647 Cormier Y, Kashima H, Summer W, Menkes H.
     Chest 1979; 75: 423–7.

648 Cornwell AC, Pollack MA, Kravath RE, Llena J,
     Nathenson G, Weitzman ED. Int J Neurosci
     1981; 15: 155–62.

649 Cornwell JB, Davis HN. Respir Ther 1979; 9:
     87–90.

650 Corson JA, Grant JL, Moulton DP, Green RL,
     Dunkel PT. Chest 1979; 76: 543–5.

651 Coryllos E. Arch Pediatr 1953; 70: 122–34.

652 Costa JL da. Med J Aust 1972; 1: 373–6.

653 Cote M, Bureau M, Leger C, Martin J, Gattiker
     H, Cimon M, Larose A, Lemieux B. Can J
     Neurol Sci 1979; 6: 151–7.

654 Cote M, Davignon A, Pecko–Drouin K, et al.
     Can J Neurol Sci 1976; 3: 319–21.

655 Cotes JE. Thorax 1960; 15: 244–51.

656 Cotes JE, Gilson JC. Lancet 1956; 1: 872–6.

657 Cotton RT. Arch Otolaryngol 1983; 109: 502.

658 Couch AHC. Thorax 1953; 8: 326–8.

659 Council on Physical Medicine. J Am Med Assoc
     1947; 135: 715.

660 Council on Physical Medicine. J Am Med Assoc
     1948; 137: 867.

661 Council on Physical Medicine. J Am Med Assoc
     1949; 141: 658.

662 Council on Physical Medicine. J Am Med Assoc
     1949; 139: 1273.

663 Council on Physical Medicine. J Am Med Assoc
     1949; 139: 1001.

664 Council on Physical Medicine. J Am Med Assoc
     1950; 144: 1181.

665 Council on Physical Medicine. J Am Med Assoc
     1950; 143: 1157.

666 Counihan TB. Br Heart J 1956; 18: 425–6.

667 Cournand A. Circulation 1950; 2: 641–57.

668 Cournand A, Berry FB. Ann Surg 1942; 116:
     532–52.

669 Cournand A, Himmelstein A, Riley RL, Lester
     CW. J Thorac Surg 1947; 16: 30–49.

670 Cournand A, Richards DW Jnr. Am Rev Tuberc
     1941; 44: 123–72.

671 Cournand A, Richards DW Jnr, Maier HC. Am
     Rev Tuberc 1941; 44: 272–87.

672 Cournand A, Riley RL, Himmelstein A,
     Austrian R. J Thorac Surg 1950; 19: 80–116.

673 Courtenay Evans RJ, Benson MK, Hughes
     DTD. Br Med J 1971; 1: 530–1.

674 Coutts KD, Rhodes EC, McKenzie DC. J Appl
     Physiol 1983; 55: 479–82.

675 Covelli HD, Black JW, Olsen MS, Beekman JF.
     Ann Intern Med 1981; 95: 579–81.

676 Covelli HD, Weled BJ, Beekman JF. Chest 1982;
     81: 147–50.

677 Cox MA, Schiebler GL, Taylor WJ, Wheat MW
     Jnr, Krovetz LJ. J Pediatr 1965; 67: 192–7.

678 Craddock WL, Barracks J. J Am Med Assoc
     1951; 146: 1315–6.

679 Crane MG, Affeldt JE, Austin E, Bower AG. J
     Appl Physiol 1956; 9: 11–18.

680 Creese BJ, Land A, Fielden R. Br J Prev Soc
     Med 1977; 31: 116–21.

681 Creese R. J Physiol 1950; 110: 450–7.

682 Criner G, Make B, Celli B. Chest 1987; 91:
     139–41.

683 Croft CB, McKelvie P, Fairley JW, Hol–Allen
     RTJ, Shaheen O. J R Soc Med 1986; 79: 473–5.

684 Crofton J. Br Med J 1959; 1: 1610–4.

685 Cronin RE, Ferguson ER, Shannon WA Jnr,
     Knochel JP. Am J Physiol 1982; 243: F113–20.

686 Cropp AJ, diMarco AF, Altose MD. Am Rev
     Respir Dis 1984; 129: A34.

687 Cropp A, DiMarco AF. Am Rev Respir Dis
     1987; 135: 1056–61.

688 Cross AB, Webber RH. Br Med J 1985; 291:
     532–4.

689 Cross KW. Proc R Soc Med 1950; 43: 445–6.

690 Cullen DJ, Ferrara LC, Briggs BA, Walker PF, Gilbert J. N Engl J Med 1976; 294: 982–7.

691 Cullen JH, Brum VC, Reidt WU. Am J Med 1959; 27: 551–7.

692 Cullen JH, Formel PF. Am J Med 1962; 32: 525–31.

693 Cummiskey J, Lynne–Davies P, Guilleminault C. In: Guilleminault C, Dement WC eds. Sleep Apnea Syndromes. New York: AR Liss Inc; 1978: 295–308.

694 Cummiskey J, Williams TC, Krumpe PE, Guilleminault C. Am Rev Respir Dis 1982; 126: 221–4.

695 Cundy JM. Anaesthesia 1980; 35: 35–41.

696 Curran FJ. Arch Phys Med Rehabil 1981; 62: 270–4.

697 Curtis DJ, Cruess DF, Berg T. Am J Roentgenol 1984; 142: 497–500.

698 Curtis JK, Bauer H, Rasmussen HK, Mendenhall JT. J Thorac Surg 1959; 37: 598–605.

699 Curtis JK, Liska AP, Rasmussen HK, Cree EM. J Am Med Assoc 1968; 206: 1037–40.

700 Cushing H. Brain 1909; 32: 44–53.

701 Cutting WC. Stanford Med Bull 1944; 2: 172–5.

702 Czorniak MA, Gilmartin ME, Make BJ. Am Rev Respir Dis 1987; 135: Suppl A194.

703 Da Costa JL. Med J Aust 1972; 1: 373–6.

704 Daher YH, Lonstein JE, Winter RB, Bradford DS. Clin Orth Rel Res 1986; 202: 219–22.

705 Dail CW. Calif Med 1951; 75: 217–8.

706 Dail CW. Med Arts Sci 1956; 10: 64–70.

707 Dail CW. Arch Phys Med Rehabil 1965; 46: 655–75.

708 Dail CW, Affeldt JE, Collier CR. J Am Med Assoc 1955; 158: 445–9.

709 Dail CW, Bennett VR, Bower AG. Arch Phys Med 1950; 31: 276–80.

710 Daley R. Br Heart J 1945; 7: 101–3.

711 Daly MdeB, Angell–James JE. Lancet 1979; 1: 764–7.

712 Dalziel J. Br Assoc Adv Sci 1838; 2: 127–8.

713 D'Angelo E, Sant'Ambrogio G, Agostoni E. J Appl Physiol 1974; 37: 311–5.

714 Danon J, Druz WS, Goldberg NB, Sharp JT. Am Rev Respir Dis 1979; 119: 909–19.

715 Daras M, Spiro AJ, Swerdlow M. NY State J Med 1984; 84: 570–2.

716 Darwish RY, Fairshter RD, Vaziri ND, Rooney J, Schwartz G. Western J Med 1985; 143: 383–5.

717 Datey KK, Deshmukh MM, Engineer SD, Dalvi CP. Br Heart J 1964; 26: 614–9.

718 Dau PC. Chest 1984; 85: 721–2.

719 Dau PC, Lindstrom JM, Cassel CK, Denys EH, Sher EE, Spitler LE. N Engl J Med 1977; 297: 1134–40.

720 Davenport PW, Thompson FJ, Reep RL, Freed AN. Brain Res 1985; 328: 150–3.

721 Davidson JT, Whipp BJ, Wasserman K, Koyal SN, Lugliani R. N Engl J Med 1974; 290: 819–22.

722 Davies AG, Dingle HR. J Neurol Neurosurg Psychiatr 1972; 35: 176–9.

723 Davies CE, MacKinnon J. Lancet 1949; 2: 883–5.

724 Davies CTM, Godfrey S, Light M, Sargeant AJ, Zeidifard E. J Appl Physiol 1975; 38: 373–6.

725 Davies G, Reid L. Arch Dis Childh 1971; 46: 623–32.

726 Davies H. Br J Dis Chest 1959; 53: 151–8.

727 Davies H, Williams J, Wood P. Br Heart J 1962; 24: 129–38.

728 Davies HM. Pulmonary Tuberculosis. Medical and surgical treatment. London: Cassell Co Ltd, 1933: 323–6.

729 Davies HW, Haldane JS, Priestley JG. J Physiol 1919; 53: 60–9.

730 Davies SF, Iber C. Am Rev Respir Dis 1983; 127: 245–7.

731 D'Avignon P, Sundell L, Werneman H. Acta Med Scand 1956; Suppl 316: 107–10.

732 Davis CJF, Gallai V. Acta Neurol 1979; 34: 365–70.

733 Davis H 2nd, Lefrak SS, Miller D, Malt S. J Am Med Assoc 1980; 243: 43–5.

734 Davis JN. Arch Neurol 1974; 30: 480–3.

735 Davis JN, Goldman M, Loh L, Casson M. Q J Med 1976; 45: 87–100.

736 Davis JN, Loh L. Bull Europ Physiopath Resp 1979; 15: Suppl 45–51.

737 Daw E, Chandler G. Postgrad Med J 1976; 52: 492–6.

738 De Backer M, Bergmann P, Perissino A, Gottignies P, Kahn RJ. Eur J Intensive Care Med 1967; 2: 63–7.

739 de Ramirez AF, Aguirre AU, Ancira FP, Mata MR. Rev Invest Clin (Mex) 1981; 33: 25–8.

740 De Troyer A. Respir Physiol 1983; 53: 341–53.

741 De Troyer A. Bull Eur Physiopath Respir 1984; 20: 409–13.

742 De Troyer A, Bastenier–Geens J. J Appl Physiol 1979; 47: 1162–8.

743 De Troyer A, Borenstein S. Am Rev Respir Dis 1979; 119: Suppl 303.

744 De Troyer A, Borenstein S. Am Rev Respir Dis 1980; 121: 629–38.

745 De Troyer A, Borenstein S, Cordier R. Thorax 1980; 35: 603–10.

746 De Troyer A, de Beyl DZ, Thirion M. Am Rev Respir Dis 1981; 123: 631–2.

747 De Troyer A, Deisser P. Am Rev Respir Dis 1981; 124: 132–7.

748 De Troyer A, Estenne M. Thorax 1981; 36: 169–74.

749 De Troyer A, Estenne M. J Appl Physiol 1984; 57: 899–906.

750 De Troyer A, Estenne M, Heilporn A. N Engl J Med 1986; 314: 740–4.

751 De Troyer A, Estenne M, Ninane V. Am Rev Respir Dis 1985; 132: 793–9.

752 De Troyer A, Estenne M, Vincken W. Am Rev Respir Dis 1986; 133: 1115–9.

753 De Troyer A, Heilporn A. Am Rev Respir Dis 1980; 122: 591–600.

754 De Troyer A, Kelly S. J Appl Physiol 1984; 56: 326–32.

755 De Troyer A, Kelly S, Zin WA. Science 1983; 220; 87–8.

756 De Troyer A, Sampson M, Sigrist S, Kelly S. J Appl Physiol 1983; 54: 465–9.

757 De Troyer A, Sampson M, Sigrist S, Macklem PT. Science 1981; 213: 237–8.

758 De Troyer A, Sampson M, Sigrist S, Macklem PT. J Appl Physiol 1982; 53: 30–9.

759 De Troyer A, Yernault J–C, Englert M, Baran D, Paiva M. J Appl Physiol 1978; 44: 521–7.

760 DeBusk FL, O'Connor S. Pediatrics 1972; 50: 328–9.

761 DeCramer M, de Troyer A, Kelly S, Zocchi L, Macklem PT. J Appl Physiol 1984; 57; 1682–7.

762 Dee PM, Suratt PM, Bray ST, Rose CE Jnr. Chest 1984; 85: 363–6.

763 Deedwania PC, Swiryn S, Dhingra RC, Rosen KM. Chest 1979; 76: 319–21.

764 Degat OR, Camus P, Vanoli A, Sorokaty JM, Jeamin L. Lyon Med 1981; 245: 547–9.

765 Delhez L, Petit J–M. Rev Fra Etudes Clin Biol 1961; 6: 580–4.

766 Demedts M, Beckers J, Rochette F, Bulcke J. Eur J Respir Dis 1982; 63: 62–7.

767 Dement WC, Carskadon MA, Richardson G. In: Guilleminault C, Dement WC, eds. Sleep Apnea Syndromes. New York: AR Liss Inc, 1978; 23–46.

768 D'Empaire G, Hoaglin DC, Perlo VP, Pontoppidan H. J Thorac Cardiovasc Surg 1985; 89: 592–6.

769 Dempsey JA. Chest 1976; 70: 114–8.

770 Dempsey JA, Skatrud JB. Am Rev Respir Dis 1986; 133: 1163–70.

771 Denison DM, Bellamy D, Pierce RJ. In: Zorab PA, Siegler D, eds. Scoliosis, 1979; London: Academic Press, 1980: 137–47.

772 Denison DM, Peacock AJ, Morgan MDL, Branthwaite MA, Gourlay AR. Br J Dis Chest 1982; 76: 20–34.

773 Deonna T, Arczynska W, Torrado A. J Pediatr 1974; 84: 710–4.

774 Department of Health and Social Security. Non-contributory benefits for disabled people. London: HMSO, 1985.

775 Derenne J–PH, Macklem PT, Roussos C. Am Rev Respir Dis 1978; 118: 119–33, 373–90, 581–601.

776 deReuck J, de Coster W, Inderadjaja N. J Neurolog Sci 1977; 33: 453–60.

777 DeRosa GP. Spine 1985; 10: 618–22.

778 Derveaux L, Lacquet LM. Thorax 1982; 37: 870–1.

779 Desert R, Chevre A, Desriaux D, Guilloux J le. Rev Tuberculose 1969; 33: 424–35.

780 Desmarais MHL, Alcock AJW, Hildes JA. Can Med Assoc J 1956; 75: 654–7.

781 deSouza RFX, Longo AM. Bull Europ Physiopath Respir 1986; 20: 22s.

782 Dessertine A. In: Olson DA, Henig E, eds. Proceedings of an international symposium. Whatever happened to the polio patient? Chicago, 1979: 151–4.

783 Devathasan G, Tong HI. Aust NZ J Med 1980; 10: 188–91.

784 Deveraux MW, Keane JR, Davis RL. Arch Neurol 1973; 29: 46–55.

785 DeVilliers R, Nose Y, Meier W, Kantrowitz A. Trans Am Soc Artif Intern Organs 1964; 10: 357–65.

786 Dewhurst CJ. J Obstet Gynaecol Br Empire 1953; 60: 76–9.

787 Di Maria G. Poumon Coeur 1962; 18: 539–64.

788 Diagnostic classification of sleep and arousal disorders. First edition. Sleep Disorders Classification Committee. Roffwarg HB, Chairman. Sleep 1979; 2: 1–137.

789 Diamond E, Druz W, D'Souza V, Sharp JT. Am Rev Respir Dis 1982; 125: 235.

790 Diaz FV, Pelous AN, Valdes FG, Grande FGG, Granados A. Am J Cardiol 1962; 10: 272–7.

791 DiBenedetto RJ, Firth M, Ham E, Causey D. South Med J 1983; 76: 1312–4.

792 Dickson RA. Br Med J 1984; 289: 269–70.

793 Diessner GR, Howard FM Jnr, Winkelmann RK, Lambert EH, Mulder DW. Arch Intern Med 1966; 117: 757–63.

794 DiMarco AF, Kelling J, Sajovic M, Jacobs I, Shields R, Altose MD. Clin Res 1982; 30: 427A.

795 DiMarco AF, Nochomovitz M, Dimarco MS, Altose MD, Kelsen SG. Am Rev Respir Dis 1985; 132: 800–5.

796 DiMarco AF, Wolfson DA, Gottfried SB, Altose MD. J Appl Physiol 1982; 53: 1481–6.

797 Dimase JD, Groover R, Allen JE. N Engl J Med 1959; 261: 553–5.

798 DiMauro S, Stern LZ, Mehler M, Nagle RB, Payne C. Muscle Nerve 1978; 1: 27–36.

799 Dingemans LM, Hawn JM. Paraplegia 1978; 16: 175–83.

800 DiRocco J, Breed AL, Carlin JI, Reddan WG. Arch Phys Med Rehabil 1983; 64: 476–8.

801 Djallilian M, Kern EB, Brown HA, et al. Mayo Clin Proc 1975; 50: 11–14.

802 Dobie RA, Tobey DN. J Am Med Assoc 1979; 242: 2197–201.

803 Dodge PR, Gamstorp I, Byers RK, Russell P. Pediatrics 1965; 35: 3–19.

804 Doe OW. Bost Med Surg J 1889; 120: 9.

805 Doekel RC, Zwillich CW, Scoggin CH, Kryger M, Weil JV. N Engl J Med 1976; 295: 358–61.

806 Dollery CT, Gillam PMS, Hugh–Jones P, Zorab PA. Thorax 1965; 20: 175–81.

807 Dolly FR, Block AJ. Am J Med 1982; 73: 239–43.

808 Dolly FR, Block AJ. Chest 1983; 84: 394–8.

809 Domm BM, Vassallo CL. Am Rev Respir Dis 1973; 107: 123–6.

810 Domm BM, Vassallo CL. Am Rev Respir Dis 1973; 107: 842–5.

811 Donald K. Lancet 1949; 2: 1056–7.

812 Donner MW, Silbiger ML. Am J Med Sci 1966; 251: 600–16.

813 Donoghue FE, Winkelmann RK, Moersch HJ. Ann Otol 1960; 69: 1139–45.

814 Donovan WH, Taylor N. Arch Phys Med Rehabil 1973; 54: 485–8.

815 D'Orbcastel OR, de Fenoyl O. Rev Med 1983; 24: 602–8.

816 Dorner RA, Keil PG, Schissel DJ. J Thorac Surg 1950; 20: 444–53.

817 Dorr JR, Brown JC, Perry J. J Bone Joint Surg 1973; 55A: 436–7.

818 Douglas FG, Chong PY. J Appl Physiol 1972; 33: 559–63.

819 Douglas JG, Fergusson RJ, Crompton GK, Grant IWB. Br Med J 1983; 286: 1943–6.

820 Douglas NJ. Clin Chest Med 1985; 6: 563–75.

821 Douglas NJ, Brash HM, Wraith PK, et al. Am Rev Respir Dis 1979; 119: 311–3.

822 Douglas NJ, Calverley PMA, Leggett RJE, Brash HM. Lancet 1979; 1: 1–4.

823 Douglas NJ, Connaughton JJ, Morgan AD, Shapiro CM, Pardy N, Flenley DC. Bull Eur Physiopath Respir 1983; 19: 631.

824 Douglas NJ, White DP, Weil JV, et al. Am Rev Respir Dis 1982; 125: 286–9.

825 Douglas NJ, White DP, Weil JV, Pickett CK, Zwillich CW. Thorax 1982; 37: 791.

826 Douglas NJ, White DP, Weil JV, Pickett CK, Zwillich CW. Am Rev Respir Dis 1982; 126: 758–62.

827 Douglass BE, Clagett OT. Dis Chest 1960; 37: 294–7.

828 Douglass PS, Rosen RL, Butler PW, Bone RC. Chest 1987; 91: 413–7.

829 Dowell AR, Buckley CE 3rd, Cohen R, Whalen RE, Sieker HO. Arch Int Med 1971; 127: 712–26.

830 Dowell AR, Heyman A, Sieker HO, Tripathy K. N Engl J Med 1965; 273: 1447–53.

831 Dowling PC, Menonna JP, Cook SD. J Am Med Assoc 1977; 238: 317–8.

832 Dowman CE. J Am Med Assoc 1927; 88: 95–7.

833 Downs JB, Perkins HM, Sutton WW. Anesthesiology 1974; 40: 602–3.

834 Drachman DA, Tuncbay TO. Neurology 1965; 15: 1127–35.

835 Drachman DB, Gumnit RJ. Arch Neurol 1962; 6: 471–7.

836 Draper MH, Ladefoged P, Whitteridge D. Br Med J 1960; 1: 1837–43.

837 Dressler W, Kleinfeld M. Am J Med 1954; 16: 61–72.

838 Drinker P. Lancet 1931; 1: 1186–9.

839 Drinker P, McKhann CF. J Am Med Assoc 1929; 92: 1658–60.

840 Drinker P, Roy EL. J Pediatr 1938; 13: 71–4.

841 Drinker P, Shaughnessy TJ, Murphy DP. J Am Med Assoc 1930; 95: 1249–53.

842 Drinker P, Shaw LA. J Clin Invest 1929; 7: 229–47.

843 Drinker PA, McKhann CF III. J Am Med Assoc 1986; 255: 1476–80.

844 Dripps RD, Comroe JH Jnr. Am J Physiol 1947; 149: 43–51.

845 Druz WS, Danon J, Fishman HC, Goldberg NB, Moisan TC, Sharp JT. Am Rev Respir Dis 1979; 119: Suppl 145–9.

846 Dubowitz LMS, Dubowitz V. Arch Dis Childh 1964; 39: 293–6.

847 Dubowitz V. Muscle Disorders in Childhood. London: WB Saunders Co Ltd, 1978.

848 Duchenne GB. In: A treatise on localized electrization and its applications to pathology and therapeutics. (Translated by Tibbets H.) London: Robert Hardwicke, 1871: 105.

849 Duchenne GB. In: Physiology of motion demonstrated by means of electrical stimulation and clinical observation and applied to the study of paralysis and deformities. (Translated by Kaplan EB.) Philadelphia: WB Saunders 1949: 498–9.

850 Duffy PE, Ziter FA. Neurology 1964; 14: 500–9.

851 Dugan RJ, Black ME. Am J Obstet Gynecol 1957; 73: 89–93.

852 Dujovny M, Osgood CP, Segal R. Laryngoscope 1976; 86: 1397–401.

853 Dulfano MJ, Ishikawa S. Ann Intern Med 1965; 63: 829–41.

854 Dull WL, Polu JM, Sadoul P. Clin Sci 1983; 64: 25–31.

855 Dull WL, Sadoul D. Am Rev Respir Dis 1981; 123: Suppl 74.

856 Dundee JW, Gray RC, Gupta PK. Anaesthesia 1974; 29: 710–4.

857 Dunkin LJ. Anaesthesia 1983; 38: 644–9.

858 Dunn AD, Heagey FW. Am J Med Sci 1920; 160: 568–82.

859 Dunn JM. Am J Obstet Gynecol 1976; 125: 265–6.

860 Dunnell K, Adler MW, Day I, Holland WW, Ide L, Thorne S. Community Med 1972; 22: 503–6.

861 Dunnill MS. Med Thorac 1965; 22: 261–74.

862 Duranceau CA, Letendre J, Clermont RJ, Levesque H–P, Barbeau A. Can J Surg 1978; 21: 326–9.

863 Durand P, Razzi A, Mastragostino A, Gimelli FA. Min Pediatr 1965; 17: 1437–41.

864 Duron B. Acta Neurobiol Exp 1973; 33: 355–80.

865 Duron B. In: Hornbein TF, ed. Regulation of Breathing. Part 1. New York: Marcel Dekker, 1981: 473–540.

866 Duron B, Marlot D. Sleep 1980; 3: 269–80.

867 Duron B, Quichaud J, Fullana N. Bull Physiopath Respir 1972; 8: 1277–88.

868 D'Urzo AD, Lawson VG, Vassal KP, Rebuck AS, Slutsky AS, Hoffstein V. Am Rev Respir Dis 1987; 135: 392–5.

869 Dutt AK. Am Rev Respir Dis 1970; 101: 755–8.

870 Duvoisin RC, Marsden CD. J Neurol Neurosurg Psychiatr 1975; 38: 787–93.

871 Dwight T. Am J Med Sci 1900; 120: 429–35.

872 Dye JP. N Engl J Med 1983; 308: 1167–8.

873 Dyke SC. Lancet 1918; 1: 570.

874 Easton PA, Fleetham JA, Rocha A de la, Anthonisen NR. Am Rev Respir Dis 1983; 127: 125–8.

875 Eberle E, Brink J, Azen S, White D. J Pediatr 1975; 86: 356–9.

876 Economo C von. Encephalitis Lethargica. Its Sequelae and Treatment. (Trans Newman KO.) London: Oxford Medical Publications, 1931.

877 Edelman J, Stewart–Wynne EG. Br Med J 1981; 283: 275–6.

878 Edelman NH, Cherniack NS, Lahiri S, Richards E, Fishman AP. J Clin Invest 1970; 49: 1153–65.

879 Edelman NH, Lahiri S, Braudo L, Cherniack NS, Fishman AP. N Engl J Med 1970; 282: 405–11.

880 Edelman NH, Richards EC, Fishman AP. J Clin Invest 1967; 46: 1051.

881 Edelman NH, Rucker RB, Peavy HH. Am Rev Respir Dis 1986; 134: 347–52.

882 Edelman NH, Santiago TV, eds. Breathing Disorders of Sleep. New York: Churchill Livingstone, 1986.

883 Ederli A, Figa–Talamanca L, Vesentini G, Carratelli D. Riv Neurobiol 1978; 24: 67–71.

884 Edison B, Kerth JD. Arch Otolaryngol 1973; 98: 205–7.

885 Edmondson RS, Flowers MW. Br Med J 1979; 1: 1401–4.

886 Edstrom L, Kugelberg E. J Neurol Neurosurg Psychiatr 1968; 31: 424–33.

887 Edwards C, Heath D, Harris P. J Pathol 1971; 104: 1–13.

888 Edwards G, Leszczynski SO. Lancet 1967; 2: 226–9.

889 Edwards RHT. Clin Sci Molec Med 1978; 54: 463–70.

890 Edwards RHT, Griffiths RD, Hayward M, Helliwell T. J R Coll Physicians 1986; 20: 49–55.

891 Edwards RHT, Hill DK, Jones DA, Merton PA. J Physiol 1977; 272: 769–78.

892 Edwards RHT, Round JM, Jones DA. Muscle Nerve 1983; 6: 676–83.

893 Edwards WM. Calif Med 1948; 69: 367–74.

894 Efron R, Kent DC. Arch Neurol 1957; 77: 575–87.

895 Efthimiou J, Belman MJ, Holman RAE, Edwards RHT, Spiro SG. Am Rev Respir Dis 1986; 133: 667–71.

896 Efthimiou J, Fleming J, Gomes C, Spiro SG. Thorax 1987; 42: 227.

897 Egbert LD, Laver MB, Bendixen HH. Anesthesiology 1963; 24: 57–60.

898 Eichenhorn MS, Dossantos CJ, Harper PA. Am Rev Respir Dis 1983; 128: 765–7.

899 Eisele J, Trenchard D, Burki N, Guz A. Clin Sci 1968; 35: 23–33.

900 Eisele JH, Cross CE, Rausch DC, Kurpershoek CJ, Zelis RF. N Engl J Med 1971; 285: 366–8.

901 Eisenberg H, Dubois EL, Sherwin RP, Balchum OJ. Ann Intern Med 1973; 79: 37–45.

902 Eisenkraft JB, Papatestas AE, Kahn CH, Mora CT, Fagerstrom R, Genkins G. Anesthesiol 1986; 65: 79–82.

903 Eisenmenger R. Wien Klin Wschr 1929; 47: 1502–3.

904 Eisenmenger R. Wien Med Wschr 1939; 44: 1032–6.

905 Elam JO, Hemingway A, Gullickson G, Visscher MB. Arch Intern Med 1948; 81: 649–65.

906 Eldridge FL. J Appl Physiol 1975; 39: 567–74.

907 Eldridge FL. Chest 1978; 73 Suppl: 256–8.

908 Eldridge FL, Millhorn DE, Waldrop TG, Kiley JP. Respir Physiol 1983; 53: 239–61.

909 Eldridge FL, Vaughn KZ. J Appl Physiol 1977; 43: 312–21.

910 Eliaschar I, Lavie P, Halperin E, Gordon C, Alroy G. Arch Otolaryngol 1980; 106: 492–6.

911 Elliott CG, Hill TR, Adams TE, Crapo RO, Neitzeba RM, Gardner RM. Bull Eur Physiopath Respir 1985; 21: 363–8.

912 Ellis ER, Bye PTP, Bruderer JW, Sullivan CE. Am Rev Respir Dis 1987; 135: 148–52.

913 Emerson JH. The Evolution of Iron Lungs. JH Emerson Co, 1978.

914 Emery AEH, Skinner R. Clin Genet 1976; 10: 189–201.

915 Emirgil C, Sobol BJ. Am Rev Respir Dis 1973; 108: 831–42.

916 Emmanuel GE, Smith WM, Briscoe WA. J Clin Invest 1966; 45: 1221–33.

917 Engel AG. Brain 1970; 93: 599–616.

918 Engel AG, Gomez MR, Seybold ME, Lambert EH. Neurology 1973; 23: 95–106.

919 Engel LA, Ritchie B. J Appl Physiol 1971; 30: 173–7.

920 Engel WK, Gold GN, Karpati G. Arch Neurol 1968; 18: 435–44.

921 Enghoff H, Holmdahl MH, Risholm L. Acta Soc Med Upsal 1952; 57: 61–9.

922 Engstrom C–G. Br Med J 1954; 2: 666–9.

923 Epstein SW, Vanderlinden RG, Man SFP, et al. Can Med Assoc J 1979; 120: 1360–8.

924 Erikson H, Hauge M. Acta Orthop Scand 1963; 33: 395–6.

925 Esau SA, Bye PTP, Pardy RL. J Appl Physiol 1983; 55: 731–5.

926 Escher DJW, Furman S, Solomon N, Schwedel JB. Am Heart J 1966; 72: 283–4.

927 Escourrou P, Harf A, Simonneau G, Atlan G, Lemaire F, Laurent D. Bull Europ Physiopath Resp 1981; 17: 187–95.

928 Estenne M, Borenstein S, de Troyer A. Am Rev Respir Dis 1984; 130: 681–4.

929 Estenne M, de Troyer A. Am Rev Respir Dis 1985; 132: 53–9.

930 Estenne M, De Troyer A. Am Rev Respir Dis 1986; 134: 121–4.

931 Estenne M, de Troyer A. Am Rev Respir Dis 1987; 135: 367–71.

932 Estenne M, Heilporn A, Delhez L, Yernault J–C, de Troyer A. Am Rev Respir Dis 1983; 128: 1002–7.

933 Estes EH Jnr, Sieker HO, McIntosh HD, Kelser GA. Circulation 1957; 16: 179–87.

934 Estrup C, Lyager S, Naeraa N, Olsen C. Respiration 1986; 50: 36–43.

935 Euler C von. J Appl Physiol 1983; 55: 1647–59.

936 Euler C von, Hayward JN, Marttila I, Wyman RJ. Brain Res 1973; 61: 1–22.

937 Evans CC, Hipkin LJ, Murray GM. Thorax 1977; 32: 322–7.

938 Evans TW, Howard P. Br Med J 1984; 289: 449–50.

939 Eve FC. Lancet 1932; 2: 995–7.

940 Eve FC. Br Med J 1943; 1: 535–7.

941 Eve FC. Br Med J 1945; 1; 21–2.

942 Eve FC, Forsyth NC. Br Med J 1948; 2: 554–5.

943 Fabricius J, Davidsen HG, Hansen AT. Dan Med Bull 1957; 4: 251–7.

944 Fackler CD, Perret GE, Bedell GN. J Appl Physiol 1967; 23: 923–6.

945 Fadell EJ, Richman AD, Ward WW, Hendon JR. N Engl J Med 1962; 266: 861–3.

946 Faerber I, Liebert PB, Suskind M. J Appl Physiol 1962; 17: 289–92.

947 Faling LJ. Clin Chest Med 1986; 7: 599–618.

948 Fallat RJ, Jewitt B, Bass M, Kamm B, Norris FH Jnr. Arch Neurol 1979; 36: 74–80.

949 Fan L, Murphy S. Am J Dis Child 1981; 135: 550–2.

950 Fanta CH, Leith DE, Brown R, Scharf S, Song P, Ingram RH Jnr. Am Rev Respir Dis 1980; 121: Suppl 133.

951 Farebrother MJB. Br J Dis Chest 1979; 73: 211–29.

952 Farebrother MJB, McHardy GJR, Munro JF. Br Med J 1974; 3: 391–3.

953 Farhi LE, Rahn H. J Appl Physiol 1955; 7: 472–84.

954 Farmer W, Littner MR, Gee JBL. Arch Intern Med 1977; 137: 309–12.

955 Farmer WC, Glenn WWL, Gee JBL. Am J Med 1978; 64: 39–49.

956 Farney RJ, Walker LE, Jensen RL, Walker JM. Chest 1986; 89: 533–9.

957 Faulkner JA, Maxwell LC, Ruff GL, White TP. Am Rev Respir Dis 1979; 119: Suppl 89–92.

958 Fearl CS. West J Surg Obstet Gynecol 1951; 59: 411–22.

959 Feigelson CI, Dickinson DG, Talner NS, Wilson JL. N Engl J Med 1956; 254: 611–3.

960 Feinsilver SH, Friedman JH, Rosen JM. J Neurol Neurosurg Psych 1986; 49: 964.

961 Feldman J, Tuteur PG. Heart Lung 1982; 11: 162–5.

962 Feldman RM. Orthopedics 1985; 8: 888–9.

963 Feltman JA, Newman W, Schwartz A, Stone DJ, Lovelock FJ. J Clin Invest 1952; 31: 762–9.

964 Fencl V, Vale JR, Broch JA. J Appl Physiol 1969; 27: 67–76.

965 Fenichel GM. Arch Neurol 1978; 35: 97–103.

966 Ferdinandus J, Pederson JA, Whang R. Arch Intern Med 1981; 141: 669–70.

967 Ferguson A, Gaensler EA. Surg Clin North Am 1968; 48: 293–310.

968 Ferguson JT, Murphy RP, Lascelles RG. J Neurol Neurosurg Psychiatr 1982; 45: 217–22.

969 Ferrer MI. Med Clin North Am 1979; 63: 251–65.

970 Ferris BG Jnr, Pollard DS. J Clin Invest 1960; 39: 143–9.

971 Ferris BG Jnr, Pollard DS. N Engl J Med 1960; 263: 1048–52.

972 Ferris BG Jnr, Warren A, Beals CA. N Engl J Med 1955; 252: 618–21.

973 Ferris BG Jnr, Whittenberger JL, Affeldt JE. N Engl J Med 1952; 246: 919–23.

974 Ferris BG, Mead J, Whittenberger JL, Saxton GA. N Engl J Med 1952; 247: 390–3.

975 Ferris EB, Engel GL, Stevens CD, Webb J. J Clin Invest 1946; 25: 734–43.

976 Fielding JW, Tuul A, Hawkins RJ. J Bone Joint Surg 1975; 57A: 1000–1.

977 Filler J, Smith AA, Stone S, Dancis J. J Pediatr 1965; 66: 509–16.

978 Filley GF, Swanson GD, Kindig NB. Clin Chest Med 1980; 1: 13–32.

979 Finch CA, Miller LR, Inamdar AR, Person R, Seiler K, Mackler B. J Clin Invest 1976; 58: 447–53.

980 Findley LJ, Blackburn MR, Goldberger AL, Mandell AJ. Am Rev Respir Dis 1984; 130: 937–9.

981 Findley LJ, Wilhoit SC, Suratt PM. Chest 1985; 87: 432–6.

982 Finegold MJ, Katzew H, Genieser NB, Becker MH. Am J Dis Child 1971; 122: 153–9.

983 Fink A, Rivin A, Murray JF. Arch Intern Med 1961; 108: 427–37.

984 Fink BR. J Appl Physiol 1961; 16: 15–20.

985 Fink BR, Basek M, Epanchin V. Laryngoscope 1956; 66: 410–25.

986 Fink BR, Katz R, Reinhold H, Schoolman A. Am J Physiol 1962; 202: 217–20.

987 Finley KH. Arch Neurol Psychiatr 1931; 26: 754–83.

988 Fisch C, Evans PV. N Engl J Med 1954; 251: 527–9.

989 Fischer DA. Cleve Clin Q 1985; 52: 303–6.

990 Fischer DA, Prentice WS. Chest 1982; 82: 739–43.

991 Fischer L, Engeser J. Med Welt 1936; 47: 1664–7.

992 Fischer RA, Ellison GW, Thayer WR, Spiro HM, Glaser GH. Ann Intern Med 1965; 63: 229–48.

993 Fisher CM. Acta Neurol Scand 1969; 45: Suppl 36, 1–56.

994 Fisher SV, Gullickson G Jnr. Arch Phys Med Rehabil 1978; 59: 124–33.

995 Fishman AP, Bergofsky EH, Turino GM, Jameson AG, Richards DW. Circulation 1956; 14: 935.

996 Fishman AP, Goldring RM, Turino GM. Q J Med 1966; 35: 261–75.

997 Fishman AP, Turino GM, Bergofsky EH. Am J Med 1957; 23: 333–9.

998 Fishman LS, Samson JH, Sperling DR. Am J Dis Child 1965; 110: 155–61.

999 Fisk JR, Bunch WH. Orthop Clin North Am 1979; 10: 863–75.

1000 Flagstad AE, Kollman S. J Bone Joint Surg 1928; 10: 724–34.

1001 Flaum A. Acta Med Scand 1936; Suppl 78: 849–55.

1002 Fleetham JA, Bradley CA, Kryger MH, Anthonisen NR. Am Rev Respir Dis 1980; 122: 833–40.

1003 Fleetham JA, Clarke H, Dhingra S, Chernick C, Anthonisen NR. Am Rev Respir Dis 1980; 121: 1045–9.

1004 Fleming PJ, Bryan MH, Bryan AC. Pediatrics 1980; 66; 425–8.

1005 Flemister G, Goldberg NB, Sharp JT. Chest 1981; 79: 33–8.

1006 Flenley DC. Chest 1985; 87: 99–103.

1007 Flenley DC. J R Soc Med 1985; 78: 1031–3.

1008 Fletcher EC, Levin DC. Chest 1984; 85: 6–14.

1009 Flowers NC, Dawson JE, Horan LG. J Tenn Med Assoc 1972; 65: 804–8.

1010 Fluck TC. Clin Sci 1966; 31: 383–8.

1011 Fodstad H, Andersson G, Blom S, Linderholm H. Appl Neurophysiol 1985; 48: 351–7.

1012 Fodstad H, Blom S. Neurochirurgia 1984; 27: 115–6.

1013 Fodstad H, Blom S, Linderholm H. Scand J Rehabil Med 1983; 15: 173–81.

1014 Folgering H, Kuyper F, Kille JF. Bull Europ Physiopath Resp 1979; 15: 659–65.

1015 Follansbee WP, Curtiss EI, Rahko PS, et al. Am J Med 1985; 79: 183–92.

1016 Forbes GS, Glenn WWL, Lange RC. Surgery 1974; 75: 398–407.

1017 Forner JV. Paraplegia 1980; 18: 258–66.

1018 Forner JV, Llombart RL, Valledor MCV. Paraplegia 1977; 15: 245–51.

1019 Forster HV, Dempsey JA, Birnbaum ML, et al. Fed Proc 1969; 28: 1274–9.

1020 Foster JH, Killen DA, Rhea WG Jnr, McCracken RC, Diveley WL, Hubbard WW. Am Rev Respir Dis 1965; 92: 489–90.

1021 Foster S, Hoskins D. Pediatr Clin North Am 1981; 28: 855–7.

1022 Foulks CJ. South Med J 1981; 74: 1423–4.

1023 Fountain FF, Reynolds LB, Tickle SM. Am J Phys Med 1973; 52: 277–88.

1024 Fowler WS. J Appl Physiol 1954; 6: 539–45.

1025 Fox JL. Acta Neurochir 1968; 18: 309–17.

1026 Fox JL. Neurology 1969; 1115–8.

1027 Fraimow W, Cathcart RT, Goodman E. Am Rev Respir Dis 1960; 81: 815–22.

1028 Fraimow W, Mann JJ, Flickinger H, Cathcart RT. J Am Med Assoc 1960; 173: 1098–101.

1029 Francis RS, Curwen MP. Tubercle 1964; 45: Suppl 1–79.

1030 Francois T, Mayaud C, Carette MF, et al. Ann Med Intern 1982; 133: 553–6.

1031 Frank Y, Kravath RE, Inoue K, et al. Ann Neurol 1981; 10: 18–27.

1032 Frankel HL, Mathias CJ, Spalding JMK. Lancet 1975; 2: 1183–5.

1033 Franssen MJAM, Herwaarden CLA van, Putte LBA van de, Gribnau FWJ. J Rheumatol 1986; 13: 936–40.

1034 Fraser IM. Clin Chest Med 1986; 7: 131–9.

1035 Fraser RS, Sproule BJ, Dvorkin J. Can Med Assoc J 1963; 89: 1178–82.

1036 Frates RC Jnr, Splaingard ML, Smith EO, Harrison GM. J Pediatr 1985; 106: 850–6.

1037 Fredberg JJ, Wohl MEB, Glass GM, Dorkin HL. J Appl Physiol 1980; 48: 749–58.

1038 Freedman B. Thorax 1950; 5: 169–82.

1039 Freedman BJ. Br J Ophthalmol 1963; 47: 290–4.

1040 Freedman S. J Physiol 1966; 184: 42–4P.

1041 Freedman S. Respir Physiol 1970; 8: 230–44.

1042 Freeman WJ. Laryngoscope 1973; 83: 238–49.

1043 Fremion AS, Garg BP, Kalsbeck J. J Pediatr 1984; 104: 398–401.

1044 French LA. Lancet 1953; 73: 283–7.

1045 French SG. J R Naval Med Serv 1938; 24: 349–50.

1046 Freyschuss U, Nilsonne U, Lundgren K–D. Acta Med Scand 1968; 184: 365–72.

1047 Freyschuss U, Nilsonne U, Lundgren K–D. Acta Med Scand 1972; 192: 41–9.

1048 Friedman S, Goffin FB. Laryngoscope 1966; 76: 1520–3.

1049 Frith RW, Cant BR. Thorax 1985; 40: 45–50.

1050 Froese AB, Bryan AC. Am Rev Respir Dis 1987; 135: 1363–74.

1051 Fromm GB, Wisdom PJ, Block AJ. Chest 1977; 71: 612–4.

1052 (a) Frost EAM. J Neurosurg 1979; 50: 699–714. (b) Fruhmann G. Bull Physiopath Resp 1972; 8: 1173–9.

1053 Fugl–Meyer AR. Scand J Rehabil Med 1971; 3: 141–50.

1054 Fugl–Meyer AR. Scand J Rehabil Med 1971; 3: 168–77.

1055 Fugl–Meyer AR, Grimby G. Scand J Clin Lab Invest 1969; Suppl 110: 44.

1056 Fugl–Meyer AR, Grimby G. Scand J Rehabil Med 1971; 3: 161–7.

1057 Fugl–Meyer AR, Grimby G. Scand J Rehabil Med 1971; 3: 151–60.

1058 Fugl–Meyer AR, Linderholm H, Wilson AF. Scand J Rehabil Med 1983; Suppl 9: 118–24.

1059 Fujita S, Conway W, Zorick F, Roth T. Otolaryngol – Head Neck Surg 1981; 89: 923–4.

1060 Fujita S, Conway WA, Sicklesteel JM, et al. Laryngoscope 1985; 95: 70–4.

1061 Fulkerson WJ, Wilkins JK, Esbenshade AM, Eskind JB, Newman JH. Am Rev Respir Dis 1984; 129: 185–7.

1062 Furman RH, Callaway JJ. Dis Chest 1950; 18: 232–43.

1063 Furman S, Koerner SK, Escher DJW, Papowitz AJ, Benjamin J, Tarjan P. J Thorac Cardiovasc Surg 1971; 62: 743–51.

1064 Gacad G, Hamosh P. Am Rev Respir Dis 1973; 107: 286–9.

1065 Gadoth N, Sokol J, Lavie P. J Neurol Sci 1983; 60: 117–25.

1066 Gaensler EA. J Lab Clin Med 1952; 39: 917–34.

1067 Gaensler EA, Cugell DW. J Lab Clin Med 1952; 40: 558–78.

1068 Gaensler EA, Cugell DW, Lindgren I, Verstraeten JM, Smith SS, Strieder JW. J Thorac Surg 1955; 29: 163–87.

1069 Gaensler EA, Lindgren I. Am Rev Respir Dis 1959; 80: 185–93.

1070 Gaensler EA, Strieder JW. J Thorac Surg 1950; 20: 774–97.

1071 Gaensler EA, Strieder JW. J Thorac Surg 1951; 22: 1–34.

1072 Gaensler EA, Watson TR Jnr, Patton WE. J Lab Clin Med 1953; 41: 436–55.

1073 Gailani S, Danowski TS, Fisher DS. Circulation 1958; 17: 583–8.

1074 Gal TJ. Anesthesiology 1980; 52: 324–9.

1075 Galdston M. J Clin Invest 1952; 31: 631.

1076 Galdston M. Am J Med 1955; 19: 516–32.

1077 Galdston M, Geller J. Am J Med 1957; 23: 183–96.

1078 Galloway TC. J Am Med Assoc 1943; 123: 1096–7.

1079 Galloway TC. Arch Otolaryngol 1947; 46: 125–36.

1080 Galloway TC, Seifert MH. J Am Med Assoc 1949; 141: 1–8.

1081 Galpine JF. Lancet 1954; 1: 707–9.

1082 Galy P, Brune J, Paramelle B, et al. Rev Lyon Med 1970; 19: 361–75.

1083 Gamble CJ, Pepper OHP, Muller GP. J Am Med Assoc 1925; 85: 1485–7.

1084 Garay SM, Rapoport D, Sorkin B, Epstein H, Feinberg I, Goldring RM. Am Rev Respir Dis 1981; 124: 451–7.

1085 Garay SM, Turino GM, Goldring RM. Am J Med 1981; 70: 269–74.

1086 Gardner–Medwin D. Br Med Bull 1980; 36: 109–15.

1087 Garlind T, Linderholm H. Acta Med Scand 1958; 162: 333–49.

1088 Garrett JM, DuBose TD Jnr, Jackson JE, Norman JR. Arch Intern Med 1969; 123: 26–32.

1089 Garrison JH. Arch Phys Med Rehabil 1982; 63: 180–1.

1090 Gashi F, Kenrick MM. South Med J 1975; 68: 1524–8.

1091 Gaskell D. Physiotherapy 1970; 56: 360–4.

1092 Gaskell DV, Webber BA. The Brompton Hospital Guide to Chest Physiotherapy, 3rd ed. Oxford: Blackwell Scientific Publications, 1977.

1093 Gastaut H, Tassinari CA, Duron B. Rev Neurol 1965; 112: 568–79.

1094 Gastaut H, Tassinari CA, Duron B. Brain Res 1966; 1: 167–86.

1095 Gathier JC, Bruyn GW. In: Vinken PJ, Bruyn GW, eds. Handbook of Clinical Neurology, Volume 8. Amsterdam: North–Holland, 1970: 77–85.

1096 Gattiker H, Buhlmann A. Helv Med Acta 1966; 33: 122–38.

1097 Gaultier C. Bull Eur Physiopath Respir 1985; 21: 55–112.

1098 Gauthier GF, Padykula HA. J Cell Biol 1966; 28: 333–54.

1099 Gautier H, Lefrancois R, Pasquis P. Respir Physiol 1975; 23: 201–7.

1100 Gautier H, Remmers JE, Bartlett D Jnr. Respir Physiol 1973; 18: 205–21.

1101 Gazioglu K. Bull Physiopath Respir 1973; 9: 711–3.

1102 Gazioglu K, Goldstein LA, Femi–Pearse D, Yu PN. J Bone Joint Surg 1968; 50A: 1391–9.

1103 Geddes DM, Rudolf M, Saunders KB. Thorax 1976; 31: 548–51.

1104 Geffin B, Grillo HC, Cooper JD, Pontoppidan H. J Am Med Assoc 1971; 216: 1984–8.

1105 Geoffroy G, Barbeau A, Breton G, et al. Can J Neurol Sci 1976; 3: 279–86.

1106 George CF, Kryger MH. Am Rev Respir Dis 1985; 131: 485–6.

1107 George CF, West P, Kryger MH. Am Rev Respir Dis 1987; 135: Suppl A: 50.

1108 George RJD, Geddes DM. Br J Hosp Med 1985; 33: 344–9.

1109 George RJD, Howard RS, Geddes DM. Thorax 1984; 39: 717.

1110 George RJD, Winter RJD, Flockton SJ, Geddes DM. Thorax 1984; 39: 235.

1111 George RJD, Winter RJD, Johnson MA, Slee IP, Geddes DM. Thorax 1984; 39: 234–5.

1112 Gerard M, Robert D, Salamand J, Buffat J, Chemorin B, Bertoye A. Lyon Medical 1981; 245: 555–8.

1113 Gerlag PGG, Rooy MJ van, Booij A, Dam FE van, Coul AAW op de. Clin Neurol Neurosurg 1981; 82: 237–43.

1114 Getzen LC, Rehman I, Holloway CK. J Thorac Cardiovasc Surg 1968; 55: 169–77.

1115 Gibbons WJ, Levy RD, Deschamps A, Rotaple M, Gregory W, Marliss E, Cosio MG. Am Rev Respir Dis 1987; 135: A294.

1116 Gibson DA, Koreska J, Robertson D, Kahn A III, Albisser AM. Orthop Clin North Am 1978; 9: 437–50.

1117 Gibson DA, Wilkins KE. Clin Orthop Rel Res 1975; 108: 41–51.

1118 Gibson GJ, Clark E, Pride NB. Am Rev Respir Dis 1981; 124: 665–89.

1119 Gibson GJ, Edmonds JP, Hughes GRV. Am J Med 1977; 63: 926–32.

1120 Gibson GJ, Pride NB. Am Rev Respir Dis 1979; 119 Suppl: 119–20.

1121 Gibson GJ, Pride NB. Am Rev Respir Dis 1982; 126: 1117–8.

1122 Gibson GJ, Pride NB, Newsom Davis J, Loh LC. Am Rev Respir Dis 1977; 115: 389–95.

1123 Gibson TC. Am Heart J 1975; 90: 389–96.

1124 Gilbert R, Auchincloss JH Jnr, Brodsky J, Boden W. J Appl Physiol 1972; 33: 252–4.

1125 Gilbert R, Auchincloss JH Jnr, Peppi D. Chest 1981; 80: 607–12.

1126 Gilbert R, Auchincloss JH Jnr, Peppi D, Ashutosh K. Chest 1974; 65: 152–7.

1127 Gill PK. J Physiol 1963; 168: 239–57.

1128 Gillam PMS, Heaf PJD, Kaufman L, Lucas BGB. Thorax 1964; 19: 112–20.

1129 Gillam PMS, Mymin D. Lancet 1961; 2: 853–5.

1130 Gilmartin JJ, Gibson GJ. Am Rev Respir Dis 1986; 134: 683–7.

1131 Gilmartin JJ, Walls TJ, Stone TN, Gibson GJ. Thorax 1984; 39: 716.

1132 Gilmartin JJ, Wright AJ, Cartlidge NEF, Gibson GJ. Thorax 1984; 39: 313–4.

1133 Gilmartin ME. Clin Chest Med 1986; 7: 619–27.

1134 Gilroy J, Cahalan JL, Berman R, Newman M. Circulation 1963; 27: 484–93.

1135 Gimenez M, Pham QT, Vittoz-Polu E. Ann Med Physique 1969; 12: 9–25.

1136 Gish GB. In: Young JA, Crocker D, eds. Principles and Practice of Respiratory Therapy, 2nd ed. Chicago: Year Book Medical Publishers Inc; 1976: 453–526.

1137 Giundi GM, Bannister R, Gibson WPR, Payne JK. J Neurol Neurosurg Psych 1981; 44: 49–53.

1138 Glasser RL, Tippett JW, Davidian VA Jnr. Nature 1966; 209: 810–2.

1139 Glenn WWL. Pace 1978; 1: 357–70.

1140 Glenn WWL. Ann Thorac Surg 1980; 30: 106–9.

1141 Glenn WWL, Gee JB, Cole DR, Farmer WC, Shaw RK, Beckman CB. Am J Med 1978; 64: 50–60.

1142 Glenn WWL, Gee JBL, Schachter EN. J Thorac Cardiovasc Surg 1978; 75: 273–81.

1143 Glenn WWL, Haak B, Sasaki C, Kirchner J. Ann Surg 1980; 191: 655–63.

1144 Glenn WWL, Hogan JF, Loke JSO, Ciesielski TE, Phelps ML, Rowedder R. N Engl J Med 1984; 310: 1150–5.

1145 Glenn WWL, Hogan JF, Phelps ML. Surg Clin North Am 1980; 60: 1055–78.

1146 Glenn WWL, Holcomb WG, Gee JBL, Rath R. Ann Surg 1970; 172: 755–73.

1147 Glenn WWL, Holcomb WG, Hogan J, et al. J Thorac Cardiovasc Surg 1973; 66: 505–20.

1148 Glenn WWL, Holcomb WG, McLaughlin AJ, O'Hare JM, Hogan JF, Yasuda R. N Engl J Med 1972; 286: 513–6.

1149 Glenn WWL, Holcomb WG, Shaw RK, Hogan JF, Holschuh KR. Ann Surg 1976; 183: 566–77.

1150 Glenn WWL, Phelps ML. Neurosurgery 1985; 17: 974–84.

1151 Glenn WWL, Sairenji H. In: Roussos C, Macklem PT, eds. Thorax. Marcel Dekker Inc, 1985: 1407–40.

1152 Glogowska M, Richardson PS, Widdicombe JG, Winning AJ. Respir Physiol 1972; 16: 179–96.

1153 Gluck MC, Becker KL, Katz S. Am Rev Respir Dis 1967; 95: 676–80.

1154 Gode GR, Raju AV, Jayalakshmi TS, Kaul HL, Bhide NK. Lancet 1976; 2: 6–8.

1155 Godfrey S. Respiration 1970; 27: Suppl 67–70.

1156 Godfrey S. J Pediatr 1980; 96: 649–52.

1157 Godfrey S, Campbell EJM. Respir Physiol 1968; 5: 385–400.

1158 Gold AR, Bleecker ER, Smith PL. Am Rev Respir Dis 1985; 132: 220–3.

1159 Gold AR, Schwartz AR, Bleecker ER, Smith PL. Am Rev Respir Dis 1986; 134: 925–9.

1160 Goldberg AI. Chest 1983; 84: 365–6.

1161 Goldberg AI. Chest 1984; 86: 345–6.

1162 Goldberg AI. Chest 1986; 90: 744–8.

1163 Goldberg AI. Bull Eur Physiopath Respir 1986; 22: Suppl 99–100S.

1164 Goldberg AI, Faure EAM. Chest 1983; 86: 912–4.

1165 Goldberg AI, Faure EAM, Vaughn CJ, Snarski R, Seleny FL. J Pediatr 1984; 104: 785–95.

1166 Goldberg AI, Kettrick RG, Buzdygan D, Lis EF, Schraeder B, Vaughn C. Crit Care Med 1980; 8: 238.

1167 Goldberg SJ, Stern LZ, Feldman L, Sahn DJ, Allen HD, Valdes-Cruz LM. J Am Coll Cardiol 1983; 2: 137–42.

1168 Goldman AL, George J. Neurology 1976; 26: 815–7.

1169 Goldman JM, Morgan MDL, Denison DM. Thorax 1985; 40: 701.

1170 Goldman JM, Rose LS, Morgan MDL, Denison DM. Thorax 1986; 41: 513–8.

1171 Goldman JM, Rose LS, Williams SJ, Silver JR, Denison DM. Thorax 1986; 41: 940–5.

1172 Goldman JM, Williams SJ, Denison D, Silver JR. Thorax 1986; 41: 244.

1173 Goldman JM, Williams SJ, Denison DM. Thorax 1987; 42: 227.

1174 Goldman M. Am Rev Respir Dis 1979; 119 Suppl: 135–6.

1175 Goldman MD, Grassino A, Mead J, Sears TA. J Appl Physiol 1978; 44: 840–8.

1176 Goldman MD, Mead J. J Appl Physiol 1973; 35: 197–204.

1177 Goldring RM, Turino GM, Heinemann HO. Am J Med 1971; 51: 772–84.

1178 Goldstein RL, Hyde RW, Lapham LW, Gazioglu K, dePapp ZG. Am J Med 1974; 56: 443–9.

1179 Goldstein RS, Molotiu N, Contreras M, Skrastins R, Phillipson EA. Am Rev Respir Dis 1986; 133: A167.

1180 Goldstein RS, Molotiu N, Contreras M, Skrastins R, Jenne H. Am Rev Respir Dis 1986; 133: A167.

1181 Goldstein RS, Molotiu N, Skrastins R, et al. Am Rev Respir Dis 1987; 135: 1049–55.

1182 Goldstein RS, Ramcharan V, Bowes G, McNicholas WT, Bradley D, Phillipson EA. N Engl J Med 1984; 310: 425–9.

1183 Goldstein S, Asknazi J, Weissman C, Thomashow B, Kinney JM. Chest 1987; 91: 222–4.

1184 Gollnick PD, Piehl K, Saltin B. J Physiol 1974; 241: 45–57.

1185 Gomez–Fernandez P, Agudo LS, Calatrava JM, Escuin F, Selgas R, Martinez ME, Montero A, Sanchez–Sicilia L. Nephron 1984; 36: 219–23.

1186 Gompertz D, Bartlett K, Blair D, Stern CMM. Arch Dis Childh 1973; 48: 975–7.

1187 Goodland RL, Reynolds JG, McCoord AB, Pommerenke WT. Fertil Steril 1953; 4: 300–17.

1188 Goodman MJ. J Am Med Assoc 1941; 116: 1635–8.

1189 Goodman RS, Goodman M, Gootman N, Cohen H. Laryngoscope 1976; 86: 1367–74.

1190 Gordon A. Med J Record 1928; 127: 530–1.

1191 Gordon AS, Fainer DC, Ivy AC. J Am Med Assoc 1950; 144: 1455–64.

1192 Gordon AS, Prec O, Wedell H, et al. J Appl Physiol 1951; 4: 421–38.

1193 Gordon AS, Raymon F, Sadove M, Ivy AC. J Am Med Assoc 1950; 144: 1447–52.

1194 Gordon B. Am J Med Sci 1934; 187: 692–700.

1195 Gordon EE, Januszko DM, Kaufman L. Am J Med 1967; 42: 582–99.

1196 Gordon J, Brook R, Welles ES, Lake S. J Thorac Surg 1949; 18: 337–62.

1197 Gordon JE, Young DC, Top FH. J Pediatr 1933; 3: 580–5.

1198 Gormezano J, Branthwaite MA. Anaesthesia 1972; 27: 249–57.

1199 Gothe B, Strohl KP, Levin S, Cherniack NS. Chest 1985; 87: 11–17.

1200 Gothe R, Kunze K. In: Soulsby EJL, ed. Parasitic Zoonoses, Clinical and Experimental Studies. New York: Academic Press, 1974; 369–82.

1201 Gotoh F, Meyer JS, Takagi Y. Am J Med 1969; 47: 534–45.

1202 Gottdiener JS, Hawley RJ, Gay JA, DiBianco R, Fletcher RD, Engel WK. Am Heart J 1982; 104: 77–85.

1203 Gottdiener JS, Hawley RJ, Maron BJ, Bertorini TF, Engle WK. Am Heart J 1982; 103: 525–31.

1204 Gottdiener JS, Sherber HS, Hawley RJ, Engel WK. Am J Cardiol 1978; 41: 1141–9.

1205 Gottfried SB, Leech I, DiMarco AF, Zaccardelli W, Altose MD. J Appl Physiol 1984; 57: 989–94.

1206 Gotze HG, Sunram F, Scheele K, Klisa B. Deutsche Med Wschr 1974; 99: 1761–9.

1207 Gotze HG, Sunram F, Scheele K, Munster IW. Zeitschr Orthop 1974; 112: 832–6.

1208 Gough JH, Barlow D, Sellors TH, Thompson VC. Thorax 1957; 12: 241–57.

1209 Gould GA, Forsyth IS, Flenley DC. Thorax 1986; 41: 808–9.

1210 Gould GA, Hayhurst MD, Scott W, Flenley DC. Thorax 1985; 40: 820–4.

1211 Gould GA, Scott W, Hayhurst MD, Flenley DC. Thorax 1985; 40: 811–6.

1212 Gould L, Kaplan S, McElhinney AJ, Stone DJ. Am Rev Respir Dis 1967; 96: 812–4.

1213 Goulon M, Barois A, Lord G, et al. Arch Fr Ped 1967; 24: 667–86.

1214 Goulon M, Raphael J–C, Brunel D, Chastang C. Bull Acad Nat Med 1984; 168: 448–54.

1215 Gourie–Devi M, Ganapathy GR. J Neurol Neurosurg Psychiatr 1985; 48: 245–9.

1216 Gower DJ, Davis CH Jnr. South Med J 1985; 78: 1010–11.

1217 Graaff WB van de, Gottfried SB, Mitra J, Lunteren E van, Cherniack NS, Strohl KP. J Appl Physiol 1984; 57: 197–204.

1218 Gracey DR, Divertie MB, Howard FM Jnr. Mayo Clin Proc 1983; 58: 597–602.

1219 Gracey DR, Divertie MB, Howard FM Jnr, Payne WS. Chest 1984; 86: 67–71.

1220 Gracey DR, Gillespie D, Nobrega F, Naessens JM, Krishan I. Chest 1987; 91: 424–7.

1221 Gracey DR, Howard FM Jnr, Divertie MB. Chest 1984; 85: 739–43.

1222 Gracey DR, McMichan JC, Divertie MB, Howard FM Jnr. Mayo Clin Proc 1982; 57: 742–6.

1223 Gracey DR, Southorn PA. Chest 1987; 91: 716–8.

1224 Graham AN, Martin PD, Haas LF. Thorax 1985; 40: 635–6.

1225 Graham MD. Laryngoscope 1963; 73: 85–92.

1226 Grant IWB, Maudsley C, Crompton GK, Jellinek EH, Willey RF, Ashworth B. Thorax 1981; 36: 159–60.

1227 Grant JL, Arnold W Jnr. J Am Med Assoc 1965; 194: 119–22.

1228 Grant RP, Jenkins LC. Can Anaesth Soc J 1982; 29: 112–6.

1229 Grassino A, Goldman MD, Mead J, Sears TA. J Appl Physiol 1978; 44: 829–39.

1230 Grassino A, Gross D, Macklem PT, Roussos C, Zagelbaum G. Bull Eur Physiopath Resp 1979; 15: 105–11.

1231 Grassino AE, Bake B, Martin RR, Anthonisen NR. J Appl Physiol 1975; 39: 997–1003.

1232 Grassino AE, Derenne JP, Almirall J, Milic–Emili J, Whitelaw W. J Appl Physiol 1981; 50: 134–42.

1233 Grassino AE, Whitelaw WA, Milic–Emili J. J Appl Physiol 1976; 40: 971–5.

1234 Grau M, Leisner B, Rohloff R, Fink U, Moser E, Matzen KA, Hausinger K. Nuklearmedizin 1981; 20: 178–82.

1235 Gravelyn TR, Weg JG. J Am Med Assoc 1980; 244: 1123–5.

1236 Gray DF, Morse BS, Phillips WF. Ann Intern Med 1962; 57: 230–44.

1237 Gray FD, Field AS. Am J Med Sci 1959; 238: 146–52.

1238 Green JH, Neil E. J Physiol 1955; 129: 134–41.

1239 Green M. Bull Eur Physiopath Respir 1984; 20: 433–6.

1240 Green M, Moxham J. In: Flenley DC, Petty TL, eds. Recent Advances in Respiratory Medicine. London: Churchill, 1983: 1–20.

1241 Green M, Moxham J. Clin Sci 1985; 68: 1–10.

1242 Green RA, Coleman DJ. Anaesthesia 1955; 10: 369–73.

1243 Greenberg M, Edmonds J. Pediatr Clin North Am 1974; 21: 927–34.

1244 Greene R. South Med J 1932; 25: 392–4.

1245 Greene W, L'Hereux P, Hunt CE. Am J Dis Child 1975; 129: 1402–5.

1246 Greenfield JG, Bosanquet FD. J Neurol Neurosurg Psychiatr 1953; 16: 213–26.

1247 Gregory RJ. Acta Med Scand 1971; 189: 551–4.

1248 Grendahl H. Acta Med Scand 1966; 179: 41–5.

1249 Grendahl H, Refsum HE. Acta Med Scand 1965; 177: 539–47.

1250 Grewel F. Acta Psychiatr Neurol Scand 1957; 32: 440–9.

1251 Gribbin HR, Gardiner IT, Heinz GJ III, Gibson GJ, Pride NB. Clin Sci 1983; 64: 487–95.

1252 Griggs DE, Coggin CB, Evans N. Am Heart J 1939; 17: 681–90.

1253 Griggs RC, Donohue KM, Utell MJ, Goldblatt G, Moxley RT III. Arch Neurol 1981; 38: 9–12.

1254 Grimby G. Am Rev Respir Dis 1974; 110: Suppl 145–53.

1255 Grimby G, Bunn J, Mead J. J Appl Physiol 1968; 24: 159–66.

1256 Grimby G, Fugl–Meyer AR, Blomstrand A. Thorax 1974; 29: 179–84.

1257 Grimby G, Oxhoj H, Bake B. Clin Sci Molec Med 1975; 48: 193–9.

1258 Grimby G, Soderholm B. Acta Med Scand 1963; 173: 199–206.

1259 Grimby L, Hannerz J. J Physiol 1977; 264: 865–79.

1260 Grinman S, Whitelaw WA. Chest 1983; 84: 770–2.

1261 Gross D, Grassino A, Ross WRD, Macklem PT. J Appl Physiol 1979; 46: 1–7.

1262 Gross D, Grassino A, Scott G, Ladd H, Macklem PT. Clin Res 1977; 25: 713A.

1263 Gross D, Ladd HW, Riley EJ, Macklem PT, Grassino A. Am J Med 1980; 68: 27–35.

1264 Gross D, Riley E, Grassino A, Ladd H, Macklem PT. Am Rev Respir Dis 1978; 117: Suppl 343.

1265 Gross NJ, Hamilton JD. Br Med J 1963; 2: 1096–7.

1266 Gross PM, Whipp BJ, Davidson JT, Koyal SN, Wasserman K. J Appl Physiol 1976; 41: 336–40.

1267 Grover RF, Vogel JHK, Voigt GC, Blount SG Jnr. Am J Cardiol 1966; 18: 928–32.

1268 Gruber H, Metson R. Ann Intern Med 1980; 92: 800–2.

1269 Grulee CG Jnr, Elam JO. Pediatrics 1948; 1: 684–707.

1270 Gucker T III. J Bone Joint Surg 1962; 44A: 469–81.

1271 Gui L, Savini R, Vicenzi G, Ponzo L. Ital J Orthop Traumatol 1976; 2: 191–205.

1272 Guillain G. Proc R Soc Med 1938; 31: 1031–8.

1273 Guilleminault C. Chest 1978; 73: 293–9.

1274 Guilleminault C. Sleep 1980; 3: 227–34.

1275 Guilleminault C, Billiard M, Montplaisir J, Dement WC. J Neurol Sci 1975; 26: 377–93.

1276 Guilleminault C, Briskin JG, Greenfield MS, Silvestri R. Sleep 1981; 4: 263–78.

1277 Guilleminault C, Connolly S, Winkle R, Melvin K, Tilkian A. Lancet 1984; 1: 126–31.

1278 Guilleminault C, Connolly SJ, Winkle RA. Am J Cardiol 1983; 52: 490–4.

1279 Guilleminault C, Cummiskey J. Am Rev Respir Dis 1982; 126: 14–20.

1280 Guilleminault C, Cummiskey J, Dement WC. Adv Intern Med 1980; 26: 347–72.

1281 Guilleminault C, Cummiskey J, Motta J, Lynne–Davies P. Sleep 1978; 1: 19–31.

1282 Guilleminault C, Dement WC. In: Williams RL, Karacan I, eds. Sleep Disorders, Diagnosis and Treatment. Wiley; 1978: 9–28.

1283 Guilleminault C, Eldridge F, Dement WC. Bull Physiopath Respir 1972; 8: 1127–38.

1284 Guilleminault C, Eldridge FL, Dement WC. Science 1973; 181: 856–8.

1285 Guilleminault C, Eldridge FL, Simmons FB, Dement WC. Pediatrics 1976; 58: 23–30.

1286 Guilleminault C, Eldridge FL, Tilkian A, Simmons FB, Dement WC. Arch Intern Med 1977; 137: 296–300.

1287 Guilleminault C, Hayes B. Bull Eur Physiopath Respir 1983; 19: 632–4.

1288 Guilleminault C, Hayes B, Smith L, Simmons FB. Bull Eur Physiopath Respir 1983; 19: 595–9.

1289 Guilleminault C, Hill MW, Simmons B, Dement WC. Exp Neurol 1978; 62: 48–67.

1290 Guilleminault C, Hoed J van den. Lancet 1979; 2: 750–1.

1291 Guilleminault C, Hoed J van den, Mitler MM. In: Guilleminault C, Dement WC, eds. Sleep Apnea Syndromes. New York: AR Liss Inc, 1978; 1–12.

1292 Guilleminault C, Korobkin R, Winkle R. Lung 1981; 159: 275–87.

1293 Guilleminault C, Kurland G, Winkle R, Miles LE. Chest 1981; 79: 626–30.

1294 Guilleminault C, McQuitty J, Ariagno RL, Challamel J, Korobkin R, McClead RE Jnr. Pediatrics 1982; 70: 684–94.

1295 Guilleminault C, Mondini S, Greenfield M. Am Rev Respir Dis 1984; 129: 512–3.

1296 Guilleminault C, Motta J. In: Guilleminault C, Dement WC, eds. Sleep Apnea Syndromes. New York: AR Liss Inc, 1978: 309–15.

1297 Guilleminault C, Motta J, Mihm F, Melvin K. Chest 1986; 89: 331–4.

1298 Guilleminault C, Riley R, Powell N. Chest 1984; 86: 793–4.

1299 Guilleminault C, Riley R, Powell N. Chest 1985; 88: 776–8.

1300 Guilleminault C, Rosekind M. Bull Europ Physiopath Resp 1981; 17: 341–9.

1301 Guilleminault C, Simmons FB, Motta J, et al. Arch Intern Med 1981; 141: 985–8.

1302 Guilleminault C, Tilkian A, Dement WC. Ann Rev Med 1976; 27: 465–84.

1303 Guilleminault C, Tilkian A, Lehrman K, Forno L, Dement WC. J Neurol Neurosurg Psychiatr 1977; 40: 718–25.

1304 Guller B, Hable K. Chest 1974; 66: 165–71.

1305 Gunella G. Bull Physiopath Respir 1972; 8: 1257–76.

1306 Gupta OK, Saksena PN, Gupta NN. Indian J Pediatr 1973; 40: 93–101.

1307 Gupta PK, Dundee JW. Anaesthesia 1974; 29: 33–9.

1308 Guthrie TC, Kurtzke JF, Berlin L. Ann Intern Med 1952; 77: 1197–203.

1309 Guttmann L, Silver JR. Paraplegia 1965; 3: 1–22.

1310 Guyton AC, Crowell JW, Moore JW. Am J Physiol 1956; 187: 395–8.

1311 Guz A. In: Howell JBL and Campbell EJM, eds. Breathlessness. Oxford: Blackwell Scientific Publications, 1966: 65–71.

1312 Guz A. Ann Rev Physiol 1975; 37: 303–23.

1313 Guz A, Noble MIM, Trenchard D, Cochrane HL, Makey AR. Clin Sci 1964; 27: 293–304.

1314 Guz A, Noble MIM, Widdicombe JG, Trenchard D, Mushin WW. Respir Physiol 1966; 1: 38–40.

1315 Guz A, Noble MIM, Widdicombe JG, Trenchard D, Mushin WW, Makey AR. Clin Sci 1966; 30: 161–70.

1316 Gyllensward A, Irnell L, Michaelsson M, Qvist O, Sahlstedt B. Acta Paediatr Scand 1975; Suppl 255: 1–14.

1317 Haas A, Lowman EW, Bergofsky EH. Arch Phys Med Rehabil 1965; 46: 399–405.

1318 Haas A, Rusk HA, Pelosof H, Adam JR. Arch Phys Med Rehabil 1967; 48: 174–9.

1319 Haas H, Johnson LR, Gill TH, Armentrout TS. Am Rev Respir Dis 1981; 123: 465–7.

1320 Haber P, Kummer F. Acta Med Austriaca 1982; 9: 171–3.

1321 Haber P, Kummer F, Lukeschitsch G, Dorda W. Respiration 1982; 43: 241–8.

1322 Hackett PH, Roach RC, Harrison GL, Schoene RB, Mills WJ Jnr. Am Rev Respir Dis 1987; 135: 896–8.

1323 Hackney JD, Crane MG, Collier CC, Rokaw S, Griggs DE. Ann Intern Med 1959; 51: 541–52.

1324 Haddad GG, Akabas SR. Clin Chest Med 1986; 7: 79–89.

1325 Haddad GG, Mazza NM, Defendini R, et al. Medicine 1978; 57: 517–26.

1326 Hadorn W, Scherrer M. Schweiz Med Wschr 1959; 89: 647–52.

1327 Hagan R, Bryan AC, Bryan MH, Gulston G. Physiologist 1976; 19: 214.

1328 Hagan R, Bryan AC, Bryan MH, Gulston G. J Appl Physiol 1977; 42: 362–7.

1329 Hajiroussou V, Joshi RC. Thorax 1979; 34: 690–1.

1330 Haldane JS. Br Med J 1917; 1: 181–3.

1331 Haldane JS, Priestley JG. J Physiol 1905; 32: 225–66.

1332 Hall WJ. Adv Neurol 1977; 17: 317–24.

1333 Haller JA Jnr, Pickard LR, Tepas JJ, et al. J Pediatr Surg 1979; 14: 779–85.

1334 Hallett WY, Martin CJ. Ann Intern Med 1961; 54: 1146–55.

1335 Halpern SL, Covner AH. Arch Intern Med 1949; 84: 907–16.

1336 Hamilton EA, Nichols PJR, Tait GBW. Ann Phys Med 1970; 10: 223–9.

1337 Hamilton F, Thomas P, Peralta MM Jnr. Surg Gynecol Obstet 1970; 130: 1067–72.

1338 Hamilton JD, Gross NJ. Br Med J 1963; 2: 1092–6.

1339 Hamly FH, Timms RM, Mihn VD, Moser KM. Am Rev Respir Dis 1975; 111: 911–2.

1340 Hanissian AS, Riggs WW Jnr, Thomas DA. J Pediatr 1967; 71: 855–64.

1341 Hanley T, Platts MM, Clifton M, Morris TL. Q J Med 1958; 27: 155–71.

1342 Hanninen P, Wendelin H, Rasanen O, Panelius M. Acta Paed Scand 1972; Suppl 228: 1–32.

1343 Hanson DG, Ludlow CL, Bassich CJ. Ann Otol Rhinol Laryngol 1983; 92: 85–90.

1344 Hansotia P, Frens D. Neurology 1981; 31: 1336–7.

1345 Hapke EJ, Meek JC, Jacobs J. Chest 1972; 61: 41–7.

1346 Haponik EF, Bleecker ER, Allen RP, Smith PL, Kaplan J. Am Rev Respir Dis 1981; 124: 571–4.

1347 Haponik EF, Givens D, Angelo J. Neurology 1983, 33: 1046–9.

1348 Haponik EF, Munster AM, Wise RA, et al. Am Rev Respir Dis 1984; 129: 251–7.

1349 Haponik EF, Munster AM, Wise RA, et al. Am Rev Respir Dis 1984; 129: 251–7.

1350 Haponik EF, Smith PL, Bohlman ME, Allen RP, Goldman SM, Bleecker ER. Am Rev Respir Dis 1983; 127: 221–6.

1351 Haponik EF, Smith PL, Kaplan J, Bleecker ER. Thorax 1983; 38: 609–15.

1352 Harati Y, Niakan E, Bloom K, Casar G. J Neurol Neurosurg Psychiatr 1987; 50: 108–10.

1353 Hardie RJ, Efthimiou J, Stern GM. J Neurol Neurosurg Psychiatr 1986; 49: 1326.

1354 Hardy AE, Hewer RL. Q J Med 1983; 52: 489–502.

1355 Hardy JH, Curtis BH. J Bone Joint Surg 1971; 53A: 1021–2.

1356 Hardy RC, Perret G, Meyers R. J Neurosurg 1957; 14: 400–4.

1357 Harf A, Bertrand C, Chang HK. J Appl Physiol 1984; 56: 155–60.

1358 Harman E, Wynne JW, Block AJ, Malloy–Fisher L. Chest 1981; 79: 256–60.

1359 Harman EM, Wynne JW, Block AJ. Chest 1982; 82: 291–4.

1360 Harper PS. Myotonic Dystrophy. Vol 9. Major Problems in Neurology. Philadelphia: WB Saunders 1979: 90–115.

1361 Harper PS, Dyken PR. Lancet 1972; 2: 53–5.

1362 Harpin RP, Gignac SP, Epstein SW, Gallacher WN, Vanderlinden RG. Am Rev Respir Dis 1986; 134: 1321–3.

1363 Harries JR, Lawes WE. Br Med J 1957; 2: 1204–5.

1364 Harries JR, Tyler JM. Am J Med 1964; 36: 68–78.

1365 Harris KS, Berry AM, Mitchell PA, Sanyal SK. Heart Lung 1978; 7: 1000–5.

1366 Harrison BDW. Clin Sci 1973; 44: 563–70.

1367 Harrison BDW, Collins JV, Brown KGE, Clark TJH. Thorax 1971; 26: 579–84.

1368 Harrison BDW, Stokes TC. Br J Dis Chest 1982; 76: 313–40.

1369 Harrison GM Jnr, Mitchell MB. Arch Phys Med Rehabil 1961; 42: 590–8.

1370 Harrison VC, Heese H de V, Klein M. Pediatrics 1968; 41: 549–59.

1371 Hart FD, Bogdanovitch A, Nichol WD. Ann Rheum Dis 1949; 9: 116–31.

1372 Hart FD, Emerson PA, Gregg I. Ann Rheum Dis 1963; 22: 11–18.

1373 Hart FD, Maclagan NF. Ann Rheum Dis 1955; 14: 77–83.

1374 Hart TB, Radow SK, Blackard WG, Tucker HStG, Cooper KR. Arch Intern Med 1985; 145: 865–6.

1375 Harter JS, Overholt RH, Perkin HJ. J Thorac Surg 1938; 7: 290–301.

1376 Harvey JC, Sherbourne DH, Siegel CI. Am J Med 1965; 39: 81–90.

1377 Hasegawa M. Ann Otol 1982; 91: 112–4.

1378 Haskard DO. Ann Rheum Dis 1983; 42: 460–1.

1379 Hasleton PS, Heath D, Brewer DB. J Pathol Bacteriol 1968; 95: 431–40.

1380 Hattwick MAW, Weis TT, Stechschulte J, Baer GM, Gregg MB. Ann Intern Med 1972; 76: 931–42.

1381 Hauge BN. Scand J Respir Dis 1971; 52: 26–33.

1382 Hauge BN. Scand J Respir Dis 1971; 52: 84–99.

1383 Hauge BN. Scand J Respir Dis 1973; 54: 38–44.

1384 Hauke I. Wien Med Presse 1874; 15: 785–8, 836–7.

1385 Hawley RJ, Gottdiener JS, Gay JA, Engel K. Arch Intern Med 1983; 143: 2134–6.

1386 Haxhiu MA, Graaff WB van de, Mitra J, Salamone J, Bruce E, Cherniack NS. Clin Res 1982; 30: 784A.

1387 Haxhiu MA, Lunteren E van, Graaff WB van de, et al. Respir Physiol 1984; 57: 153–69.

1388 Haymaker W, Kernohan JW. Medicine 1949; 28: 59–141.

1389 Head H, Campbell AW. Brain 1900; 23: 353–523.

1390 Heath D. Thorax 1983; 38: 561–4.

1391 Heath D, Edwards C, Harris P. Thorax 1970; 25: 129–40.

1392 Heath D, Smith P, Hurst G. Br J Dis Chest 1986; 80: 122–30.

1393 Heath D, Smith P, Jago R. J Pathol 1982; 138: 115–27.

1394 Hebertson WM, Talbert OR, Cohen ME. Trans Am Neurol Assoc 1959; 84: 176–9.

1395 Heck AF. J Neurol Sci 1954; 1: 226–55.

1396 Heffner JE, Miller KS, Sahn SA. Chest 1986; 90: 430–6.

1397 Heimer D, Scharf SM, Lieberman A, Lavie P. Chest 1983; 84: 184–5.

1398 Heinbecker P, Bishop GH, O'Leary JL. Arch Neurol Psychiatr 1976; 35: 1233–55.

1399 Heine J, Meister R, Klempt H–W, Munster IW. Orth Grenzgebiete 1975; 113: 586–9.

1400 Heinemann HO, Goldring RM. Am J Med 1974; 57: 361–70.

1401 Hekmatpanah J. Med Clin North Am 1968; 52: 189–201.

1402 Helperin SW, Waskow WH. Anesth Analg 1959; 38: 444–50.

1403 Helperin SW, Waskow WH. Anesthesiology 1959; 20: 127–8.

1404 Hemingway A, Bors E, Hobby RP. J Clin Invest 1958; 37: 773–82.

1405 Hemingway A, Neil E. Br Med J 1944; 1: 833–6.

1406 Henche HR, Morscher E, Rutishauser M. Zeitschr Orthop 1977; 115: 816–20.

1407 Henke KG, Arias A, Skatrud J, Dempsey J. Am Rev Respir Dis 1987; 135: A54.

1408 Hensinger RM, McEwen GD. J Bone Joint Surg 1976; 58A: 13–24.

1409 Hepper NGG, Black LF, Fowler WS. Am Rev Respir Dis 1965; 91: 356–62.

1410 Hepper NGG, Ferguson RH, Howard FM. Med Clin North Am 1964; 48: 1031–42.

1411 Hernandez SF. Am J Otolaryngol 1982; 3: 229–34.

1412 Herrick CJ. An Introduction to Neurology. 5th Ed. Philadelphia: WB Saunders Co, 1934: 284–9.

1413 Hertzog AJ, Manz WR. Am Heart J 1943; 25: 399–403.

1414 Hewer RL. Br Med J 1968; 3: 649–52.

1415 Hewer RL. Br Heart J 1969; 31: 5–14.

1416 Hewer RL, Hilton PJ, Crampton Smith A, Spalding JMK. Q J Med 1968; 37: 479–91.

1417 Hey EN, Lloyd BB, Cunningham DJC, Jukes MGM, Bolton DPG. Respir Physiol 1966; 1: 193–205.

1418 Heyman A. Med Serv J Can 1960; 16: 425–8.

1419 Heyman A, Birchfield RI, Sieker HO. Neurology 1958; 8: 694–700.

1420 Heymsfield SB, McNish T, Perkins JV, Felner JM. Am Heart J 1978; 95: 283–94.

1421 Hickey RF, Severinghaus JW. In: Hornbein TF, ed. Regulation of Breathing. Part 2. New York: Marcel Dekker, 1981: 1251–312.

1422 Hierons R. Brain 1957; 80: 176–92.

1423 Higenbottam T, Allen D, Loh L, Clark TJH. Thorax 1977; 32: 589–95.

1424 Hildes JA, Schaberg A, Alcock AJW. Circulation 1955; 12: 986–93.

1425 Hill MW, Guilleminault C, Simmons FB. In: Guilleminault C, Dement WC, eds. Sleep Apnea Syndromes. New York: AR Liss Inc, 1978; 249–58.

1426 Hill NS. Chest 1986; 90: 897–905.

1427 Hill R, Martin J, Hakim A. Arch Neurol 1983; 40: 30–2.

1428 Hill R, Robbins AW, Messing R, Arora NS. Am Rev Respir Dis 1983; 127: 129–31.

1429 Hill WJ. Am Heart J 1949; 37: 435–40.

1430 Hillerdal G. Eur J Respir Dis 1983; 64: 437–41.

1431 Hilpert P. Zeitschr Orthop 1975; 113: 583–5.

1432 Hirdes JJ. Arch Chir Neerl 1960; 12: 241–61.

1433 Hirdes JJ, Bosch MW. J Thorac Surg 1955; 30: 719–40.

1434 Hirsch CS, Martin DL. Neurology 1971; 21: 682–90.

1435 Hirschfield SS, Rudner C, Nash CL Jnr, Nussbaum E, Brower EM. Pediatrics 1982; 70: 451–4.

1436 Hirshman CA, McCullough RE, Weil JV. J Appl Physiol 1975; 38: 1095–8.

1437 Hitchcock E. Excerpta Med International Congress Series 1965; 93: 78–9.

1438 Hitchcock E, Leece B. J Neurosurg 1967; 27: 320–9.

1439 Hoberman M. Am J Phys Med 1955; 34: 109–15.

1440 Hodgkins JE, Petroff PA, Hyatt RE. Am Rev Respir Dis 1972; 105: 1015–6.

1441 Hoeppner VH, Cockroft DW, Dosman JA, Cotton DJ. Am Rev Respir Dis 1984; 129: 240–3.

1442 Hoff HE, Breckenridge CG. Arch Neurol Psychiatr 1954; 72: 11–42.

1443 Hoffbrand BI, Beck ER. Br Med J 1965; 1: 1273–7.

1444 Hoffman CE, Clark RT Jnr, Brown EB Jnr. Am J Physiol 1946; 145: 685–92.

1445 Hoffman LA, Dauber JH, Ferson PF, Openbrier DR, Zullo TG. Am Rev Respir Dis 1987; 135: 153–6.

1446 Hoffstein V, Phillipson EA, Zamel N. Fed Proc 1983; 42: 1008.

1447 Hoffstein V, Slutsky AS. Am Rev Respir Dis 1987; 135: 1210–2.

1448 Hoffstein V, Taylor R. Chest 1985; 88: 145–7.

1449 Hoffstein V, Zamel N, Phillipson EA. Am Rev Respir Dis 1984; 130: 175–8.

1450 Hogan GR, Guttmann L, Schmidt R, Gilbert E. Neurology 1969; 19: 894–900.

1451 Holgate ST, Glass DN, Haslam P, Maini RN, Turner–Warwick M. Clin Exp Immunol 1976; 24: 385–95.

1452 Holinger LD, Holinger PC, Holinger PH. Ann Otol Rhinol Laryngol 1976; 85: 428–36.

1453 Hollenberg C, Desmarais MHL, Frihagen L, Dale A. Can Med Assoc J 1959; 81: 343–7.

1454 Holley HS, Milic–Emili J, Becklake MR Bates DV. J Clin Invest 1967; 46: 475–81.

1455 Holliday PL, Bauer RB. Arch Neurol 1983; 40: 56–7.

1456 Holloszy JO. Prog Cardiovasc Dis 1976; 18: 445–58.

1457 Holloszy JO, Booth FW. Ann Rev Physiol 1976; 38: 273–91.

1458 Holmes TW. Dis Chest 1967; 52: 371–5.

1459 Holtackers TR, Loosbrock LM, Gracey ER. Respir Care 1982; 27: 271–5.

1460 Holton P, Wood JB. J Physiol 1965; 181: 365–78.

1461 Homma I, Kageyama S, Nagai T, Taniguchi I, Sakai T, Abe M. Clin Sci 1981; 61: 599–603.

1462 Honda Y, Myojo S, Hasegawa S, Hasegawa T, Severinghaus JW. J Appl Physiol 1979; 46: 908–12.

1463 Honda Y, Watanabe S, Hashizume I, et al. J Appl Physiol 1979; 46: 632–8.

1464 Hoover CF. Arch Intern Med 1913; 12: 214–24.

1465 Hoover CF. Arch Intern Med 1917; 20: 701–15.

1466 Hoover CF. J Am Med Assoc 1920; 75: 1626–30.

1467 Hoover CF. Am J Med Sci 1920; 159: 633–46.

1468 Hope–Simpson RE. Proc R Soc Med 1965; 58: 9–20.

1469 Hopkins A, Neville B, Bannister R. Lancet 1974; 1: 769–71.

1470 Hopkins GO, McDougall J, Mills KR, Isenberg DA, Ebringer A. Br J Rheumatol 1983; 22: 151–7.

1471 Hopkins IJ, Lindsey JR, Ford FR. Brain 1966; 89: 299–310.

1472 Hormia AL. Am J Med Sci 1957; 233: 635–40.

1473 Houser CR, Johnson DM. Phys Ther 1971; 51: 751–9.

1474 Houser WC, Schlueter DP. J Am Med Assoc 1978; 239: 340–1.

1475 Howard FM Jnr. Proc Staff Meetings Mayo Clin 1963; 38: 203–12.

1476 Howard P. Thorax 1983; 38: 161–4.

1477 Howard RS, Lees AJ. Brain 1987; 110: 19–33.

1478 Howell S, Fitzgerald RS, Roussos C. Am Rev Respir Dis 1986; 133: 407–13.

1479 Howell S, Roussos C. Am Rev Respir Dis 1984; 129: Suppl A270.

1480 Howell S, Roussos C. Am Rev Respir Dis 1984; 129: 118–24.

1481 Hsu JD. Spine 1983; 8: 771–5.

1482 Huang CT, Lyons HA. J Thorac Cardiovasc Surg 1977; 74: 409–17.

1483 Hubmayr RD, Kaitz ES, Stivers DH, Irwin RS. Am Rev Respir Dis 1984; 129: Suppl A101.

1484 Huddleston OL. Calif Med 1947; 66: 25–7.

1485 Hudgel DW, Martin RJ, Johnson B, Hill P. J Appl Physiol 1984; 56: 133–7.

1486 Hudgel DW, Weil JV. Ann Intern Med 1974; 80: 622–5.

1487 Hudgson P, Gardner–Medwin D, Fulthorpe JJ, Walton JN. Neurology 1967; 17: 1125–42.

1488 Hudgson P, Gardner–Medwin D, Worsfold M, Pennington BJT, Walton JN. Brain 1968; 91: 435–62.

1489 Huebert HT, MacKinnon WB. J Bone Joint Surg 1969; 51B: 338–43.

1490 Huettemann U, Huckauf H. Respiration 1970; 27: 363–76.

1491 Hughes JMB. Brain 1967; 90: 675–80.

1492 Hughes RL. Chest 1984; 86: 344–5.

1493 Hukuhara T, Nakayama S, Okada H. Jpn J Physiol 1954; 4: 145–53.

1494 Huldtgren A–C, Fugl–Meyer AR, Jonasson E, Bake B. Eur J Respir Dis 1980; 61: 347–56.

1495 Hummer HP, Willital GH. Zeitschr Orthop 1983; 121: 216–20.

1496 Hung CT, Pelosi M, Langer A, Harrigan JT. Am J Obstet Gynecol 1975; 121: 287–8.

1497 Hunninghake GW, Fauci AS. Am Rev Respir Dis 1979; 119: 471–503.

1498 Hunsaker RH, Fulkerson PK, Barry FJ, Lewis RP, Leier CV, Unverfeth DV. Am J Med 1982; 73: 235–8.

1499 Hunt CE. Chest 1980; 77: 565–7.

1500 Hunt CE, Inwood RJ, Shannon DC. Am Rev Respir Dis 1979; 119: 263–9.

1501 Hunt CE, Matalon SV, Thompson TR, et al. Am Rev Respir Dis 1978; 118: 23–8.

1502 Hunt GB. Br Med J 1909; 2: 314–5.

1503 Hunter AR. Acta Anaesthesiol Scand 1966; Suppl 23 199–202.

1504 Hunter JS, Millikan CH. Obstet Gynecol 1954; 4: 147–54.

1505 Hunziker A, Frick P, Regli F, Rossier PH. Deutsch Med Wschr 1964; 89: 676–80.

1506 Huppert FA. Thorax 1982; 37: 858–60.

1507 Hurtado A, Merino C, Delgado E. Arch Intern Med 1945; 75: 284–323.

1508 (a) Huseby JS, Petersen D. Chest 1981; 80: 31–3. (b) Hussain SNA, Rabinovitch B, Macklem PT, Pardy RL. J Appl Physiol 1985; 58: 2020–26.

1509 Hutchison DCS, Flenley DC, Donald KW. Br Med J 1964; 2: 1159–66.

1510 Hutchison DCS, Rocca G, Honeybourne D. Thorax 1981; 36: 473–7.

1511 Huxley EJ, Viroslav J, Gray WR, Pierce AK. Am J Med 1978; 64: 564–8.

1512 Hwang B, Simon G, Keim HA, Krongrad E. J Electrocardiol 1982; 5: 131–6.

1513 Hwang J–C, St John WM, Bartlett D Jnr. Respir Physiol 1984; 55: 355–66.

1514 Hyland RH, Hutcheon MA, Perl A, et al. Am Rev Respir Dis 1981; 124: 180–5.

1515 Hyland RH, Jones NL, Powles ACP, Lenkie SCM, Vanderlinden RG, Epstein SW. Am Rev Respir Dis 1978; 117: 1165–72.

1516 Iacob G. Poumon Coeur 1967; 23: 439–51.

1517 Iber C, Berssenbrugge A, Skatrud JB, Dempsey JA. J Appl Physiol 1982; 52: 607–14.

1518 Iber C, Chapman R, Davies S, Mahiwald M. Am Rev Respir Dis 1985; 131: Suppl A345.

1519 Iber C, Davies SF, Chapman RC, Mahowald MM. Chest 1986; 89: 800–5.

1520 Ibsen B. Proc R Soc Med 1954; 47: 72–4.

1521 Ilbawi MN, Hunt CE, DeLeon SY, Idriss FS. Ann Thorac Surg 1981; 31: 61–5.

1522 Iliffe GD, Pettigrew NM. Br Med J 1983; 286: 337–8.

1523 Ilson J, Braun N, Fahn S. Neurology 1983; 33: Suppl 113.

1524 Imaizumi T. Am Heart J 1980; 100: 513–6.

1525 Imes NK, Orr WC, Smith RO, Rogers RM. J Am Med Assoc 1977; 237: 1596–7.

1526 Indihar FJ. Chest 1984; 86: 155–6.

1527 Indihar FJ, Forsberg DP. Chest 1982; 81: 189–92.

1528 Indihar FJ, Walker NE. Chest 1984; 86: 616–20.

1529 Ingram RH Jnr. Am Rev Respir Dis 1980; 122: Suppl 23–4.

1530 Ingram RH, Bishop JB. Am Rev Respir Dis 1970; 102: 645–7.

1531 Inkley SR, Oldenburg SC, Vignos PJ Jnr. Am J Med 1974; 56: 297–306.

1532 The Intermittent Positive Pressure Breathing Trial Group. Ann Intern Med 1983; 99: 612–20.

1533 Ip MSM, So SY, Lam WK, Mok CK. Chest 1986; 89: 727–30.

1534 Irwin M, Openbrier D, Owens G, Dauber J, Rogers R. Am Rev Respir Dis 1983; 127: Suppl 149.

1535 Irwin RS, Rosen MJ, Braman SS. Arch Intern Med 1977; 137: 1186–91.

1536 Isenberg DA, Snaith ML. J Rheumatol 1981; 8: 917–24.

1537 Ishikawa S, Mannig J, Singer W, Dupre B, Bartret E, Eldridge T. Am Rev Respir Dis 1976; 113: Suppl 139.

1538 Israel F. Z Geburtshulfe Gynakol 1927; 91: 602–22.

1539 Israel F. Zentralbl Chir 1928; 55: 331–4.

1540 Israel RH, Marino JM. Ann Neurol 1977; 2: 83.

1541 Issa FG, Costas LV, Berthon–Jones M, McCauley VJ, Bruderer J, Sullivan CE. Am Rev Respir Dis 1985; 131: Suppl A108.

1542 Issa FG, Sullivan CE. J Neurol Neurosurg Psychiatr 1982; 45: 353–9.

1543 Issa FG, Sullivan CE. J Appl Physiol 1983; 55: 1113–9.

1544 Issa FG, Sullivan CE. J Appl Physiol 1984; 57: 528–35.

1545 Issa FG, Sullivan CE. J Appl Physiol 1984; 57: 520–4.

1546 Issa FG, Sullivan CE. Chest 1986; 90: 165–71.

1547 Iverson LIG, Mittal A, Dugan DJ, Samson PC. Am J Surg 1976; 132: 263–9.

1548 Jack TM, Lloyd JW. Ann R Coll Surg Engl 1983; 65: 97–102.

1549 Jackson JH. Lancet 1895; 1; 476–8.

1550 Jackson JII. Lancet 1899; 1: 79–80.

1551 Jackson RM. Chest 1985; 88: 900–5.

1552 Jacobaeus HC. J Thorac Surg 1938; 7: 235–61.

1553 Jacobelli S, Moreno R, Massardo L, Rivero S, Lisboa C. Arthritis Rheum 1985; 28: 781–8.

1554 Jacobsen E, Dano P, Skovsted P. Scand J Respir Dis 1974; 55: 332–9.

1555 Jaeger–Denavit O, Duval–Beaupere G, Grossiord A. Rev Epidemiol Sante Publique 1978; 26: 171–81.

1556 Jager AEJ de, Meinesz AF. J Neurol 1983; 230: 105–10.

1557 James JIP. Scoliosis. 2nd ed. Churchill Livingstone: Edinburgh, 1976.

1558 James JL, Park HWJ. Lancet 1961; 2: 1281–2.

1559 James WS III, Minh V, Minteer MA, Moser KM. Chest 1977; 71: 59–64.

1560 Jameson AG, Ferrer MI, Harvey RM. Am Rev Resp Dis 1959; 80: 510–21.

1561 Jammes Y, Delpierre S, Zwirn P, Nicoli M–M. Nouv Press Med 1977; 6: 1113–6.

1562 Jardim J, Farkas G, Prefaut C, Thomas D, Macklem PT. Am Rev Respir Dis 1981; 124: 274–9.

1563 Jean N, Posteyer J, Guery J. Ann Anesth Fra 1977; 18: 303–8.

1564 Jederlinic P, Muspratt JA, Miller MJ. Chest 1984; 86: 870–3.

1565 Jeffries BF, Tarlton M, Smet AA de, Dwyer SJ III, Brower AC. Radiology 1980; 134: 381–5.

1566 Jenkins JG, Bohn D, Edmonds JF, Levison H, Barker GA. Crit Care Med 1982; 10: 645–9.

1567 Jennett S. Br Med J 1984; 289: 335–6.

1568 Jenney FS, Cohen AC. Dis Chest 1963; 43: 62–7.

1569 Jenny DB, Goris GB, Urwiller RD, Brian BA. J Am Med Assoc 1978; 240: 1378–9.

1570 Jensen NK, Schmidt WR, Garamella JJ. J Thorac Cardiovasc Surg 1962; 43: 731–41.

1571 Jensen NK, Schmidt WR, Garamella JJ, Lynch MF. J Pediatr Surg 1970; 5: 4–13.

1572 Jessen O, Kristensen HS, Rasmussen K. Lancet 1967; 2: 9–12.

1573 Jewett TC Jnr, Thomson NB Jnr. J Thorac Cardiovasc Surg 1964; 48: 861–6.

1574 Jezek V, Ourednik A, Stepanek J, Boudik F. Clin Sci 1970; 38: 549–54.

1575 Joannides M. Dis Chest 1946; 12: 89–110.

1576 Johns DP, Rochford PD, Streeton JA. Thorax 1985; 40: 806–10.

1577 Johnson BE, Westgate HD. J Bone Joint Surg 1970; 52A: 1433–9.

1578 Johnson EW, Kennedy JH. Arch Phys Med Rehabil 1971; 52: 110–4.

1579 Johnson EW, Reynolds HT, Stauch D. Arch Phys Med Rehabil 1985; 66: 260–1.

1580 Johnson RL Jnr, Lillehei JP, Miller WF. Clin Res Proc 1956; 4: 47–8.

1581 Johnson V, Eiseman B. J Thorac Cardiovasc Surg 1971; 62: 651–7.

1582 Jones DA, Howell S, Roussos C, Edwards RHT. Clin Sci 1982; 63: 161–7.

1583 Jones DH. Lancet 1964; 1: 517–20.

1584 Jones GL, Killian KJ, Summers E, Jones NL. J Appl Physiol 1985; 58: 1608–15.

1585 Jones JB, Wilhoit SC, Findley LJ, Suratt PM. Chest 1985; 88: 9–15.

1586 Jones RAK. Arch Dis Child 1981; 56: 889–91.

1587 Jones RH, MacNamara J, Gaensler EA. Am Rev Respir Dis 1960; 82: 164–85.

1588 Jones RS, Kennedy JD, Hasham F, Owen R, Taylor JF. Thorax 1981; 36: 456–61.

1589 Joos TH, Dickinson DG, Talner NS, Wilson JL. N Engl J Med 1956; 255: 1089–90.

1590 Jordan CE, White RI, Fischer KC, Neill C, Dorst JP. Am Heart J 1972; 84: 463–9.

1591 Jordanoglou J. Thorax 1969; 24: 407–14.

1592 Jordanoglou J. Respir Physiol 1970; 10: 109–20.

1593 Josenhans WT, Wang CS, Josenhans G, Woodbury JFL. Respiration 1971; 28: 331–46.

1594 Juan G, Calverley P, Talamo C, Schnader J, Roussos C. N Engl J Med 1984; 310: 874–9.

1595 Judd AR. J Thorac Surg 1947; 16: 512–23.

1596 Judson JP, Glenn WWL. J Am Med Assoc 1968; 203: 1033–7.

1597 Juhl O, Thorshauge C. Acta Anaesth Scand 1957; 1; 137–8.

1598 Julian DG, Travis DM, Bayles TB. Arthritis Rheum 1959; 2: 38–9.

1599 Jungner I, Lindhal J, Strom J. Acta Med Scand 1956; Suppl 316: 80–5.

1600 Kaada BR. Acta Physiol Scand 1951; 24: Suppl 83, 1–285.

1601 Kaada BR. In: Field J, ed. Handbook of Physiology, Neurophysiology, Vol 2. Washington: American Physiological Society, 1960: 1345–72.

1602 Kaada BR, Jasper H. Arch Neurol Psychiatr 1952; 68: 609–19.

1603 Kabat H. J Comp Neurol 1936; 64: 187–208.

1604 Kadefors R, Kaiser E, Petersen I. Electromyography 1968; 8: 39–74.

1605 Kafer ER. Am Rev Respir Dis 1974; 110: 450–7.

1606 Kafer ER. J Clin Invest 1975; 55: 1153–63.

1607 Kafer ER. J Clin Invest 1976; 58: 825–33.

1608 Kafer ER. Bull Eur Physiopath Respir 1977; 13: 300–21.

1609 Kafer ER. Anesthesiology, 1980; 52: 339–51.

1610 Kafer ER. Bull Europ Physiopath Resp 1981; 17: 1–13.

1611 Kagen LJ, Hochman RB, Strong EW. Arthritis Rheum 1985; 28: 630–6.

1612 Kalia M, Senapati JM, Parida B, Panda A. J Appl Physiol 1972; 32: 189–93.

1613 Kallenbach J, Lewis M, Zaltzman M, Fritz V, Reef H, Zwi S. South African Med J 1982; 61: 613–6.

1614 Kaltreider NL, Fray WW, Phillips EW. J Thorac Surg 1938; 7: 262–89.

1615 Kamat SR, Dulfano MJ, Segal MS. Am Rev Respir Dis 1962; 86: 360–80.

1616 Kammer GM, Hamilton CR Jnr. Am J Med 1974; 56: 464–70.

1617 Kaneyuki T, Hogan JF, Glenn WWL, Holcomb WG. J Thorac Cardiovasc Surg 1977; 74: 109–15.

1618 Kanner RE. Chest 1983; 84: 304–6.

1619 Kaplan E, Detweiler J, Kaplan BM, Baker LA. J Am Med Assoc 1954; 156: 1499–500.

1620 Kaplan S. Arch Otolaryngol 1957; 65: 495–8.

1621 Karpati G, Carpenter S, Andermann F. Arch Neurol 1971; 24: 291–304.

1622 Karpati G, Carpenter S, Eisen A, Aube M, DiMauro S. Ann Neurol 1977; 1: 276–80.

1623 Kase CS. Neurology 1980; 30: 652–5.

1624 Kattwinkel J, Fleming D, Cha CC, Fanaroff AA, Klaus MH. Pediatrics 1973; 52: 131–4.

1625 Kattwinkel J, Nearman HS, Fanaroff AA, Katona PG, Klaus MH. J Pediatr 1975; 86: 588–92.

1626 Katz JA, Kramer RW, Gjerde GE. Chest 1985; 88: 519–26.

1627 Kauffmann F, Drouet D, Brille D, Hatzfeld C, Liot F, Kompalitch M. Rev Fr Mal Resp 1979; 7: 370–6.

1628 Kaufman BJ, Ferguson MH, Cherniack RM. J Clin Invest 1959; 38: 500–7.

1629 Kaufman J, Friedman JM, Sadowsky D, Harris J. J Oral Maxillofacial Surg 1983; 41: 667–71.

1630 Kaufman L. Proc R Soc Med 1960; 53: 183–8.

1631 Kavey NB, Blitzer A, Gidro–Frank S, Korstanje K. Am J Otolaryngol 1985; 6: 373–7.

1632 Kaya N. Sleep 1984; 7: 77–8.

1633 Kearley R, Wynne JW, Block AJ, Boysen PG, Lindsey S, Martin C. Chest 1980; 78: 682–5.

1634 Keens TG, Bryan AC, Levison H, Ianuzzo CD. J Appl Physiol 1978; 44: 909–13.

1635 Keens TG, Ianuzzo CD. Am Rev Respir Dis 1979; 119: Suppl 139–41.

1636 Keens TG, Krastins IRB, Wannamaker EM, Levison H, Crozier DN, Bryan AC. Am Rev Respir Dis 1977; 116: 853–60.

1637 Keeton BR, Moosa A. Arch Dis Childh 1976; 51: 636–8.

1638 Kehoe RF, Bauernfeind R, Tommaso C, Wyndham C, Rosen KM. Arch Intern Med 1981; 94: 41–3.

1639 Kelleher WH. Lancet 1961; 2: 1113–6.

1640 Kelleher WH, Kinnier–Wilson AB, Ritchie–Russell W, Stott FD. Br Med J 1952; 2: 413–5.

1641 Kelleher WH, Parida RK. Br Med J 1957; 2: 740–3.

1642 Kelley WO. J Thorac Surg 1950; 19: 923–8.

1643 Kelling JS, DiMarco AF, Gottfried SB, Altose MD. J Appl Physiol 1985; 59: 1752–6.

1644 Kellogg RH. In: Hornbein TF, ed. Regulation of Breathing. Part 1. New York: Marcel Dekker, 1981: 3–66.

1645 Kelly DH, Krishnamoorthy KS, Shannon DC. Pediatrics 1980; 66: 429–31.

1646 Kelly SM, Rosa A, Field S, Coughlin M, Shizgal HM, Macklem PT. Am Rev Respir Dis 1984; 130: 33–7.

1647 Kelsen SG. Clin Chest Med 1986; 7: 101–10.

1648 Keltz H. Am Rev Respir Dis 1965; 91: 934–8.

1649 Kendrick AH, O'Reilly JF, Laszlo G. Thorax 1986; 41: 243.

1650 Kennedy RH, Danielson MA, Mulder DW, Kurland LT. Mayo Clin Proc 1978; 53: 93–9.

1651 Kenyon GS, Apps MCP, Traub M. Laryngoscope 1984; 94: 1106–8.

1652 Kepes ER, Martinez LR, Andrews IC, et al. NY State J Med 1972; 72: 1051–3.

1653 Kerby GR, Mayer LS, Floreani A, Pingleton SK. Am Rev Respir Dis 1986; 133: A168.

1654 Kerby GR, Mayer LS, Pingleton SK. Am Rev Respir Dis 1987; 135: 738–40.

1655 Kerr WJ, Lagen JB. Ann Intern Med 1936; 10: 569–95.

1656 Kerridge PMT. Lancet 1934; 1: 786–8;

1657 Kerridge PMT. Lancet 1936; 1: 504.

1658 Keswani NH, Hollinshead WH. Anat Rec 1956; 125: 683–700.

1659 Kety SS, Schmidt CF. J Clin Invest 1948; 27: 484–92.

1660 Khoo MCK, Kronauer RE, Strohl KP, Slutsky AS. J Appl Physiol 1982; 53: 644–59.

1661 Kiker JD, Woodside JR, Jelinek GE. J Urol 1982; 128: 1038–9.

1662 Kilburn KH. Arch Intern Med 1965; 116: 409–15.

1663 Kilburn KH, Eagan JT, Heyman A. Am J Med 1959; 26: 929–35.

1664 Kilburn KH, Eagan JT, Sieker HO, Heyman A. N Engl J Med 1959; 261: 1089–96.

1665 Killian KJ, Gandevia SC, Summers E, Campbell EJM. J Appl Physiol 1984; 57: 686–91.

1666 Killick EM. J Physiol 1935; 84 162–72.

1667 Killick EM, Cowell EM, Crowden GP. Lancet 1939; 2: 897–9.

1668 Killick EM, Eve FC. Lancet 1933; 2; 740–2.

1669 Kim JH, Manuelidis EE, Glenn WWL, Kaneyuki T. J Thorac Cardiovasc Surg 1976; 72: 602–8.

1670 Kim MJ, Druz WS, Danon J, Machnach W, Sharp JT. J Appl Physiol 1976; 41: 369–82.

1671 Kim R. J Neurol Neurosurg Psychiatr 1968; 31: 393–8.

1672 Kimura H, Hayashi F, Yoshida A, Watanabe S, Hashizume I, Honda Y. J Appl Physiol 1984; 56: 1627–32.

1673 King EG, Jacobs H. Can Med Assoc J 1971; 104: 393–400.

1674 King M, Gleeson M, Rees J. Br Med J 1987; 294: 1605–6.

1675 Kinnear WJM. MD Thesis, London: submitted 1987.

1676 Kinnear WJM, Harvey J, Shneerson JM. Bull Europ Physiopath Resp 1986; 20: 66s.

1677 Kinnear WJM, Hockley S, Harvey J, Shneerson JM. Eur Resp J 1988; 1: (In press).

1678 Kinnear WJM, Phillips MS, Gough S, Shaw DG, Shneerson JM. Unpublished observations.

1679 Kinnear WJM, Phillips MS, Shneerson JM. Thorax 1986; 41: 244.

1680 Kinnear WJM, Shaw DG, Jones DK, Higenbottam T, Shneerson JM. Bull Europ Physiopath Resp 1986; 20: 162s.

1681 Kinnear WJM, Shneerson JM. Thorax 1985; 40: 677–81.

1682 Kinnear WJM, Shneerson JM. Thorax 1985; 40: 150–1.

1683 Kinnear WJM, Shneerson JM. Br J Dis Chest 1985; 79: 313–51.

1684 Kinnear WJM, Shneerson JM. Thorax 1986; 41: 710.

1685 Kinnear WJM, Petch M, Taylor G, Shneerson JM. Eur Resp J 1988; 1: (In press).

1686 Kinnear WJM, Shneerson JM. Am Rev Respir Dis 1987; 135: A423.

1687 Kinnear WJM, Shneerson JM. Am Rev Respir Dis 1987; 135: A231.

1688 Kinnear WJM, Shneerson JM, Anderson JR. Unpublished observations.

1689 Kinnear WJM, Shneerson JM, Shaw GD, Higenbottam T. Thorax 1985; 40: 701.

1690 Kinnear WJM, Talonen P, Shneerson JM. Thorax 1987; 42: 229.

1691 Kira S, Hukushima Y. J Appl Physiol 1968; 25: 42–7.

1692 Kirby NA, Barnerias MJ, Siebens AA. Arch Phys Med Rehabil 1966; 47: 705–10.

1693 Kirby RR, Smith RA, Desautels TA, eds. Mechanical Ventilation. New York: Churchill Livingston, 1985.

1694 Kirchner JC, Sasaki CT. Otolaryngol Clin North Am 1984; 17: 49–56.

1695 Kirilloff LH, Owens GR, Rogers RM, Mazzocco MC. Chest 1985; 88: 436–44.

1696 Kirk BW. Univ Manitoba Med J 1980; 50: 93–7.

1697 Kirkwood WD, Myers B. Lancet 1923; 2: 65–8.

1698 Kirsch WM, Duncan BR, Black FO, Stears JC. J Neurosurg 1968; 28: 207–14.

1699 Kiss GT, Rao K. Chest 1980; 78: 353–4.

1700 Kitagawa M, Hislop A, Boyden EA, Reid L. Br J Surg 1971; 58: 342–6.

1701 Kitahata LM. Br J Anaesth 1971; 43: 1187–90.

1702 Kittredge P. Chest 1977; 71: 118.

1703 Klassen AC, Heaney LM, Lee MC, Kronenberg RS. Neurology 1980; 30: 951–5.

1704 Klassen KP, Morton DR, Curtis GM. J Thorac Surg 1950; 20: 552–70.

1705 Klein M, Reynolds LG. Lancet 1986; 1: 935–9.

1706 Klineberg PL, Rehder K, Hyatt RE. J Appl Physiol 1981; 51: 26–32.

1707 Kluin KJ, Maynard F, Bogdasarian RS. Otolaryngol – Head Neck Surg 1984; 92: 625–7.

1708 Knill R, Bryan AC. J Appl Physiol 1976; 40: 352–6.

1709 Knochel JP. Arch Intern Med 1977; 137: 203–20.

1710 Knochel JP, Schlein EM. J Clin Invest 1972; 51: 1750–8.

1711 Knoedler JP, Niewohner DE. Chest 1981; 80: 119–20.

1712 Knudson RJ, Mead J, Knudson DE. J Appl Physiol 1974; 36: 653–67.

1713 Koepke GH, Murphy AJ, Rae JW Jnr, Dickinson DG. Arch Phys Med Rehabil 1955; 36: 217–22.

1714 Kohn NN, Faires JS, Rodman T. N Engl J Med 1964; 271: 1179–83.

1715 Kohn RM. Circulation, 1959; 20: 721–2.

1716 Kohorst WR, Schonfeld SA, Altman M. Chest 1984; 85: 65–8.

1717 Kokal KC, Dastur FD, Mahashur AA, Kolhatkar VP. J Assoc Physicians India, 1984; 32: 691–5.

1718 Kokkola K, Moller A, Lehtonen T. Ann Clin Res 1975; 7: 77–9.

1719 Kolb LC, Kleyntjens F. Brain 1937; 60: 259–74.

1720 Kolton M. Can Anaesth Soc J 1984; 31: 416–29.

1721 Komajda M, Frank R, Vedel J, Fontaine G, Petitot J–C, Grosgogeat Y. Br Heart J 1980; 43: 315–20.

1722 Kompalitch M, Diaz M, Abdelaoui A, Brille D, Decroix G. Rev Fr Mal Resp 1977; 5: 458–60.

1723 Konig G, Albrecht J, Attenberger E, Fruhmann G. Munch Med Wschr 1982; 124: 903–6.

1724 Koninck J de, Gagnon P, Lallier S. Sleep 1983; 6: 52–9.

1725 Konno A, Mead J. J Appl Physiol 1968; 24: 544–8.

1726 Konno A, Togawa K, Hoshino T. Laryngoscope 1980; 90: 699–707.

1727 Konno K, Mead J. J Appl Physiol 1967; 22: 407–22.

1728 Koopmann CF Jnr, Feld RA, Coulthard SW. Otolaryngol – Head Neck Surg 1981; 89: 949–52.

1729 Kopelman PG, Apps MCP, Cope T, Empey DW. Br Med J 1983; 287: 859–61.

1730 Kopenhager T. Br J Obstet Gynaecol 1977; 84: 585–7.

1731 Korczyn AD, Carel RS, Bruderman I. J Neurol 1977; 215: 67–71.

1732 Korczyn AD, Leibowitz U, Bruderman I. Neurology 1969; 19: 97–100.

1733 Korner AF, Guilleminault C, Hoed J van den, Baldwin RB. Pediatrics 1978; 61: 528–33.

1734 Korner AF, Kraemer HC, Haffner ME, Cosper LM. Pediatrics 1975; 56: 361–7.

1735 Kory RC. J Am Med Assoc 1957; 165: 448–50.

1736 Koskenvuo M, Kaprio J, Telakivi T, Partinen M, Heikkila K, Sarna S. Br Med J 1987; 294: 16–19.

1737 Kozlowski K, Masel J. Pediatr Radiol 1976; 5: 30–3.

1738 Kramer LI, Pierpont ME. J Pediatrics 1976; 88: 297–9.

1739 Kramer P, Atkinson M, Wyman SM, Ingelfinger FJ. J Clin Invest 1957; 36: 589–95.

1740 Kravath RE, Pollak CP, Borowiecki B. Pediatrics 1977; 59: 865–71.

1741 Kravath RE, Pollak CP, Borowiecki B, Weitzman ED. J Pediatr 1980; 96: 645–8.

1742 Kreitzer SM, Feldman NT, Saunders NA, Ingram RH Jnr. Am J Med 1978; 65: 89–95.

1743 Kreitzer SM, Saunders NA, Tyler HR, Ingram RH Jnr. Am Rev Respir Dis 1978; 117: 437–47.

1744 Kreitzer SM, Saunders NA, Tyler HR, Ingram RH Jnr. Chest 1978; 73: Suppl 266–7.

1745 Krieger AJ. Heart Lung 1973; 2: 546–51.

1746 Krieger AJ. In: Guilleminault C, Dement WC, eds. Sleep Apnea Syndromes. New York: A R Liss Inc, 1978: 273–94.

1747 Krieger AJ, Christensen HD, Sapru HN, Wang SC. J Appl Physiol 1972; 33: 431–5.

1748 Krieger AJ, Christensen HD, Wang SC. Physiologist 1969; 12: 277.

1749 Krieger AJ, Danetz I, Wu SZ, Spatola M, Sapru HN. J Neurosurg 1983; 59: 262–7.

1750 Krieger AJ, Detwiler J, Trooskin S. Neurology 1974; 24: 1064–7.

1751 Krieger AJ, Detwiler JS, Fandozzi R. Crit Care Med 1974; 2: 155–8.

1752 Krieger AJ, Detwiler JS, Trooskin SZ. Laryngoscope 1976; 86: 718–23.

1753 Krieger AJ, Rosomuff HL. J Neurosurg 1974; 40: 168–80.

1754 Krieger AJ, Rosomuff HL. J Neurosurg 1974; 40: 181–5.

1755 Krieger AJ, Standish MS, Rosomuff HL. Crit Care Med 1974; 2: 91–5.

1756 Krieger AJ, Trooskin SZ. Postgrad Med 1976; 59: 239–43.

1757 Krieger J. Clin Chest Med 1985; 6: 577–94.

1758 Krieger J. Bull Eur Physiopath Respir 1986; 22: 147–89.

1759 Krieger J, Kurtz D, Roeslin N. Nouv Presse Med 1976; 5: 2890.

1760 Krieger J, Mangin P, Kurtz D. Rev Electroencephalogr Neurophysiol 1979; 9: 250–7.

1761 Krieger J, Mangin P, Kurtz D. Curr Ther Res 1982; 32: 697–705.

1762 Krieger J, Mangin P, Kurtz D. Bull Eur Physiopath Respir 1983; 19: 630.

1763 Krieger J, Racineux JL, Huber P, et al. Bull Eur Physiopath Respir 1986; 22: 393–7.

1764 Krieger J, Sautegau A, Sauder P, Weitzenblum E, Kurtz D. Presse Med 1984; 13: 2559–62.

1765 Krieger J, Turlot J–C, Mangin P, Kurtz D. Sleep 1983; 6: 108–20.

1766 Krieger J, Weitzenblum E, Monassier J–P, Stoeckel C, Kurtz D. Lancet 1983; 2: 1429–30.

1767 Krieger MH, Mezon BJ, Acres JC, West P, Brownell L. Arch Intern Med 1982; 142: 956–8.

1768 Kronenberg R, Hamilton FN, Gabel R, Hickey R, Read DJC, Severinghaus J. Respir Physiol 1972; 16: 109–25.

1769 Kronenberg RS, Drage CW. J Clin Invest 1973; 52: 1812–9.

1770 Kronenberg RS, Gabel RA, Severinghaus JW. Am J Med 1975; 59: 349–53.

1771 Kryger M, Quesney LF, Holder D, Gloor P, MacLeod P. Am J Med 1974; 56: 531–9.

1772 Kryger MH. Arch Intern Med 1982; 142: 1793–4.

1773 Kryger MH. Arch Intern Med 1983; 143: 2301–3.

1774 Kryger MH. Clin Chest Med 1985; 6: 555–62.

1775 Kuhara H, Wakabayashi T, Kishimoto H, Yanagi T. Jpn J Thorac Dis 1980; 18: 381–6.

1776 Kuitunen P, Rapola J, Noponen A–L, Donner M. Acta Paediatr Scand 1972; 61: 353–61.

1777 Kumano K, Tsuyama N. J Bone Joint Surg 1982; 64A: 242–8.

1778 Kumashiro H, Sato M, Hirata J, Baba O, Otsuki S. Folia Psychiatr Neurol Jpn 1971; 25: 41–9.

1779 Kummer F. Wien Zeitschr Inn Med 1973; 54: 524–43.

1780 Kummer F, Meznik F, Pfluger G. Zeitschr Orthop 1975; 113: 275–9.

1781 Kuo PC, West RA, Bloomquist DS, McNeil RW. Oral Surg, Oral Med, Oral Pathol 1979; 48: 385–92.

1782 Kuperman AS, Krieger AJ, Rosomuff HL. Chest 1971; 59: 128–32.

1783 Kuroiwa Y, Yamada A, Ikebe K, Kosaka K, Sugita H, Murakami T. J Neurol Neurosurg Psychiatr 1981; 44: 173–5.

1784 Kurtz D, Krieger J. In: Guilleminault C, Dement WC, eds. Sleep Apnea Syndromes. New York: AR Liss Inc, 1978: 145–59.

1785 Kurz LT, Mubarak SJ, Schultz P, Park SM, Leach J. J Pediatr Orthop 1983; 3: 347–53.

1786 Kuypers HGJM. J Anat 1958; 92: 198–218.

1787 Laaban JP, D'Orbcastel OR. Poumon Coeur 1980; 36: 335–43.

1788 Labelle H, Tohme S, Duhaime M, Allard P. J Bone Joint Surg 1986; 68A: 564–72.

1789 Labrid C, Regnier G, Laubie M. Eur J Respir Dis 1983; 64: Suppl 126: 185–9.

1790 Lack EE. Hum Pathol 1977; 8: 39–51.

1791 Lack EE. Am J Pathol 1978; 91: 497–507.

1792 Lack W, Haber P, Lukeschitsch G, Kummer F. Acta Med Austriaca 1981; 8: 145–9.

1793 Lahiri S, Kao FF, Velasquez T, Martinez C, Pezzia W. Respir Physiol 1969; 6: 360–74.

1794 Lahuerta J, Lipton S, Wells JCD. Ann R Coll Surg Engl 1985; 67: 41–4.

1795 Lakshminarayan S, Sahn SA, Weil JV. Am Rev Respir Dis 1978; 117: 33–8.

1796 Lamarre A, Hall JE, Weng TR, Aspin N, Levison H. J Bone Joint Surg 1971; 53A: 195.

1797 Lancaster JF, Tomashefski JF. Am Rev Respir Dis 1963; 87: 435–7.

1798 Landauer KS, Stickle G. Arch Phys Med Rehabil 1958; 39: 145–51.

1799 Landis FB, Weisel W. J Thorac Surg 1954; 27: 336–48.

1800 Landon JF. J Pediatr 1934; 5: 1–8.

1801 Lands L, Zinman R. Chest 1986; 89: 757–60.

1802 Landtman B. Ann Paediatr Fenn 1958; 4: 181–90.

1803 Lane DJ, Hazleman B, Nichols PJR. Q J Med 1974; 43: 551–68.

1804 Lane DJ, Rout NW, Williamson DH. Br Med J 1971; 3: 9–12.

1805 Lange LS, Laszlo G. J Neurol Neurosurg Psychiatr 1965; 28: 317–9.

1806 Lange RL, Botticelli JT, Carlisle RP, Tsagaris TJ, Horgan JD. Circulation 1968; 37: 331–44.

1807 Lange RL, Hecht HH. J Clin Invest 1962, 41: 42–52.

1808 Langer H, Woolf CR. Am Rev Respir Dis 1971; 104: 440–2.

1809 Langou RA, Cohen LS, Sheps D, Wolfson S, Glenn WWL. Am Heart J 1978; 95: 295–300.

1810 Lanigan C, Borzone G, Brophy C, Moxham J. Bull Eur Physiopath Respir 1986; 20: 163s.

1811 Larmi TKI, Patiala J, Karvonen MJ. Ann Med Intern Fenn 1955; 44: 57–69.

1812 Laroche CM, Mier AK, Green M. Thorax 1987; 42: 228.

1813 Laroche CM, Moxham J, Stanley NN, Courtenay–Evans RJ, Green M. Thorax 1987; 42: 744.

1814 Larsen PD, Snyder EW, Matsuo F, Watanabe S, Johnson LP. Arch Neurol 1983; 40: 769.

1815 Larson EB, Roach RC, Schoene RB, Hornbein TF. J Am Med Assoc 1982; 248: 328–32.

1816 Larson RK, Evans BH. Am Rev Respir Dis 1963; 87: 753–6.

1817 Lassen HCA. Lancet 1953; 1; 37–41.

1818 Lassen HCA. Dan Med Bull 1961; 8: 115–20.

1819 Lassen HCA, ed. Management of life–threatening poliomyelitis Copenhagen 1952–56 with a survey of autopsy findings in 115 cases. Livingstone: Edinburgh 1956.

1820 Laubie M, Schmitt H. Eur J Pharmacol 1980; 61: 125–36.

1821 Laughlin GM, Wynne JW, Victorica BE. J Pediatr 1981; 98: 435–7.

1822 Laurie G. In: Olson DA, Henig E, eds. Proceedings of an international symposium. Whatever happened to the polio patient? Chicago, 1979: 37–41.

1823 Laurie G. Rehabil Gazette 1980; 23: 3–10.

1824 Lavie CJ, Messerli FH. Chest 1986; 90: 275–9.

1825 Lavie P. Sleep 1983; 6: 244–6.

1826 Lavie P. Arch Intern Med 1984; 144: 2025–8.

1827 Lavie P, Fischel N, Zomer J, Eliaschar I. Acta Otolaryngol 1983; 95: 161–6.

1828 Lavie P, Gertner R, Zomer J, Podoshin L. Acta Otolaryngol 1981; 92: 529–33.

1829 Lavie P, Halperin E, Zomer J, Alroy G. Sleep 1981; 4: 279–82.

1830 Lavie P, Zomer J, Eliaschar I, et al. Arch Otolaryngol 1982; 108: 373–7.

1831 Lavietes MH, Clifford E, Silverstein D, Stier F, Reichman LB. Respiration 1979; 38: 121–6.

1832 Lawes WE, Harries JR. Br Med J 1957; 2: 1205–6.

1833 Lawrence LT. Am Rev Respir Dis 1959; 80: 575–84.

1834 Lawyer T Jnr, Netsky MG. Arch Neurol Psychiatr 1953; 69: 171–92.

1835 Layon J, Bannen MJ, Jaeger MJ, Peterson CV, Gallagher TJ, Modell JH. Chest 1986; 89: 517–21.

1836 Leach W. J Laryngol Otol 1962; 76: 237–40.

1837 Leak LV. Am Rev Respir Dis 1979; 119: Suppl 3–21.

1838 Lebo CP, U KS, Norris FH Jnr. Laryngoscope 1976; 66: 862–8.

1839 Leden H von, Isshiki N. Arch Otolaryngol 1965; 81: 616–25.

1840 Lederer DH, Water JM van der, Indech RB. Chest 1980; 77: 610–3.

1841 Ledsome JR, Sharp JM. Am Rev Respir Dis 1981; 124: 41–4.

1842 Lee FI, Hughes DTD. Brain 1964; 87: 521–36.

1843 Lee FS, Guenther AE, Meleney HE. Am J Physiol 1916; 40: 446–73.

1844 Lee H, Criner G, Rassulo J, Make B, Celli B. Am Rev Respir Dis 1986; 133: A168.

1845 Lee MC, Klassen AC, Heaney LM, Resch JA. Stroke 1976; 7: 382–5.

1846 Lee MC, Klassen AC, Resch JA. Stroke 1974; 5: 612–6.

1847 Leech JA, Ernst P, Rogala E, Becklake MR. Am Rev Respir Dis 1983; 127: Suppl 225.

1848 Leech JA, Ernst P, Rogala EJ, Gurr J, Gordon I, Becklake MR. J Pediatr 1985; 106: 143–9.

1849 Lefcoe NM, Paterson NAM. Am J Med 1973; 54: 343–50.

1850 Leger P, Madelon J, Jennequin J, Gerard M, Robert D. Am Rev Respir Dis 1987; 135: Suppl A193.

1851 Leggett RJ, Cooke NJ, Clancy L, Leitch AG, Kirby BJ, Flenley DC. Thorax 1976; 31: 414–8.

1852 Leggett RJE, Flenley DC. Br Med J 1977; 2: 84–6.

1853 Lehner WE, Ballard IM, Figueroa WG, Woodruff DS. J Fam Pract 1980; 10: 39–42.

1854 Lehrman KL, Guilleminault C, Schroeder JS, Tilkian A, Forno LN. Arch Intern Med 1978; 138: 206–9.

1855 Leigh RJ, Shaw DA. Arch Neurol 1976; 33; 356–61.

1856 Leiter JC, Doble EA, Knuth SL, Bartlett D Jnr. Am Rev Respir Dis 1987; 135: 383–6.

1857 Leiter JC, Knuth SL, Bartlett D Jnr. Am Rev Respir Dis 1985; 132: 1242–5.

1858 Leith DE. J Appl Physiol 1983; 55: 1932–5.

1859 Leith DE, Bradley M. J Appl Physiol 1976; 41: 508–16.

1860 Leith TE, Mead J. J Appl Physiol 1967; 23: 221–7.

1861 Lenard HG, Goebel HH. Neuropadiatrie 1975; 6: 220–31.

1862 Leon AC de, Perloff JK, Twigg H, Majd M. Circulation 1965; 32: 193–203.

1863 Lepeschkin E. Am J Med 1954; 16: 73–9.

1864 Lertzman MM, Cherniack RM. Am Rev Respir Dis 1976; 114: 1145–65.

1865 Lesoin F, Delandsheer E, Lozes G, Hurtevent JF, Jomin M, Guieu JD. Lancet 1983; 1: 1385–6.

1866 Lester CW. J Thorac Surg 1950; 19: 507–22.

1867 Lester CW. Ann Surg 1953; 137: 482–9.

1868 Lester CW. J Thorac Surg 1957; 34: 1–10.

1869 Lester CW, Cournand A, Riley RL. J Thorac Surg 1942; 11: 529–53.

1870 Leeuwenhoek A. Philos Trans 1723; 32: 341–3.

1871 Leventhal SR, Orkin FK, Hirsh RA. Anesthesiology 1980; 53: 26–30.

1872 Levin BE, Margolis G. Ann Neurol 1977; 1: 583–6.

1873 Levine BE, Bigelow DB, Hamstra RD, et al. Ann Intern Med 1957; 66: 639–50.

1874 Levine DB. Orthop Clin North Am 1979; 10: 761–8.

1875 Levine DB, Bredin CP, King TKC, Briscoe WA, Smith JP. Orthop Trans 1978; 2: 264.

1876 Levine S, Gillen JS, Huntley SK, Crawford J, Beverly J. Am Rev Respir Dis 1983; 127: Suppl 126.

1877 Levine S, Weiser P, Gillen J. Am Rev Respir Dis 1986; 133: 400–6.

1878 Levinsky L. Dis Chest 1961; 40: 564–71.

1879 Levi–Valensi P, Duwoos H, Echter E, et al. Poumon Coeur 1970; 26: 1219–35.

1880 Levi–Valensi P, Duwoos H, Giroulle H, Muir JF, Rousselin L, Vonachen P. Poumon Coeur 1977; 33: 51–8.

1881 Levy AM, Tabakin BS, Hanson JS, Narkewicz RM. N Engl J Med 1967; 277: 506–11.

1882 Levy RD, Esau SA, Bye PTP, Pardy RL. Am Rev Respir Dis 1984; 130: 38–41.

1883 Levy RD, Martin JG, Bradley TD, Macklem PT, Newman SL. Am Rev Respir Dis 1986; 133: A168.

1884 Lewins. Edinburgh Med Surg J 1840; 54: 255–6.

1885 Lewis L, Hirschberg GG, Adamson JP. Arch Phys Med Rehabil 1957; 38: 243–9.

1886 Lewis LJ, Brookhart JM. Am J Physiol 1951; 166: 241–54.

1887 Lewis MI, Belman MJ, Sieck GC. Am Rev Respir Dis 1986; 133: 672–5.

1888 Lewis TD, Daniel EE. Gastroenterology 1981; 81: 145–9.

1889 Leygonie–Goldenberg F, Perrier M, Duizabo P, Bouchareine A, Harf A, Barbizet J, Degos JD. Rev Neurol (Paris) 1977; 133: 255–70.

1890 Leznoff A, Haight JS, Hoffstein V. Am Rev Respir Dis 1986; 133: 935–6.

1891 Libby DM, Briscoe WA, Boyce B, Smith JP. Am J Med 1982; 73: 532–8.

1892 Libby DM, Schley S, Smith JP. Chest 1981; 80: 641–3.

1893 Lieberman A. NY State J Med 1954; 54: 2737.

1894 Lieberman AN, Horowitz L, Redmond P, Pachter L, Lieberman I, Leibowitz M. Am J Gastroenterol 1980; 74: 157–60.

1895 Lieberman AT. J Am Med Assoc 1942; 120: 1209–11.

1896 Lieberman DA, Faulkner JA, Craig AB Jnr, Maxwell LC. J Appl Physiol 1973; 34: 233–7.

1897 Lieberman JS, Corkill G, Nayak NN, French BN, Taylor RG. Arch Phys Med Rehabil 1980; 61: 528–31.

1898 Liggins GC, Vilos GA, Campos GA, Kitterman JA, Lee CH. J Dev Physiol 1981; 3: 267–74.

1899 Liggins GC, Vilos GA, Campos GA, Kitterman JA, Lee CH. J Dev Physiol 1981; 3: 275–82.

1900 Lightman NI, Schooley RT. Chest 1977; 72: 250–2.

1901 Liljestrand A. Physiol Rev 1958; 38: 691–708.

1902 Lilker ES, Woolf CR. Can Med Assoc J 1968; 99: 752–7.

1903 Lin HY, Nash CL, Herndon CH, Andersen NB. J Bone Joint Surg 1974; 56A: 1173–9.

1904 Lindahl J, Strom J. Acta Med Scand 1956; Suppl 316: 63–7.

1905 Lindahl T. Thorax 1954; 9: 285–90.

1906 Linderholm H, Lindgren U. Acta Orthop Scand 1978; 49: 469–78.

1907 Linderholm H, Werneman H. Acta Med Scand 1956; Suppl 316: 135–57.

1908 Lindh M. Spine 1978; 3: 313–8.

1909 Lindh M. Spine 1978; 3: 122–34.

1910 Lindh M, Bjure J. Acta Orthop Scand 1975; 46: 934–48.

1911 Lindskog GE, Felton WL II. Surg Gynecol Obstet 1952; 95: 615–22.

1912 Lindskog GE, Friedman I. Am Rev Tuberc 1936; 34: 505–26.

1913 Lisboa C, Moreno R, Fava M, Ferreti R, Cruz E, Am Rev Respir Dis 1985; 132: 48–52.

1914 Lisboa C, Pare PD, Pertuze J, et al. Am Rev Respir Dis 1986; 134: 488–92.

1915 Lissac J, Fardeau M, Contamin F, Poenaru L, Agopian P der, Salmona JP. Nouv Presse Med 1982; 11: 3797.

1916 Lissac J, Labrousse J, Mignon A, Bonnet Y, Marsac J, Gaubert J. Reanimation et Med D'Urgence 1972; 1: 277–92.

1917 Lissac J, Labrousse J, Mignon A, Bonnet Y, Marsac J, Gaubert J. Nouv Presse Med, 1972; 1: 2903.

1918 Little GM. Tubercle 1956; 37: 172–6.

1919 Littler WA, Brown IK, Roaf R. Thorax 1972; 27: 420–8.

1920 Littler WA, Reuben SR, Lane DJ. Thorax 1973; 28: 209–13.

1921 Littlewood R, Bajada S. Br Med J 1981; 282: 778–9.

1922 Liu HM, Loew JM, Hunt CE. Neurology 1978; 28: 1013–9.

1923 Loach AB, Young AC, Spalding JMK, Crampton Smith A. Br Med J 1975; 1: 309–12.

1924 Lockwood AH. Arch Neurol 1976; 33: 292–5.

1925 Loeser WD. Am J Med Sci 1956; 231: 487–93.

1926 Loffel NB, Rossi LN, Mumenthaler M, Lutschg J, Ludin H–P. J Neurol Sci 1977; 33: 71–9.

1927 Logue V, Edwards MR. J Neurol Neurosurg Psychiatr 1981; 411: 273–84.

1928 Loh L. Anaesthesia 1983; 38: 621–2.

1929 Loh L Goldman M, Newsom Davis J. Medicine 1977; 56: 165–9.

1930 Loh L, Hughes JMB, Newsom Davis J. Bull Europ Physiopath Resp 1979; 15: Suppl 137–41.

1931 Loh L, Hughes JMB, Newsom Davis J. Am Rev Respir Dis 1979; 119 Suppl: 121.

1932 Loke J, Anthonisen NR. Am Rev Respir Dis 1974; 110: Suppl 178–82.

1933 Loke J, Mahler DA, Virgulto JA. J Appl Physiol 1982; 52: 821–4.

1934 Long KJ, Allen N. Arch Neurol 1984; 41: 1109–10.

1935 Longo AM, Moser KM, Luchsinger PC. Am Rev Respir Dis 1971; 103: 690–7.

1936 Longobardo GS, Gothe B, Goldman MD, Cherniack NS. Respir Physiol 1982; 50: 311–33.

1937 Lonsdale D, Mercer RD. Lancet 1982; 2; 487.

1938 Lopata M, Freilich RA, Onal E, Pearle J, Lourenco RV. Am Rev Respir Dis 1979; 119: 165–8.

1939 Lopata M, Lourenco RV. Clin Chest Med 1980; 1: 33–45.

1940 Lopata M, Onal E. Am Rev Respir Dis 1982; 126: 640–5.

1941 Lopes J, Russell DM, Whitwell J, Jeejeebhoy KN. Am J Clin Nutr 1982; 36: 602–10.

1942 Lopes JN, Muller NL, Bryan MH, Bryan AC. J Appl Physiol 1981; 51: 547–51.

1943 Loring SH, Mead J. J Appl Physiol 1982; 53: 756–60.

1944 Lourenco RV. J Clin Invest 1969; 48: 1609–14.

1945 Lourenco RV, Cherniack NS, Malm JR, Fishman AP. J Appl Physiol 1966; 21: 527–33.

1946 Lovejoy FW, Yu PNG, Nye RE, Joos HA, Simpson JH. Am J Med 1954; 16: 4–11.

1947 Loynes RD. J Bone Joint Surg 1972; 54B: 484–98.

1948 Lozewicz S, Potter DR, Costello JF, Moyle JB, Maccabe JJ. Br Med J 1981; 283: 1015–6.

1949 Lucci B, Ortaggio F, Toffanetti R, Mosti A. Acta Neurol (Naples) 1983; 38: 109–17.

1950 Luce JM. Chest 1980; 78: 626–31.

1951 Luce JM. Crit Care Med 1985; 13: 126–31.

1952 Luce JM, Culver BH. Chest 1982; 81: 82–90.

1953 Ludman H. J Laryngol Otol 1962; 76: 234–6.

1954 Lugaresi E, Cirignotta F, Coccagna G, Piana C. Sleep 1980; 3: 221–4.

1955 Lugaresi E, Coccagna G, Ceroni GB, Mantovani M, Pazzaglia P. Electroencephologr Clin Neurophysiol 1969; 27: 99.

1956 Lugaresi E, Coccagna G, Farneti P, Mantovani M, Cirignotta F. Electroencephalogr Clin Neurophysiol 1975; 39: 59–64.

1957 Lugaresi E, Coccagna G, Mantovani M, Lebrun R. Electroencephalogr Clin Neurophysiol 1972; 32: 701–5.

1958 Lugliani R, Whipp BJ, Seard C, Wasserman K. N Engl J Med 1971; 285: 1105–11.

1959 Lugliani R, Whipp BJ, Wasserman K. Chest 1979; 76: 414–9.

1960 Lugliani R, Whipp BJ, Winter B, Tanaka KR, Wasserman K. N Engl J Med 1971; 285: 1112–4.

1961 Lukas DS, Plum F. Am J Med 1952; 12: 388–96.

1962 Luke MJ, McDonnell EJ. J Pediatr 1968; 73: 725–33.

1963 Luke MJ, Mehrizi A, Folger GM Jnr, Rowe RD. Pediatrics 1966; 37: 762–8.

1964 Lund WS. J Laryngol Otol 1968; 82: 353–67.

1965 Lundsgaard C, Slyke DD van. Medicine 1923; 2: 1–76.

1966 Lunteren E van, Graaff WB van de, Parker DM, et al. J Appl Physiol 1984; 56: 746–52.

1967 Lunteren E van, Strohl KP. Clin Chest Med 1986; 7: 171–88.

1968 Lussier JJ, Rushton WAH. J Physiol 1952; 117: 87–108.

1969 Lyager S, Naeraa N, Pedersen OF. Respiration 1984; 45: 89–99.

1970 Lynn AM, Jenkins JG, Edmonds JF, Burns JE. Crit Care Med 1982; 11: 280–2.

1971 Lyons HA, Huang CT. Am J Med 1968; 44: 881–8.

1972 Lyons HA, Zuhdi MN, Kelly JJ Jnr. Am Heart J 1955; 50: 921–2.

1973 Maayan C, Springer C, Armon Y, Bar-Yishay E, Shapira Y, Godfrey S. Pediatrics 1986; 77: 390–5.

1974 McAlpine D, Compston N. Q J Med 1952; 21: 135–67.

1975 McBride B, Whitelaw WA. J Appl Physiol 1981; 51: 1189–97.

1976 McCaffrey TV, Kern EB. Ann Otol 1979; 88: 247–52.

1977 McCleave DJ, Fletcher J, Cruden LC. Anaesth Intensive Care 1976; 4: 46–52.

1978 McClement JH, Christianson LC, Hubaytar RT, Simpson DG. Ann NY Acad Sci 1965; 121: 746–50.

1979 McComb RD, Markesbury WR, O'Connor WN. J Pediatr 1979; 94: 47–51.

1980 McConnell DH, Maloney JV, Buckberg GD. J Thorac Cardiovasc Surg 1974; 68; 944–52.

1981 McCool FD, McCann DR, Leith DE, Hoppin FG Jnr. J Appl Physiol 1986; 60: 299–303.

1982 McCool FD, Mayewski RF, Shayne DS, Gibson CJ, Griggs RC, Hyde RW. Chest 1986; 90: 546–52.

1983 McCool FD, Pichurko BM, Slutsky AS, Sarkarati M, Rossier A, Brown R. J Appl Physiol 1986; 60: 1198–202.

1984 McCormack WM, Spalter HF. J Am Med Assoc 1966; 197: 957–60.

1985 McCredie M, Lovejoy FW, Kaltreider NL. Thorax 1962; 17: 213–7.

1986 McDonald DM. In: Hornbein TF, ed. Regulation of Breathing. Part 1. New York: Marcel Dekker, 1981: 105–319.

1987 McDonald WI, Kocen RS. In: Dyck PJ, Thomas PK, Lambert EH, Bunge R, eds. Peripheral Neuropathy, 2nd ed. Philadelphia: WB Saunders 1984: 2010–7.

1988 McDowell F, Wolff HG. J Am Med Assoc 1953; 151: 1160–63.

1989 McEvoy RD, Sharp DJ, Thornton AT. Am Rev Respir Dis 1986; 133: 662–6.

1990 McEvoy RD, Thornton AT. Sleep 1984; 7: 313–25.

1991 McFadden RG, Craig ID, Paterson NAM. Br J Dis Chest 1984; 78: 187–91.

1992 McFarland HR, Heller GL. Arch Neurol 1966; 14: 196–201.

1993 MacGregor MI, Brock AJ, Wall WC Jnr. Johns Hopkins Med J 1970; 126: 279–95.

1994 McGuirt WF, Blalock D. Laryngoscope 1980; 90: 1496–501.

1995 McIlroy MB, Marshall R, Christie RV. Clin Sci 1954; 13: 127–36.

1996 McIntosh CA. Ann Surg 1935; 102: 961–71.

1997 MacIntosh RR. Lancet 1940; 2: 745–6.

1998 Macintosh RR. Practitioner 1940; 145: 275–81.

1999 Macintosh RR. Br Med J 1943; 2: 493–4.

2000 MacIntosh RR, Mushin WW. Br Med J 1946; 1: 908–9.

2001 Mackay AD, Cooper RA, Bradbury S, et al. Am Rev Respir Dis 1982; 125: Suppl 246.

2002 McKinley AC, Auchincloss JH Jnr, Nicholas JJ. Am Rev Respir Dis 1969; 100: 526–32.

2003 Macklem PT. Respir Physiol 1979; 38: 153–71.

2004 Macklem PT. Chest 1980; 78: 753–8.

2005 Macklem PT. Thorax 1981; 36: 161–3.

2006 Macklem PT. Chest 1984; 85: Suppl 60–2S.

2007 Macklem PT. Am Rev Respir Dis 1986; 134: 812–5.

2008 Macklem PT, Cohen C, Zagelbaum G, Roussos C. In: CIBA Foundation Symposium 82. Human Muscle Fatigue: Physiological Mechanisms. London: Pitman Medical, 1981, 249–63.

2009 Macklem PT, Roussos CS. Clin Sci Molec Med 1977; 53: 419–22.

2010 MacLean IC, Mattioni TA. Arch Phys Med Rehabil 1981; 62: 70–3.

2011 McLean WT Jnr, McKone RC, Salem W. Arch Neurol 1973; 29: 223–6.

2012 McLellan PA, Goldstein RS, Ramcharan V, Rebuck AS. Am Rev Respir Dis 1981; 124: 199–201.

2013 McLeod JG, Walsh JC, Prineas JW, Pollard JD. J Neurol Sci 1976; 27: 145–62.

2014 McMichael J, McGibbon JP. Clin Sci 1939; 4: 175–83.

2015 McMichan JC, Michel L, Westbrook PR. J Am Med Assoc 1980; 243: 528–31.

2016 McMichan JC, Piepgras DG, Gracey DR, Marsh HM, Sittipong R. Mayo Clin Proc 1979; 54: 662–8.

2017 McNamara JJ, Paulson DL, Urschel HC Jnr, Razzuk MA. Surgery 1968; 64: 1013–21.

2018 MacNee W, Connaughton JJ, Hayhurst MD, Rhind GB, Muir AL, Flenley DC. Respiration 1984; 46: Suppl 157–8.

2019 McNichol MW, Pride NB. Lancet 1961; 1: 906–8.

2020 McNicholas WT, Carter JL, Rutherford R, Zamel N, Phillipson EA. Am Rev Respir Dis 1982; 125: 773–5.

2021 McNicholas WT, Coffey M, Boyle T, Fitzgerald MX. Thorax 1986; 41: 243.

2022 McNicholas WT, Coffey M, McDonnell T, O'Regan R, Fitzgerald MX. Am Rev Respir Dis 1987; 135: 1316–9.

2023 McNicholas WT, Rutherford R, Grossman R, Moldofsky H, Zamel N, Phillipson EA. Am Rev Respir Dis 1983; 128: 429–33.

2024 McNicholas WT, Tarlo S, Cole P, et al. Am Rev Respir Dis 1982; 126: 625–8.

2025 McNicol MW, Pride NB. Thorax 1965; 20: 53–65.

2026 MacRae DM, Hiltz JE, Quinlan JJ. Am Rev Tuberc 1950; 61: 355–68.

2027 Macrae J, Campbell AMG. Lancet 1954; 1: 704–7.

2028 Macrae J, Walley RV, Lucas HK. Lancet 1959; 1: 452.

2029 McSweeney CJ. Lancet 1936; 2: 1093–4.

2030 McSweeney CJ. Br Med J 1938; 1: 1206–7.

2031 McWilliam RC, Gardner–Medwin D, Doyle D, Stephenson JBP. Arch Dis Childh 1985; 60: 145–9.

2032 Maddern GJ, Horowitz M, Jamieson GG, Chatterton BE, Collins PJ, Roberts–Thomson P. Gastroenterology 1984; 87: 922–6.

2033 Magyar P, Szathmary I, Szobor A. Eur Neurol 1979; 18: 59–65.

2034 Mahadevia AK, Onal E, Lopata M. Am Rev Respir Dis 1983; 128: 708–11.

2035 Majid PA, Zienkowicz BS, Roos JP. Thorax 1979; 34: 74–8.

2036 Make B, Dayno S, Gertman P. Am Rev Respir Dis 1986; 133: A167.

2037 Make B, Gilmartin M, Brody JS, Snider GL. Am Rev Respir Dis 1982; 125: Suppl 139.

2038 Make B, Gilmartin M, Brody JS, Snider GL. Chest 1984; 86: 358–65.

2039 Make BJ. Chest 1985; 87: 412.

2040 Make BJ. Clin Chest Med 1986; 7: 519–40.

2041 Make BJ, Gilmartin ME. Clin Chest Med 1986; 7: 679–91.

2042 Make BJ, O'Brien R. In: Brody JS, Snider GL, eds. Current Topics in the Management of Respiratory Diseases, 2nd ed. Edinburgh: Churchill Livingstone, 1985: 71–104.

2043 Makley JT, Herndon CH, Inkley S, et al. J Bone Joint Surg 1968; 50A: 1379–90.

2044 Makley JT, Herndon CH, Inkley SR, Doershuk CF, Post RH. J Bone Joint Surg 1968; 50A: 845.

2045 Malcolm AD. Br Heart J 1985; 53: 353–62.

2046 Maloney FP. Arch Phys Med Rehabil 1979; 60: 261–5.

2047 Maloney JV, Elam JO, Handford SW, et al. J Am Med Assoc 1953; 152: 212–6.

2048 Maloney JV Jnr, Handford SW. J Appl Physiol 1954; 6: 453–9.

2049 Maloney JV, Whittenberger JL. Am J Med Sci 1951; 221: 425–30.

2050 Mamdani MB, Masdeu J, Ross E, Ohara R. Electroencephalogr Clin Neurophysiol 1983; 55: 411–6.

2051 Man GCW, Jones RL, MacDonald GF, King EG. Chest 1979; 76: 219–21.

2052 Mangat D, Orr WC, Smith RO. Arch Otolaryngol 1977; 103: 383–6.

2053 Mankin HJ, Graham JJ, Schack J. J Bone Joint Surg 1964; 46A: 53–62.

2054 Manning CW, Prime FJ, Zorab PA. Lancet 1967; 2: 792–5.

2055 Manning CW, Prime FJ, Zorab PA. J Bone Joint Surg 1973; 55B: 521–7.

2056 Marcos JJ, Grover FL, Trinkle JK. J Surg Res 1974; 16: 523–6.

2057 Margolis ML, Hill AR. Am Rev Respir Dis 1986; 134: 328–31.

2058 Marino W. Am Rev Respir Dis 1986; 133: A167.

2059 Marino W, Braun NMT. Am Rev Respir Dis 1982; 125: Suppl 85.

2060 Markand ON, Kincaid JC, Pourmand RA, et al. Neurology 1984; 34: 604–14.

2061 Markand ON, Moorthy SS, Mahomed Y, King RD, Brown JW. Ann Thorac Surg 1985; 39: 68–73.

2062 Marks A, Bocles J, Morganti L. N Engl J Med 1963; 268: 61–8.

2063 Marriott WM. J Am Med Assoc 1920; 75: 668–9.

2064 Marsac J, Bouchoucha S, Ruff F. Bull Eur Physio Path Respir 1979; 15: Suppl 265–77.

2065 Marschke G, Beall GN, Stern WE, Murray JF. J Am Med Assoc 1965; 191: 397.

2066 Marsden CD, Duvoisin R. Arch Neurol 1980; 37: 253–4.

2067 Marsh ML, Aidinis SJ, Shapiro HM. Anesth Analg 1977; 56: 216–8.

2068 Martens J, Demedts M, Vanmeenen MT, Dequeker J. Chest 1983; 84: 170–5.

2069 Martin AJ, Stern L, Yeats J, Lepp D, Little J. Dev Med Child Neurol 1986; 28: 314–8.

2070 Martin B, Heintzelman M, Chen H–I. J Appl Physiol 1982; 52: 1581–5.

2071 Martin CJ, Hallett WY. Ann Intern Med 1961; 54: 1156–64.

2072 Martin L, Chalmers IM, Dhingra S, McCarthy D, Hunter T. J Rheumatol 1985; 12: 104–7.

2073 Martin LW, Helmsworth JA. J Am Med Assoc 1962; 179: 82–4.

2074 Martin RJ, Pennock BE, Orr WC, Sanders MH, Rogers RM. J Appl Physiol 1980; 48: 432–7.

2075 Martin RJ, Rogers RM, Gray BA. Am Rev Respir Dis 1980; 122: Suppl 105–7.

2076 Martin RJ, Sanders MH, Gray BA, Pennock BE. Am Rev Respir Dis 1982; 125: 175–80.

2077 Martin RJ, Sufit RL, Ringel SP, Hudgel DW, Hill PL. Muscle Nerve 1983; 6: 201–3.

2078 Masland WS, Yamamoto WS. Am J Physiol 1962; 203: 789–95.

2079 Massam M, Jones RS. Thorax 1980; 35: 557–8.

2080 Massumi RA, Sarin RK, Pooya M, et al. Dis Chest 1969; 55: 110–4.

2081 Massumi RA, Winnacker JL. Am J Med 1964; 36: 876–82.

2082 Master AM, Stone J. Am J Med Sci 1949; 217: 392–400.

2083 Mathew OP, Abu–Osba YK, Thach BT. J Appl Physiol 1982; 52: 445–50.

2084 Mathew OP, Abu–Osba YK, Thach BT. J Appl Physiol 1982; 52: 438–44.

2085 Mathew OP, Farber JP. Respir Physiol 1983; 54: 259–68.

2086 Mathias CJ. Eur J Intensive Care Med 1976; 2: 147–56.

2087 Mathru M, Venus B, Smith RA. Chest 1985; 87: 137–8.

2088 Matson RW. Am Rev Tuberc 1930; 22: 1–34.

2089 Matthews AW, Howell JBL. Clin Sci Molec Med 1976; 50: 199–205.

2090 Matthews HR, Hopkinson RB. Br J Surg 1984; 71: 147–50.

2091 Mauer KW, Staats BA, Olsen KD. Mayo Clin Proc 1983; 58: 349–53.

2092 Maxwell DL, Cover D, Hughes JMB. Am Rev Respir Dis 1985; 132: 1233–7.

2093 Mayer J, Fuchs E, Penzel T, Peter JH, Schnell H, Wichert PVM. Respiration 1984; 46: Suppl 158.

2094 Mayer PJ, Dove J, Ditmanson M, Young–Shung S. Spine 1981; 6: 573–82.

2095 Maynard FM. In: Olson DA, Henig E, eds. Proceedings of an international symposium. Whatever happened to the polio patient? Chicago, 1979: 159–67.

2096 Mazar A, Belman MJ, King R, Sieck GC. Am Rev Respir Dis 1983; 127: Suppl 231.

2097 Mazza FG, DiMarco AF, Altose MD, Strohl KP. Chest 1984; 85; 638–40.

2098 Mazzara JT, Ayres SM, Grace WJ. Am J Med 1974; 56: 450–6.

2099 Mead J. Am Rev Respir Dis 1979; 119: Suppl 31–2.

2100 Mead J, Banzett RB, Lehr J, Loring SH, O'Cain CF. Am Rev Respir Dis 1984; 130: 320–1.

2101 Mead J, Collier C. J Appl Physiol 1959; 14: 669–78.

2102 Mead J, Peterson N, Grimby G, Mead J. Science 1967; 156: 1383–4.

2103 Mead J, Sly P, Souef P le, Hibbert M, Phelan P. Am Rev Respir Dis 1985; 132: 1223–8.

2104 Mead J, Turner JM, Macklem PT, Little JB. J Appl Physiol 1967; 22: 95–108.

2105 Mead WJ, Collins VP. Medicine 1954; 71: 864–6.

2106 Mearns AJ. Br J Surg 1977; 64: 558–60.

2107 Medd WE, French EB, Wyllie VM. Thorax 1959; 14: 247–50.

2108 Medical Research Council. "Breathing Machines" and their use in Treatment. Report of the Respirators (Poliomyelitis) Committee. No 237: 1940.

2109 Medical Research Council. Aids to the examination of the peripheral nervous system. Memorandum No 45, 1976.

2110 Medsger TA Jnr, Robinson H, Masi AT. Arthritis Rheum 1971; 14: 249–58.

2111 Mehta AD, Wright WB, Kirby BJ. Br Med J 1978; 1: 1456–7.

2112 Mehta MH. J Bone Joint Surg 1973; 55B: 513–20.

2113 Meisner H, Schober JG, Struck E, Lipowski B, Mayser P, Sebening F. Thoracic Cardiovasc Surg 1983; 31: 21–5.

2114 Meister R. Prax Klinik Pneumol 1980; 34: 273–81.

2115 Meister R. Prax Pneumologie 1981; 35: 523–7.

2116 Meister R, Heine J. Zeitschr Orthop 1973; 111: 749–55.

2117 Meister R, Heine J. Prax Pneumol 1975; 29: 219–26.

2118 Meister R, Klempt H–W. Pneumonologie 1976; 153: Suppl 115–24.

2119 Meister R, Klempt H–W, Heine J. Med Welt 1975; 26: 1397–9.

2120 Meister R, Klempt H–W, Most E, Heine J. Med Klinik 1975; 70: 1969–75.

2121 Meister R, Merkel T. Prax Klin Pneumol 1983; 37: 691–4.

2122 Mellins RB, Balfour HH Jnr, Turino GM, Winters RW. Medicine 1970; 49: 487–504.

2123 Mellins RB, Hays AP, Gold AP, Berdon WE, Bowdler JD. Pediatrics 1974; 53: 33–40.

2124 Melot C, Naeije R, Rothschild T, Mertens P, Mols P, Hallemans R. Chest 1983; 83: 528–33.

2125 Menashe VD, Farrehi C, Miller M. J Pediatr 1965; 67: 198–203.

2126 Mendelsohn HJ, Zimmerman HA, Adelman A. J Thorac Surg 1950; 20: 366–73.

2127 Mendelson WB, Garnett D, Gillin JC. J Nerv Ment Dis 1981; 169: 261–4.

2128 Mendenhall JT, Cree E, Rasmussen HK, Bauer H, Curtis JK. J Thorac Cardiovasc Surg 1960; 39: 189–93.

2129 Menzies F. Med Officer 1938; 2: 231–2.

2130 Merav AD, Attai LA, Condit DT. Chest 1983; 84: 642–4.

2131 Mertens DJ, Shephard RJ, Kavanagh T. Respiration 1978; 35: 96–107.

2132 Metcalf VA. J Am Phys Ther Assoc 1966; 46: 835–8.

2133 Meulders M, Massion J, Colle J. Arch Ital Biol 1960; 98: 430–40.

2134 Meunier–Carus J, Lonsdorfer J, Lampert E. Poumon Coeur 1974; 30: 13–19.

2135 Meyer A, Lissac J, Labrousse J. Bull Acad Nat Med 1971; 155: 111–6.

2136 Meyer JS, Gotham J, Tazaki Y, Gotoh F. Neurology 1961; 11: 950–8.

2137 Meyer JS, Herndon RM. Neurology 1962; 12: 637–42.

2138 Meyer JS, Sakai F, Karacan I, Derman S, Yamamoto M. Ann Neurol 1980; 7: 479–85.

2139 Meyer O, Dusser D, Aubier M, Chretien J, Ryckewaert A. Presse Med 1986; 15: 844.

2140 Meyrignac C, Beriel P, Laporte JP, Degos JD. Nouv Presse Med 1982; 11: 1569.

2141 Mezon B, West P, Kryger M. Am Rev Respir Dis 1979; 119: Suppl 336.

2142 Mezon BJ, West P, Maclean JP, Kryger MH. Am J Med 1980; 69: 615–8.

2143 Mezon BL, West P, Israels J, Kryger M. Am Rev Respir Dis 1980; 122: 617–21.

2144 Michet CJ Jnr, McKenna CH, Luthra HS, O'Fallon WM. Ann Intern Med 1986; 104: 74–8.

2145 Midgren B, Petersson K, Hansson L, Eriksson L, Airikkala P., Elmqvist D. Br J Dis Chest 1988 (In press).

2146 Mier A, Brophy C, Estenne M, Moxham J, Green M, Troyer A de. J Appl Physiol 1985; 58: 1438–43.

2147 Mier A, Brophy C, Moxham J, Green M. Bull Eur Physiopath Respir 1986; 20: 163s.

2148 Mier A, Brophy C, Moxham J, Green M. Bull Eur Physiopath Respir 1986; 20: 31s.

2149 Mier A, Brophy C, Wass J, Green M. Thorax 1986; 41: 710.

2150 Mier A, Miller J, Brophy C, Moxham J, Green M. Thorax 1985; 40: 701.

2151 Mier AK, Brophy C, Green M. Br Med J 1986; 292: 1495–6.

2152 Mier M. J Am Geriatr Soc 1967; 15: 230–8.

2153 Mier M, Boshes B, Canter G. Q Bull NW Univ Med School 1960; 34: 226–31.

2154 Miki H, Hida W, Nishimaki C, Inoue H, Takishima T. Am Rev Respir Dis 1987; 135: Suppl A135.

2155 Milic–Emili J. Am Rev Respir Dis 1986; 134: 1107–8.

2156 Milic–Emili J, Grassino AE, Whitelaw WA. In: Hornbein TF, ed. Regulation of Breathing. Part 2. New York: Marcel Dekker, 1981: 675–743.

2157 Milic–Emili J, Grunstein MM. Chest 1976; 70: 131–3.

2158 Miller A, Bader RA, Bader ME. Am J Med 1962; 33: 309–18.

2159 Miller FL, Zerbi–Ortiz A, Elkins JT Jnr. N Engl J Med 1960; 262: 1264–6.

2160 Miller HG, Stanton JB. Q J Med 1954; 23: 1–27.

2161 Miller J, Moxham J, Green M. Thorax 1983; 38: 232.

2162 Miller JM, Moxham J, Green M. Clin Sci 1985; 69: 91–6.

2163 Miller JM, Sproule BJ. Am Rev Respir Dis 1964; 90: 376–82.

2164 Miller RD. Proc Mayo Clin 1957; 32: 436–7.

2165 Miller RD, Bridge EV Jnr, Fowler WS, Helmsholz HF Jnr, Ellis H Jnr, Allen GT. J Thorac Surg 1958; 35: 651–61.

2166 Miller RD, Hyatt RE. Am Rev Respir Dis 1973; 108: 475–81.

2167 Miller RD, Mulder DW, Fowler WS, Olsen AM. Ann Intern Med 1957; 46: 119–25.

2168 Miller WF. Am J Med 1954; 17: 471–7.

2169 Miller WF. Am J Med 1958; 24: 929–40.

2170 Miller WF, Archer RK, Taylor HF, Ossenfort WF. J Am Med Assoc 1962; 180: 905–11.

2171 Miller WP. Am J Med 1982; 73: 317–21.

2172 Millhorn DE, Eldridge FL, Waldrop TG. Respir Physiol 1983; 51: 219–28.

2173 Millman RP. Chest 1986; 89: 621–2.

2174 Millman RP, Bevilacqua J, Peterson DD, Pack AI. Am Rev Respir Dis 1983; 127: 504–7.

2175 Mills CP. J Laryngol Otol 1964; 78: 963–4.

2176 Mills JN. J Physiol 1946; 105: 95–116.

2177 Mills JN. J Physiol 1953; 122: 66–80.

2178 Minh V–D, Dolan GF, Konopka RF, Moser KM. J Appl Physiol 1976; 40: 67–73.

2179 Minh V–D, Friedman PJ, Kurihara N, Moser KM. J Appl Physiol 1974; 37: 505–9.

2180 Minh V–D, Kurihara N, Friedman PJ, Moser KM. J Appl Physiol 1974; 37: 496–504.

2181 Minh V–D, Moser KM. Clin Res 1971; 19: 192.

2182 Ministry of Health. Breathing Machines RHB (53) 56: 1953.

2183 Minot GR, Rackemann FM. Am J Med Sci 1915; 150; 571–82.

2184 Minz M, Autret A, Laffont F, Beillevaire T, Cathala HP, Castaigne P. Biomedicine 1979; 30: 40–6.

2185 Miserocchi G, Trippenbach T. Respir Physiol 1981; 43: 275–85.

2186 Mitchell MM, Ali HH, Savarese JJ. Anesthesiology 1978; 49: 44–8.

2187 Mitchell RA. Clin Chest Med 1980; 1: 3–12.

2188 Mitchell RA, Berger AJ. Am Rev Respir Dis 1975; 111: 206–24.

2189 Mitchell RA, Berger AJ. In: Hornbein TF, ed. Regulation of Breathing. Part 1. New York: Marcel Dekker, 1981: 541–620.

2190 Mitchell RA, Herbert DA. Anesthesiology 1975; 42: 559–66.

2191 Mitchell RA, Loeschcke HH, Massion WH, Severinghaus JW. J Appl Physiol 1963; 18: 523–33.

2192 Mitchell RA, Sinha AK, McDonald DM. Brain Res 1972; 43: 681–5.

2193 Mitchell SW. Am J Med Sci 1890; 100: 109–27.

2194 Mitchinson AG, Yoffey JM. J Anat 1947; 81: 118–20.

2195 Mithoefer JC. In: Fenn WO, Rahn H, ed. Handbook of Physiology. Vol 11, Sec 3, Respiration, 1965: Chapt 38: 1011–25.

2196 Mittman C, Edelman NH, Norris AH, Shock NW. J Appl Physiol 1965; 20: 1211–6.

2197 Mixsell HR, Giddings E. J Am Med Assoc 1921; 77: 590–4.

2198 Moersch FP, Woltman HW. Proc Staff Meetings Mayo Clin 1956; 31: 421–7.

2199 Moignetau C, Ordronneau JR, Chailleux E. Rev Fr Mal Resp 1979; 7: 381–2.

2200 Molho M, Katz I, Schwartz E, Shemesh Y, Sadeh M, Wolf E. Chest 1987; 91: 466–7.

2201 Mollaret P, Pocidalo J–J, Bonnet Y. Presse Med 1958; 66: 460–3.

2202 Molloy DW, Dhingra S, Solven F, Wilson A, McCarthy DS. Am Rev Respir Dis 1984; 129: 497–8.

2203 Montero JC, Feldman DJ, Montero D. Arch Phys Med Rehabil 1967; 48: 650–3.

2204 Montero JC, Rosenberg D. Med Times 1961; 89: 699–703.

2205 Montgomery WW. N Engl J Med 1975; 292: 1390–1.

2206 Moore GC, Zwillich CW, Battaglia JD, Cotton EK, Weil JV. N Engl J Med 1976; 295: 861–5.

2207 Moore NR, Phillips MS, Shneerson JM, Flower CDR, Dixon AK. Thorax 1986; 41: 717.

2208 Moore NR, Phillips MS, Shneerson JM, Smith ML, Flower CDR, Dixon AK. Br J Radiol 1988 (In press).

2209 Moore P, James O. Crit Care Med 1981; 9: 549–55.

2210 Moore–Gillon JC, Cameron IC. Clin Sci 1985; 69: 595–9.

2211 Moore–Gillon JC, George RJD, Geddes DM. Thorax 1985; 40: 817–9.

2212 Moore–Gillon JC, Treacher DF, Gaminara EJ, Pearson TC, Cameron IR. Br Med J 1986; 293: 588–90.

2213 Moorthy SS, Gibbs PS, Losasso AM, Lingeman RE. Laryngoscope 1983; 93: 642–4.

2214 Moorthy SS, Markand ON, Mahomed Y, Brown JW. Chest 1985; 88: 211–4.

2215 Morch ET, Saxton GA Jnr, Gish G. J Am Med Asssoc 1956; 160: 864–7.

2216 Morgan AD, Bartley TD, Swenson EW. Dis Chest 1967; 51: 221–6.

2217 Morgan MDL, de Troyer A. Bull Eur Physiopath Resp 1984; 20: 547–52.

2218 Morgan MDL, Gourlay AR, Silver JR, Wiliiams SJ, Denison DM. Thorax 1985; 40: 613–7.

2219 Morley AR. Dev Med Child Neurol 1969; 11: 471–4.

2220 Morris LK, Cuetter AC, Gunderson H. Stroke 1982; 13: 93–4.

2221 Morriston Davies H. Br Med J 1926; 1: 315–20.

2222 Mortola JP, Saetta M, Fox G, Smith B, Weeks S. J Appl Physiol 1985; 59: 295–304.

2223 Mortola JP, Sant'Ambrogio G. Clin Sci 1978; 54: 25–32.

2224 Mortola JP, Sant'Ambrogio G. Am Rev Respir Dis 1979; 119: Suppl 131–4.

2225 Moruzzi G. J Neurophysiol 1940; 3: 20–32.

2226 Moser KM, Luchsinger PC, Adamson JS, et al. N Engl J Med 1973; 288: 427–31.

2227 Moser KM, Rhodes PG, Kwaan PL. Fed Proc 1965; 24: 273.

2228 Moser KM, Shibel EM, Beamon AJ. J Am Med Assoc 1973; 225: 705–7.

2229 Moses FM, Buscemi JH. West J Med 1981; 134: 69–70.

2230 Moskowitz MA, Fisher JN, Simpser MD, Strider DJ. Ann Intern Med 1976; 84: 171–3.

2231 Motley HL, Lang LP, Gordon B. Am J Med 1948; 5: 853–6.

2232 Motta J, Guilleminault C. In: Guilleminault C, Dement WC, eds. Sleep Apnea Syndromes. New York: AR Liss Inc, 1978; 137–44.

2233 Motta J, Guilleminault C, Schroeder JS, Dement WC. Ann Intern Med 1978; 89: 454–8.

2234 Moulton A, Silver JR. Clin Sci 1970; 39: 407–22.

2235 Mountain R, Zwillich C, Weil J. N Engl J Med 1978; 298: 521–5.

2236 Moxham J. Bull Eur Physiopath Respir 1984; 20: 437–44.

2237 Moxham J, Miller J, Wiles CM, Newham D, Edwards RHT. Thorax 1983; 38: 232.

2238 Moxham J, Morris AJR, Spiro SG, Edwards RHT, Green M. Thorax 1981; 36: 164–8.

2239 Moxham J, Wiles CM, Newham D, Edwards RHT. Clin Sci 1980; 59: 463–8.

2240 Moxham J, Wiles CM, Newham D, Edwards RHT. In: CIBA Foundation Symposium 82. Human Muscle Fatigue: Physiological Mechanisms. London: Pitman Medical, 1981: 197–212.

2241 Moyer JH, Miller SI, Tashnek AB, Bowman R. J Clin Invest 1952; 31: 267–72.

2242 Mucciardi N, Miller MJ. Am Rev Respir Dis 1984; 129: Suppl A270.

2243 Mudge BJ, Taylor BB, Vanderspek AFL. Anaesthesia 1980; 35: 492–5.

2244 Mugica J, Dejean D, Bourgeois I, Smits K, Bisson A. Presse Med 1985; 14: 1919–20.

2245 Muiesan G, Sorbini CA, Grassi V, et al. Dis Chest 1969; 55: 18–24.

2246 Muir JF, Hermant A, Laroche D, Levi–Valensi P, Duwoos H. Rev Fr Mal Respir 1979; 7: 421–3.

2247 Muirhead A, Conner AN. J Bone Joint Surg 1985; 67B; 699–702.

2248 Mullan S. Surg Clin North Am 1966; 46: 3–12.

2249 Mullan S, Hosobuchi Y. J Neurosurg 1968; 28: 291–7.

2250 Mullan S, Raimondi AJ. J Neurosurg 1962; 19: 675–8.

2251 Muller N, Gulston G, Cade D, Whitton J, Froese AB, Bryan MH, Bryan AC. J Appl Physiol 1979; 46: 688–95.

2252 Muller N, Volgyesi G, Bryan MH, Bryan AC. J Pediatr 1979; 95: 793–7.

2253 Muller R. Acta Psychiatr Neurolog Scand 1952; 27: 137–56.

2254 Munsat TL, Thompson LR, Coleman RF. Arch Neurol 1969; 20: 120–31.

2255 Murakami Y, Kirchner JA. Laryngoscope 1972; 82: 454–67.

2256 Murphy AJ, Talner NS, Dickinson DG. Arch Phys Med Rehabil 1956; 37: 631–6.

2257 Murphy DP, Bowman JE, Wilson RB. Am J Dis Child 1931; 42: 1075–8.

2258 Murphy NP, Davidson TC, Bouton J. Arch Dis Childh 1985; 60: 495.

2259 Murray JF. Am Rev Respir Dis 1965; 92: 435–49.

2260 Murray JF. N Engl J Med 1979; 300: 1155–7.

2261 Murray JF. Am Rev Respir Dis 1980; 122: Suppl 121–5.

2262 Mushin WW, Faux N. Lancet 1944; 2: 685–6.

2263 Myhre JR. Acta Med Scand 1959; 165: 55–60.

2264 Nachemson A. Acta Orthop Scand 1968; 39: 466–76.

2265 Naef AP. Ann Thorac Surg 1976; 21: 53–66.

2266 Naeije N, Melot C, Naeije R, Sergysels R. Eur J Respir Dis 1982; 63: 342–6.

2267 Naeye RL. Am J Cardiol 1961; 8: 416–9.

2268 Naeye RL. Am J Pathol 1961; 38: 561–74.

2269 Naeye RL, Fisher R, Ryser M, Whalen P. Science 1976; 191: 567–9.

2270 Naiditch MJ, Bower AG. Am J Med 1954; 17: 229–45.

2271 Naimark A, Brodovsky DM, Cherniack RM. Am J Med 1960; 28: 368–75.

2272 Naimark A, Cherniack RM. J Appl Physiol 1960; 15: 377–82.

2273 Nakamura F, Uyeda Y, Sonada Y. Laryngoscope 1958; 68: 109–19.

2274 Nakano KK, Bass H, Tyler HR. Arch Intern Med 1972; 130: 346–8.

2275 Nakano KK, Bass H, Tyler HR, Carmel RJ. Dis Nerv Syst 1976; 57: 32–5.

2276 Nakayama K. Dis Chest 1961; 40: 595–604.

2277 Namba T, Brown SB, Grob D. Pediatrics 1970; 45: 488–504.

2278 Nash CL, Nevins K. J Bone Joint Surg 1974; 56A: 440.

2279 Nathan PW. J Neurol Neurosurg Psychiat 1963; 26: 487–99.

2280 Nathan PW, Sears TA. J Neurol Neurosurg Psychiatr 1960; 23: 10–22.

2281 Nattie EE, Bartlett D Jnr, Rozycki AA. Am Rev Respir Dis 1975; 112: 259–66.

2282 Nattie EE, Doble EA. Respir Physiol 1984; 56: 253–9.

2283 Naughton J, Block R, Welch M. Am Rev Respir Dis 1971; 103: 557–65.

2284 Neil JF, Reynolds CF III, Spiker DG, Kupfer DJ. Br Med J 1980; 280: 19.

2285 Nelson DA, Ray CD. Arch Neurol 1968; 19: 199–207.

2286 Nemet G, Rosenblatt MB. Am Rev Tuberc 1937; 35: 713–29.

2287 Neu HC, Connolly JJ Jnr, Schwertley FW, Ladwig HA, Brody AW. Am Rev Respir Dis 1967; 95: 33–47.

2288 Neu HN, Ladwig HA. J Chronic Dis 1955; 1: 160–7.

2289 Neustadt JE, Levy RC, Spiegel IJ. J Am Med Assoc 1964; 187: 616–7.

2290 Newball HH, Menkes HA, Permutt S, Ball WC Jnr. Am Rev Respir Dis 1976; 114: 639–45.

2291 Newman JH, Neff TA, Ziporin P. N Engl J Med 1977; 296: 1101–3.

2292 Newman PP, Wolstencroft JH. J Neurophysiol 1959; 22: 516–23.

2293 Newman W, Feltman JA, Devlin B. Am J Med 1951; 11: 706–14.

2294 Newsom Davis J. In: Howell JBL and Campbell EJM, eds. Breathlessness. Oxford: Blackwell Scientific Publications, 1966: 73–82.

2295 Newsom Davis J. J Neurol Neurosurg Psychiatr 1967; 30: 420–6.

2296 Newsom Davis J. Brain 1970; 93: 851–72.

2297 Newsom Davis J. Bull Eur Physiopath Respir 1975; 11: 111–3P.

2298 Newsom Davis J. Am Rev Respir Dis 1979; 119 Suppl: 115–7.

2299 Newsom Davis J. Br Med Bull 1980; 36; 135–8.

2300 Newsom Davis J, Loh L, Casson M. INSERM, Duron B, ed. 1976; 59: 199–202.

2301 Newsom Davis J, Plum F. Exp Pathol 1972; 34: 78–94.

2302 Newsom Davis J, Stagg D. J Physiol 1975; 245: 481–98.

2303 Newsum JK, Smith RM, Crocker D. J Am Med Assoc 1979; 242: 1650–1.

2304 Newton DAG, Bone I. Br J Dis Chest 1979; 73: 399–404.

2305 Newton–John H. Med J Aust 1985; 142: 444–5.

2306 Nicholas JJ, Gilbert R, Gabe R, Auchincloss JH Jnr. Am Rev Respir Dis 1970; 102: 1–9.

2307 Nickel VL, Perry J, Affeldt JE, Dail CW. J Bone Joint Surg 1957; 39A: 989–1001.

2308 Nickerson BG, Keens TG. J Appl Physiol 1982; 52: 768–72.

2309 Nickerson JF, Hill SR Jnr, McNeil JH, Barker SB. Ann Intern Med 1960; 53: 475–93.

2310 Nielsen EM. Ugeskr Laeger 1946; 48: 1341–8.

2311 Nielsen M, Smith H. Acta Physiol Scand 1952; 24: 293–313.

2312 Nightingale S, Bateman DE, Ellis DA, Bates D, Hudgson P, Gibson GJ. Lancet 1982; 1: 933–5.

2313 Nilsonne U, Lundgren K–D. Acta Orthop Scand 1968; 59: 456–65.

2314 Nilsson DE. Am J Obst Gynecol 1953; 65: 1334–7.

2315 Nilsson S, Staff PH, Pruett EDR. Scand J Rehabil Med 1975; 7: 51–6.

2316 Nisbet HIA, Lamarre A, Levison H, Relton JES, Hall JE. J Bone Joint Surg 1973; 55A: 1721–5.

2317 Nishino T, Yonezawa T, Honda Y. Am Rev Respir Dis 1985; 132: 1219–22.

2318 Noble MIM, Eisele JH, Frankel HL, Else W, Guz A. Clin Sci 1971; 41: 275–83.

2319 Noble–Jamieson CM, Heckmatt JZ, Dubowitz V, Silverman N. Arch Dis Child 1986; 61: 178–81.

2320 Nochomovitz ML, Cherniack NS, eds. Noninvasive Respiratory Monitoring. New York: Churchill Livingstone, 1986.

2321 Nochomovitz ML, diMarco AF, Mortimer JT, Cherniack NS. Am Rev Respir Dis 1982; 125: Suppl 209.

2322 Nochomovitz ML, Goldman M, Mitra J, Cherniack NS. J Appl Physiol 1981; 51: 1150–6.

2323 Nochomovitz ML, Hopkins M, Brodkey J, Montenegro H, Mortimer JT, Cherniack NS. Am Rev Respir Dis 1984; 130: 685–8.

2324 Nocturnal Oxygen Therapy Trial Group. Ann Intern Med 1980; 93: 391–8.

2325 Noda S, Umezaki H. Arch Neurol 1982; 39: 132.

2326 Noerhen TH, Klauber MR. Chest 1978; 73: 782–3.

2327 Nogueras A, Sobrepere G, Aguilar M, Ripoli E. Med Clin 1985; 84: 333–4.

2328 Nogues MA, Newman PK, Male VJ, Foster JB. Brain 1982; 105: 835–49.

2329 Noonan JA. Circulation 1965; 32: Suppl 2: 164.

2330 Nordgren RE, Markesbery WR, Fukuda K, Reeves AG. Neurology 1971; 21: 1140–8.

2331 Nordqvist P, Dhuner K–G, Stenberg K, Orndahl G. Acta Med Scand 1960; 166: 189–94.

2332 Norio R, Kaaviainen H, Rapola J, Herva R, Kekomaki M. Am J Med Gen 1984; 17: 471–83.

2333 North JB, Jennett S. Arch Neurol 1974; 31: 338–44.

2334 Norton PG, Dunn EV. Br Med J 1985; 291: 630–2.

2335 Nowak TV, Ionasescu V, Anuras S. Gastroenterology 1982; 82: 800–10.

2336 Nugent CA, Harris HW, Cohn J, Smith CC, Tyler FH. Am Rev Tuberc Pulm Dis 1958; 78: 682–91.

2337 Nunn JF. Applied Respiratory Physiology, 2nd ed. London: Butterworths, 1977.

2338 Nunn JF. J R Soc Med 1985; 78: 983–4.

2339 Nunn JF, Milledge JS, Singaraya J. Br Med J 1979; 1: 1525–7.

2340 Nyquist RH. Calif Med 1965; 103: 417–9.

2341 Oakes DD, Wilmot CB, Halverson D, Hamilton RD. Ann Thorac Surg 1980; 30: 118–21.

2342 Obenour WH, Stevens PM, Cohen AA, McCutchen JJ. Am Rev Respir Dis 1972; 105: 382–7.

2343 Oberklaid F, Danks DM, Mayne V, Campbell P. Arch Dis Childh 1977; 52: 758–65.

2344 Oberklaid F, Hopkins IJ. Arch Dis Childh 1976; 51: 719–21.

2345 O'Brien JP. Clin Orthop Rel Res 1977; 128: 56–64.

2346 O'Brien T, Harper PS, Newcombe RG. Clin Genet 1983; 23: 422–6.

2347 Ochsner A, DeBakey M. J Thorac Surg 1939; 8: 469–511.

2348 Oda T, Glenn WWL, Fukuda Y, Hogan JF, Gorfien J. J Surg Res 1981; 30: 142–53.

2349 O'Donohue WJ Jnr. Chest 1985; 87: 76–80.

2350 O'Donohue WJ Jnr, Baker JP, Bell GM, Muren O, Parker CL, Patterson JL Jnr. J Am Med Assoc 1976; 235: 733–5.

2351 O'Donohue WJ Jnr, Giovannoni RM, Goldberg AI, et al. Chest 1986; 90: 1–37S.

2352 Ogle WS, French LA, Peyton WT. J Neurosurg 1956; 13: 81–7.

2353 Ohresser P, Autran P, Leonardeli M, Fogliani JJ, Charpin J. Poumon Coeur 1970; 26: 165–82.

2354 Ohry A, Molho M, Rozin R. Paraplegia 1975; 13: 101–8.

2355 Ohta K. Bull Chest Dis Res Inst Kyoto Univ 1979; 12: 62–74.

2356 Olafson RA, Mulder DW, Howard FM Jnr. Mayo Clin Proc 1964; 39: 131–44.

2357 O'Leary J, King R, Leblanc M, Moss R, Liebhaber M, Lewiston N. J Pediatr 1979; 94: 419–21.

2358 Olgiati R, Jacquet J, Prampero PE di. Am Rev Respir Dis 1986; 134: 1005–10.

2359 Olgiati R, Levine D, Smith JP, Briscoe WA, King TKC. Am Rev Respir Dis 1982; 126: 229–34.

2360 Oliva PB, Williams MH, Park SS. Am Rev Respir Dis 1967; 96: 805–11.

2361 Oliven A, Kelsen SG, Deal EC, Cherniack NS. J Clin Invest 1983; 71: 1442–9.

2362 Oliver LC. Parkinson's disease and its surgical treatment. London: HK Lewis and Co Ltd, 1953.

2363 Olsen CR. Am Rev Respir Dis 1962; 86: 37–40.

2364 Olsen KD, Kern EB, O'Connell EJ. Laryngoscope 1980; 90: 832–7.

2365 Olsen KD, Kern EB, Westbrook PR. Otolaryngol – Head Neck Surg 1981; 89: 804–10.

2366 Olsen KD, Suh KW, Staats BA. Otolaryngol – Head Neck Surg 1981; 89: 726–31.

2367 Olson LG, Strohl KP. Am Rev Respir Dis 1987; 135: 356–9.

2368 Onal E, Leech JA, Lopata M. Chest 1985; 87: 437–41.

2369 Onal E, Lopata M. Am Rev Respir Dis 1982; 126: 676–80.

2370 Onal E, Lopata M, O'Connor T. Am Rev Respir Dis 1982; 125: 167–74.

2371 Onal E, Lopata M, O'Connor TD. Am Rev Respir Dis 1981; 124: 215–7.

2372 Onal E, Lopata M, O'Connor TD. J Appl Physiol 1981; 50: 1052–5.

2373 Opie LH, Smith AC, Spalding JMK. J Physiol 1959; 149: 494–9.

2374 Orem J, Netick A, Dement WC. Electroencephalogr Clin Neurophysiol 1977; 43: 14–22.

2375 Orem J, Norris B, Lydic R. Chest 1978; 73: 300–1.

2376 Oren J, Newth CJL, Hunt CE, Brouillette RT, Bachand RT, Shannon DC. Am Rev Respir Dis 1986; 134: 917–9.

2377 Orenstein DM, Boat TF, Owens RP, et al. J Pediatr 1980; 97: 765–7.

2378 Orlowski JP, Lonsdale D, Nodar RH, Williams GW. Clin Electroencephalogr 1982; 13: 226–32.

2379 Orr WC, Imes NK, Martin RJ. Arch Intern Med 1979; 139: 109–11.

2380 Orr WC, Imes NK, Martin RJ, Rogers RM. Clin Res 1978; 26: 38A.

2381 Orr WC, Males JL, Imes NK. Am J Med 1981; 70: 1061–6.

2382 Orr WC, Martin RJ. Arch Intern Med 1981; 141: 990–2.

2383 Orr WC, Martin RJ, Imes NK, Rogers RM, Stahl ML. Chest 1979; 75: 418–22.

2384 Orr WC. Chest 1986; 89: 1–2.

2385 Orzalesi MM, Cook CD. J Pediatr 1965; 66: 898–900.

2386 Osler W. The Principles and Practice of Medicine. 6th ed. London: Appleton, 1907: 431.

2387 Osserman KE, Genkins G. Mt Sinai J Med NY 1971; 38: 497–537.

2388 Osterholm JL, Hooker T, Pyneson J. J Neurosurg 1968; 28: 298–304.

2389 Osterholm JL, Lemmon WM, Hooker TB, Pyneson J. Surg Forum 1966; 17: 421–3.

2390 Otis AB, Fenn WO, Rahn H. J Appl Physiol 1950; 2: 592–607.

2391 (a) Otis AB, Guyatt AR. Respir Physiol 1968; 5: 118–29.
(b) Overholt EL, Richert JH, Gilliland PF. Dis Chest 1967; 52: 553–7.

2392 Owange–Iraka JW, Harrison A, Warner JO. Eur J Pediatr 1984; 142: 198–200.

2393 Owens GR, Fino GJ, Herbert DL, et al. Chest 1983; 84: 546–50.

2394 Owens GR, Follansbee WP. Chest 1987; 91: 118–27.

2395 (a) Page MM, Watkins PJ. Lancet 1978; 1: 14–16.
(b) Paine CJ, Hargrove MD Jnr. Chest 1973; 63: 854–5.

2396 Palmer ED. J Am Med Assoc 1974; 229: 1349.

2397 Palmer ED. Gastroenterology 1976; 71: 510–9.

2398 Papasozomenos S, Roessmann U. Neurology 1981; 31: 97–100.

2399 Papatestas AE, Alpert LI, Osserman KE, Osserman RS, Kark AE. Am J Med 1971; 50: 465–74.

2400 Paramelle B, Parent B, Rigaud D, Dimitriou R, Hohn B. Rev Fr Mal Respir 1979; 7: 413–5.

2401 Pardy RL, Bye PJP. J Appl Physiol 1985; 58: 738–42.

2402 Pardy RL, Rivington RN, Despas PJ, Macklem PT. Am Rev Respir Dis 1981; 123: 426–33.

2403 Pardy RL, Rivington RN, Despas PJ, Macklem PT. Am Rev Respir Dis 1981; 123: 421–5.

2404 Pare P, Lowenstein L. Blood 1956; 11: 1077–84.

2405 Parent B, Paramelle B, Dimitriou R, Brambilla C, Wolf JE. Rev Fr Mal Resp 1979; 7: 356–8.

2406 (a) Parhad IM, Clark AW, Barron KD, Staunton SB. Neurology 1978; 28: 18–22.
(b) Parisi RA, Croce SA, Edelman NH, Santiago TV. Chest 1987; 91: 922–4.

2407 Parisi RA, Neubauer JA, Frank MM, Edelman NH, Santiago TV. Am Rev Respir Dis 1987; 135: 378–82.

2408 Parker GW, Ramos ED. J Am Med Assoc 1962; 180: 408–10.

2409 Parkes JD. Sleep and its Disorders. Eastbourne: WB Saunders, 1985.

2410 Parkin A, Robinson PJ, Hickling P. Br J Radiol 1982; 55: 833–6.

2411 Passerini L, Cosio MG, Newman SL. Am Rev Respir Dis 1985; 132: 1366–7.

2412 Pasteur W. Am J Med Sci 1890; 100: 242–57.

2413 Patel C, Miller SM, Chalon J, Turndorf H. Bull NY Acad Med 1978; 54: 924–30.

2414 Paterson IS. Br J Anaesth 1962; 34: 340–2.

2415 Pather M, Hariparsad D, Wesley AG. Intensive Care Med 1985; 11: 30–2.

2416 Patterson JL, Heyman A, Duke TW. Am J Med 1952; 12; 382–7.

2417 Patterson JL Jnr, Heyman A, Battey LL, Ferguson RW. J Clin Invest 1955; 34: 1857–64.

2418 Patton TJ, Thawley SE, Vandermeer PJ, Waters RC, Ogura JH. Laryngoscope 1983; 93: 1387–96.

2419 Patton WE, Abelmann WH, Frank R, Badger TL, Gaensler EA. Am Rev Tuberc 1953; 67: 755–78.

2420 Patton WE, Watson TR Jnr, Gaensler EA. Surg Gynecol Obstet 1952; 95: 470–96.

2421 Paul GR, Appenzeller O. Dis Chest 1962; 42: 558–62.

2422 Paul KS, Lye RH, Strang FA, Dutton J. J Neurosurg 1983; 58: 183–7.

2423 Paul RW. Proc R Soc Med 1934; 28: 436–8.

2424 Paulson GD, Tafrate RH. Neurology 1970; 20: Suppl 14–17.

2425 Payne CA, Greenfield JC. Am Heart J 1963; 65: 436–40.

2426 Pearn JH, Gardner–Medwin D, Wilson J. J Neurol Sci 1978; 38: 23–37.

2427 Pearn JH, Wilson J. Arch Dis Childh 1973; 48: 425–30.

2428 Pecak F, Trontelj JV, Dimitrijevic MR. Int Orthop 1980; 3: 323–8.

2429 Pecorelli F, Grassi V, Ferrini L, Todisco T. Ital J Orthop Traumatol 1983; 9: 75–89.

2430 Peet MM, Kahn EA, Allen SS. J Am Med Assoc 1933; 100: 488–9.

2431 Peled R, Pratt H, Scharf B, Lavie P. Neurology (Cleveland) 1983; 33: 419–23.

2432 Peltier LF. J Appl Physiol 1953; 5: 614–8.

2433 Pena A, Perez L, Nurko S, Dorenbaum D. Am Surg 1981; 47: 215–8.

2434 Penfield W. Proc Assoc Res Nerv Dis 1943; 23: 416–33.

2435 Penfield W, Boldrey E. Brain 1937; 60: 389–443.

2436 Pengelly LD, Alderson AM, Milic–Emili J. J Appl Physiol 1971; 30: 797–805.

2437 Penner A, Druckerman LJ. Am J Dig Dis 1942; 9: 282–7.

2438 Pentland B, Fox K. J Neurol Neurosurg Psychiatr 1983; 46: 1138–42.

2439 Perez–Trullen A, Marin JM, Larraga R, Herrero I, Pasamar JA. Bull Eur Physiopath Respir 1986; 20: 32s.

2440 Perks WH, Cooper RA, Bradbury S, et al. Thorax 1980; 35: 81–5.

2441 Perks WH, Horrocks PM, Cooper RA, et al. Br Med J 1980; 280: 894–7.

2442 Perloff JK, de Leon AC Jnr, O'Doherty D. Circulation 1966; 33: 625–48.

2443 Perloff JK, Stevenson WG, Roberts NK, Cabeen W, Weiss J. Am J Cardiol 1984; 54: 1074–81.

2444 Perry TL, Bratty PJA, Hansen S, Kennedy J, Urquhart N, Dolman CL. Arch Neurol 1975; 32: 108–13.

2445 Peters RM, Roos A, Black H, Burford TH, Graham EA. J Thorac Surg 1950; 20: 484–93.

2446 Peterson RJ, Young WG Jnr, Godwin JD, Sabiston DC Jnr, Jones RH. J Thorac Cardiovasc Surg 1985; 90: 251–60.

2447 Peterson RL, Ward RC. Arch Otolaryngol 1948; 48: 156–8.

2448 Petheram IS, Branthwaite MA. Anaesthesia 1980; 35: 467–73.

2449 Petit JM, Delhez L. Arch Int Physiol 1961; 69: 413–7.

2450 Petit JM, Milic–Emili G, Delhez L. J Appl Physiol 1960; 15: 1101–6.

2451 Petren K, Sjovall E. Acta Med Scand 1926; 64: 260–91.

2452 Pettay O, Makisara P, Runeberg B. Acta Med Scand 1965; 177: 257–62.

2453 Petty TL, Filley GF, Mitchell RS. Am Rev Respir Dis 1961; 84: 572–8.

2454 Petty TL, Nett LM, Finigan MM, Brink GA, Corsello PR. Ann Intern Med 1969; 70: 1109–20.

2455 Phelan JP, Dainer MJ, Cowherd DW. South J Med 1978; 71:

2456 Phemister JC, Small JM. J Neurol Neurosurg Psychiatr 1961; 24: 173–5.

2457 Phillips BA, Okeson J, Paesani D, Gilmore R. Chest 1986; 90: 424–9.

2458 Phillips JR, Eldridge FL. N Engl J Med 1973; 289: 1390–5.

2459 Phillips MS, Kinnear WJM, Shaw D, Moore NR, Shneerson JM. Unpublished observations.

2460 Phillips MS, Kinnear WJM, Shneerson JM. Thorax 1986; 41: 719.

2461 Phillips MS, Kinnear WJM, Shneerson JM. Thorax 1987; 42: 445–51.

2462 Phillips MS, Miller MR, Kinnear WJM, Gough SE, Shneerson JM. Thorax 1987; 42: 348–52.

2463 Phillips MS, Moore NR, Kinnear WJM, Shneerson JM. Unpublished observations.

2464 Phillips MS, Stewart S, Anderson JR. J Neurol Neurosurg Psychiatr 1984; 47: 492–5.

2465 Phillips YY, Joyner LR. Am Rev Respir Dis 1978; 117: Suppl 165.

2466 Phillipson EA. Am Rev Respir Dis 1978; 118: 909–39.

2467 Phillipson EA. Am Rev Respir Dis 1980; 121: 781–2.

2468 Phillipson EA, Bowes G, Sullivan CE, Woolf GM. Sleep 1980; 3: 281–8.

2469 Phillipson EA, Sullivan CE. Am Rev Respir Dis 1978; 118; 807–9.

2470 Phipps RJ, Richardson PS. J Physiol 1976; 261: 563–81.

2471 PHLS. Communicable Disease Surveillance Centre. Br Med J 1985; 291: 41–2.

2472 Pianetto MB, Harris HA, Sweet HC. Am Rev Respir Dis 1967; 95: 189–99.

2473 Pichlmayr I, Lehmkuhl P, Pichlmayr R. Anasth Intens Notfallmed 1984; 19: 14–18.

2474 Pichurko B, McCool FD, Scanlon P, et al. Am Rev Respir Dis 1985; 131: A337.

2475 Piehler JM, Pairolero PC, Gracey DR, Bernatz PE. J Thorac Cardiovasc Surg 1982; 84: 861–4.

2476 Pierce AK, Paez PN, Miller WF. Am Rev Respir Dis 1965; 91: 653–9.

2477 Pierce JW, Creamer B, MacDermot GV. Gut 1965; 6: 392–5.

2478 Pilapil VR, Day LH, Watson DG. Surg Forum 1967; 18: 493–5.

2479 Pilsbury D, Hibbert G. Bull Eur Physiopath Respir 1987; 23: 9–13.

2480 Pinals RS, Gould LV. Arch Phys Med Rehabil 1979; 60: 133–5.

2481 Pinkerton HH. Br J Anaesthesia 1957; 29: 421–4.

2482 Pinner M, Leiner G, Zavod WA. J Thorac Surg 1942; 11: 241–65.

2483 Pitt B, Alkalay I, Sweet R, Stein M. Arch Intern Med 1965; 115: 714–7.

2484 Pitts RF. J Comp Neurol 1940; 72: 605–25.

2485 Planas RF, McBrayer RH, Koen PA. J Appl Physiol 1985; 59: 269–73.

2486 Plasse HM, Lieberman AN. Arch Otolaryngol 1981; 107: 252–3.

2487 Pleasure DE, Lovelace RE, Duvoisin RC. Neurology 1968; 18: 1143–8.

2488 Plowman PN, Stableforth DE. Proc R Soc Med 1977; 70: 738–40.

2489 Plum F. Arch Neurol 1960; 3: 484–7.

2490 Plum F. In: Howell JBL, and Campbell EJM, eds. Breathlessness. Oxford: Blackwell Scientific Publications, 1966: 203–20.

2491 Plum F. In: Porter R, ed. Breathing: Hering–Breuer Centenary Symposium. Churchill: London, 1970: 159–81.

2492 Plum F, Alvord EC Jnr. Arch Neurol 1964; 10: 101–12.

2493 Plum F, Brown HW. J Appl Physiol 1963; 18: 1139–45.

2494 Plum F, Brown HW. Ann NY Acad Sci 1963; 109: 915–31.

2495 Plum F, Brown HW, Snoep E. J Am Med Assoc 1962; 181: 1050–5.

2496 Plum F, Leigh RJ. In: Hornbein TF, ed. Regulation of Breathing. Part 2. New York: Marcel Dekker, 1981: 989–1067.

2497 Plum F, Lukas DS. Am J Med Sci 1951; 221: 417–24.

2498 Plum F, Posner JB. The Diagnosis of Stupor and Coma, 3rd ed. Philadelphia: F and J Davis Co., 1980.

2499 Plum F, Swanson AG. Arch Neurol Psychiatr 1958; 80: 267–85.

2500 Plum F, Swanson AG. Arch Neurol Psychiatr 1959; 81: 535–49.

2501 Plum F, Whedon GD. N Engl J Med 1951; 245: 235–41.

2502 Plum F, Wolff HG. J Am Med Assoc 1951; 146: 442–6.

2503 Pluto LA, Fahey PJ, Sorensen L, Chandrasekhar AJ. Am Rev Respir Dis 1985; 131: A64.

2504 Poe RH, Reisman JL, Rodenhouse TG. J Trauma 1978; 18: 71–3.

2505 Poewe W, Willeit H, Sluga E, Mayr U. J Neurol Neurosurg Psychiatr 1985; 48: 887–93.

2506 Poitras B, Rosenthal A, Hall JE. J Pediatr 1975; 86: 476–7.

2507 Polatty RC, Cooper KR. Southern Med J 1986; 79: 897–9.

2508 Polgar G, Koop CE. Pediatrics 1963; 32: 209–15.

2509 Pollard JD, Selby G. J Neurol Sci 1978; 37: 113–25.

2510 Pollock LJ. Arch Intern Med 1912; 9: 406–8.

2511 Polnitsky CA, Sherter CB, Sugar JO. Arch Otolaryngol 1981; 107: 629–30.

2512 Poloni M, Mento SA, Mascherpa C, Ceroni M. Ital J Neurol Sci 1983; 4: 39–46.

2513 Polu JM, Desmeules M, Sadoul P. Rev Tuberc Pneumolog 1972; 36: 1105–20.

2514 Pontoppidan H. Am Rev Respir Dis 1980; 122: Suppl 109–19.

2515 Pontoppidan H, Geffin B, Lowenstein E. N Engl J Med 1972; 287: 743–52.

2516 Pontoppidan H, Geffin B, Lowenstein E. N Engl J Med 1972; 287: 799–806.

2517 Pontoppidan H, Laver MB, Geffin B. Adv Surg 1970; 4: 163–254.

2518 Pool JL, Ransohoff J. J Neurophysiol 1949; 12: 385–92.

2519 Poppel MA, Jacobson HG, Shapiro JH, Adler H, Stern J. Am J Dig Dis 1956; 1: 116–25.

2520 Poppius H, Varpela E, Korhonen O. Scand J Respir Dis 1969; 50: 68–75.

2521 Porter WT. J Physiol 1895; 17: 455–85.

2522 Poulton EP. Lancet 1936; 2: 981–3.

2523 Pourriat JL, Lamberto C, Hoang BH, Fournier JL, Vasseur B. Chest 1986; 90: 703–7.

2524 Powell N, Guilleminault C, Riley R, Smith L. Bull Eur Physiopath Respir 1983; 19: 607–10.

2525 Power WR, Mosko SS, Sassin JF. Neurology 1982; 32: 763–6.

2526 Powers SR Jnr, Himmelstein A. J Thorac Surg 1951; 22: 45–51.

2527 Powner DJ, Hoffman LG. Chest 1978; 74: 469–71.

2528 Priest RE, Boies LR, Goltz NF. Ann Otol Rhinol Laryngol 1947; 56: 250–63.

2529 Prime FJ. In: Zorab PA, ed. Proceedings of a Symposium on Scoliosis. London: National Fund for Research into Poliomyelitis and other Crippling Diseases, 1965: 57–60.

2530 Prime FJ. In: Zorab PA, ed. Scoliosis. Proceedings of a 5th Symposium. London: Academic Press, 1977: 329–38.

2531 Primiano FP Jnr, Nussbaum E, Hirschfield SS, et al. J Pediatr Orthop 1983; 3: 475–81.

2532 Prinzmetal M, Kountz WB. Medicine 1935; 14: 457–98.

2533 Proctor DF. Bull Hist Med 1974; 48: 352–76.

2534 Proctor DF. Eur J Respir Dis 1983; 64: Suppl 128, 89–96.

2535 Prowse CM, Gaensler EA. Anesthesiology 1965; 26: 381–92.

2536 Pruzanski W. Dis Chest 1962; 42: 608–10.

2537 Pruzanski W. Brain 1966; 89: 563–8.

2538 Pruzanski W, Profis A. Am Rev Respir Dis 1965; 91: 874–9.

2539 Pryor JA, Webber BA, Hodson ME, Batten JC. Br Med J 1979; 2: 417–8.

2540 Pryor WW. Circulation 1951; 4: 233–8.

2541 Purcell M. Arch Dis Childh 1976; 51: 602–7.

2542 Purdy A, Hahn A, Barnett HJM, et al. Ann Neurol 1979; 6: 523–31.

2543 Putnam JS, Kaufman LV, Michaels RM, Canter HG, Katz S. Chest 1973; 64: 137–40.

2544 Pye IF, Blandford RL. Postgrad Med J 1977; 53: 704–9.

2545 Quast U, Hennessen W, Widmark RM. Dev Biolog Stand 1979; 43: 25–32.

2546 Radecki LL, Tomatis LA. J Pediatr 1976; 88: 969–71.

2547 Raetzo MA, Junod AF, Kryger MH. Bull Eur Physiopath Respir 1987; 23: 171–5.

2548 Raff H, Shinsako J, Keil LC, Dallman MF. Am J Physiol 1983; 244: E453–8.

2549 Rahn H, Otis AB, Chadwick LE, Fenn WO. Am J Physiol 1946; 146: 161–78.

2550 Raininko R. Ann Clin Res 1986; 18: 93–8.

2551 Rajagopal KR, Abbrecht PH, Jabbari B. Chest 1986; 90: 815–21.

2552 Rajagopal KR, Abbrecht PH, McCumber TR, Hunt KK Jnr. Am Rev Respir Dis 1982; 125: 128.

2553 Rajagopal KR, Abbrecht PH, Zwillich CW. Am Rev Respir Dis 1984; 129: Suppl A247.

2554 Rajagopal KR, Bennett LL, Dillard TA, Tellis CJ, Tenholder MF. Chest 1986; 90: 172–6.

2555 Raman TK, Blake JA, Harris TM. Chest 1971; 60: 555–7.

2556 Ramirez AF, Aguirre AU, Ancira FP, Mata MR. Riv Invest Clin 1981; 33: 25–8.

2557 Ramsay ID. Lancet 1966; 2: 931–5.

2558 Ranson SW, Magoun HW. Arch Neurol Psychiatr 1933; 29: 1179–94.

2559 Raper AJ, Thompson WT Jnr, Shapiro W, Patterson JL Jnr. J Appl Physiol 1966; 21: 497–502.

2560 Rapoport DM, Garay SM, Epstein H, Goldring RM. Chest 1986; 89: 627–35.

2561 Rapoport DM, Garay SM, Goldring RM. Bull Eur Physiopath Respir 1983; 19: 616–20.

2562 Rapoport DM, Sorkin B, Garay SM, Goldring RM. N Engl J Med 1982; 307: 931–3.

2563 Rapoport S, Watkins PB. Ann Neurol 1984; 16: 359–61.

2564 Ratcheson RA, Wirth FP Jnr, Li C–L, Buren JM van. Acta Neurochir 1971; 24: 169–77.

2565 Rattenborg C. Acta Anaesth Scand 1961; 5: 129–40.

2566 Ratto O, Briscoe WA, Morton JW, Comroe JH. Am J Med 1955; 19: 958–65.

2567 Ravichandran G, Silver JR. Paraplegia 1982; 20: 264–9.

2568 Ravin M, Newmark Z, Savielle G. Anesth Analg 1975; 54: 216–8.

2569 Ravina A. Annee Ther 1962; 33: 111–3.

2570 Ravitch MM. Surgery 1951; 30: 178–94.

2571 Ravn H. Acta Neurol Scand 1967; 43: Suppl 30: 1–64.

2572 Rawlings MS. Am J Cardiol 1960; 5: 333–8.

2573 Rawlings MS. Dis Chest 1961; 39: 435–43.

2574 Ray CS, Sue DY, Bray G, Hansen JE, Wasserman K. Am Rev Respir Dis 1983; 128: 501–6.

2575 Razzi A, Rosso C, Durand P. Min Pediatr 1965; 17: 1823–7.

2576 Read D, Young A. Postgrad Med J 1983; 59: 520–1.

2577 Read DJC. Aust NZ J Med 1967; 16: 20–32.

2578 Rebuck AS, Campbell EJM. Am Rev Respir Dis 1974; 109: 345–50.

2579 Rebuck AS, Chapman KR, D'Urzo A. Chest 1983; 83: 860–4.

2580 Rebuck AS, Slutsky AS. In: Hornbein TF, ed. Regulation of Breathing. Part 2. New York: Marcel Dekker, 1981: 745–72.

2581 Rechavia E, Rotenberg Z, Fuchs J, Strasberg B. Chest 1985; 88: 309–11.

2582 Reckles LN, Peterson HA, Bianco AJ Jnr, Weidman WH. J Bone Joint Surg 1975; 57A: 449–55.

2583 Redgate ES. Am J Physiol 1960; 198: 1299–303.

2584 Redgate ES. Ann NY Acad Sci 1963; 109: 606–18.

2585 Rees PJ, Clark TJH. Lancet 1979; 2: 1315–7.

2586 Rees PJ, Prior JG, Cochrane GM, Clark TJH. J R Soc Med 1981; 74: 192–5.

2587 Reeve P, Harvey G, Seaton D. Br Med J 1985; 291: 331–2.

2588 Reeves WC, Griggs R, Nanda NC, Thomson K, Gramiak R. Arch Neurol 1980; 37: 273–7.

2589 Refsum HE. Clin Sci 1963; 25: 361–7.

2590 Reichel J. Clin Chest Med 1980; 1: 119–24.

2591 Reid L. In: Zorab PA, ed. Proceedings of a Symposium on Scoliosis. London: National Fund for Research into Poliomyelitis and other Crippling Diseases, 1965: 71–8.

2592 Reid WD. J Am Med Assoc 1930; 94: 483.

2593 Reis DJ, McHugh PR. Am J Physiol 1968; 214: 601–10.

2594 Remmers JE. Respir Physiol 1970; 10: 358–83.

2595 Remmers JE, Anch AM, deGroot WJ. Clin Chest Med 1980; 1: 57–71.

2596 Remmers JE, Anch AM, deGroot WJ, Baker JP Jnr, Sauerland EK. Sleep 1980; 3: 447–53.

2597 Remmers JE, deGroot WJ, Sauerland EK, Anch AM. J Appl Physiol 1978; 44: 931–8.

2598 Remmers JE, Sterling JA, Thorarinsson B, Kuna ST. Am Rev Respir Dis 1984; 130: 1152–5.

2599 Renshaw TS. J Am Med Assoc 1982; 248: 922–3.

2600 Renzetti AD Jnr, Nicholas W, Dutton RE Jnr, Jivoff L. N Engl J Med 1960; 262: 215–8.

2601 Report by the British Orthopaedic Association and the British Scoliosis Society. Br Med J 1983; 287: 963–4.

2602 Report of the Medical Research Council for the year 1956–57. Cmnd. 453. London: HMSO, 1958.

2603 Report of the Medical Research Council Working Party. Lancet 1981; 1: 681–6.

2604 Report of the Surgeon General's Workshop on Children with Handicaps and their Families. US Department of Health and Human Services. Public Health Service 1983.

2605 Reusch CS. Circulation 1961; 24: 1143–50.

2606 Reynolds CF III, Coble PA, Black RS, Holzer B, Carroll R, Kupfer DJ. J Am Geriatr Soc 1980; 28: 164–70.

2607 Reynolds CF III, Coble PA, Spiker DG, Neil JF, Holzer BC, Kupfer DJ. J Nerv Ment Dis 1982; 170: 565–7.

2608 Rice D. Otolaryngol Clin North Am 1986; 19: 135–40.

2609 Richards DGB, Whitfield AGW, Arnoff WM, Waterhouse JAH. Br Heart J 1953; 15: 83–6.

2610 Richards J, Chevalier V, Capelle R, Cavrot E, Content J, Delforge J. Arch Fra Ped 1957; 14: 563–98.

2611 Richardson RR, Johnson N, Cerullo LJ. Neurosurgery 1978; 3: 75–8.

2612 Richardson RR, Roseman B, Singh N. Neurosurg 1981; 9: 317–9.

2613 Richmond GH. J Appl Physiol 1949; 2: 16–23.

2614 Richter T, West JR, Fishman AP. N Engl J Med 1957; 256: 1165–70.

2615 Riddick MF, Winter RB, Lutter LD. Spine 1982; 7: 476–83.

2616 Rideau Y, Glorion B, Delaubier A, Tarle O, Bach J. Muscle Nerve 1984; 7: 281–6.

2617 Rideau Y, Jankowski LW, Grellet J. Muscle Nerve 1981; 4: 155–64.

2618 Ridyard JB, Steward RM. Thorax 1976; 31: 438–42.

2619 Ries AL, Farrow JT, Clausen JL. Am Rev Respir Dis 1985; 132: 685–9.

2620 Ries AL, Moser KM. Chest 1986; 90: 285–90.

2621 Rigatto M, Medeiros NP de. Am J Med 1962; 32: 103–9.

2622 Rigaud D, Dubois F, Godart J, Paramelle B. Am Rev Respir Dis 1981; 123: Suppl 112.

2623 Riley CM. Adv Pediatr 1957; 9: 157–90.

2624 Riley CM, Moore RH. Pediatrics 1966; 37: 435–46.

2625 Riley DA, Berger AJ. Exp Neurol 1979; 66: 636–49.

2626 Riley DJ, Santiago TV, Daniele RP, Schall B, Edelman NH. Am J Med 1977; 63: 459–66.

2627 Riley EA. Am J Med 1962; 32: 404–16.

2628 Riley R, Guilleminault C, Herran J, Powell N. Sleep 1983; 6: 303–11.

2629 Riley R, Guilleminault C, Powell N, Derman S. Sleep 1984; 7: 79–82.

2630 Riley RL. Ann Intern Med 1954; 41: 172–6.

2631 Ringqvist I, Ringqvist T. Acta Med Scand 1971; 190: 499–508.

2632 Ringqvist I, Ringqvist T. Acta Med Scand 1971; 190: 509–18.

2633 Ringqvist T. Scand J Clin Lab Invest 1966; 18: Suppl 88, 1–179.

2634 Rinow ME, Saltzman AR. Chest 1986; 90: 204–8.

2635 Riordan JF, Sillett RW, McNichol MW. Br J Dis Chest 1975; 69: 57–62.

2636 Riseborough EJ. Isr J Med Sci 1973; 9: 787–90.

2637 Ritzmann LW, Morris JF, Bristow JD, Pitcairn DE, Griswold HE. Circulation 1963; 28: 790.

2638 Rivlin J, Hoffstein V, Kalbfleisch J, McNicholas W, Zamel N, Bryan AC. Am Rev Respir Dis 1984; 129: 355–60.

2639 Rivlin J, McNicholas WT, Kalbfleisch J, Zamel N, Hoffstein V, Bryan AC. Physiologist 1982; 25: 211.

2640 Rizvi SS, Ishikawa S, Faling LJ, Schlessinger L, Satia J, Seckel B. Am J Med 1974; 56: 433–6.

2641 Roa NL, Moss KS. Anesthesiol 1984; 60: 71–3.

2642 Roaf R. J Bone Joint Surg 1966; 48B: 786–92.

2643 Robert D, Chemorin B, Gerard M, et al. Rev Fr Mal Resp 1979; 7: 408–12.

2644 Robert D, Fournier G, Thomas L, Gerard M, Chemorin B, Bertoye A. Rev Fr Mal Resp 1979; 7: 353–5.

2645 Robert D, Gerard M, Leger L, Salamand J, Gaussorgues P, Buffat J. Agressologie 1985; 26: 753–5.

2646 Robert D, Gerard M, Leger P, et al. Chest 1982; 82: 258–9.

2647 Robert D, Gerard M, Leger P, et al. Rev Fr Mal Resp 1983; 11: 923–36.

2648 Robert D, Gerard M, Leger P, Salamand J, Buffat J. Am Rev Respir Dis 1985; 131: Suppl A100.

2649 Robert D, Leger P, Gerard M, Fournier G, Bertoye A. Am Rev Respir Dis 1980; 121: Suppl 183.

2650 Robert D, Salamand J, Chemorin B, et al. Rev Fr Mal Resp 1979; 7: 377–80.

2651 Roberts DF, Bradley WG. J Med Genet 1977; 14: 16–19.

2652 Robertson CH Jnr, Foster GH, Johnson RL Jnr. J Clin Invest 1977; 59: 31–42.

2653 Robertson CH Jnr, Pagel MA, Johnson RL Jnr. J Clin Invest 1977; 59: 43–50.

2654 Robertson HF, Varmus F. Milit Surg 1944; 95: 129–32.

2655 Robicsek F, Sanger PW, Taylor FH, Thomas MJ. J Thorac Cardiovasc Surg 1963; 45: 691–701.

2656 Robin ED. N Engl J Med 1963; 268: 917–22.

2657 Robin ED, Abuabara F, Myers C, et al. West J Med 1979; 130: 522–30.

2658 Robin ED, Crump CH, Wagman RJ. N Engl J Med 1960; 262: 758–61.

2659 Robin ED, Whaley RD, Crump CH, Travis DM. J Clin Invest 1958; 37: 981–9.

2660 Robin GC. Isr J Med Sci 1976; 13: 203–6.

2661 Robin GC, Brief LP. J Bone Joint Surg 1971; 53A: 466–76.

2662 Robin IG. Proc R Soc Med 1968; 61: 575–82.

2663 Robinson PK, Mosberg WH Jnr, Lowe RCW. J Neurol Neurosurg Psychiatr 1950; 13: 296–306.

2664 Robinson RW, White DP, Zwillich CW. Am Rev Respir Dis 1985; 132: 1238–41.

2665 Robinson RW, Zwillich CW. Clin Chest Med 1985; 6: 603–14.

2666 Robinson RW, Zwillich CW, Bixler EO, Cadieux RJ, Kales A, White DP. Chest 1987; 91: 197–203.

2667 Robotham JL. Crit Care Med 1979; 7: 563–6.

2668 Robotham JL, Chipps BE, Shermeta DW. Anesthesiology 1980; 52: 167–70.

2669 Robotham JL, Scharf SM. Clin Chest Med 1983; 4: 161–87.

2670 Rochester DF. Am J Med 1974; 57: 402–20.

2671 Rochester DF. Am J Med 1980; 68: 803–5.

2672 Rochester DF. N Engl J Med 1981; 305: 278–9.

2673 Rochester DF. Am Rev Respir Dis 1986; 134: 646–8.

2674 Rochester DF. Clin Chest Med 1986; 7: 91–9.

2675 Rochester DF, Arora NS. Med Clin North Am 1983; 67: 573–97.

2676 Rochester DF, Arora NS, Braun NMT, Goldberg SK. Bull Eur Physiopath Respir 1979; 15: 951–75.

2677 Rochester DF, Bettini G. J Clin Invest 1976; 57: 661–72.

2678 Rochester DF, Braun NMT. Am Rev Respir Dis 1979; 119: Suppl 77–80.

2679 Rochester DF, Braun NMT. Am Rev Respir Dis 1985; 132: 42–7.

2680 Rochester DF, Braun NMT, Laine S. Am J Med 1977; 63: 223–32.

2681 Rochester DF, Goldberg SK. Am Rev Respir Dis 1980; 122: Suppl 133–46.

2682 Rochester DF, Pradel-Guena M. J Appl Physiol 1973; 34: 68–74.

2683 Rockwell GH, Greene NM. Clin Pharmacol Ther 1963; 4: 728–33.

2684 Rodenstein DO, Cuttita G, Hoeven C, Stanescu DC. Bull Europ Physiopath Resp 1986; 20: 53s.

2685 Rodenstein DO, Stanescu DC. Am Rev Respir Dis 1986; 134: 311–25.

2686 Rodgers RS, Ellwood PM, Ratelle AE. J Urol 1956; 76: 447–52.

2687 Rodman T, Close HP. Am J Med 1959; 26: 808–17.

2688 Rodman T, Fennelly JF, Kraft AJ, Close HP. N Engl J Med 1962; 267: 1279–85.

2689 Rodman T, Resnick ME, Berkowitz RD, Fennelly JF, Oliva J. Am J Med 1962; 32: 208–17.

2690 Rodrigues JF, York EL, Nair CPV. Chest 1984; 86: 147–8.

2691 Rodriguez J, Weissman C, Askanazi J, Damask MC, Milic–Emili J, Kinney JM. Anesthesiology 1982; 57: A119.

2692 Roehrs T, Conway W, Wittig R, Zorick F, Sicklesteel J, Roth T. Am Rev Respir Dis 1985; 132: 520–3.

2693 Roesler H. Am J Roentgenol Radium Ther 1934; 32: 464–86.

2694 Rogan MC, Needham CD, McDonald I. Ann Rheum Dis 1955; 14: 452.

2695 Rogan MC, Needham CD, McDonald I. Clin Sci 1955; 14: 91–6.

2696 Rohatgi N, Fields A, Sly RM. Ann Allergy 1980; 45: 177–9.

2697 Rojewski TE, Schuller DE, Clark RW, Schmidt HS, Potts RE. Laryngoscope 1982; 92: 246–50.

2698 Roland LP, Hoefer PFA, Aranow H Jnr, Merritt HH. Neurology 1956; 6: 307–26.

2699 Rolbin SH, Levinson G, Shnider SM, Wright RG. Anesth Analg 1978; 57: 441–7.

2700 Rom WN, Miller A. Thorax 1978; 33: 106–10.

2701 Romanczuk BJ. Otolaryngology 1978; 86: 897–903.

2702 Romanul FCA, Meulen JP van der. Arch Neurol 1967; 17: 387–402.

2703 Romet TT, MacHattie CF, Crawford JS, Wright TA. Orthop Trans 1981; 5: 299.

2704 Rosenberg HS, Williams RL. Arch Dis Child 1975; 50: 667.

2705 Rosenblueth A, Alanis J, Pilar G. Arch Int Physiol Bioch 1961; 69: 19–25.

2706 Rosenow EC, Engel AG. Am J Med 1978; 64: 485–91.

2707 Rosenow EC III, Strimlan CV, Muhm JR, Ferguson RH. Mayo Clin Proc 1977; 52: 641–9.

2708 Rosenzweig MS, Huang MTC. NY State J Med 1982; 82: 1097–9.

2709 Rosomuff HL, Krieger AJ, Kuperman AS. J Neurosurg 1969; 31: 620–7.

2710 Ross BB, Gramiak R, Rahn H. J Appl Physiol 1955; 8: 264–8.

2711 Rossi GF, Brodal A. J Anat 1956; 90: 42–62.

2712 Rostand RA, Block AJ, Hunt LA, Boysen PG, Wynne JW. Chest 1978; 74: 349.

2713 Roth A, Rosenthal A, Hall JE, Mizel M. Clin Orthop Rel Res 1973; 93: 95–102.

2714 Rotherham EB, Safar P, Robin ED. J Am Med Assoc 1964; 189: 993–6.

2715 Rothstein E, Strzelczyk RPT. Ann Intern Med 1951; 34: 401–6.

2716 Roussos C. Lung 1982; 160: 59–84.

2717 Roussos C. Chest 1985; 88: Suppl 124S–32S.

2718 Roussos C, Fixley M, Gross D, Macklem PT. J Appl Physiol 1979; 46: 897–904.

2719 Roussos C, Macklem PT. N Engl J Med 1982; 307: 786–97.

2720 Roussos C, Macklem PT, eds. The Thorax, Vol 29 Part B. New York: Marcel Dekker, 1985.

2721 Roussos C, Macklem PT, eds. The Thorax, Vol 29, Part A. New York: Marcel Dekker, 1985.

2722 Roussos CS, Macklem PT. J Appl Physiol 1977; 43: 189–97.

2723 Rout MW, Lane DJ, Wollner L. Br Med J 1971; 3: 7–9.

2724 Rovner RN, Barron KD. Neurology 1966; 16: 328.

2725 Royal College of Physicians Report. J R Coll Physicians 1981; 15: 69–87.

2726 Rubin A–HE, Eliaschar I, Joachim Z, Alroy G, Lavie P. Bull Eur Physiopath Respir 1983; 19: 612–5.

2727 Rubin LA, Urowitz MB. J Rheumatol 1983; 10: 973–6.

2728 Rullan A. Arch Otolaryngol 1956; 64: 207–12.

2729 Rushton WAH. J Physiol 1927; 63: 357–77.

2730 Russell DC, Maloney A, Muir AL. Thorax 1981; 36: 219–20.

2731 Russell WR, Schuster E, Smith AC, Spalding JMK. Lancet 1956; 1: 539–41.

2732 Sackner JD, Nixon AJ, Davis B, Atkins N, Sackner MA. Am Rev Respir Dis 1980; 122: 867–71.

2733 Sackner MA. Arthritis Rheum 1962; 5: 184–94.

2734 Sackner MA. Am Rev Respir Dis 1974; 110: 25–34.

2735 Sackner MA. J Am Med Assoc 1975; 231: 295–6.

2736 Sackner MA, Akgun N, Kimbel P, Lewis DH. Ann Intern Med 1964; 60: 611–30.

2737 Sackner MA, Gonzalez H, Rodriguez M, Belsito A, Sackner DR, Grenvik S. Am Rev Respir Dis 1984; 130: 588–93.

2738 Sackner MA, Landa J, Forrest T, Greeneltch D. Chest 1975; 67: 164–71.

2739 Sackner MA, Silva G, Banks JM, Watson DD, Smoak WM. Am Rev Respir Dis 1974; 109: 331–7.

2740 Sacks OW, Kohl M, Schwartz W, Messeloff C. Lancet 1970; 1: 1006.

2741 Sadoul P. Ann NY Acad Sci 1965; 121: 836–48.

2742 Sadoul P, Cardinaud JP. Bull Eur Physiopath Respir 1986; 22: Suppl 1–6S.

2743 Sadoul P, Cherrier F. J Fr Med Chir Thor 1963; 17: 167–80.

2744 Sahebjami H. Clin Chest Med 1986; 7: 111–26.

2745 Saheki B, Fukuyama K, Miyoshi M, Tani J, Koshiyama K. Iryo 1967; 21: 794–9.

2746 Sahlin B. Acta Med Scand 1932; 79: 76–124.

2747 Said SI. Ann Intern Med 1960; 53: 1121–9.

2748 Said SI, Banerjee CM. Am J Med 1962; 33: 845–51.

2749 Sainsbury HSK. Lancet 1947; 2: 615–6.

2750 St John WM, Bartlett D Jnr, Knuth KV, Knuth SL, Daubenspeck JA. Am Rev Respir Dis 1986; 133: 46–8.

2751 Sainton P. Rev Neurol 1901; 9: 297–300.

2752 Sakai DN, Hsu JD, Bonnett CA, Brown JC. Clin Orthop Rel Res 1977; 128: 256–60.

2753 Salih MAM. Ann Trop Paediatr 1981; 1: 97–101.

2754 Salih MAM, Ekmejian A, Ibrahim M. Ann Trop Paediatr 1984; 4: 45–8.

2755 Salkin D, Cadden AV, Edson RC. Am Rev Tuberc 1943; 47: 351–69.

2756 Salmeron G, Greenberg SD, Lidsky MD. Arch Intern Med 1981; 141: 1005–10.

2757 Salmoiraghi GC. Ann NY Acad Sci 1963; 109: 571–86.

2758 Salmoiraghi GC, Burns BD. J Neurophysiol 1960; 23: 2–13.

2759 Salmons S. Trends Neurosci 1980; 3: 134–7.

2760 Salmons S, Gale DR, Sreter FA. J Anat 1978; 127: 17–31.

2761 Salmons S, Henriksson J. Muscle Nerve 1981; 4: 94–105.

2762 Salomon J, Shah PM, Heinle RA. Am J Cardiol 1975; 36: 32–6.

2763 Saltz SA, Banner AS. Am Rev Respir Dis 1984; 129: A107.

2764 Saltzman HA, Salzano JV. J Appl Physiol 1971; 30: 228–31.

2765 Sambrook MA, Hutchinson EC, Aber GM. Brain 1973; 96: 171–90.

2766 Samet P, Fierer EM, Bernstein WH. J Appl Physiol 1960; 15: 826–8.

2767 Sanders JS, Berman TM, Bartlett MM, Kronenberg RS. Chest 1980; 78: 279–82.

2768 Sanders MH. Chest 1984; 86: 839–44.

2769 Sanders MH, Gruendl CA, Rogers RM. Chest 1986; 90: 330–3.

2770 Sanders MH, Holzer BC. Clin Res 1984; 32: 436A.

2771 Sanders MH, Holzer BC, Pennock BE. Chest 1983; 84: 336.

2772 Sanders MH, Martin RJ, Pennock BE, Rogers RM. J Am Med Assoc 1981; 245: 2414–8.

2773 Sanders MH, Moore SE, Eveslage J. Chest 1983; 83: 144–5.

2774 Sanders MH, Rogers RM. Chest 1985; 88: 320–1.

2775 Sanders MH, Rogers RM, Pennock BE. Am Rev Respir Dis 1985; 131: 401–8.

2776 Sandham JD, Shaw DT, Guenter CA. Chest 1977; 72: 96–8.

2777 Sandhu HS. Clin Chest Med 1986; 7: 629–42.

2778 Santamaria J, Prior J, Fleetham JA. Am Rev Respir Dis 1985; 131: Suppl A105.

2779 Sant'Ambrogio G, Frazier DT, Wilson MF, Agostoni E. J Appl Physiol 1963; 18: 43–6.

2780 Sant'Ambrogio G, Mathew OP. Clin Chest Med 1986; 7: 211–22.

2781 Santiago TV, Remolina C, Scoles V III, Edelman NH. N Engl J Med 1981; 304: 1190–5.

2782 Sanyal SK, Bernal R, Hughes WT, Feldman S. J Am Med Assoc 1976; 236: 1727–8.

2783 Sanyal SK, Johnson WW. Circulation 1982; 66: 853–63.

2784 Sanyal SK, MacGaw D, Hughes WT. J Pediatr 1974; 85: 230–2.

2785 Sanyal SK, Mitchell C, Hughes WT, Feldman S, Caces J. Chest 1975; 68: 143–8.

2786 Saoyama N, Harada K, Shimada Y. Rinsho Kyobu Geka 1984; 4: 153–7.

2787 Sarnoff FJ, Whittenberger JL, Affeldt JE. J Am Med Assoc 1951; 147: 30–4.

2788 Sarnoff LC, Sarnoff SJ. Arch Phys Med 1950; 31: 448–52.

2789 Sarnoff SJ, Gaensler EA, Maloney JV Jnr. J Thorac Surg 1950; 19: 929–37.

2790 Sarnoff SJ, Hardenbergh E, Whittenberger JL. Am J Physiol 1948; 155: 1–9.

2791 Sarnoff SJ, Hardenbergh E, Whittenberger JL. Science 1948; 108: 482.

2792 Sarnoff SJ, Maloney JV Jnr, Sarnoff LC, Ferris BG Jnr, Whittenberger JL. J Am Med Assoc 1950; 143: 1383–90.

2793 Sarnoff SJ, Sarnoff LC, Whittenberger JL. Surg Gynecol Obstet 1951; 93: 190–6.

2794 Sarnoff SJ, Whittenberger JL, Hardenbergh E. Am J Physiol 1948; 155: 203–7.

2795 Sasaki K, Inoue S–I, Yoshida A, Hayashi F, Masuda Y, Honda Y. Tohoku J Exp Med 1982; 137: 145–51.

2796 Sauerbruch F, O'Shaughnessy L. Thoracic Surgery. London: Edward Arnold and Co, 1937.

2797 Sauerland EK, Harper RM. Exp Neurol 1976; 51: 160–70.

2798 Saunders NA, Kreitzer SM. Am Rev Respir Dis 1979; 119: Suppl 127–30.

2799 Saunders NA, Sullivan CE, eds. Sleep and Breathing. New York: Marcel Dekker, 1984.

2800 Sautegau A, Hannhart B, Begin P, Polu JM, Schrijen F. Bull Eur Physiopath Respir 1984; 20: 541–5.

2801 Savini R, Parisini P, Vicenzi G. Ital J Orthop Traumatol 1976; 2: 247–59.

2802 Sawicka EH, Branthwaite MA, Spencer GT. Thorax 1982; 37: 791.

2803 Sawicka EH, Branthwaite MA, Spencer GT. Thorax 1983; 28: 433–5.

2804 Sawicka EH, Loh L, Branthwaite MA. Thorax 1985; 40: 209.

2805 Sawicka EH, Spencer GT, Branthwaite MA. Br J Dis Chest 1986; 80: 191–6.

2806 Scadding GK, Havard CWH, Lange MJ, Domb I. J Neurol Neurosurg Psychiatr 1985; 48; 401–6.

2807 Scales JT, Kinnier–Wilson AB, Holmes–Sellors T, Stevenson FH, Stott FD. Lancet 1953; 1: 671–4.

2808 Scharenberg K. J Neuropathol Exp Neurol 1955; 14: 297–304.

2809 Scharf SM, Feldman NT, Goldman MD, Haut HZ, Bruce E, Ingram RH Jnr. Am Rev Respir Dis 1978; 117: 391–7.

2810 Schaub F, Buhlmann A, Kalin R, Wegmann T. Schweiz Med Wschr 1954; 84: 1147–50.

2811 Schechter DC. Bull NY Acad Med 1970; 46: 932–51.

2812 (a) Scherrer M. Bibl Tuberk 1956; 11: 83–101.
(b) Schiavi EA, Roncoroni AJ, Puy RJM. Am Rev Respir Dis 1984; 129: 337–9.

2813 Schiffman PL. Chest 1985; 87: 124–6.

2814 Schmalstieg EJ, Peters BH, Schochet SS, Findlay SR. Arch Neurol 1977; 34: 473–6.

2815 Schmidt CD, Elliott CG, Carmelli D, et al. Crit Care Med 1983; 11: 407–11.

2816 Schmidt HS. Bull Eur Physiopath Respir 1983; 19: 625–9.

2817 Schmidt HS, Clark RW, Hyman PR. Am J Psychiatr 1977; 134: 183–5.

2818 Schmidt K, Kaniak G. Neurochirurg 1960; 3: 182–93.

2819 Schmidt–Nowara WW, Marder EJ, Feil PA. Arch Neurol 1984; 41: 567–8.

2820 Schmitt N, Bowmer EJ, Gregson JD. Can Med Assoc J 1969; 100: 417–21.

2821 Schneider PD, Wise RA, Hochberg MC, Wigley FM. Am J Med 1982; 73: 385–94.

2822 Schochat SJ, Csongradi JJ, Hartman GE, Rinsky LA. J Pediatr Surg 1981; 16: 353–7.

2823 Schock CC. Orthop Trans 1978; 2: 269.

2824 Schoenen J, Hadjoudj H, Dumont M, Reznik M. Rev Med Liege 1981; 22: 830–5.

2825 Schonfield T, O'Neal MH, Platzker ACG, Weitzman JJ, Fishman LS, Whiteman S, Keens TG. Thorax 1980; 35: 631–2.

2826 Schroeder JS, Motta J, Guilleminault C. In: Guilleminault C, Dement WC, eds. Sleep Apnea Syndromes. New York: AR Liss Inc, 1978; 177–96.

2827 Schuster E, Fischer–Williams M. Lancet 1953; 2: 1074–6.

2828 Schwartz AR, Avram R, Gold MD, Smith PL. Am Rev Respir Dis 1985; 131: Suppl A102.

2829 Schwartz AR, Gold AR, Smith PL. Am Rev Respir Dis 1985; 131: A102.

2830 Schwartz MZ, Filler RM. J Pediatr Surg 1978; 13: 259–63.

2831 Schwartz OA, Campbell NA, Walsh JK. Am Rev Respir Dis 1987; 135: A231.

2832 Schwartzstein R, Leith D, Scharf S, Brown R. Am Rev Respir Dis 1985; 131: A337.

2833 Schwatt H. Am J Med Sci 1934; 187: 338–47.

2834 Schwentker EP, Gibson DA. J Bone Joint Surg 1976; 58A: 32–8.

2835 Scobie BA. Br Med J 1971; 4: 560.

2836 Scott E, leFever H, Oliver M. Ohio State J Med 1934; 30: 213–23.

2837 Scott R. Thorax 1965; 20: 357–61.

2838 Scott RM, Whitwam JG, Chakrabarti MK. Br J Anaesth 1977; 49: 227–31.

2839 Scrima L, Broudy M, Nay KN, Cohn MA. Sleep 1982; 5: 318–28.

2840 Sears TA, Berger AJ, Phillipson EA. Nature 1982; 299: 728–30.

2841 Seay AR, Ziter FA, Thompson JA. J Pediatr 1978; 93: 88–90.

2842 Secher NH, Madsen F, Bjerre–Jepsen K, et al. Lancet 1980; 2: 858.

2843 Secker–Walker RH, Ho JE, Gill IS. Respiration 1979; 38: 194–203.

2844 Sedwitz JL, Christoph R, Thomas BD. Int Surg 1972; 57: 467–9.

2845 Segal AM, Calabrese LH, Ahmad M, Tubbs RR, White CS. Sem Arthritis Rheum 1985; 14: 202–24.

2846 Sehnal E, Haber P, Lack W. Respiration 1981; 44: 376–81.

2847 Seide MJ. N Engl J Med 1957; 257: 1227–30.

2848 Seiler J. De la Galvanisation par Influence. Paris: Bailliere, 1860.

2849 Sellors TH. Thorax 1947; 2: 216–23.

2850 Selzer A. Am J Med 1951; 10: 334–55.

2851 Semb C, Erikson H, Refsum HE. Acta Chir Scand 1961; Suppl 283: 39–44.

2852 Seriff NS. Ann NY Acad Sci 1965; 121: 691–705.

2853 Serisier DE, Mastaglia FL, Gibson GJ. Thorax 1980; 35: 710.

2854 Serisier DE, Mastaglia FL, Gibson GJ. Q J Med 1982; 51: 205–26.

2855 Serpick AA, Baker EL, Woodward TE. Arch Intern Med 1965; 115: 192–7.

2856 Serratto M, Kezdi P. Ann Intern Med 1963; 58: 938–45.

2857 Sethi G, Reed WA. J Thorac Cardiovasc Surg 1971; 62: 138–43.

2858 Setliff RC III, Puyau FA, Ward PH. Laryngoscope 1968; 78: 845–56.

2859 Sevastikoglou JA, Linderholm H, Lindgren U. Acta Orthop Scand 1976; 47: 540–5.

2860 Severinghaus JW. Ann Rev Physiol 1962; 24: 421–70.

2861 Severinghaus JW, Mitchell RA. Clin Res 1962; 10: 122.

2862 Shafiq SA, Dubowitz V, Peterson H de C, Milhorat AT. Brain 1967; 90: 817–28.

2863 Shambaugh GE Jnr, Harrison WG Jnr, Farrell JI. J Am Med Assoc 1930; 94: 1371–3.

2864 Shanks C, Kafer ER. Respiratory aspects of anaesthesia for the operative correction of scoliosis. Australia: Butterworths, 1970: 376–81.

2865 Shannon DC. Sleep 1980; 3: 343–9.

2866 Shannon DC, Kelly DH, O'Connell K. N Engl J Med 1977; 297: 747–50.

2867 Shannon DC, Marsland DW, Gould JB, Callahan B, Todres ID, Dennis J. Pediatrics 1976; 57: 342–6.

2868 Shannon DC, Riseborough EJ, Kazemi H. J Am Med Assoc 1971; 217: 579–84.

2869 Shannon DC, Riseborough EJ, Laercio MV, Kazemi H. J Bone Joint Surg 1970; 52A: 131–44.

2870 Shapiro CM, Douglas NJ. Thorax 1987; 42: 722.

2871 Shapiro F, Bresnan MJ. J Bone Joint Surg 1982; 64A: 949–53.

2872 Shapiro J, Strome M, Crocker AC. Ann Otol Rhinol Laryngol 1985; 94: 458–61.

2873 Sharp JT. Chest 1985; 88: Suppl 118–23S.

2874 Sharp JT, Barrocas M, Chokroverty S. Clin Chest Med 1980; 1: 103–18.

2875 Sharp JT, Danon J, Druz WS, Goldberg NB, Fishman H, Machnach W. Am Rev Respir Dis 1974; 110; Suppl 154–67.

2876 Sharp JT, Druz WS, D'Souza V, Diamond E. Am Rev Respir Dis 1982; 125: Suppl 233.

2877 Sharp JT, Druz WS, D'Souza V, Diamond E. Chest 1985; 87: 619–24.

2878 Sharp JT, Druz WS, Kondragunta VR. Am Rev Respir Dis 1986; 133: 32–7.

2879 Sharp JT, Druz WS, Moisan T, Foster J, Machnach W. Am Rev Respir Dis 1980; 122: 201–11.

2880 Sharp JT, Goldberg NB, Druz WS, Danon J. J Appl Physiol 1975; 39: 608–18.

2881 Sharp JT, Goldberg NB, Druz WS, Fishman HC, Danon J. Am Rev Respir Dis 1977; 115: 47–56.

2882 Sharp JT, Henry JP, Sweany SK, Meadows WR, Pietras RJ. J Appl Physiol 1964; 19: 959–66.

2883 Sharp JT, Henry JP, Sweany SK, Meadows WR, Pietras RJ. J Clin Invest 1964; 43: 728–39.

2884 Sharp JT, Lith P van, Nuchprayoon C vej, Briney R, Johnson FN. Am J Med 1968; 44: 39–46.

2885 Sharp JT, Sweany SK, Henry JP, et al. J Lab Clin Med 1964; 63: 254–63.

2886 Shaw LA, Drinker P. J Clin Invest 1930; 8: 33–46.

2887 Shaw RK, Glenn WWL, Hogan JF, Phelps ML. J Neurosurg 1980; 53: 345–54.

2888 Shaw RK, Glenn WWL, Holcomb WG. Surg Forum 1975; 26: 195–7.

2889 Shearer MO, Banks JM, Silva G, Sackner MA. Phys Ther 1972; 52: 139–48.

2890 Shee CD, Ploy–Song–Sang Y, Milic–Emili J. J Appl Physiol 1985; 58: 1859–65.

2891 Sheldon GP. Medicine 1963; 42: 197–227.

2892 Sheldon GP. Chest 1976; 69: 133–4.

2893 Shelton RL, Bosma JF. J Appl Physiol 1962; 17: 209–14.

2894 Shepard JW, Garrison MW, Grither DA, Dolan GF. Chest 1985; 88: 335–40.

2895 Shephard RJ. Clin Sci 1967; 32: 167–76.

2896 Shepherd MP. Thorax 1985; 40: 328–40.

2897 Sherrington C. Proc R Soc Lond 1929; Series B: 105: 332–62.

2898 Shils ME. Medicine 1969; 48: 61–85.

2899 Shimomura S, McHugh BP, Flatow FA Jnr, Bell ALL Jnr. Am Rev Respir Dis 1967; 95: 576–83.

2900 Shneerson JM. Med Hist 1977; 21: 397–410.

2901 Shneerson JM. Clin Allergy 1977; 7: 203.

2902 Shneerson JM. Thorax 1978; 33: 457–63.

2903 Shneerson JM. Thorax 1978; 33: 747–54.

2904 Shneerson JM. Thorax 1980; 35: 347–50.

2905 Shneerson JM, Edgar MA. Thorax 1979; 34: 658–61.

2906 Shneerson JM, Madgwick R. Acta Orthop Scand 1979; 50: 303–6.

2907 Shneerson JM, Sutton GC, Zorab PA. Clin Orthop Rel Res 1978; 135: 52–7.

2908 Shneerson JM, Venco A, Prime FJ. Thorax 1977; 32: 700–5.

2909 Shore T, Millman RP. Arch Intern Med 1983; 143: 1278.

2910 Sieben RL, Hamida MB, Shulman K. Neurology 1971; 21: 673–81.

2911 Siebens AA, Kirby NA, Poulos DA. Arch Phys Med Rehabil 1964; 45: 1–8.

2912 Siebens AA, Pietraszek CF, Weaver J, Storey CF. Am Rev Tuberc 1954; 70; 672–88.

2913 Siebens AA, Storey CF, Newman MM, Frank NR, Swenson EW. Am Rev Tuberc Pulm Dis 1955; 71: 676–92.

2914 Sieck GC, Mazar A, Belman MJ. Respir Physiol 1985; 61: 137–52.

2915 Siegel IM. Clin Orthop Rel Res 1973; 93: 235–8.

2916 Siegel IM. Phys Ther 1975; 55: 160–2.

2917 Siegel JS, Schechter E. Am J Med 1967; 42: 309–13.

2918 Siegfried J, Pitteloud J–J. Confin Neurol 1965; 25: 227–33.

2919 Siegler D, Zorab PA. Br J Dis Chest 1981; 75: 367–70.

2920 Siegler D, Zorab PA. Br J Dis Chest 1982; 76: 44–50.

2921 Sieker HO, Estes EH Jnr, Kelser GA, McIntosh HD. J Clin Invest 1955; 34: 916.

2922 Sieker HO, Hickam JB. Medicine 1956; 35: 389–423.

2923 Sigrist S, Thomas D, Howell S, Roussos C. Am Rev Respir Dis 1982; 126: 46–50.

2924 Silbestein SL, Barland P, Grayzel AI, Koerner SK. J Rheumatol 1980; 7: 187–95.

2925 Silbiger ML, Pikielney R, Donner MW. Invest Radiol 1967; 2: 442–8.

2926 Silver JR. Paraplegia 1963; 1: 204–14.

2927 Silver JR, Abdel–Halim RE. Paraplegia 1971; 9: 123–31.

2928 Silver JR, Gibbon NOK. Br Med J 1968; 4: 79–83.

2929 Silver JR, Lehr RP. J Neurol Neurosurg Psychiatr 1981; 44: 837–42.

2930 Silver JR, Lehr RP. J Neurol Neurosurg Psychiatr 1981; 44: 842–5.

2931 Silverstein A, Gilbert H, Wasserman LR. Ann Intern Med 1962; 57: 909–16.

2932 Simmons FB, Guilleminault C, Dement WC, Tilkian AG, Hill M. Laryngoscope 1977; 87: 326–38.

2933 Simmons FB, Guilleminault C, Silvestri R. Arch Otolaryngol 1983; 109: 503–7.

2934 Simon G. In: Zorab PA, ed. Proceedings of a Symposium on Scoliosis. London: National Fund for Research into Poliomyelitis and other Crippling Diseases, 1965: 65–70.

2935 Simonds AK, Branthwaite MA. Thorax 1985; 40: 213.

2936 Simonds AK, Parker RA, Branthwaite MA. Thorax 1986; 41: 244–5.

2937 Simonds AK, Parker RA, Sawicka EH, Branthwaite MA. Thorax 1985; 40: 702.

2938 Simonds AK, Sawicka EH, Carroll N, Branthwaite MA. Thorax 1987; 42: 713–4.

2939 Simonneau G, Denjean A, Raffestin B, et al. Am Rev Respir Dis 1981; 123: Suppl 88.

2940 Simonneau G, Meignan M, Denjean A, Raffestin B, Harf A, Prost J–F. Chest 1986; 89: 174–9.

2941 Simonneau G, Vivien A, Sartene R, et al. Am Rev Respir Dis 1983; 128: 899–903.

2942 Simpser MD, Strieder DJ, Wohl ME, Rosenthal A, Rockenmacher S. Pediatrics 1977; 60: 290–3.

2943 Simpson K. Arch Dis Childh 1975; 50: 569–71.

2944 Simpson T. Br Med J 1948; 2: 639–41.

2945 Simpson T. Br Med J 1954; 1: 297–301.

2946 Singh BN. NZ Med J 1965; 64: 392–4.

2947 Sinha R, Bergofsky EH. Am Rev Respir Dis 1972; 106: 47–57.

2948 Sink J, Bliwise DL, Dement WC. Chest 1986; 90: 177–80.

2949 Sivak ED, Cordasco EM, Celmer EF. Chest 1980; 78: 540–1.

2950 Sivak ED, Cordasco EM, Gipson WT. Respir Care 1983; 28: 42–9.

2951 Sivak ED, Cordasco EM, Gipson WT, Stelmak K. Cleve Clin Q 1983; 50: 219–25.

2952 Sivak ED, Gipson WT, Hanson MR. Ann Neurol 1982; 12: 18–23.

2953 Sivak ED, Gipson WT, Stelmak K. Chest 1983; 84: 239.

2954 Sivak ED, Mehta A, Hanson M, Cosgrove DM. Cleve Clin Q 1984; 51: 585–9.

2955 Sivak ED, Razavi M, Groves LK, Loop FD. Crit Care Med 1983; 11: 438–40.

2956 Sivak ED, Salanga VD, Vilbourn AJ, Mitsumoto H, Golish J. Ann Neurol 1981; 9: 613–5.

2957 Sivak ED, Streib EW. Ann Neurol 1980; 7: 188–91.

2958 Skatrud J, Iber C, Ewart R, Thomas G, Rasmussen H, Schultze B. Am Rev Respir Dis 1981; 124: 325–9.

2959 Skatrud J, Iber C, McHugh W, Rasmussen H, Nichols D. Am Rev Respir Dis 1980; 121: 587–93.

2960 Skatrud JB, Dempsey JA. Am Rev Respir Dis 1983; 127: 405–12.

2961 Skatrud JB, Dempsey JA, Bhansali P, Irvin C. J Clin Invest 1980; 625: 813–21.

2962 Skatrud JB, Dempsey JA, Iber C, Berssenbrugge A. Am Rev Respir Dis 1981; 124: 260–8.

2963 Skatrud JB, Dempsey JA, Kaiser DG. J Appl Physiol 1978; 44: 939–44.

2964 Sleath GE, Graves HB. Can Anaesth Soc J 1958; 5: 330–6.

2965 Slonim AE, Coleman RA, McElligot MA, et al. Neurology 1983; 33: 34–8.

2966 Slotkin EA, Loeser WD, Ament R. J Urol 1956; 76: 499–507.

2967 Slutsky AS, Strohl KP. Am Rev Respir Dis 1980; 121: 893–5.

2968 Smallwood R, Giblin E, Ralph D, Vitiello M, Prinz P. Sleep Res 1984; 13: 166.

2969 Smallwood RG, Vitiello MV, Giblin EC, Prinz PN. Sleep 1983; 6: 16–22.

2970 Smirne S, Comi G. Sleep Res 1976; 4: 237.

2971 Smith AC. Proc R Soc Med 1958; 51: 1006–8.

2972 Smith B. Pediatrics 1972; 49: 449–51.

2973 Smith E. J Am Med Assoc 1933; 100; 1666–70.

2974 Smith E, Harris IL, Rosenblatt P. J Paediatr 1953; 43: 9–20.

2975 Smith HL. Am Heart J 1928; 4: 79–93.

2976 Smith HP, Smith HP Jnr. Am J Med 1955; 19: 808–13.

2977 Smith JP Jnr, Falk GA, Perry JA. Ann Intern Med 1971; 74: 841.

2978 Smith LH. Am Pract Dig Treatm 1956; 7: 1165–72.

2979 Smith M. Am Rev Respir Dis 1964; 89: 450–2.

2980 Smith PEM, Edwards RHT, Calverley PMA. Am Rev Respir Dis 1987; 135: Suppl A185.

2981 Smith PL, Haponik EF, Allen RP, Bleecker ER. Am Rev Respir Dis 1983; 127: 8–13.

2982 Smith PL, Haponik EF, Bleecker ER. Am Rev Respir Dis 1984; 130: 958–63.

2983 Smith RE. Lancet 1953; 1: 674–6.

2984 Smith SL. J Am Med Assoc 1939; 113: 1806–7.

2985 Smith SL. J Am Med Assoc 1952; 149: 654–5.

2986 Smith TH, Baska RE, Francisco CB, McCray GM, Kunz S. J Pediatr 1978; 93: 891–2.

2987 Smith W. Lancet 1931; 1: 1267–8.

2988 Smith WK. J Neurophysiol 1938; 1: 55–68.

2989 Smorto MP, Vigneri MR, Fierro B. Riv Neurobiol 1973; 18: 48–54.

2990 Smyth RJ, Chapman KR, Rebuck AS. Chest 1984; 86: 568–72.

2991 Smyth RJ, Chapman KR, Wright TA, Crawford JS, Rebuck AS. Thorax 1984; 39: 901–4.

2992 Smyth RJ, Chapman KR, Wright TA, Crawford JS, Rebuck AS. Pediatrics 1986; 77: 690–7.

2993 Sneddon DG, Bedbrook G. Paraplegia 1982; 20: 201–7.

2994 Snider TH, Stevens JP, Wilner FM. J Am Med Assoc 1959; 170: 1631–2.

2995 Snyderman NL, Johnson JT, Moller M, Thearle PB. Ann Otol Rhinol Laryngol 1982; 91: 597–8.

2996 Soderstrom N. Acta Med Scand 1945; 122: 95–102.

2997 Soffer D, Feldman S, Alter M. J Neurol Sci 1978; 37: 135–43.

2998 Soldatos CR, Kales JD, Scharf MB, Bixler EO, Kales A. Science 1980; 207: 551–3.

2999 Solliday NH, Gaensler EA, Schwaber JR, Parker TF. Respiration 1974; 31: 177–92.

3000 Sonne LJ. Chest 1984; 86: 939.

3001 Sonne LJ, Davis JA. Chest 1982; 81: 436–9.

3002 Sorensen AWS, With TK. Acta Med Scand 1971; 190: 219–22.

3003 Sorensen SC. Acta Physiol Scand 1971; Suppl 361: 1–72.

3004 Sorensen SC, Severinghaus JW. J Appl Physiol 1968; 25: 211–6.

3005 Sorensen SC, Severinghaus JW. J Appl Physiol 1968; 25: 221–3.

3006 Sorensen SC, Severinghaus JW. J Appl Physiol 1968; 25: 217–20.

3007 Souadjian JV, Cain JC. Postgrad Med 1968; 43: 72–7.

3008 Spain DM, Thomas AG. Ann Intern Med 1950; 32: 152–61.

3009 Spalding JMK, Opie L. Lancet 1958; 1: 613–5.

3010 Spector S, Bautista AG. NY State J Med 1956; 56: 2118–9.

3011 Speizer FE, Frank NR. J Appl Physiol 1964; 19: 176–8.

3012 Spencer G. In: Zorab PA, ed. Scoliosis. London: Academic Press, 1977: 315–28.

3013 Spencer GT. In: Olson DA, Henig E, eds. Proceedings of an international symposium. Whatever happened to the polio patient? Chicago, 1979: 129–35.

3014 Spencer WA, Vallbona C. J Appl Physiol 1959; 14: 279–83.

3015 Spencer WG. Phil Trans R Soc (B) 1894; 185: 609–57.

3016 Spier S, Rivlin J, Rowe RD, Egan T. Chest 1986; 90: 711–5.

3017 Spiers ASD. Med J Aust 1963; 1: 850–3.

3018 Spillane JD. Br Heart J 1951; 13: 343–7.

3019 Spiller WG, Martin E. J Am Med Assoc 1912; 58: 1489–90.

3020 Spire JP, Kuo PC, Campbell N. Bull Eur Physiopath Respir 1983; 19: 604–6.

3021 Spiteri MA, Mier AK, Brophy CJ, Pantin CFA, Green M. Thorax 1985; 40: 631–2.

3022 Spitz A. Deutsches Arch Klin Med 1937; 181: 286–304.

3023 Spitzer SA, Korczyn AD, Kalaci J. Chest 1973; 64: 355–7.

3024 Splaingard ML, Frates RC, Harrison GM, Carter RE, Jefferson LS. Chest 1983; 84: 376–82.

3025 Splaingard ML, Frates RC Jnr, Jefferson LS, Rosen CL, Harrison GM. Arch Phys Med Rehabil 1985; 66: 239–42.

3026 Splaingard ML, Jefferson LS, Harrison GM. Am Rev Respir Dis 1982; 125: Suppl 139.

3027 Staehelin R. Handbuch der inneren Medizin. Vol 2. Berlin: Julius Springer, 1930; 1713.

3028 Stafford N, Youngs R, Waldron J, Baer S, Randall C. J Laryngol Otol 1986; 100: 861–3.

3029 Stain JP, Morere P, Lefrancois R, Lemercier JP, Pasquis P, Nouvet G. Poumon Coeur 1972; 28: 45–8.

3030 Stanbury JB. Am Practitioner 1948; 2: 761–5.

3031 Stanley NN, Galloway JM, Flint KC, Campbell DB. Br J Dis Chest 1983; 77: 136–46.

3032 Stanley NN, Galloway JM, Gordon B, Pauly N. Thorax 1983; 38: 200–4.

3033 Stauffer ES, Bell GD. Orthop Clin North Am 1978; 9: 1081–9.

3034 Stauffer ES, Mankin JH. J Bone Joint Surg 1966 48A: 339–48.

3035 Stauffer JL, Olson DE, Petty TL. Am J Med 1981; 70: 65–76.

3036 Stauffer JL, Silvestri RC. Respir Care 1982; 27: 417–34.

3037 Steegman AT. J Nerv Ment Dis 1951; 114: 35–65.

3038 Stein M, Kimbel P, Johnson RL. J Clin Invest 1961; 40: 348–63.

3039 Steinbach HL, Feldman R, Goldberg MB. Radiology 1959; 72: 535–49.

3040 Steiner WR. Boston Med Surg J 1908; 159: 720–3.

3041 Steinmann EP. Zeitschr Orthop 1951; 80: 202–26.

3042 Stella G. J Physiol 1939; 96: 26P.

3043 Stella G, Stevan G. Arch Int Pharmacodyn Ther 1962; 136: 1–11.

3044 Stemmer EA, Crawford DW, List JW, Heber RE, Connolly JE. J Thorac Cardiovasc Surg 1967; 54: 649–57.

3045 Stepanski E, Lamphere J, Badia P, Zorick F, Roth T. Sleep 1984; 7: 18–26.

3046 Stephenson SE Jnr, Young W, Montgomery LH, Batson R. Dis Chest 1961; 39: 363–71.

3047 Stern L, Ramos AD, Outerbridge EW, Beaudry PH. Can Med Assoc J 1970; 102: 595–601.

3048 Stern M, Hellwege HH, Gravinghoff L, Lambrecht W. Acta Paediatr Scand 1981; 70: 121–4.

3049 Stern MM. J Nerv Ment Dis 1949; 109: 48–53.

3050 Steuart W. Med J South Africa 1918; 13: 147–50.

3051 Stevenson FH. J Bone Joint Surg 1952; 34B: 256–65.

3052 Stevenson FH, Wilson ABK, Bottomley AH, Airey DM. J Bone Joint Surg 1963; 45B: 326–36.

3053 Stewart RM, Ridyard JB, Pearson JD. Thorax 1976; 31: 433–7.

3054 Steyer BJ, Quan SF, Morgan WJ. Am Rev Respir Dis 1985; 131: 592–5.

3055 Stigol LC, Cuello AC. J Appl Physiol 1966; 21: 1911–2.

3056 Stirling AJ, Smith RM, Dickson RA. Br Med J 1986; 292: 1305–6.

3057 Stoboy H, Speierer B. Arch Orthopad Unfall–Chirurgie, 1975; 81: 247–54.

3058 Stokes DC, Phillips JA, Leonard CO, et al. J Pediatr 1983; 102: 534–41.

3059 (a) Stone DJ, Keltz H. Am Rcv Respir Dis 1963; 88: 621–9.
     (b) Stone DJ, Schwartz A, Newman W, Feltman JA, Lovelock FJ. Am J Med 1953; 14: 14–22.

3060 Stookey B. Arch Neurol Psychiatr 1931; 26: 443.

3061 Storstein O. Exp Med Surg 1964; 22: 13–23.

3062 Stradling JR. Br Med J 1982; 285: 407–8.

3063 Stradling JR. Thorax 1983; 38: 237–8.

3064 Stradling JR. Lung 1986; 164: 17–31.

3065 Stradling JR, Barnes P, Pride NB. Clin Sci 1982; 63: 401–4.

3066 Stradling JR, Chadwick GA, Frew AJ. Thorax 1985; 40; 364–70.

3067 Stradling JR, Chadwick GA, Quirk C, Phillips T. Bull Eur Physiopath Respir 1985; 21: 317–24.

3068 Stradling JR, Huddart S, Arnold AG. Thorax 1981; 36: 634–5.

3069 Stradling JR, Lane DJ. Thorax 1981; 36: 321–5.

3070 Stradling JR, Nicholl CG, Cover D, Davies EE, Hughes JMB, Pride NB. Clin Sci 1984; 66: 435–42.

3071 Stradling JR, Phillipson EA. Q J Med 1986; 59: 3–18.

3072 Strang FA. Proc R Soc Med 1971; 64: 484–9.

3073 Strasberg B, Kanakis C, Dhingra RC, Rosen KM. Chest 1980; 78: 845–8.

3074 Strauss JF. Arch Otolaryngol 1943; 38: 225–9.

3075 Streeten EA, Monte SM de la, Kennedy TP. Chest 1986; 89: 760–2.

3076 Striano S, Meo R, Bilo L, Vitolo S. Electroencephalogr Clin Neurophysiol 1983; 56: 323–5.

3077 Strieder DJ, Baker WG, Baringer JR, Kazemi H. Am Rev Respir Dis 1967; 96: 501–7.

3078 Strohl KP, Brown R, Hensley MJ, Hallett M, Saunders NA, Ingram RH Jnr. Am Rev Respir Dis 1979; 119: Suppl 173.

3079 Strohl KP, Cherniack NS, Gothe B. Am Rev Respir Dis 1986; 134: 791–802.

3080 Strohl KP, Gottfried SB, Graaff WB van de, Fouke JM. Clin Res 1982; 30: 751A.

3081 Strohl KP, Hensley MJ, Hallett M, Saunders NA, Ingram RH Jnr. J Appl Physiol 1980; 49: 638–42.

3082 Strohl KP, Hensley MJ, Saunders NA, Scharf SM, Brown R, Ingram RH Jnr. J Am Med Assoc 1981; 245: 1230–2.

3083 Strohl KP, Redline S. Am Rev Respir Dis 1986; 134: 555–8.

3084 Strohl KP, Saunders NA, Feldman NT, Hallett M. N Engl J Med 1978; 299: 969–73.

3085 Strom J. Acta Med Scand 1956; Suppl 316: 40–6.

3086 Strumpf IJ, Reynolds SF, Vash P, Tashkin DP. Am Rev Respir Dis 1978; 117: Suppl 183.

3087 Stuart FS, Henry M, Holley HL. Arthritis Rheum 1960; 3: 229–32.

3088 Stubbs SE, Hyatt RE. J Appl Physiol 1972; 32: 325–31.

3089 Sugar O. J Am Med Assoc 1978; 240: 236–7.

3090 Sugerman HJ, Fairman P, Baron PL, Kwentus JA. Chest 1986; 90: 81–6.

3091 Sukumalchantra Y, Dinakara P, Williams MH Jnr. Am Rev Respir Dis 1966; 93: 215–22.

3092 Sukumalchantra Y, Park SS, Williams MH Jnr. Am Rev Respir Dis 1965; 92: 885–93.

3093 Sukumalchantra Y, Tongmitr V, Tanphaichitr V, Jumbala B. Am Rev Respir Dis 1968; 98: 1037–43.

3094 Sullivan CE. Chest 1980; 78: 354.

3095 Sullivan CE, Berthon–Jones M, Issa FG. Am Rev Respir Dis 1982; 125: Suppl 107.

3096 Sullivan CE, Berthon–Jones M, Issa FG. Am Rev Respir Dis 1983; 128: 177–81.

3097 Sullivan CE, Berthon–Jones M, Issa FG. N Engl J Med 1983; 309: 112–3.

3098 Sullivan CE, Issa FG. Clin Chest Med 1985; 6: 633–50.

3099 Sullivan CE, Issa FG, Berthon–Jones M, Eves L. Lancet 1981; 1: 862–5.

3100 Sullivan CE, Issa FG, Berthon–Jones M, McCauley VB, Costash JV. Bull Eur Physiopath Respir 1984; 20: 49–54.

3101 Sullivan CE, Murphy E, Kozar LF, Phillipson EA. J Appl Physiol 1978; 45: 681–9.

3102 Sullivan KN. Arch Intern Med 1969; 123: 598.

3103 Sullivan KN, Manfredi F, Behnke RH. Arch Intern Med 1968; 122: 116–21.

3104 Sullivan SF, Patterson RW, Papper EM. J Appl Physiol 1966; 21: 247–50.

3105 Sundberg M, Hirsjarvi E, Tarvala R. Acta Allergol 1965; 21: 254–60.

3106 Sundermeyer JF, Gudbjarnason S, Wendt VE, den Bakker PB, Bing RJ. Circlation 1961; 24: 1348–55.

3107 Sunderrajan EV, Davenport J. Medicine 1985; 64: 333–41.

3108 Supinski GS, Deal EC Jnr, Kelsen SG. Am Rev Respir Dis 1984; 130: 429–33.

3109 Supinski GS, Deal EC Jnr, Kelsen SG. Am Rev Respir Dis 1986; 133: 809–13.

3110 Supinski GS, Kelsen SG. Am Rev Respir Dis 1983; 127: Suppl 231.

3111 Suratt PM, Dee P, Atkinson RL, Armstrong P, Wilhoit SC. Am Rev Respir Dis 1983; 127: 487–92.

3112 Suratt PM, McTier RF, Wilhoit SC. Am Rev Respir Dis 1985; 132: 967–71.

3113 Suratt PM, Turner BL, Wilhoit SC. Chest 1986; 90: 324–9.

3114 Suratt PM, Wilhoit SC, Brown ED, Findley LJ. Bull Eur Physiopath Respir 1986; 22: 127–31.

3115 Sussman MD. Dev Med Child Neurol 1985; 27: 522–4.

3116 Sutton FD Jnr, Zwillich CW, Creagh CE, Pierson DJ, Weil JV. Ann Intern Med 1975; 83: 476–9.

3117 Sutton JR, Houston CS, Mansell AL, et al. N Engl J Med 1979; 301: 1329–31.

3118 Sutton MGStJ, Olukotun AY, Tajik AJ, Lovett JL, Giuliani ER. Br Heart J 1980; 44: 309–16.

3119 Sutton PP, Parker RA, Webber BA, et al. Eur J Respir Dis 1983; 64: 62–8.

3120 Svanberg L. Acta Chir Scand 1956; 111: 169–96.

3121 Swai EA. Cent Afr J Med 1982; 28: 213–6.

3122 Swank SM, Winter RB, Moe JH. Spine 1982; 7: 343–54.

3123 Swanson GD, Whipp BJ, Kaufman RD, Aqleh KA, Winter B, Bellville JW. J Appl Physiol 1978; 45: 971–7.

3124 Swartz MA, Marino PL. Chest 1985; 88: 726–39.

3125 Swick HM, Werlin SL, Dodds WJ, Hogan WJ. Ann Neurol 1981; 10: 454–7.

3126 Switzer JL. Gastroenterology 1956; 31: 79–82.

3127 Sybrecht GW, Garrett L, Anthonisen NR. J Appl Physiol 1975; 39: 707–13.

3128 Sykes MK. Thorax 1985; 40: 161–5.

3129 Taasan V, Wynne JW, Cassisi N, Block AJ. Laryngoscope 1981; 91: 1163–72.

3130 Taasan VC, Block AJ, Boysen PG, Wynne JW, White C, Lindsey S. Am J Med 1981; 71: 240–5.

3131 Tabary JC, Tabary C, Tardieu C, Tardieu G, Goldspink G. J Physiol 1972; 224: 231–44.

3132 Tait GB. Ann Phys Med 1967; 9: 172.

3133 Taitz LS, Redman CWG. Proc R Soc Med 1971; 64: 1222.

3134 Talbert OR, Currens JH, Cohen ME. Trans Am Neurol Assoc 1954; 79: 226–8.

3135 Talbot AR, Robertson LW. Arch Otolaryngol 1973; 98: 277–81.

3136 Talbot S. Br J Clin Pract 1971; 25: 491–4.

3137 Talmage EA, McKechnie FB. Anesthesiology 1959; 20: 717–9.

3138 Tamaya S, Kondo T, Yamabayashi H. Jpn J Med 1983; 22: 45–9.

3139 Tammelin BR, Wilson AF, Borowiecki BdeB, Sassin JF. Am Rev Respir Dis 1983; 128: 712–5.

3140 Tammeling GJ, Laros CD. J Thorac Surg 1959; 37: 148–65.

3141 Tassinari CA, Bernadina BD, Cirignotta F, Ambrosetto G. Bull Physiopath Respir 1972; 8: 1087–102.

3142 Taterka JH, O'Sullivan ME. J Am Med Assoc 1943; 122: 737–9.

3143 Taylor A. J Physiol 1960; 151: 390–402.

3144 Taylor N. N Engl J Med 1972; 286: 1267–8.

3145 Tempo CP bon, Ronan JA Jnr, Leon AC de Jnr, Twigg HL. Am J Cardiol 1975; 36: 27–31.

3146 Tenicela R, Rosomuff HL, Feist J, Safar P. Anesthesiology 1968; 29: 7–16.

3147 Tenney SM, Miller RM. Am J Med 1955; 19: 498–508.

3148 Tenney SM, Reese RE. Respir Physiol 1968; 5: 187–201.

3149 Thibeault DW, Poblete E, Auld PAM. Paediatrics 1968; 41: 574–87.

3150 Thomas JN. J Laryngol Otol 1978; 92: 41–6.

3151 Thomas NE, Passamonte PM, Sunderrajan EV, Andelin JB, Ansbacher LE. Am Rev Respir Dis 1984; 129: 507–9.

3152 Thompson PJ, Dhillon DP, Ledingham J, Turner–Warwick M. Am Rev Respir Dis 1985; 132: 926–8.

3153 Thompson WT Jnr, Patterson JL Jnr, Shapiro W. Arch Intern Med 1964; 113: 856–65.

3154 Thoren C. Acta Paediatr 1964; 53: Suppl 153 1–136.

3155 Thoren C. Acta Paediatr 1964; 53: Suppl 153, 388–9.

3156 Thornton G. Lancet 1899; 2: 79–82.

3157 Thornton JA, Darke CS, Herbert P. Anaesthesia 1974; 29: 44–9.

3158 Thorpy MJ, Schmidt–Nowara WW, Pollak CP, Weitzman ED. Ann Neurol 1982; 12: 308–11.

3159 Thunberg T. Klin Wschr 1925; 4: 536–8.

3160 Thunberg T. Scand Arch Physiol 1926; 48: 80–94.

3161 Tiep BL, Carter R, Nicotra B, Berry J, Phillips RE, Otsap B. Chest 1987; 91: 15–19.

3162 Tilkian AG, Guilleminault C, Schroeder JS, Lehrman KL, Simmons FB, Dement WC. Ann Intern Med 1976; 85: 714–9.

3163 Tilkian AG, Guilleminault C, Schroeder JS, Lehrman KL, Simmons FB, Dement WC. Am J Med 1977; 63: 348–58.

3164 Tilkian AG, Motta J, Guilleminault C. In: Guilleminault C, Dement WC, eds. Sleep Apnea Syndromes. New York: AR Liss Inc, 1978; 197–210.

3165 Timms RM, Khaja FU, Williams GW and the Nocturnal Therapy Trial Group. Ann Intern Med 1985; 102: 29–36.

3166 Ting EY, Hong SK, Rahn H. J Appl Physiol 1960; 15: 557–60.

3167 Ting EY, Hong SK, Rahn H. J Appl Physiol 1960; 15: 554–6.

3168 Ting EY, Karliner JS, Williams MH Jnr. Am Rev Respir Dis 1963; 88: 833–8.

3169 Ting EY, Lyons HA. Am Rev Respir Dis 1964; 89: 379–86.

3170 Tirlapur VG, Mir MA. Lancet 1984; 1: 514–5.

3171 Tobin MJ, Perez W, Guenther SM, et al. Am Rev Respir Dis 1986; 134: 1111–8.

3172 Tobin MJ, Snyder JV. Crit Care Med 1984; 12: 882–7.

3173 Todesco JM. Lancet 1942; 1: 261.

3174 Toker P. South African Med J 1955; 29: 40–1.

3175 Tolo VT. Spine 1983; 8: 373–77.

3176 Tomori Z, Widdicombe JG. J Physiol 1969; 200: 25–49.

3177 Toriello HV, Higgins JV, Jones AS, Radecki LL. Am J Med Gen 1985; 21: 87–92.

3178 Tornow P. Deutsche Med Wschr 1969; 94: 1032–3.

3179 Torre R de la, Mier M, Boshes B. Q Bull NW Univ Med School 1960; 34: 232–6.

3180 Torres G, Lyons HA, Emerson P. Am J Med 1960; 29: 946–54.

3181 Torvik A, Brodal A. Anat Rec 1957; 128: 113–38.

3182 Tourniaire A, Tartulier M, Deyrieux F. Arch Mal Coeur 1962; 55: 1042–59.

3183 Tourreau A, Collin A, Molina N, Abraham D, Roche G. Rev Fr Mal Resp 1978; 6: 373–6.

3184 Towers MK, Zorab PA. In: Zorab PA, ed. Scoliosis. London: Heinemann Medical Books Limited, 1969: 54–66.

3185 Travis DM, Cook CD, Julian DG, et al. Am J Med 1960; 29: 623–32.

3186 Trend PStJ, Wiles CM, Spencer GT, Morgan–Hughes JA, Lake BD, Partrick AD. Brain 1985; 108: 845–60.

3187 Tsairis P, Dyck PJ, Mulder DW. Arch Neurol 1972; 27: 109–17.

3188 Tsanaclis A, Grassino AE. Am Rev Respir Dis 1979; 119: Suppl 366.

3189 Tsigelnik AV, Volkova KV. Prob Tuberk 1973; 51: 35–8.

3190 Tsitouris G, Fertakis A. Am J Med 1965; 39: 173–8.

3191 Tsou E, O'Connor RJ, Waldhorn RE, Rustgi V. Am Rev Respir Dis 1983; 127: Suppl 125.

3192 Tuck RR, McLeod JG. J Neurol Neurosurg Psychiatr 1981; 44: 983–90.

3193 Tuck SJ, Monin P, Duvivier C, May T, Vert P. Arch Dis Child 1982; 57: 475–7.

3194 Tucker CR, Foules RE, Calin A, Popp RL. Am J Cardiol 1982; 49: 680–6.

3195 Tucker DH, Sieker HO. Am Rev Respir Dis 1960; 82: 787–91.

3196 Tumulty PA. J Am Med Assoc 1954; 156: 947–53.

3197 Tunstall ME, Bolton MP. Anaesthesia 1977; 32: 177–8.

3198 Turino GM, Goldring RM, Fishman P. Bull NY Acad Sci 1965; 41: 959–80.

3199 Turner EA. Brain 1954; 77: 448–86.

3200 Turner WA, Critchley M. Brain 1925; 48: 72–104.

3201 Turner WA, Critchley M. J Neurol Psychopathol 1928; 8: 191–208.

3202 Turner-Stokes L, Turner-Warwick M. Clin Rheum Dis 1982; 8: 229–42.

3203 Tusiewicz K, Moldofsky H, Bryan AC, Bryan MH. J Appl Physiol 1977; 43: 600–2.

3204 Tweeddale PM, Douglas NJ. Thorax 1985; 40: 825–7.

3205 Tyler HR. Otolaryngol Clin North Am 1984; 17: 75–9.

3206 Tyler JM. J Clin Invest 1960; 39: 34–41.

3207 Uddman R, Sundler F. Clin Chest Med 1986; 7: 201–9.

3208 Uggla L–G. Acta Tuberc Scand 1957; Suppl 41: 1–179.

3209 Unger M, Atkins M, Briscoe WA, King TKC. J Appl Physiol 1977; 43: 662–7.

3210 Urciuoli R, Nivoli GC. Min Neurochir 1969; 13: 57–8.

3211 Urich H, Norman RM, Lloyd OC. Confin Neurol 1957; 17: 360–71.

3212 Urmey WF, Loring SH, Mead J, et al. Physiologist 1981; 24: 97.

3213 Urmey W, Loring S, Mead J, et al. J Appl Physiol 1986; 60: 618–22.

3214 Vaccarezza RF, Soubrie A, Rey JC. Dis Chest 1948; 14: 580–4.

3215 Valentinuzzi ME, Geddes LA. Cardiovasc Res Cent Bull 1974; 12: 87–103.

3216 Valero A, Alroy G. Arch Intern Med 1965; 115: 307–10.

3217 Vallbona C, Harrington PR, Harrison GM, Freire RM, Reese WO. Arch Phys Med Rehabil 1969; 50: 68–74.

3218 Vallbona C, Spencer WA. J Chronic Dis 1959; 9: 617–35.

3219 van Heeckeren DW, Glenn WWL. J Thorac Cardiovasc Surg 1966; 52: 655–65.

3220 Vandenbergh E, Woestijne KEP van de, Gyselen A. Am Rev Respir Dis 1967; 95: 556–66.

3221 Vapalahti M, Troupp H. Br Med J 1971; 3: 404–7.

3222 Varkey B, Funahashi A. Chest 1982; 82: 132.

3223 Vas CJ, Parsonage M, Lord OC. J Neurol Neurosurg Psychiatr 1965; 28: 401–3.

3224 Vaughan RW, Cork RC, Hollander D. Anesthesiology 1981; 54: 325–8.

3225 Veale E, Cooper BG, Gilmartin JJ, et al. Thorax 1986; 41: 710–1.

3226 Vella LM, Hewitt PB, Jones RM, Adams AP. Anaesthesia 1984; 39: 108–12.

3227 Vellody VP, Nassery M, Druz WS, Sharp JT. J Appl Physiol 1978; 45: 581–9.

3228 Venus B, Jacobs HK, Lim L. Chest 1979; 76: 257–61.

3229 Versano S, Treves TH, Bruderman I, Bechar M, Korczyn AD. Harefuah 1982; 103: 93–6.

3230 Vesian F de. MD Thesis 1884; A Parent, Paris.

3231 Vignos BJ, Spencer GE Jnr, Archibald KC. J Am Med Assoc 1963; 184: 89–96.

3232 Vignos PJ. J Am Med Assoc 1966; 197: 843–8.

3233 Vignos PJ Jnr. Isr J Med Sci 1976; 13: 207–14.

3234 Viires N, Aubier M, Murciano D, Fleury B, Talamo C, Pariente R. Am Rev Respir Dis 1984; 129: 396–402.

3235 Vincken W, Cosio MG. Chest 1985; 86: 480.

3236 Vincken W, Dollfuss R, Cosio M. Am Rev Resir Dis 1983; 127: Suppl 143.

3237 Vincken W, Elleker G, Cosio M. Am Rev Respir Dis 1983; 127: Suppl 142.

3238 Vincken W, Elleker G, Cosio MG. Chest 1986; 90: 52–7.

3239 Vincken W, Gauthier S, Dollfuss R, Cosio M. Am Rev Respir Dis 1983; 127: Suppl 115.

3240 Vincken W, Gauthier S, Dollfuss R, Hanson RE, Darauay CM, Cosio MG. N Engl J Med 1984; 311: 438–42.

3241 Vincken W, Guilleminault C, Silvestri L, Cosio M, Grassino A. Am Rev Respir Dis 1987; 135: 372–7.

3242 Visser HKA, Veenstra HW, Pik C. Arch Dis Childh 1964; 39: 397–402.

3243 Voelkel NF. Am Rev Respir Dis 1986; 133: 1186–93.

3244 Voisin M, Dimeglio A, Grolleau R, Pous JG, Dumas R, Jean R. Arch Mal Coeur 1983; 76: 568–74.

3245 Vyas MN, Banister EW, Morton JW, Grzybowski S. Am Rev Respir Dis 1971; 103: 390–400.

3246 Wachtel FW, Ravitch MM, Grishman A. Am Heart J 1956; 52: 121–37.

3247 Wade JG, Larson CP, Hickey RF, Ehrenfeld WK, Severinghaus JW. N Engl J Med 1970; 282: 823–9.

3248 Wade OL. J Physiol 1954; 124: 193–212.

3249 Wade OL, Gilson JC. Thorax 1951; 6: 103–26.

3250 Wadia RS, Wadgaonkar SU, Amin RB, Sardesai HV. J Med Genet 1976; 13: 352–6.

3251 Wagner DR, Pollak CP, Weitzman ED. N Engl J Med 1983; 308: 461–2.

3252 Waldenburg L. Die pneumatische behandlung der Respirations – und Circulationskrankheiten im Anschluss an die Pneumatometrie und Spirometrie. Berlin: A Hirschwald, 1880, 420.

3253 Wallace G, Webb EL, Becker WH, Coppolino CA. Anesth Analg 1961; 40: 505–8.

3254 Walley RV. Br Med J 1959; 2: 82–5.

3255 Walsh RE, Michaelson ED, Harkleroad LE, Zighelboim A, Sackner MA. Ann Intern Med 1972; 76: 185–92.

3256 Walters DL, Dickinson DG, Wilson JL. Am J Dis Child 1955; 89: 2–6.

3257 Walton J, ed. Disorders of Voluntary Muscle, 4th ed. Edinburgh: Churchill Livingstone, 1981.

3258 Wang CS, Josenhans WT. J Appl Physiol 1971; 31: 576–80.

3259 Ward M. Ann R Coll Surg 1973; 52: 330–4.

3260 Warrell DA. Trans R Soc Trop Med Hyg 1976; 70: 188–95.

3261 Warwick R, Mitchell GAG. J Anat 1955; 89: 562–3.

3262 Wasserman HP. South African Med J 1962; 36: 985–9.

3263 Wasserman K, Whipp BJ, Koyal SN, Cleary MG. J Appl Physiol 1975; 39: 354–8.

3264 Waterhouse JC, Howard P. Thorax 1983; 28: 302–6.

3265 Waters RM, Bennett JH. Anesth Analg 1936; 15: 151–4.

3266 Watts JM. Br J Surg 1963; 50: 954–75.

3267 Waud RA. Nature 1937; 140: 849.

3268 Webb P. J Appl Physiol 1974; 37: 899–903.

3269 Weber B, Smith JP, Briscoe WA, Friedman SA, King TKC. Am Rev Respir Dis 1975; 111: 389–97.

3270 Weber FA. J Bone Joint Surg 1974; 56B: 589.

3271 Wechsler RL, Kleiss LM, Kety SS. J Clin Invest 1950; 29: 28–30.

3272 Wedzicha JA, Rudd RM, Apps MCP, Cotter FE, Newland AC, Empey DW. Br Med J 1983; 286: 511–4.

3273 Weg JG, Krumholz A, Harkleroad LE. Am Rev Respir Dis 1967; 96: 936–45.

3274 Wegria R, Capeci N, Kiss G, Glaviano VV, Keating JH, Hilton JG. Am J Med 1955; 19: 509–15.

3275 Weil JV, Byrne–Quinn E, Sodal IE, Filley GF, Grover RF. J Clin Invest 1971; 50: 186–95.

3276 Weil MH. J Am Med Assoc 1955; 159: 1592–5.

3277 Weimann RL, Gibson DA, Moseley CF, Jones DC. Spine 1983; 8: 776–80.

3278 Weinberg B, Bosma AF. J Speech Hear Disord 1970; 35: 25–32.

3279 Weiner D, Mitra J, Salamone J, Cherniack NS. J Appl Physiol 1982; 52: 530–6.

3280 Weiner D, Mitra J, Salamone J, Nochomovitz M, Cherniack NS. Am Rev Respir Dis 1980; 121: Suppl 418.

3281 Weiner M, Chausow A, Szidon P. Br J Dis Chest 1986; 80: 391–5.

3282 Weinstein L, Shelokov A, Seltzer R, Winchell GD. N Engl J Med 1952; 246: 296–302.

3283 Weinstein SL, Zavala DC, Ponseti IV. J Bone Joint Surg 1981; 63A: 702–12.

3284 Weiss E, Kronzon I, Winer HE, Berger AR. Am J Med Sci 1981; 282: 136–40.

3285 Weisse AB, Moschos CB, Frank MJ, Levinson GE, Cannilla JE, Regan TJ. Am J Med 1975; 58: 92–8.

3286 Weitzenblum E, Moyses B, Hirth C, Kuissu S, Methlin G. Bull Eur Physiopath Respir 1977; 13: 749–61.

3287 Weitzenblum E, Sautegeau A, Ehrhart M, Mammoser M, Pelletier A. Am Rev Respir Dis 1985; 131: 493–8.

3288 Weitzman ED, Pollak CP, Borowiecki B, Burack B, Shprintzen R, Rakoff S. In: Guilleminault C, Dement WC, eds. Sleep Apnea Syndromes. New York: AR Liss Inc, 1978; 235–48.

3289 Wells HH, Kattwinkel J, Morrow JD. J Pediatr 1980; 96: 865–7.

3290 Wells WA. Am J Med Sci 1898; 116: 677–92.

3291 Welsh JD, Haase GR, Bynum TE. Arch Intern Med 1964; 114: 669–79.

3292 Weng TR, Schultz GE, Chang CH, Nigro MA. Chest 1985; 88: 488–95.

3293 Wepsic JG. Clin Neurosurg 1975; 23: 454–64.

3294 Werner WI. J Am Med Assoc 1930; 95: 1162–4.

3295 Wesselhoeft C, Smith EC. N Engl J Med 1932; 207: 559–63.

3296 West P, Kryger MH. Clin Chest Med 1985; 6: 691–712.

3297 Westbrook PR, Stubbs SE, Sessler AD, Rehder K, Hyatt RE. J Appl Physiol 1973; 34: 81–6.

3298 Westcott RN, Fowler NO, Scott RC, Hauenstein VD, McGuire J. J Clin Invest 1951; 30: 957–70.

3299 Westgate HD. Am Rev Respir Dis 1967; 96: 147.

3300 Westgate HD. J Bone Joint Surg 1968; 50A: 845–6.

3301 Westgate HD, Moe JH. J Bone Joint Surg 1969; 51A: 935–46.

3302 Westlake EK, Kaye M. Br Med J 1954; 1: 302–4.

3303 Westlake EK, Simpson T, Kaye M. Q J Med 1955; 24: 155–73.

3304 Wexler HA, Poole CA. Am J Roentgenol 1976; 127: 617–22.

3305 Whatley JL, Rehman I. US Navy Med 1971; 57: 28–34, 37.

3306 Whedon GD, Deitrick JE, Shorr E. Am J Med 1949; 6: 684–711.

3307 Whipp BJ, Ward SA. In: Wilson AF, ed. Pulmonary Function Testing. Indications and Interpretations. Orlando: Grune and Stratton 1985: 201–19.

3308 Whipp BJ, Wasserman K. Fed Proc 1980; 39: 2668–73.

3309 White DP. Clin Chest Med 1985; 6: 623–32.

3310 White DP, Cadieux RJ, Lombard RM, Bixler EO, Kales A, Zwillich CW. Am Rev Respir Dis 1985; 132: 972–5.

3311 White DP, Douglas NJ, Pickett CK, Zwillich CW, Weil JV. Am Rev Respir Dis 1983; 128: 984–6.

3312 White DP, Miller F, Erickson RW. Am Rev Respir Dis 1983; 127: 132–3.

3313 White DP, Weil JV, Zwillich CW. J Appl Physiol 1985; 59: 384–91.

3314 White DP, Zwillich CW, Pickett C, Hudgel DW, Weil JV. Am Rev Respir Dis 1981; 123: Suppl 177.

3315 White DP, Zwillich CW, Pickett CK, Douglas NJ, Findley LJ, Weil JV. Ann Intern Med 1982; 142: 1816–9.

3316 White JC, Sweet WH, Hawkins R, Nilges RG. Brain 1950; 73: 346–67.

3317 White RI, Jordan CE, Fischer KC, Lampton L, Neill CA, Dorst JP. Am J Roentgenol Radiother Nucl Med 1972; 116: 531–8.

3318 Whitehouse AC, Petty TL. Lancet 1969; 1: 1029–30.

3319 Whitelaw WA, Derenne J–P, Milic–Emili J. Respir Physiol 1975; 23: 181–99.

3320 Whitfield AGW. Br J Dis Chest 1959; 53: 28–40.

3321 Whittenberger JL. Physiol Rev 1955; 35: 611–28.

3322 Whittenberger JL, Ferris BG Jnr. Am J Phys Med 1952; 31: 226–37.

3323 Whittenberger JL, Sarnoff SJ, Hardenbergh E. J Clin Invest 1949; 28: 124–8.

3324 Whitty CWM. Proc R Soc Med 1955; 48: 463–9.

3325 Wicks AB, Menter RR. Chest 1986; 90: 406–10.

3326 Wicks JM, Davison R, Belic N. Chest 1978; 74: 303–5.

3327 Widdicombe JG. In: Hornbein TF, ed. Regulation of Breathing. Part 1. New York: Marcel Dekker, 1981: 429–72.

3328 Widdicombe JG. Clin Chest Med 1986; 7; 159–70.

3329 Wiers PWJ, Coultre R le, Dallinga OT, Dijl W van, Meinesz AF, Sluiter HJ. Thorax 1977; 32: 221–8.

3330 Wightman HB, Shaughnessy TJ. J Am Med Assoc 1929; 93: 456–7.

3331 Wiles CM, Edwards RHT. Clin Physiol 1982; 2: 485–97.

3332 Wiles CM, Moxham J, Newham D, Edwards RHT. Clin Sci 1983; 64: 547–50.

3333 Wiles CM, Young A, Jones DA, Edwards RHT. Clin Sci 1979; 56: 47–52.

3334 Wiles CM, Young A, Jones DA, Edwards RHT. Clin Sci 1979; 57: 375–84.

3335 Wilhoit C, Suratt PM. Chest 1987; 91: 654–8.

3336 Wilhoit SC, Brown ED, Suratt PM. Chest 1984; 85: 170–3.

3337 Wilkins KE, Gibson DA. J Bone Joint Surg 1976; 58A: 24–32.

3338 Wilkinson AR, McCormick MS, Freeland AP, Pickering D. Br Med J 1981; 282: 1579–81.

3339 Willeput R, Vachaudez JP, Lenders D, Nys A, Knoops T, Sergysels R. Respiration 1983; 44: 204–14.

3340 Williams A, Hanson D, Calne DB. J Neurol Neurosurg Psychiatr 1979; 42: 151–3.

3341 Williams B. Brain 1978; 101: 223–50.

3342 Willis WH, Weaver DF. Arch Otolaryngol 1968; 87: 468–70.

3343 Wilson AF, Fugl–Meyer AR. Clin Res 1975; 23: 139A.

3344 Wilson AS, Krcek JP. Exp Neurol 1975; 47: 490–502.

3345 Wilson DO, Rogers RM, Hoffman RM. Am Rev Respir Dis 1985; 132: 1347–65.

3346 Wilson DO, Rogers RM, Openbrier D. Clin Chest Med 1986; 7: 643–56.

3347 Wilson DO, Rogers RM, Sanders MH, Pennock BE, Reilly JJ. Am Rev Respir Dis 1986; 134: 672–7.

3348 Wilson JL. Am J Dis Child 1932; 43: 1433–54.

3349 Wilson NJ, Armada O, Vindzberg WV, O'Brien WB. J Thorac Surg 1956; 32: 797–819.

3350 Wilson SAK, Bruce AN. Neurology. 2nd ed. London: Butterworth and Co, 1954.

3351 Wilson SH, Cooke NT, Edwards RHT, Spiro SG. Thorax 1984; 39: 535–8.

3352 Wilson SH, Cooke NT, Moxham J, Spiro SG. Am Rev Respir Dis 1984; 129: 460–4.

3353 Wilson SL, Thach BT, Brouillette RT, Abu–Osba YK. J Appl Physiol 1980; 48: 500–4.

3354 Wilson WR, Bedell GN. J Clin Invest 1960; 39: 42–55.

3355 Winnie AP. Acta Anaesthesiol Scand 1973; Suppl 51: 1–32.

3356 Winter B. N Engl J Med 1970; 283: 661.

3357 Winter B. Int Surg 1972; 57: 458–66.

3358 Winter JH, Neilly JB, Henderson AF, et al. Q J Med 1986; 61: 1171–8.

3359 Winter RB, Lovell WW, Georgia D, Moe JH. J Bone Joint Surg 1975; 57A: 972–7.

3360 Winter RJD, George RJD, Moore–Gillon JC, Geddes DM. Lancet 1984; 2: 1371–2.

3361 Wislicki L. Br Med J 1954; 2: 672–4.

3362 Woillez M. Bull l'Acad Med 1876; 5: 611–27.

3363 Wojtulewski JA, Sturrock RD, Branfoot AC, Hart FD. Br Med J 1973; 3: 145–6.

3364 Wolf E, Mossery M, Berlin B, Vilozni D. Harefuah 1954; 106: 120–2.

3365 Wolf E, Shochina M, Ferber I, Gonen B. Electromyogr Clin Neurophysiol 1981; 21: 35–53.

3366 Wolf E, Shochina M, Gordin M. Isr J Med Sci 1983; 19: 568–70.

3367 Wolkove N, Altose MD, Kelsen SG, Cherniack NS. Am Rev Respir Dis 1980; 122: 163–7.

3368 Wood JB, Frankland AW, Eastcott HHG. Thorax 1965; 20: 570–3.

3369 Woodcock AA, Gross ER, Geddes DM. Lancet 1981; 1: 907–9.

3370 Woolf CR. Chest 1970; 58: 49–53.

3371 Woolf CR, Suero JT. Dis Chest 1969; 55: 37–44.

3372 Woollam CHM. Anaesthesia 1976; 31: 537–47.

3373 Woollam CHM. Anaesthesia 1976; 31: 666–85.

3374 Wright CD, Williams JG, Ogilvie CM, Donnelly RJ. J Thorac Cardiovasc Surg 1985; 90: 195–8.

3375 Wright GW, Place R, Prince F. Am Rev Tuberc 1949; 60: 706–14.

3376 Wright J. Am J Nurs 1947; 47: 454–5.

3377 Wright WD, Niebauer JJ. J Bone Joint Surg 1956; 38A: 1131–6.

3378 Wurmser P, Kaeser HE. Schweiz Med Wschr 1963; 93: 1393–6.

3379 Wyler AR, Weymuller EA Jnr. Ann Neurol 1981; 9: 403–4.

3380 Wynne JW. Chest 1982; 82: 657–8.

3381 Wynn–Williams N. Thorax 1954; 9: 299–303.

3382 Yamada H, Nakamura S, Tajima M, Kageyama N. J Neurosurg 1981; 54: 49–57.

3383 Yamamoto T, Hirose N, Miyoshi K. Eur Neurol 1977; 15: 188–93.

3384 Yang G–FW, Alba A, Lee M. Arch Phys Med Rehabil 1984; 65: 556–8.

3385 Yap C–B, Mayo C, Barron K. Arch Neurol 1968; 18: 304–10.

3386 Yau ACMC, Hsu LCS, O'Brien JP, Hodgson AR. J Bone Joint Surg 1974; 56A: 1419–34.

3387 Yernault JC, Gibson GJ. Bull Eur Physiopath Respir 1982; 18: 395–401.

3388 York EL, Jones RL, Menon D, Sproule BJ. Am Rev Respir Dis 1980; 121: 813–8.

3389 Young RF. Neurosurgery 1978; 2: 43–6.

3390 Young RR, Asbury AK, Corbett JL, Adams RD. Brain 1975; 98: 613–36.

3391 Younger DS, Braun NMT, Jaretzki A III, Penn AS, Lovelace RE. Neurology 1984; 34: 336–40.

3392 Yousefzadeh TK, Agha AS, Reinertson J. Pediatr Radiol 1979; 8: 45–7.

3393 Zakopoulos KS, Tsatas AT. Dis Chest 1965; 47: 109–10.

3394 Zalman F, Perloff JK, Durant NN, Campion DS. Am Heart J 1983; 105: 510–11.

3395 Zampollo A, Galbiati D, Spreafico A. Ateneo Parmense (Acta Biomed) 1978; 49: 401–8.

3396 Zeilhofer R, Sroka W. Beitr Klin Tuberk 1960; 122: 48–70.

3397 Zidulka A, Gross D, Minami H, Vartian V, Chang HK. Am Rev Respir Dis 1983; 127: 709–13.

3398 Zifroni A, Bruderman I, Rosenberg M. Harefuah 1972; 83: 57–9.

3399 Zimmerman HA. J Thorac Surg 1951; 22: 94–8.

3400 Zocche GP, Fritts HW Jnr, Cournand A. J Appl Physiol 1960; 15: 1073–4.

3401 Zorab PA. Q J Med 1962; 31: 267–80.

3402 Zorab PA, Harrison A, Harrison WJ. Lancet 1964; 2: 1063.

3403 Zorab PA, Prime FJ, Harrison A. Lancet 1963; 1: 195–6.

3404 Zorab PA, Prime FJ, Harrison A. Spine 1979; 4: 22–8.

3405 Zorick F, Roehrs T, Conway W, Fujita S, Wittig R, Roth T. Bull Eur Physiopath Respir 1983; 19: 600–3.

3406 Zorick F, Roth T, Kramer M, Flessa H. Chest 1980; 77: 689–90.

3407 Zwillich C, Devlin T, White D, Douglas N, Weil J, Martin R. J Clin Invest 1982; 69: 1286–92.

3408 Zwillich CW, Pickett C, Hanson FN, Weil JV. Am Rev Respir Dis 1981; 124: 158–60.

3409 Zwillich CW, Pierson DJ, Hofeldt FD, Lufkin EG, Weil JV. N Engl J Med 1975; 292: 662–5.

3410 Zwillich CW, Sahn SA, Weil JV. J Clin Invest 1977; 60: 900–6.

3411 Zwillich CW, Sutton FD, Pierson DJ, Creagh EM, Weil JV. Am J Med 1975; 59: 343–8.

3412 Zwillich CW, Weil JV. Clin Res 1976; 24: 103A.

Index

Page numbers in italic refer to figures and/or tables